Lippincott® *Q&A Certification Review*

EMERGENCY NURSING (CEN)

THIRD EDITION

Patricia L. Clutter, RN, MEd, CEN, FAEN
Emergency Department Staff Nurse
Mercy Hospital Lebanon
Lebanon, Missouri
Independent Educator and Journalist
Strafford, Missouri

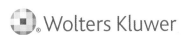 Wolters Kluwer

Philadelphia • Baltimore • New York • London
Buenos Aires • Hong Kong • Sydney • Tokyo

Acquisitions Editor: Nicole Dernoski
Developmental Editor: Maria M. McAvey
Editorial Coordinator: Blair Jackson
Production Project Manager: Barton Dudlick
Design Coordinator: Holly Reid McLaughlin
Manufacturing Coordinator: Kathleen Brown
Marketing Manager: Linda Wetmore
Prepress Vendor: S4Carlisle Publishing Services

Third edition

Library of Congress Cataloging-in-Publication Data

ISBN-13: 978-1-9751-1455-8

ISBN-10: 1-9751-1455-8

Library of Congress Control Number: 2019943323

CCS0719

This book is dedicated to the profession of emergency nursing and to all those who understand its intricacies, its craziness, and its poignant moments that keep us coming back. Each day brings with it new and exciting situations along with a few tears—both joyful and sorrowful—excitement, adrenaline, the thrill of a save, and a few laughs to keep us strong. We who work in this specialty field know the true meaning of the phrase, "You can't make this up!" We work hard, and we make friendships that withstand so much. Without each other, we would not make it through! Thank goodness for each other and the work we do that makes us whole and gives our lives meaning.

Contributors

Nancy Mannion Bonalumi, DNP, RN, CEN, FAEN
Clinician, Educator, Nurse Leader
President and Founder
NMB Global Leadership, LLC
Lancaster, Pennsylvania

Patricia L. Clutter, RN, MEd, CEN, FAEN
Emergency Department Staff Nurse
Mercy Hospital Lebanon
Lebanon, Missouri
Independent Educator and Journalist
Strafford, Missouri

Jaime Dahm, MSN, RN, CEN
Clinical Educator
Mercy Hospital Lebanon
Lebanon, Missouri

Debra Delaney, DNP, MHA, RN, CEN
President
Delaney Healthcare Consultants, LLC
West Boylston, Massachusetts

Terry Foster, RN, MSN, FAEN, CCRN, CPEN, TCRN, CEN
Ambassador and Clinical Nurse Specialist
Six Emergency Departments
St. Elizabeth Healthcare
Edgewood, Kentucky

Cathy C. Fox, RN, CEN, CPEN, TCRN, FAEN
Quality Nurse Consultant
Emergency Department, Cath Lab and Cardiovascular Service Lines
Naval Medical Center
Portsmouth, Virginia

Monta Rae Glaser, RN, CEN
Registered Nurse
Emergency Department Staff Nurse
Orthopedic Hospital Staff Nurse
Mercy Hospital
Springfield, Missouri

Bill Light, MSN, RN, CEN, CPEN, TCRN
Vice President and Chief Nursing Officer
Solheim Enterprises
West Linn, Oregon

Geraldine F. Muller, MSN, RN, CEN, TCRN
Nurse Practice Specialist
Emergency Department
Henry Ford Health System
Detroit, Michigan

Joan Somes, PhD, RN-BC, CEN, CPEN, FAEN, NRP
Critical Care Educator
EMS, Regions Hospital
St. Paul, Minnesota

Tiffany Strever, BSN, RN, CEN, TCRN, FAEN
Trauma Program Manager
Trauma Services
Abrazo West Campus
Goodyear, Arizona

Melissa L. Weir, MS, BSN, RN, CEN, CPEN
Professor
Department of Nursing
Howard University
Washington, District of Columbia

Aaron Wolff, RN, BSN, CEN
Director of Emergency Services
Mercy Medical Center—Redding
Redding, California

Previous Edition Contributors

Kelly Allen, RN, MSN, CEN

Susan Barnason, PhD, APRN-CNS, CEN, CCRN

Beth Ann Broering, MSN, RN, CEN, CCRN, CPEN, CCNS, FAEN

Cheyenne Brown, RN, BS, CEN

Laurie Donaghy, BSN, RN, CEN

Laura Favand, RN, MS, CEN

Andi Foley, MSN, RN, CEN

Wm. Bryan Gibboney, MSN, APRN, FNP-C, ACNP-BC, CEN, CPEN, CCRN

Molly Groban, MS, MAEd, RN, CEN, CCRN, LNC, MICN, SANE

Jill Johnson, DNP, APRN, FNP-BC, CCRN, CEN, CFRN

Charles Kunkle, MSN, CEN, CCRN, BC-NA

Sharon L. G. Lee, MSN, FNP-C, ARNP, CEN, CCRN

Charles L. Mandelin, RN, BA, BSN, CEN

Cheryl Schmitz, MS, RN, BC, CNS-BC, CEN

Dawn M. Specht, MSN, PhD, RN, APRN, CEN, CCRN, CCNS

Polly Gerber Zimmermann, RN, MS, MBA, CEN, FAEN

Preface

The world of emergency nursing is more than just a job—it's a passion. The energy that we derive from this fast-paced venue is hard to describe, and even on our toughest days, we go home and end up coming back . . . and back . . . and back. It runs thick in our veins and becomes the essence of our being—the very identity of ourselves.

Congratulations on pursuing your certification in our specialty field! As someone who has been certified since its inception in 1980, I know how important it is to me to have these initials, and I pass on to you the joy of that feeling. During your preparation time, you will have many long days—and nights—of studying ahead of you, but the reward is great and the feeling of accomplishment will fuel your spirit.

As you embark on this next phase of your career, take heart that many have done this before you and survived! Those of us who are on the verge of closing out our own careers are excited to have a new group that feel compelled to take on the task of certification. It's part of the pride you will carry with you knowing that you proved to yourself, your colleagues, and your patients that the excellent level of care that you have always provided is now validated.

We hope this book will help you in your preparation for this goal. This book includes questions from every aspect of your upcoming test. The rationales are intended to teach as well as scoring yourself. And we included bits and pieces of other information pertinent to the question that was just presented, test-taking tips, and some things we have simply learned along the way that have helped us in our day-to-day practice. It's all about the sharing you know!

When you place the initials, CEN, after your name, do so with pride, a feeling of extreme accomplishment, and a renewed hunger for even more knowledge. In our world, there is no end to the search for knowledge and every day that we step through those doors marked "Emergency Department," we end up learning something new and exciting. It makes it all worth it—every step of the way.

When you are weary and feel like you cannot go into one more room, remember what you mean to all those patients who you have cared for. Remember the good ones who held your hand, thanked you, and appreciated your kindness and skills. Remember the hard ones who were difficult and yet you stuck with them and made a difference in their lives too. And most of all, remember that in the end, this is what, and who, we are there for—each and every one who comes to us trusting us to know our stuff and to advocate for their well-being. Knowledge is strength, and it helps us all to be the best emergency nurse we can be! May you each enjoy your own professional journey as much as I have mine.

Patricia L. Clutter

Acknowledgments

My deepest gratitude to everyone who helped me in making this book a reality. First of all, I so appreciate everyone at Wolters Kluwer for having faith in me to put this book together. Each and every individual whom I have corresponded with has shown utmost kindness and professionalism on every aspect. From my initial discussions with Nicole Dernoski, who started me on this journey, to all the individuals at the office who have helped me through every step of the way, I thank you. My deepest gratitude to Kayla Smull, Julie Kostelnik, Maria McAvey, Blair Jackson, LaPorsche Rogers, Bharathi Sanjeev, and Barton Dudlick for keeping me straight and providing me with all the right answers and encouragement.

Thanks is not enough for the contributors of each chapter in this book. For those who have not had the opportunity to write test items, trust me when I tell you that it is very difficult and takes a great amount of time! I appreciate every moment that each of you spent on each and every question, tweaking it until it was just right.

I also want to acknowledge my family who steadfastly stand by me every time I take on a project like this. My husband, Randy, is my total soul mate who takes care of me and encourages me through everything. Thank you for the computer side snacks and short talks that kept me sane and also for your smiling and understanding every time I stayed up late, got up early, and worked steadfastly throughout the day instead of spending time with you.

Thanks also to my children and their families—Justace, Huan, and Axton and Ben, Melanie, Kaylie, Brittany, Jordan, Madison, Briana, and Koty—my sister and brothers, and my mom, Celia who saw me work on this a great deal instead of watching TV and sharing a conversation with her. And, of course, to all of my friends who understood and listened to me patiently when I was behind in my work. I really appreciated it.

And, of course, I must acknowledge all the patients who have taught all of us so much through the years. Every patient is unique, and they have made these words that make up the art and science of emergency nursing real and meaningful. Without our patients, our lives would not be filled with this significant intrinsic worth that satisfies our inner being.

Thanks also to the team that I work with in Lebanon, Missouri—you are awesome and keep me grounded. And to all of my dear ENA friends and colleagues—you bolster me and help me be who I am today. I am indebted to each of you.

Contributor Monta Rae Glaser, RN, CEN, was a first-time author, a great nurse and educator, and a proud CEN. Unfortunately, she lost her life in a tragic accident before the publication of this book. She will be missed forever and remembered fondly for her daily contributions to our specialty area. Rest in peace, good and faithful servant.

Contents

Part II   Sample Tests and Appendices 305

Part I
Clinical Practice

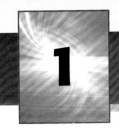

1 Understanding the Certified Emergency Nurse Examination

Patricia L. Clutter, RN, MEd, CEN, FAEN

Congratulations on your decision to pursue certification in Emergency Nursing! This journey will reward you in many ways, certainly the most important being the self-satisfaction that will fill you with pride each time you write those initials after your name! Your patients also appreciate the extra effort and are happy to be taken care of by someone who has proven himself/herself. It certainly does help with your marketability and, of course, some institutions provide monetary incentives for your hard work.

According to the National Specialty Nursing Certifying Organization, certification is the process by which a nongovernmental agency or association validates, on the basis of predetermined standards, a registered nurse's qualifications and knowledge for practice in a defined functional or clinical area of nursing. To enhance your performance on the Certified Emergency Nurse (CEN) examination, review the answers to the following commonly asked questions.

Who sponsors the CEN examination?

The Board of Certification for Emergency Nurses (BCEN) sponsors the CEN examination. The BCEN evaluates and recognizes nurses who have attained a defined body of emergency nursing knowledge needed to function at a competent level. The website for this organization is important to the test taker. It is located at www.bcencertifications.org.

Is the CEN examination as difficult as the National Council Licensure Examination (NCLEX)?

Health care professionals who take a certification examination for a specialty area of practice already have the knowledge required by the basic licensure examination. Because the knowledge measured by the CEN examination is specialized for emergency nursing, the CEN examination is at least as difficult as or more challenging than the NCLEX. This is also an individual viewpoint, with individual nurses varying in their ability to take the test and in how they view the questions. For some emergency nurses taking the test, it may seem easy, and for others, it will be very hard.

If I have been an emergency nurse for years, do I need to study?

As an emergency nurse, you have probably mastered complex technical skills related to the care of emergency patients as well as the theoretical knowledge that underlies these skills. You have also probably developed the ability to make sound nursing judgments in crises that often determine whether a patient lives or dies. Despite such advanced knowledge, skill mastery, and decision-making ability, many emergency nurses experience high levels of test-taking anxiety that may prevent them from seeking certification. This book can help alleviate test-taking anxiety and provide a level of confidence to the reader by providing a thorough review of the material contained in the CEN examination. It is the hope of this author and contributors to provide the tools that will help you successfully pass this test. Included among the questions are helpful hints about emergency care issues that are coordinated with the question and the answer. This provides additional information that might not otherwise be dealt with in the test questions themselves.

Also, keep in mind that all nurses should study for the examination because it is impossible for every nurse to care for every kind of patient or to remember every nuance about disease processes and interventions. It is highly recommended that each nurse study for at least 1 month before sitting for the examination. Everyone has high spots and low spots in their knowledge base. Reminding yourself of some of the points of care of patient disease processes and injuries that you may not have cared for in the past is essential to the success of the emergency nurse taking this examination.

What are the eligibility requirements?

The BCEN establishes criteria for eligibility to take the CEN examination. Current criteria are listed here.

- You must possess a current unrestricted license or nursing certificate as a registered nurse in the United States.

- Nurses from other countries must possess licensure, registration, or certification to practice as a registered nurse in that country. An additional international testing fee will be assessed at the time of application.
- Any restriction, suspension, or probation, or any order arising from a Nursing License Authority that limits your ability to function in an emergency nurse setting and perform those tasks normally associated with emergency nursing practice will disqualify you to sit for the examination unless you are a qualified individual with a disability who can perform the essential functions of emergency nursing with or without reasonable accommodation.
- Although not a requirement, the BCEN recommends that you have 2 years of experience in emergency nursing practice.
- Membership in the Emergency Nurses Association (ENA) qualifies you for a reduced CEN examination application fee. This reduction is usually substantial. To become a member of the ENA, go to its website, www.ena.org.
- A new voucher system that your hospital can take advantage of for employees is available. Contact the BCEN for information.

How many questions are on the examination?

The CEN examination consists of 175 multiple-choice questions, of which 150 are scored. A candidate is allotted 3 hours to complete the examination. Twenty-five questions on the examination are present to test the question itself, not the test taker. This is the process by which a potential test item becomes an official test item because it is the only way to test that item for reliability and validity. The test taker will not know which questions are pretest questions. This will help gain the best information about each test item. These questions are embedded among the "real" questions to gain the best knowledge about their usefulness.

How is the examination administered?

The CEN examination is administered by computer. Upon special request, a pencil-and-paper test may be available. When the emergency nurse requests to sit for the examination, she/he will be given a list of test sites in the area of choice. The nurse will be able to sign up at the time of the application for the time and location. One of the nice things now is that each nurse takes this examination individually, unlike in the beginning when everyone sat in the same room with paper and pencil. This means that the test taker is the only one who knows when that person is taking the test. No one need know about the day of your test except for those you choose to tell. At the time

of application, the nurse has 90 days to take the examination. That gives ample time to start the studying process and gives the emergency nurse a deadline to work with.

Where do these questions come from?

Each question on the test has gone through a rigorous system to become an actual test item. To begin with, nurses from all over the country are invited to become item writers. Each year, this group of nurses is chosen according to their perceived ability to write questions, their geographic location, and the size of the hospital in which they work. The BCEN makes sure that all nurses are represented—throughout the country—and that all sizes of hospitals are included. After these nurses attend classes on item writing, they are given their assignments. When these assigned questions are completed, they are then reviewed by another group of nurses called the Examination Construction and Review Committee (ECRC). These nurses, who were prior item writers, review these questions and start the rewrite process. The final process is from the testing company who then edits the questions and places them on your test. So, in the end, the test items are written by nurses, for nurses.

What topics does the examination cover?

The content of the CEN examination, based on recognized standards and practices for emergency nursing, is divided into two major areas: clinical practice and professional issues.

Clinical practice

The questions in Chapters 2 to 13 of this book approximate the content areas shown later. The sample tests at the end of the book reflect the blueprint of the actual examination. This blueprint can be found on the BCEN website and includes the breakdown according to the number of questions for each area and also provides some insight into possible topics that may be on the test.

In 2017, after the last Role Delineation Study (RDS), a survey sent out to thousands of emergency nurses that helps keep the test up to date with current nursing practice, the blueprint was changed a great deal. These surveys help drive the major changes that occur in the test itself over the years. The content is usually changed in minor ways, that is, removing content; however, the test may see other major changes happening. For instance, in 2011, the focus of the test items moved from task oriented to disease process oriented, which made the test a bit harder. This was complemented by reducing the number of correct answers that were required for successful completion. The test taker had to answer 105 questions correctly. In 2017, the blueprint of the test was changed

Test Area	Number of Questions
Cardiovascular Emergencies	20
Respiratory Emergencies	16
Neurologic Emergencies	16
Gastrointestinal (GI)/Genitourinary/ Gynecologic/Obstetric Emergencies	21
Psychosocial/Medical Emergencies	25
Maxillofacial/Ocular/Orthopedic/Wound Management Emergencies	21
Environmental/Toxicological/ Communicable Disease Emergencies	15
Professional Issues	16

and the categories were restructured with several of them combined. The blueprint went from 13 categories to 8 categories. All body systems and emergencies were maintained, they were just redistributed. You might notice that there is not a category for shock. All of the shock states have been incorporated into the other appropriate categories, that is, cardiogenic shock is included in the cardiovascular section. The test taker now must answer 106 questions correctly to be successful.

This book has maintained separate chapters for each body system, including a separate chapter for shock because we believe it is easier to study for the potential questions in this way. The content did not change, it was simply moved around. Also, on the test, sections are not presented; instead, all questions are mixed throughout the test.

Once the categories are established with the correct number of questions on the test, these questions are further divided by the nursing process. These are as follows: Assessment, Analysis, Intervention, and Evaluation. So, on the test there will be 32 assessment, 34 analysis, 43 intervention, and 25 evaluation questions. Regarding the professional issues category, these questions are further divided by cognitive level—Recall (3), Application (10), and Analysis (3). Another item of interest is that nursing diagnoses have been removed from test items.

Assessment questions
These questions test your ability to collect data. They focus on such nursing behaviors as:
- assessing the patient's physiologic and psychosocial health as well as safety needs.

- collecting information from the patient, family, friends, hospital records, and health team members.
- recognizing symptoms and findings.
- challenging orders and decisions by health team members, as appropriate.

Analysis questions
These questions test your ability to understand disease processes and their related testing modalities. They focus on such nursing behaviors as:
- organizing, interpreting, and validating assessment data.
- gathering additional data when necessary.
- understanding the pathophysiology of the process.
- relating laboratory and radiographic results to the problem.

Intervention
These questions test your ability to initiate and complete actions that provide nursing care for the patient. They focus on such nursing behaviors as:
- selecting the best nursing measures to deliver effective care.
- prioritizing interventions to ensure optimal outcomes.
- identifying community resources to assist the patient and family.
- coordinating the patient's care with other health care providers.
- delegating care responsibilities to other health care providers.
- supervising and validating the activities of other health team members.
- formulating outcomes of nursing interventions.

Evaluation
These questions test your ability to measure goal achievement. They focus on such nursing behaviors as:
- comparing actual outcomes with expected outcomes.
- evaluating the patient's compliance with the prescribed plan of care.
- documenting the patient's response to care.
- revising the plan of care and reordering priorities as needed.
- making sure the patient understood the discharge information.

What is the best way to study?

Although individual study is highly recommended, the "best" way to study is a matter of personal preference. Remember that some people are visual learners and some are auditory learners. Figure out how you learn best and make sure you utilize that! Some test candidates prefer to study alone, whereas others opt for group study, and still others enjoy a combination of the two.

Individual study

No matter what other study strategies you use, individual preparation for the CEN examination is highly recommended. This preparation can take several forms.

- Read review books such as this one to help you pinpoint areas that need improvement. You can then concentrate on reviewing materials in those areas.
- Consult emergency nursing textbooks and study guides. As you read the material, ask yourself multiple-choice questions about the information. Consider how the CEN examination might test your knowledge of this material.
- Answer practice questions similar to those on the test. Spend about 30 minutes each day answering 10 to 20 questions (do not try to answer 100 questions on your day off). After you answer the questions, compare your answers with the correct answers listed in the review book; also review the rationales provided. In this book, we have included the rationale for the correct answer and for the incorrect answers as well. If you answer some questions incorrectly and are not sure why, return to the textbook or review book to find the rationale. By doing this, you will become more familiar and comfortable with the examination's format while reinforcing the information you have studied.
- If you have not attended an Advanced Cardiac Life Support (ACLS) course, Pediatric Advanced Life Support (PALS) course, Trauma Nursing Care Course (TNCC), or an Emergency Nursing Pediatric Course, consider attending these courses or review the course provider manuals for these courses. Content covered in these courses is often found in the CEN examination. These manuals are often used as reference material. Expect to have a few rhythm strips and emergency medication questions on the test.

Group study

Studying with others can effectively prepare you for the CEN examination. To get the most from your sessions, follow these guidelines:

- Be choosy about whom to include in your study group. Limit the number of people (the recommended size is four to six people); larger groups can disrupt study.
- Ask each member to prepare one section of the study topic before the group meets. For example, have one person discuss anatomy and physiology, another to review the drugs used for treatments, and a third to cover key elements of emergency nursing care.
- Meet regularly (once or twice weekly) to maintain a studious atmosphere.
- Limit each study session to 2 hours. Longer sessions invite participants to wander off the topic and promote a negative attitude toward the examination.

- Avoid turning study sessions into a party. Although snacks and refreshments can help maintain the group's energy, a party atmosphere will render the session ineffective.

How can I master a multiple-choice test?

Multiple-choice questions are one of the most commonly used test formats for such standardized tests as the CEN examination. After you have mastered these test-taking strategies, you will be able to score better on multiple-choice tests.

- Read the question and all options carefully and completely. This is really important. Take your time and read every word. Missing one word can make a big difference in how you answer the question.
- Treat each question individually. Use only the information provided for that question, and avoid reading into a question any information that is not provided.
- Monitor your time. You will have approximately 60 seconds per question; because most test takers average 45 seconds per question, you may finish well before the time limit. You are given 3 hours to complete the test. Before the test, you will be given a 10-minute time period to "practice." Take this time to get settled in and start answering questions. The 3-hour period does not start until the actual test is opened.
- Narrow your choices using the process of elimination. If you can identify even one option as incorrect, you can focus your attention on the more plausible answers (and improve your chances of answering correctly). If something in any of the options seems to not match with the stem of the question, toss that one out. Usually, the test taker (myself included) can eliminate two of the answers, which now gives you an advantage of a 50/50 chance!
- Do not change your answers. Studies show that test takers who change an answer on a multiple-choice examination usually change it from a correct answer to an incorrect one or from one incorrect answer to another incorrect answer. Rarely do they change to a correct answer. This is super important!
- Look for qualifying words in the question (such as *first, best, most, better,* and *highest*) that ask you to judge the priority of the options; then select the answer that has the highest priority. Be careful with questions that actually give you the first intervention and ask you to choose the "next" intervention!
- Look for negative words in the question (such as *not, least, unlikely, inappropriate, unrealistic, lowest, contraindicated, except, inconsistent, all but, atypical,* and *incorrect*). In general, when you are asked a negative question, three of the choices are appropriate actions, and one is inappropriate. You are being asked to select

the inappropriate choice as your answer. These can be tricky! On the test, these negative words will be capitalized, bolded, and underlined. Be on the lookout for them!

- Avoid selecting answers that contain absolute words (including *always, every, only, all, never,* and *none*); these options usually are incorrect.
- Never choose an option that refers the patient to a physician/provider. Because the CEN examination is for nurses and includes conditions and problems that nurses should be able to solve independently, an answer that refers a patient to the physician/provider usually is incorrect and can be eliminated from consideration.
- Do not look for a pattern (such as C, C, A, B, C, C, A, B) when selecting answers. The questions and answers on the examination are randomly arranged.
- Do not panic if you read a question that you do not understand. Some questions may refer to diseases, drugs, or laboratory tests that you are unfamiliar with. In such cases, remember that nursing care is similar in many situations, even when disease processes differ markedly. Just select the answer that seems logical and involves general nursing care. Also, utilize your understanding of pathophysiology and normal anatomy and physiology. When you get to these questions, stop and take a deep breath. You can probably work your way through it.
- If necessary, skip a question and come back to it later. Sometimes something will jog your memory or otherwise help you with the question. Just be sure to go back and answer it! Blank answers are wrong answers!
- Remember that there are no zebras on the test! Every situation is classic textbook picture. Thousands of emergency nurses across the country are taking this test. The questions have to be uniform!
- Be careful about how "things are done in my ER." Again, this test is universal. Understand the importance of knowing the "book way" just in case there is a question about a procedure.
- Another good point is to cover up the answers, and when the stem is read, figure out what answer you are looking for. Then reveal the options and see if that answer is there.
- If something seems bizarre, it is! If an answer just does not make sense, consider it as wrong and move on.
- Questions now are much "cleaner" and there are not as many scenarios that include things like, "A 55-year-old male was involved. . .." If there is an actual age or gender in the question, it is there for a reason.
- When taking practice examinations, please remember that you do not have to be getting 100% or even close

to that to be prepared! On the test, you have to answer 106 questions out of 150 correctly! That is not even 80%! Do not be so hard on yourself and think you have to be making extremely high scores on all of the practice examinations!

- Remember that things that you might have learned to help you "take a test" will not be on this test! There are no answers on the test that use the words, "All of the above" or "None of the above." There will be four distinct answers for you to choose from. Also, words that are used in the stem of the question are not repeated in the one correct answer. And the best one of all! All answers are the same length! You will not be able to choose the correct answer depending on the length of the option. This is a test of your emergency nursing ability, not your test-taking ability!
- Think positively about the examination. People who have a positive attitude score higher than those who do not.

Are there any other tips I should know?

Proper planning can go a long way toward ensuring your success on the CEN examination. Try these suggestions.

Before examination day

- A week or so before the examination, drive to the test site to familiarize yourself with parking facilities and to locate the test room. Knowing where to go will greatly reduce your anxiety on the day of the examination.
- Follow as normal a schedule as possible on the day before the examination. If you need to travel to the test site and stay away from home overnight, try to follow your usual nightly routine; avoid the urge to do something different.
- The night before the test, avoid drinking alcoholic beverages. Alcohol, a central nervous system (CNS) depressant, interferes with your ability to concentrate. Avoid eating foods you have never eaten before, which may cause adverse GI effects the next day.
- Avoid taking sleep medications you have never taken before. Like alcohol, most sleep aids are CNS depressants; some have a hangover effect, while others produce drowsiness for an extended period.
- Do not stay up late to study; this will make you tired during the test, which will decrease your ability to concentrate. Besides, you are probably as prepared as you can be. Review formulas, charts, and lists for no more than 1 hour. Then relax, perhaps by watching television or reading a magazine or book. These activities will help decrease your anxiety. In reality, try not to study the night before!
- Go to bed at your usual time.

Examination day

- On the morning of the examination, do not attempt a major review of the material. The likelihood of learning something new is slim, and intensive study may only increase your anxiety.
- Do not drink excessive amounts of coffee, tea, or caffeine-containing beverages. Caffeine will increase your nervousness and stimulate your renal system.
- Eat breakfast, even if you usually do not, and include foods high in glucose and protein to maintain your energy level and help you think! Shun greasy, heavy foods, which tend to form an uncomfortable knot in your stomach and may decrease your ability to concentrate.
- Dress in comfortable, layered clothing. Jogging suits are popular. Many rooms are air-conditioned in the summer and may be cool even if it is hot outside. Be prepared by taking a sweater or sweatshirt.
- Arrive at the test site 30 to 45 minutes early, and make sure you have the required papers and documents for admittance to the test room. Latecomers are not admitted to the examination. They are now requiring two photo IDs. The paperwork you are provided with will let you know which to bring.

- Do not bring pencils, pens, note paper, calculators, calipers, or other resources. Nothing is permitted to be taken into the testing room.
- At the testing center, you will be given a pencil and a blank piece of paper for notes and calculations. You will be asked to turn in that paper at the completion of the test.
- Think positively about how you will do. Taking the CEN examination shows confidence in your knowledge of emergency nursing. When you receive your passing results, plan to celebrate your success, a significant achievement in your professional life that deserves to be rewarded.
- RELAX! Try not to get too stressed! It is normal to have some anxiety, but make sure it stays in the mild stage where it will help keep you on your toes and not become a liability!

Who can I contact for more information?

Contact the Board of Certification of Emergency Nursing with any questions. They are now located at 1900 Spring Road, Suite 501, Oak Brook, Illinois. Phone number is 1-877-302-2236 (BCEN). Website: www.bcencertifications.org

- YOU ARE AN EMERGENCY NURSE!

- YOU SAVE LIVES FOR A LIVING!

- IT DOES NOT GET ANY HARDER THAN THAT!

- THIS TEST IS SIMPLY WORDS ON A PIECE OF PAPER!

- YOU GOT THIS!

GOOD LUCK!!!!

2 Professional Issues

Debra Delaney, DNP, MHA, RN, CEN

Emergency nurses are faced with many challenges that extend beyond physical illnesses. Professional issues on the Certified Emergency Nurse (CEN) examination include 16 questions regarding legal and ethical issues; stabilization and transfer of patients; cultural diversity; safety, and other situations faced by the emergency nurse such as disaster preparedness and domestic violence. This chapter includes those challenges that are not specific to a disease process, but rather focuses on these other issues that emergency nurses deal with every day.

The practice questions in this chapter, as well as the rationale and details in the answer section, are meant to provide you with the tools to understand the professional issues faced by emergency nurses. Rationales for each of the correct answers as well as those that are NOT true will help the emergency nurse comprehend the knowledge of professional issues needed to earn certification in Emergency Nursing. Additional information has been supplied throughout the chapter.

1. During a disaster, surge capacity is the hospital's ability to manage a sudden influx of patients. Which of the following should the emergency department nurse do first in this situation?
[ ] A. Initiate activation of the Emergency Operations Plan (EOP).
[ ] B. Keep patients and visitors informed of the plan.
[ ] C. Activate relevant specialty procedures (e.g., active shooter).
[ ] D. Prioritize hazards, safety, and health issues.

2. The Joint Commission sentinel event alert related to preventing restraint deaths identified all of the following risks **EXCEPT**:
[ ] A. placing a restrained patient in a supine position could increase aspiration risk.
[ ] B. placing a restrained patient in a prone position could increase suffocation risk.
[ ] C. a restraint may cause further psychological trauma or traumatic memories.
[ ] D. appropriate alternatives to restraints are to be used only as a last resort.

3. When the emergency nurse approaches the patient to draw blood and the patient rolls up his sleeve and holds out his arm, this type of consent would be considered to be:
[ ] A. express consent.
[ ] B. implied consent.
[ ] C. involuntary consent.
[ ] D. informed consent.

4. After a disaster has occurred, emergency department nurses assist with arranging counseling and looking for suitable housing for the victims. Which of the following would this type of prevention be considered?
[ ] A. Primary
[ ] B. Secondary
[ ] C. Tertiary
[ ] D. Primordial

5. The ENA Code of Ethics believes that the emergency nurse should collaborate with other health professionals and the public to do all of the following **EXCEPT**:
[ ] A. protect human rights.
[ ] B. promote health diplomacy.
[ ] C. document restraints appropriately.
[ ] D. reduce health disparities.

6. Several victims have arrived from a chemical plant after a bomb exploded. The victims are covered with a strong-smelling liquid and have labored respirations. Which of the following actions should the emergency nurse responding take first?
[ ] A. Prioritize patients based on degree of respiratory distress
[ ] B. Assess identity of chemicals the victims were exposed to
[ ] C. Don personal protective garments
[ ] D. Remove the victims' clothing

7. The following four patients arrive at triage at the same time. Which patient should be taken to a treatment room first?
[ ] **A.** A 7-year-old with a history of asthma with wheezing before arrival who now has increased respiratory rate but diminished wheezing
[ ] **B.** A 33-year-old with sickle cell anemia complaining of joint pain and lower back pain after a recent bacterial illness
[ ] **C.** A 12-year-old with a 1" (2.5 cm) laceration on his left foot from stepping on a piece of glass with bleeding controlled
[ ] **D.** A 16-year-old soccer player with a tibia-fibula deformity who has pedal and posterior tibialis pulses and capillary refill of 2 seconds

8. The signs and symptoms of critical incident stress can be physical, emotional, cognitive, or behavioral. Which of the following is a physical manifestation of this stress?
[ ] **A.** Fatigue
[ ] **B.** Confusion
[ ] **C.** Fear
[ ] **D.** Anorexia

9. When communicating with someone whose primary language is other than English, it is important to do all of the following **EXCEPT**:
[ ] **A.** avoid slang, professional jargon, and acronyms.
[ ] **B.** have the patient rephrase what he thinks he heard you say.
[ ] **C.** pause to allow enough time for the patient to process what you said.
[ ] **D.** simplify for him by asking more yes or no questions.

10. The Emergency Medical Treatment and Active Labor Act (EMTALA) requires that a patient with no insurance:
[ ] **A.** should be transferred to a teaching hospital that receives federal funds.
[ ] **B.** must be transferred to a Level I trauma center as soon as possible.
[ ] **C.** should be transferred if the receiving hospital can provide additional care.
[ ] **D.** cannot be transferred to another facility, as defined by the COBRA law.

11. Which of the following is **NOT** a component of the transfer system between facilities?
[ ] **A.** Communications with the receiving hospital
[ ] **B.** Following your hospital's policies and procedures
[ ] **C.** Available transportation resources in the community
[ ] **D.** Cost of the transfer to the appropriate location

12. Standards of Emergency Nursing Practice incorporate patient education as an expectation. Which of the following is **NOT** an expectation regarding this aspect?
[ ] **A.** Most state nurse practice acts
[ ] **B.** The Joint Commission (formerly JCAHO)
[ ] **C.** Quality assurance/quality improvement (QA/QI) criteria
[ ] **D.** Health Insurance Portability and Accountability Act (HIPAA)

13. Teaching a patient with diabetes the symptoms of hyperglycemia and hypoglycemia is an example of which type of learning?
[ ] **A.** Cognitive
[ ] **B.** Affective
[ ] **C.** Psychomotor
[ ] **D.** Social

14. Which of the following observations would indicate that a depressed patient is becoming suicidal?
[ ] **A.** The patient slams the phone after speaking to a loved one.
[ ] **B.** The patient refuses to eat a turkey sandwich.
[ ] **C.** The patient spits on the security officer.
[ ] **D.** The patient gives the nurse her favorite watch.

15. A registered nurse reads a journal's research study. The study taught fever control measures to first-time parents. Which of the following is most important to determine before attempting to apply the same project in the nurse's emergency department?
[ ] **A.** Was the study approved by an Institutional Review Board (IRB)?
[ ] **B.** What was the actual content that the researcher taught to the parents?
[ ] **C.** Are the researcher's and nurse's settings similar enough for transferability?
[ ] **D.** Did the researcher statistically verify the data results with an analysis of variance (ANOVA)?

16. The Joint Commission in 2018 released a Quick Safety alert on "Identifying Human Trafficking Victims" and pinpointed several red flags of a potential victim. All of the following would be examples of human trafficking victims **EXCEPT**:

[ ] **A.** acting fearful, anxious, depressed, submissive, tense, nervous or paranoid, and avoiding eye contact.

[ ] **B.** requesting additional follow-up treatment at a separate appointment in order to see another provider.

[ ] **C.** showing reluctance or refusing to change into a gown and/or to cooperate with the physical examination.

[ ] **D.** exhibiting behavior or demeanor not in alignment with injury or complaint (that is, acts like it is "no big deal").

17. All of the following populations are commonly targeted for human trafficking **EXCEPT**:

[ ] **A.** Native Americans, Native Hawaiians, and Pacific Islanders.

[ ] **B.** lesbian, gay, bisexual, transgender and questioning (LGBTQ) individuals.

[ ] **C.** employees involved in the foster care and juvenile justice system.

[ ] **D.** migrant workers, undocumented immigrants, and racial and ethnic minorities.

18. Screening questions to identify human trafficking must be brief and limited because the perpetrator will not leave the victim alone for long. Simple screening questions include all of the following **EXCEPT**:

[ ] **A.** "Are doors and windows locked so you cannot leave?"

[ ] **B.** "Has your ID or documentation been taken from you?"

[ ] **C.** "Have you been denied food, water, sleep, or medical care?"

[ ] **D.** "What is your cell phone number so we can reach you?"

19. In 2018, The Joint Commission's Quick Safety alert on "Identifying Human Trafficking Victims" stated all of the following **EXCEPT**:

[ ] **A.** human trafficking should only be addressed by the ED RN caring for the victim.

[ ] **B.** anyone working in a hospital or clinic should be trained to notice the red flags.

[ ] **C.** support staff such as transporters or technicians might seem less intimidating to victims.

[ ] **D.** medical care is often necessary for trafficking victims and we must be vigilant.

20. The emergency nurse is triaging a patient who has a fear of leaving his house. He only comes outside when accompanied by his spouse. The nurse determines the patient is experiencing which of the following?

[ ] **A.** Social phobia

[ ] **B.** Agoraphobia

[ ] **C.** Claustrophobia

[ ] **D.** Hypochondriasis

21. Benzodiazepines such as lorazepam (Ativan) are no longer considered a first-line treatment for insomnia, agitation, and delirium in older adults. According to guidelines published in 2013, "elderly patients are significantly more sensitive to the sedative effects of benzodiazepines." Emergency nurses know that benzodiazepines can cause which of the following?

[ ] **A.** Respiratory depression

[ ] **B.** Hypoxemia

[ ] **C.** Delirium

[ ] **D.** Alcohol withdrawal

22. Which level trauma center must have a trauma surgeon, trauma director, operating suite, and in-house operating room staff on duty 24 hours per day?

[ ] **A.** Level I trauma center only

[ ] **B.** Level I, II, and III trauma centers

[ ] **C.** Level I and II trauma centers

[ ] **D.** Level IV trauma center

23. A multisystem trauma victim is being transferred to a trauma center. The receiving physician insists that the patient be intubated before transfer. Who is legally responsible for ensuring that the patient is intubated before transfer?

[ ] **A.** The receiving physician

[ ] **B.** The referring physician

[ ] **C.** The referring ED nurse

[ ] **D.** The transport team

24. Before an air lift transfer, the emergency nurse recalls that air expands in the altitude of any aircraft; therefore, the nurse recalls issues related to gas-filled organs and medical equipment before transport. Which of the following is **NOT** an appropriate statement regarding this understanding?

[ ] **A.** Air splints will expand and are encouraged.

[ ] **B.** Chest tubes should be in place for pneumothoraces.

[ ] **C.** Decompress the stomach with a gastric tube.

[ ] **D.** Insert a urinary catheter to monitor urinary output.

25. Increased emergency department patient length of stay (LOS) across hospitals in the United States increases risk for patients and leads to patient and staff frustration. Which of the following is **NOT** a way to improve throughput to avoid increased LOS?

[ ] **A.** Timely testing and obtaining test results
[ ] **B.** Direct (or immediate) bedding whenever possible
[ ] **C.** Holding inpatients (boarding) in the ED
[ ] **D.** Placing a provider at triage during peak hours

26. The American Nurses Association (ANA) defines bullying as "repeated, unwanted, harmful actions intended to humiliate, offend, and cause distress in the recipient." Which of the following is a true statement regarding bullying?

[ ] **A.** Some acts of aggression may be verbal and are entirely acceptable because of the stress of the ED.
[ ] **B.** ED nurses may not defend against violence because the perpetrator is a patient or visitor.
[ ] **C.** Bullying occurs in all work sectors, with the health care industry having much higher incidents.
[ ] **D.** Bullying is less common than either sexual harassment or racial discrimination on the job.

27. An emergency nurse delegates the responsibility of taking and recording a patient's blood pressure to the unlicensed assistive personnel (nurse's aide). Later, the nurse notes that there is no blood pressure recorded on the patient's chart. Which of the following options is the best response for this situation?

[ ] **A.** Take the blood pressure now himself and speak to the UAP at the end of the shift.
[ ] **B.** Talk to the involved unlicensed assistive personnel (nurse aide/technician) now.
[ ] **C.** Ask the patient whether anyone took his blood pressure today.
[ ] **D.** Discuss the matter with the charge nurse and proceed accordingly.

28. A patient in the triage area is yelling and becoming increasingly agitated; he throws his bottle of water on the floor. The family states this agitated and aggressive behavior is new over the past few hours. Which of the following is the best response for the triage nurse at this time?

[ ] **A.** Approach the patient and directly confront him to control him through authority.
[ ] **B.** Inform the patient that this is not acceptable behavior in the emergency department.
[ ] **C.** Reassure the patient that the nurse is here to help him.
[ ] **D.** Shout for security to call the police immediately.

29. Which of the following is an advantage of ground transport over helicopter transport?

[ ] **A.** Better radio communications with hospitals
[ ] **B.** More space inside
[ ] **C.** Faster speed
[ ] **D.** Fewer traffic and road factors

30. A patient is pacing and agitated, with rapid speech and is becoming belligerent. Which of the following should be the first priority?

[ ] **A.** Provide immediate safety for the patient.
[ ] **B.** Offer the patient a less stimulated area to calm down.
[ ] **C.** Change the subject by offering the patient food.
[ ] **D.** Assist the staff in caring for the other patients' safety.

31. A patient arrives in the emergency department with signs and symptoms consistent with a non-ST elevation myocardial infarction (NSTEMI). His vital signs are as follows: blood pressure, 100/68 mm Hg; pulse, 46 beats/minute; and respirations, 24 breaths/minute. The physician decides to transfer him to another facility by air. After stabilizing the patient with oxygen, an arterial line, intravenous line placement, and appropriate medication therapy, which of the following should be considered before transport via aircraft?

[ ] **A.** Nothing; the patient is ready to be transported.
[ ] **B.** The effect of air transport on the arterial line pressure bag
[ ] **C.** The ability of the patient's family to accompany the patient
[ ] **D.** Ensuring that vital signs are documented just before departure

32. When planning care for a patient in a crisis state, which of the following is a true statement?

[ ] **A.** All individuals experiencing a crisis have the same crisis symptoms.
[ ] **B.** Individuals in crisis state are displaying signs of severe mental illness.
[ ] **C.** There is an underlying emotional illness exacerbating crisis state.
[ ] **D.** Each person reacts uniquely and differently to a crisis situation.

33. Quantitative studies are important in nursing research and utilize numeric findings for quantification. Which of the following is a true statement regarding quantitative studies?
[ ] A. These studies compare the results of one form of treatment against a control group.
[ ] B. This type of research gathers insight into a person's motivations and opinions.
[ ] C. This particular research study follows subjects with a particular disease process.
[ ] D. This study examines relationships and determines the cause and effect of variables.

34. The PICO acronym is often used in quantitative studies to help researchers ask focused clinical questions. The "P" in PICO refers to the "Population" or "Problem" being considered. What do the "I" and "C" represent?
[ ] A. Intervention and Control group
[ ] B. Intervention and Comparison
[ ] C. Implementation and Considerations
[ ] D. Implementation and Consultation

35. The Health Insurance Portability and Accountability Act (HIPAA) includes protected information in public venues. However, protected health information can be shared without patient consent in which of the following situations?
[ ] A. Insurance companies for billing purposes
[ ] B. To an ex-spouse for legal recovery of information
[ ] C. EMS to determine patient's marital status
[ ] D. To share with neighbors or friends who call

36. When caring for a case involving forensics, which of the following is an important concept?
[ ] A. Cut off clothing through holes and stains.
[ ] B. Place all clothing together in one neat pile.
[ ] C. Package each piece of clothing in a plastic airtight bag.
[ ] D. Use paper bags with tamper-resistant seal for evidence.

37. An elderly patient with stroke-like symptoms has an active DNR (Do Not Resuscitate) order. In caring for this patient, the understanding would be which of the following options?
[ ] A. Should not initiate labs or an IV line as the patient does not want further treatment
[ ] B. May not provide care for this patient until family arrives and gives consent
[ ] C. An intravenous line may be established, but no medications should be given.
[ ] D. Should initiate care for this patient's stroke symptoms regardless of the DNR wishes

38. A research study involves asking a group of nurses questions regarding perception of the value of an ED-specific preceptor program versus a hospital-based preceptor program. This type of research is considered to be:
[ ] A. qualitative.
[ ] B. quantitative.
[ ] C. systematic.
[ ] D. retrospective.

39. A behavioral health patient is behaving bizarrely and is considered a danger to himself and others. His hold is based on which of the following types of consent?
[ ] A. Express consent
[ ] B. Implied consent
[ ] C. Involuntary consent
[ ] D. Informed consent

40. An 86-year-old patient is being prepared for surgery. Which of the following approaches best ensures he will understand the risks and benefits?
[ ] A. Give him enough time to process the information.
[ ] B. Ask family members to make these decisions.
[ ] C. Ask patient to respond immediately so he does not forget.
[ ] D. Give the patient reading material to review postoperatively.

41. An elderly patient has decided to discontinue treatment. It would be recognized that the patient is competent to make this decision and support the decision based on which of the following ethical principles?
[ ] A. Justice
[ ] B. Fidelity
[ ] C. Autonomy
[ ] D. Confidentiality

42. Which of the following would the nurse avoid placing in the medical record when an error has occurred with a patient?
[ ] A. Nurses involved in the care of this patient
[ ] B. Interventions that have been performed
[ ] C. Physician notifications
[ ] D. Incident report submitted

43. The common adage of being unable to show anger to someone at work, therefore you go home and "kick the cat" is a way to describe the defense mechanism known as:
[ ] **A.** displacement.
[ ] **B.** denial.
[ ] **C.** repression.
[ ] **D.** projection.

44. Which of the following would **NOT** be involved in the assessment of a patient's motivation for learning?
[ ] **A.** Patient's verbal response to instructions
[ ] **B.** Patient's nonverbal feedback
[ ] **C.** Patient's interest during teaching
[ ] **D.** Patient's education level

45. Which of the following organizations provides a nationwide template to enable federal, state, local, and tribal governments to work together for a range of domestic incidents?
[ ] **A.** Federal Response Plan (FRP)
[ ] **B.** Federal Bureau of Investigation (FBI)
[ ] **C.** National Incident Management System (NIMS)
[ ] **D.** Disaster Relief and Emergency Assistance Act

46. Based on the relationship and time frame commonly available for patient education in the emergency department, which of the following kinds of learning goals are best established with a patient in this setting?
[ ] **A.** Long term
[ ] **B.** Short term
[ ] **C.** Middle range
[ ] **D.** Tertiary range

47. Which of the following is the best method for the emergency department staff to protect themselves against possible negligence or malpractice litigation?
[ ] **A.** Document your actions with a difficult family member in the medical record.
[ ] **B.** Document the nurse-to-patient ratio to defend your caseload.
[ ] **C.** Provide and document care provided within accepted hospital standards.
[ ] **D.** Provide the best care you can and describe what you were not able to complete as well.

48. What does the plaintiff have to prove in litigation for negligence?
[ ] **A.** Intent to cause harm
[ ] **B.** Substandard care delivery
[ ] **C.** Mitigating circumstances
[ ] **D.** Lack of intent

49. Which of the following is the most common unintentional tort involving health care personnel?
[ ] **A.** Malpractice
[ ] **B.** Negligence
[ ] **C.** Assault
[ ] **D.** Battery

50. Which of the following is a true statement regarding breach of duty?
[ ] **A.** Willful violation of an oath or code of ethics regarding patient care
[ ] **B.** Failure to meet accepted standards in providing care for a patient
[ ] **C.** Threatening a patient with withholding pain medication
[ ] **D.** Confining a patient to a psychiatric unit without a physician's order

51. It is the plaintiff's responsibility to prove certain elements in a negligence lawsuit. Which of the following is **NOT** one of these elements?
[ ] **A.** A duty was owed to the patient.
[ ] **B.** The defendant breached the duty.
[ ] **C.** This breach of duty was the cause of the plaintiff's injury.
[ ] **D.** The plaintiff was at risk for an injury because of the breach of duty.

52. "The protective privilege ends where the public peril begins" indicates the duty of the emergency nurse when a patient threatens another person with bodily injury or harm. What does the quoted statement mean?
[ ] **A.** Confidentiality between patient and nurse does not relieve staff of the duty to warn the threatened person and authorities.
[ ] **B.** Confidentiality between nurse and patient is as sacred as the attorney–client privilege and is never broken.
[ ] **C.** The emergency nurse must weigh the seriousness of the threat before breaking the confidentiality of that patient.
[ ] **D.** Warning the patient not to commit a felony covers the emergency nurse as duty to warn and is sufficient.

53. With regard to the phrase "The protective privilege ends where the public peril begins," which of the following patient situations would be subject to this quoted phrase?
[ ] **A.** The discharge of a child with his parents to a new home
[ ] **B.** The discharge of a single mother and her neonate
[ ] **C.** The discharge of a psychiatric patient threatening to kill his wife
[ ] **D.** The discharge of a woman with a gunshot wound to her apartment

54. When triaging a woman of childbearing age, it is important to gather which assessment data?
[ ] **A.** Number of pregnancies and live births
[ ] **B.** Date of last menstrual period
[ ] **C.** Known sexual partners
[ ] **D.** Gynecologic health of her siblings

55. A mother brings her 3-year-old to the emergency department because of blood in the child's underwear. The examination by the sexual assault nurse examiner (SANE nurse) reveals sexual assault and felonious penetration. The mother wants to leave. Which action should the nurse take?
[ ] **A.** No action is necessary because the mother is the child's legal guardian and her decisions are final.
[ ] **B.** Immediately report the findings to Child Protective Services and the police.
[ ] **C.** Encourage the mother to reconsider her decision and refer her to a child psychologist.
[ ] **D.** Have the emergency department physician talk to the mother and try to persuade her to stay.

56. Child Protective Services has decided to remove a child from the mother's care pending further investigation of a sexual assault on the child. The mother becomes upset and is afraid the child's father will beat her. The nurse can refer the mother to several social service agencies. Which one of the following agencies would be most appropriate in this situation?
[ ] **A.** Local women's shelter
[ ] **B.** The welfare bureau
[ ] **C.** A homeless shelter
[ ] **D.** A soup kitchen

57. Which of the following is true regarding the Emergency Medical Treatment and Active Labor Act (EMTALA) mandate for a patient having labor contractions?
[ ] **A.** If the contractions are 5 (or more) minutes apart, she should be referred to a hospital that offers maternity services.
[ ] **B.** All patients having contractions must be medically screened and stabilized before transport to another facility.
[ ] **C.** Only women in obvious active labor need to be medically screened before transport to another facility.
[ ] **D.** The emergency department has the right to refuse patients when it does not offer the needed services.

58. Which of the following is a true statement regarding the Emergency Medical Treatment and Active Labor Act (EMTALA) mandate regarding a patient presenting without insurance?
[ ] **A.** Medical screening examination cannot be delayed pending insurance coverage or the ability to pay.
[ ] **B.** The patient must present proof of ability to pay before services are rendered.
[ ] **C.** Every hospital must maintain inpatient beds for patients who are not able to pay for services.
[ ] **D.** The ability to pay for services should not be part of the admission procedure.

59. Several sources of law affect the emergency department nurse. Which source of law would Medicare laws fall under?
[ ] **A.** Ordinances
[ ] **B.** Common law
[ ] **C.** Constitutional law
[ ] **D.** Statutory law

60. A 44-year-old patient with a broken right ankle refuses morphine for pain. The nurse notices that the patient continues to grimace after a cast has been applied. The patient still refuses the morphine, but the nurse decides the patient would obtain relief from the morphine and gives it intravenously, planning to tell the patient after she sees how well it worked. This is an example of which of the following?
[ ] **A.** Assault
[ ] **B.** Breach of duty
[ ] **C.** Proximate cause
[ ] **D.** Battery

61. A patient who slashed his wrist is placed on a suicidal hold and security is called to observe him, although the patient wants to leave the emergency department. Which of the following types of consent would allow staff to keep this patient and provide treatment?

[ ] **A.** Implied
[ ] **B.** Informed
[ ] **C.** Involuntary
[ ] **D.** Express

62. A patient took an overdose of Valium and requests that the incident not be reported because he could lose his job. It is a mandatory reportable situation. The physician states that he will not report it this time, but if it occurs again, he will. Which of the following options should the emergency nurse execute?

[ ] **A.** Confront the physician as to whether he is reporting the incident.
[ ] **B.** Assume the physician will report it because it is mandatory.
[ ] **C.** Report the incident regardless of the physician's promise to the patient.
[ ] **D.** It is none of the nurse's business; it is between the doctor and the patient.

63. Appropriate RN staffing in the emergency department requires that the nurse manager must:

[ ] **A.** know and utilize the patient volume and acuity levels by hour of the day and take into consideration variability by day of the week and/or time of year.
[ ] **B.** be aware of The Joint Commission (TJC) standard that emergency services shall be appropriately integrated with other units and departments within the organization.
[ ] **C.** realize that patient visits in the emergency department are too unpredictable to appropriately staff on an everyday basis.
[ ] **D.** for the sake of standardization, ensure that emergency department staffing is designed to mimic the rest of the organization.

64. A team of nurses, physicians, and registration clerks meet to address a departmental goal of decreasing total length of stay (LOS) in the department. First, they collect and review data (sorted by triage category) on the length of time patients wait to be seen. This is an early step in:

[ ] **A.** descriptive qualitative research.
[ ] **B.** indicator relevance testing.
[ ] **C.** collaborative scientific research.
[ ] **D.** quality improvement process.

65. Which of the following factors should determine the composition of the intrahospital transport team?

[ ] **A.** Patient's acuity level
[ ] **B.** Medications needed
[ ] **C.** Patient's weight
[ ] **D.** Unit receiving the patient

66. Brainstorming is a problem-solving method whereby a group rapidly generates which of the following types of solutions?

[ ] **A.** As many as possible
[ ] **B.** As practical as possible
[ ] **C.** As wild and crazy as possible
[ ] **D.** As high-quality as possible

67. Which of the following grade levels is usually the best for written discharge instructions?

[ ] **A.** First
[ ] **B.** Third
[ ] **C.** Fourth
[ ] **D.** Fifth

68. Which of the following is a manager allowed to do in response to a collective bargaining initiative?

[ ] **A.** Prevent employees from engaging in recruiting activities during nonworking hours.
[ ] **B.** Prevent employees from participating in informal union activities in patient care areas.
[ ] **C.** Withhold desirable assignments from those nurses who are union organizers.
[ ] **D.** Provide special considerations to discourage employees from joining the union.

69. Which of the following would be an appropriate technique to employ to enhance recall for the patient receiving discharge instructions?

[ ] **A.** Use a passive voice.
[ ] **B.** Be general in explanations.
[ ] **C.** Announce topics.
[ ] **D.** Utilize medical terms.

70. Many emergency departments have customer service committees whose charge is to improve customer relations. Effectiveness is most likely to occur in which of these scenarios?

[ ] **A.** An all-nurse committee because nurses have the most patient contact
[ ] **B.** A committee that includes all disciplines and levels of staff and management
[ ] **C.** A small committee of managers who can respond most effectively to complaints
[ ] **D.** A multidisciplinary staff-level committee that closely monitors complaints against staff

71. An applicant for an emergency department nursing position is qualified depending on personal qualities, education, experience, and credentials. An applicant's (ENPC) (Emergency Nursing Pediatric Course),TNCC (Trauma Nursing Core Course), ACLS (Advanced Cardiac Life Support), and CEN (Certified Emergency Nurse) certification as well as RN (Registered Nurse) licensure are examples of which qualifications?
[ ] **A.** Personal qualities
[ ] **B.** Experience
[ ] **C.** Educational preparation
[ ] **D.** Credentials

72. A department with a shared governance model would more likely have which of these scheduling processes?
[ ] **A.** Self-scheduling of staff, by the staff
[ ] **B.** Management scheduling of staff
[ ] **C.** Designated staff leader scheduling of staff
[ ] **D.** A centralized computer-generated scheduling system

73. What is the purpose of research in emergency nursing?
[ ] **A.** To enhance the professional status of emergency nursing
[ ] **B.** To generate a scientific knowledge base for validating and improving practice
[ ] **C.** To evaluate new medical devices, tools, and medications
[ ] **D.** To help nurses identify problems in their clinical setting

74. Research that aims to examine the feelings and perceptions of emergency nurses working with battered female patients is which of the following types of study?
[ ] **A.** Qualitative
[ ] **B.** Quasi-scientific
[ ] **C.** Quantitative
[ ] **D.** Experimental

75. A registered nurse is the preceptor for a new graduate nurse. The graduate nurse tells the nurse preceptor that his patient has an order for a urinary catheter insertion but he does not know how to perform this procedure. Which of the following actions is best for the preceptor nurse?
[ ] **A.** Refer him to the policy and procedure book.
[ ] **B.** Do the procedure for him but require him to chart it.
[ ] **C.** Tell him to call the clinical nurse educator.
[ ] **D.** Perform the procedure with him.

Answers/Rationales

1. Answer: A

Cognitive Level: Application

Rationale: **Although each of these items is important in safely and effectively managing surge, keeping patients and visitors informed, activating relevant procedures, and prioritizing hazards, safety, and health issues cannot be done unless (or until) the charge nurse activates the plan.**

2. Answer: D

Cognitive Level: Recall

Rationale: **Appropriate alternatives are to be considered *first* always before the application of any type of restraints.** The goal is to use the least restrictive restraint possible and only after unsuccessful use of alternatives. Restraint use should not be part of any routine protocol. There are many risks associated with physically restraining an individual, including risk of aspiration/suffocation and increased psychological trauma and traumatic memories. Another issue with long-term restraint use is the development of deep vein thrombosis/pulmonary embolus.

CENsational Pearl of Wisdom!

Interactions that are calm, respectful, and collaborative can diminish the need for restraints. There are three distinct types of restraints; physical, chemical, and seclusion. Reduction of restraint use is a focus for many hospitals and health care facilities, and many hospitals now prohibit the use of medications for chemical restraint.

It is important that ED nurses receive training in the application of each type of restraint as well as in ongoing competencies and review of new research regarding the use of restraints.

3. Answer: B

Cognitive Level: Application

Rationale: **This voluntary physical action by the patient indicates his acceptance of the procedure and willingness to have it performed, which is considered to be implied consent.**

CENsational Pearl of Wisdom!

Express consent *can be expressed verbally or in writing when the patient arrives. The patient may simply say "I consent."*

Implied consent *occurs through the actions or conduct of the patient, for example, by showing up at the agreed upon time for surgery. In the ED, it can be said that arriving to the triage window requesting care displays the patient's implied consent or providing the arm for phlebotomy or to have a laceration repaired.*

Informed consent *means that the patient has been informed of the risks and dangers involved in a treatment and that the patient consents to this treatment. It is typically an agreement in writing, in which the patient's signature is considered consent. The provider performing the procedure has the responsibility to inform the patient regarding the abovementioned information.*

Involuntary consent *occurs when a patient is incapable of making prudent medical decisions because of injury or illness.*

4. Answer: C

Cognitive Level: Application

Rationale: **The only possible answer is tertiary because the disaster has already happened.** Tertiary prevention aims to minimize the ongoing lasting effects of the injury or illness to improve the quality of life and life expectancy. In disaster preparedness, this phase is designed to support the long-term effects of the catastrophe and help the community to "rebuild" both physically and psychologically. Primordial, primary, and secondary measures would no longer be relevant. **Primordial** prevention involves minimizing and or mitigation of the social, economic, and cultural patterns of living that contribute to an elevated risk of disease. Working to improve lifestyles to decrease obesity, smoking, and so on is an example of primordial prevention. This is done through individual and mass education. **Primary** prevention refers to risk reduction. It is concerned with preventing the onset of disease/disasters and to reduce the incidence of disease or disasters such as with vaccinations or banning the use of asbestos. **Secondary** prevention aims to reduce the impact of a disease or injury that has already occurred. Examples include routine mammograms, low-dose aspirin daily regimen, and light duty for workers to get back to work.

5. Answer: C

Cognitive Level: Recall

Rationale: **Although documentation is always important (especially with restraints!), this answer is not included in the ENA Code of Ethics.** Protecting human rights, promoting health diplomacy, and working to reduce disparities in the health care realm are all parts of the Code of Ethics.

CENsational Pearl of Wisdom!

The American Nurses Association (ANA) recognizes the Nursing Code of Ethics to be a nonnegotiable and ethical standard of the nursing profession. This document serves as an expression of nursing's commitment to society. Within the code, there are nine provisions. The Emergency Nurses Association (ENA) is recognized by the ANA as a specialty body of nursing.

The nine provisions are as follows:
Provision 1: The nurse practices with compassion and respect for the inherent dignity, worth, and unique attributes of every person.
Provision 2: The nurse's primary commitment is to the patient, whether an individual, family, group, community, or population.

Provision 3: The nurse promotes, advocates for, and protects the rights, health, and safety of the patient.
Provision 4: The nurse has authority, accountability, and responsibility for nursing practice; makes decisions; and takes action consistent with the obligation to promote health and to provide optimal care.
Provision 5: The nurse owes the same duties to self as to others, including the responsibility to promote health and safety, preserve wholeness of character and integrity, maintain competence, and continue personal and professional growth.
Provision 6: The nurse, through individual and collective effort, establishes, maintains, and improves the ethical environment of the work setting and conditions of employment that are conducive to safe, quality health care.
Provision 7: The nurse, in all roles and settings, advances the profession through research and scholarly inquiry, professional standards development, and the generation of both nursing and health policy.
Provision 8: The nurse collaborates with other health professionals and the public to protect human rights, promote health diplomacy, and reduce health disparities.
Provision 9: The profession of nursing—collectively, through its professional organizations—must articulate nursing values, maintain the integrity of the profession, and integrate principles of social justice into nursing and health policy.

This Code of Ethics relates to the specialty of emergency nursing and serves as a point of reference for the emergency nurse to guide professional practice.
For more details and interpretive statements about each provision, see the "Nursing Code of Ethics: Provisions and Interpretative Statements for Emergency Nurses" at www.ena.org

6. Answer: C

Cognitive Level: Application

Rationale: **The emergency nurse should be donning personal protective garments for protection before caring for these patients.** All of the other answers are appropriate, but not without the nurse being safe enough to deliver care.

7. Answer: A

Cognitive Level: Analysis

Rationale: **The patient with asthma is most emergent.** This child may not be wheezing as air movement significantly decreases. Any problems in airway and breathing are considered life-threatening and should be seen

immediately. In most cases, a patient presenting with sickle cell anemia is considered stable but urgent; this patient would be seen second. The 16-year-old with the fracture would most likely be seen third and a small foot laceration with controlled bleeding, fourth.

8. Answer: A

Cognitive Level: Application

Rationale: Although all of the answers are manifestations of critical incident stress responses, the only one categorized as *physical* is fatigue.

 CENsational Pearl of Wisdom!

According to the Occupational Safety and Health Administration (OSHA) Critical Incident Stress Debriefing (CISD) guidelines, the following critical incident stress manifestations often occur:

Physical	Cognitive	Emotional	Behavioral
Fatigue	Uncertainty	Grief	Inability to rest
Chills	Confusion	Fear	Withdrawal
Unusual thirst	Nightmares	Guilt	Antisocial behavior
Chest pain	Poor attention	Intense anger	Increased alcohol consumption
Headaches	Decreased decision-making ability	Apprehension and depression	Change in communications
Dizziness	Poor concentration and memory	Irritability	Loss/increase in appetite
	Poor problem-solving ability	Chronic anxiety	

9. Answer: D

Cognitive Level: Application

Rationale: **Asking more yes and no questions does not simplify the information for the patient. It is important *to minimize* the use of yes/no questions.** Avoiding slang and jargon is important for any communication with patients. Pausing allows the patient to "translate"/comprehend what was just said, and asking the patient to rephrase is important for the nurse to see that the person did understand the information given.

10. Answer: C

Cognitive Level: Application

Rationale: **EMTALA is a federal law that requires hospital emergency departments to medically screen every patient who seeks emergency care and to stabilize or transfer those with medical emergencies, regardless of health insurance status or ability to pay.** This law has been an unfunded mandate since it was enacted in 1986. Transferring to a teaching hospital is not part of the process. Patients should be transferred to an appropriate hospital relative to the illness or injury and must be stabilized before the transfer.

11. Answer: D

Cognitive Level: Recall

Rationale: **The components of a transfer system are communications, transport resources, and policies and procedures.** Although financial issues may influence where and how the patient is transferred, it is not a component of the transfer itself.

12. Answer: D

Cognitive Level: Recall

Rationale: **The Health Insurance Portability and Accountability Act (HIPAA) ensures the appropriate transfer of medical information and protection of the patient's privacy, not the patient's education.** Patient education is the responsibility of the emergency department nurse, especially upon discharge, and the need for patient education is recognized and stated in all other documents cited.

13. Answer: A

Cognitive Level: Application

Rationale: **Understanding of the signs and symptoms of a disease process utilizes cognitive learning skills. This type of learning requires thinking and reasoning in order to integrate the concepts.** Affective learning involves feelings and attitudes. Psychomotor learning requires the coordination of the brain and extremities to complete a task. Social learning requires the ability to interact with others in a social setting.

14. Answer: D

Cognitive Level: Application

Rationale: **Giving away prized possessions is an indication that the person may be considering suicide.**

The other options could be signs of violence, increasing hostility, or depression but do not necessarily indicate suicidal intent.

CENsational Pearl of Wisdom!

According to the Harvard University website, some suicides have absolutely no forewarning and are completely unpredictable. Many suicides and suicide attempts, however, do have warning signs.

A few behaviors that may put friends and family on notice that the risk of suicide is increased would be as follows:

- *Talking about suicide: statements like "I'd be better off dead" or "If I see you again. . ."*
- *Seeking the means: trying to get access to guns, pills, or other objects that could be used in a suicide attempt.*
- *No hope for the future: feelings of helplessness, hopelessness, and a feeling of being trapped (no way out), or believing that things will never get better.*
- *Self-loathing: feelings of worthlessness, guilt, shame, and self-hatred.*
- *Getting affairs in order: giving away prized possessions or making arrangements for family members.*
- *Saying goodbye: unusual or unexpected visits or calls to family and friends; saying goodbye to people as if they will not be seen again.*

People who exhibit these signs are often communicating their distress, hoping to get a response. This is very useful information that should not be ignored.

National Suicide Prevention Lifeline at 800-273-TALK. Counselors are available 24 hours a day, 7 days a week. The service is available to anyone. All calls are confidential.

15. Answer: C

Cognitive Level: Application

Rationale: **To apply the study, the two settings need to be similar enough to allow transferability.** It would not be as effective, for instance, if the emergency department in the study was an inner-city teaching facility treating 200 patients a day and the nurse reading the study worked at a small community hospital with 20 patients a day. An Institutional Review Board (IRB) is a type of committee that applies research ethics by reviewing the methods proposed for research to ensure that they are ethical. They also ensure the rights of the subjects. Such boards are formally designated to approve (or reject), monitor, and review biomedical and behavioral research involving humans. It is essential to know the content of the teaching so it can be implemented, but transferability needs to be determined first. ANOVA is one statistical option for testing differences among three or more group means.

16. Answer: B

Cognitive Level: Recall

Rationale: **Option B is the exception to behaviors related to human trafficking victims because the patient will not request additional follow-up or treatment; the patient will most likely refuse any follow-up if provided.** Each of the other answers describes behaviors that may indicate the patient is a victim of trafficking.

17. Answer: C

Cognitive Level: Analysis

Rationale: **The key word in this answer is "employees" because all of the other answers include populations commonly targeted.** The children in foster care and juvenile facilities are, in fact, also considered targeted populations as well as members of all the other options.

18. Answer: D

Cognitive Level: Analysis

Rationale: **Asking for a cell phone number may trigger fear in the victim that the perpetrator will find out and/ or that the victim "said too much."** All of the other questions are brief, appropriate, and can be answered quickly.

 CENsational Pearl of Wisdom!

For more information on human trafficking, see The Joint Commission Resource entitled Quick Safety 42: Identifying human trafficking victims.

"The United States is one of the largest markets and destinations for human trafficking victims in the world.[1]" and that "Knowing how to identify victims of human trafficking, when to involve law enforcement, and what community resources are available to help the individual is important information for all health care professionals." Identifying and helping victims of human trafficking can be difficult and can further endanger the victim. Most human trafficking victims or their families have been threatened

with harm if the victim reveals their exploitation. In some cases, victims from different countries or cultures do not realize that their exploitation is unusual or criminal. Also, some human trafficking victims have bonded with their exploiter, a condition called trauma bonding that is similar to Stockholm syndrome. Victims may keep silent about their exploitation from shame or fear of being humiliated. Since medical care is occasionally necessary for trafficking victims, health care professionals are in a unique position to help these unfortunate victims.

19. Answer: A

Cognitive Level: Analysis

Rationale: **RNs are important caregivers who should be trained to identify victims; however, *ALL* health care providers are able to assist and intervene with appropriate education.** All of the other responses are appropriate.

20. Answer: B

Cognitive Level: Recall

Rationale: **Agoraphobia is a fear of open spaces and the fear of being trapped in a situation from which there may not be an escape.** Patients fear a sense of helplessness or embarrassment and results in minimizing social and professional interactions. Social phobias include specific situations, such as the fear of speaking, performing, or eating in public. Claustrophobia is a fear of closed places. Hypochondriacs focus their anxiety on physical complaints and are hyper-focused on their own health.

21. Answer: A

Cognitive Level: Application

Rationale: **Benzodiazepines can cause respiratory depression as well as systemic hypotension in elderly adults with agitation and/or delirium.** Hypoxemia, delirium, and alcohol withdrawal are all potential causes of agitation/delirium in elders that the emergency nurse should rule out.

22. Answer: C

Cognitive Level: Recall

Rationale: **Level I and Level II trauma centers must have a trauma surgeon, trauma director, and staffed operating room available around the clock.** Level III trauma centers are excused from the staffed operating room requirement. Level IV trauma centers are excused from all the above requirements.

CENsational Pearl of Wisdom!

Trauma Center Levels

There are five different levels of trauma centers in the United States (this can vary by state—some states do not recognize all five levels). According to the American Trauma Society, the five levels are as follows:

Level I provides total care, from prevention through rehabilitation. These also offer a teaching program for medical residents, as well as for ongoing research.

Level II is similar to a Level I trauma center but does not necessarily offer teaching or research. Both Levels I and II can treat either children or adults.

Level III is smaller than Level I and II centers but can provide prompt care to injured patients.

Level IV has demonstrated an ability to provide advanced trauma life support (ATLS) before transfer of patients to a higher level trauma center. It provides evaluation, stabilization, and diagnostic capabilities for injured patients.

Level V provides initial evaluation, stabilization, and diagnostic capabilities and prepares patients for transfer to higher levels of care.

23. Answer: B

Cognitive Level: Application

Rationale: **The transferring hospital is legally responsible for performing those treatment and diagnostic studies requested by the receiving facility.** The referring physician is legally responsible for ensuring that tests and procedures are completed.

24. Answer: A

Cognitive Level: Application

Rationale: **Air splints are to be used with caution (if at all) and always loosened to accommodate the effects of altitude.** The other responses are appropriate for air transport.

25. Answer: C

Cognitive Level: Analysis

Rationale: **The longer a patient waits in the emergency department for a bed in an inpatient unit, the higher the potential exists for the patient to have an adverse event or poor health outcome.** Obtaining specimens and test results in a timely manner, direct bedding when possible, and utilizing a provider in triage during peak times are all ways to help decrease both length of stay (LOS) and frustrations.

 CENsational Pearl of Wisdom!

Emergency department (ED) boarders is another name for patients who have been admitted under an in-patient service but remain in the ED. The literature describes how ED boarders have worse outcomes than do their counterparts who are admitted quickly to inpatient beds. Some of the issues include increased medication delays, increased mortality and morbidity, hospital expense, and overall hospital length of stay (LOS), as well as decreasing patient and staff satisfaction. In addition, the literature relates that ED boarders have a detrimental effect on other ED patients because ED nurses are caring for patients who would be better cared for by the expert nurses on their appropriate unit.

26. Answer: C

Cognitive Level: Analysis

Rationale: **Bullying has long been health care's dirty little secret, with more incidents than in other work place venues. Acts of aggression may be verbal; however, they are NOT acceptable in the ED or in any other health care setting.** ED nurses should defend against violence in the workplace no matter who the perpetrator is, and bullying is more common than sexual harassment and racial discrimination.

 CENsational Pearl of Wisdom!

As described in The Joint Commission (TJC) safety issue brief 24 (June 2016):

Civility is a system value that improves safety in health care settings. The link between civility, workplace safety and patient care is not a new concept. The 2004 Institute of Medicine report, "Keeping Patients Safe: Transforming the Work Environment of Nurses," emphasizes the importance of the work environment in which nurses provide care. Workplace incivility that is expressed as bullying behavior is at epidemic levels. A recent Occupational Safety and Health Administration (OSHA) report on workplace violence in health care highlights the magnitude of the problem:

while 21 percent of registered nurses and nursing students reported being physically assaulted, over 50 percent were verbally abused (a category that included bullying) in a 12-month period. In addition, 12 percent of emergency nurses experienced physical violence, and 59 percent experienced verbal abuse during a seven-day period.

CENsational Pearl of Wisdom!

The ED nurse should always be on the alert for abnormal psychosocial behavior that may have a pathophysiologic etiology. Aggressive behavior in an individual that does not usually demonstrate this type of behavior could be from an intracranial basis or a diagnosis that creates hypoxia. Always be concerned about this possibility.

27. Answer: B

Cognitive Level: Analysis

Rationale: **The unlicensed assistive personnel (UAP) may have taken the blood pressure and forgotten to chart it. Even if the task was not done, it is important to follow up to reinforce responsibility for the future.** Taking the blood pressure himself may be duplication of work, and the matter should be cleared up now, not at the end of the shift. The patient could be mistaken about the blood pressure being taken if asked, and it still does not give the results even if it was done. More information should be clarified and the UAP dealt with directly before bringing in management. Management can be brought in if there is a repetitive pattern.

CENsational Pearl of Wisdom!

Remember!!! When the nurse is delegating tasks, the nurse is ultimately responsible for that task! The nurse should be providing follow through on all of the tasks that are asked of others to perform.

28. Answer: C

Cognitive Level: Application

Rationale: **The patient is exhibiting excessive agitation, which has a potential for violence; therefore, reassuring the patient and his family is the most therapeutic response.** The nurse should avoid being within the patient's physical reach to reduce the risk of being hit. Taking an authoritative stance is likely to further agitate the patient. He may not be able to cognitively take verbal cueing or instructions because of an underlying pathologic process. Shouting that outside authorities should be called will also likely incite further agitation.

29. Answer: B

Cognitive Level: Analysis

Rationale: **Ground vehicles have more space inside.** However, helicopter transport has the advantages of having better radio communication with hospitals, traveling at faster speeds, and contending with fewer traffic and road factors.

30. Answer: A

Cognitive Level: Application

Rationale: **The nurse's own and the patient's safety first is paramount.** A less stimulating environment, offering food as a distraction, and assisting other staff members in caring for other emergency patients' safety and well-being can be important; however, scene safety is the first priority.

31. Answer: B

Cognitive Level: Analysis

Rationale: **Altitude changes will cause changes in air pressure, causing a hypobaric environment, whereby the pressure decreases as altitude increases. There will be enough of a pressure change to cause an arterial line pressure bag to lose some pressure, which may result in an inaccurate arterial blood pressure reading.** The patient is not ready to be transported as of yet. The arterial line must be considered and any other altitudinal changes that might impact the patient. Family cannot accompany the patient on board the aircraft. Documenting vital signs is important, but only after the arterial line pressure bag is stabilized.

32. Answer: D

Cognitive Level: Recall

Rationale: **All individuals experiencing a crisis respond in their own way. There is no right or wrong response.** People do not all respond the same and individuals in crisis do not necessarily have an underlying mental illness nor is there an underlying emotional illness that is exacerbating the problem.

33. Answer: D

Cognitive Level: Application

Rationale: **Quantitative research (think *QUANTITY*) uses measurable data to formulate facts and uncover patterns; it examines the data to determine cause and effect.** A study that compares treatments against a control group would be classified as a randomized control study in which participants are compared to a control group. Quantitative research does not necessarily follow all subjects of a specific disease process. Cohort studies follow patients over time and qualitative research (think *QUALITY*) utilizes small groups and individual insights to gather greater understanding of peoples' opinions and motivations. It provides insights into the problem. *QUALITATIVE* studies can be used to develop ideas or hypotheses for potential quantitative research.

 CENsational Pearl of Wisdom!

Case series and case reports *consist of collections of reports on the treatment of individual patients or a report on a single patient. Because they are reports of cases and use no control groups to compare outcomes, they have little statistical validity.*

Case control studies *are studies in which patients who already have a specific condition are compared with people who do not have the condition. The researcher looks back to identify factors or exposures that might be associated with the illness. They often rely on medical records and patient recall for data collection. These types of studies are often less reliable than randomized controlled trials and cohort studies because showing a statistical relationship does not mean than one factor necessarily caused the other.*

Cohort studies *identify a group of patients who are already taking a particular treatment or have an exposure, follow them forward over time, and then compare their outcomes with a similar group that has not been affected by the treatment or exposure being studied. Cohort studies are observational and not as reliable as randomized controlled studies, because the two groups may differ in ways other than in the variable study.*

Randomized controlled clinical trials *are carefully planned experiments that introduce a treatment or exposure to study its effect on real patients. They include methodologies that reduce the potential for bias (randomization and blinding) and that allow for comparison between intervention groups and control (no intervention) groups. A randomized controlled trial is a planned experiment and can provide sound evidence of cause and effect.*

Systematic reviews *focus on a clinical topic and answer a specific question. An extensive literature search is conducted to identify studies with sound methodology. The studies are reviewed, assessed for quality, and the results summarized according to the predetermined criteria of the review question.*

A **meta-analysis** *will thoroughly examine a number of valid studies on a topic and mathematically combine the results using accepted statistical methodology to report the results as if it were one large study.*

Cross-sectional studies *describe the relationship between diseases and other factors at one point in time in a defined population. Cross-sectional studies lack any information on timing of exposure and outcome relationships and include only prevalent cases. They are often used for comparing diagnostic tests. Studies that show the efficacy of a diagnostic test are also called prospective, blind comparison to a gold standard study. This is a controlled trial that looks at patients with varying degrees of an illness and administers both diagnostic tests—the test under investigation and the "gold standard" test—to all of the patients in the study group. The sensitivity and specificity of the new test are compared to that of the gold standard to determine potential usefulness.*

A retrospective cohort (or historical cohort) *follows the same direction of inquiry as a cohort study. Subjects begin with the presence or absence of an exposure or risk factor and are followed up until the outcome of interest is observed. However, this study design uses information that has been collected in the past and kept in files or databases. Patients are identified for exposure or nonexposures and the data are followed forward to an effect or outcome of interest.*

Qualitative research *answers a wide variety of questions related to human responses to actual or potential health problems. The purpose of qualitative research is to describe, explore, and explain the health-related phenomena being studied.*

34. Answer: B

Cognitive Level: Recall

Rationale: **Evidence-based models use a framework with the acronym PICO(T). These elements include the following: Problem/Patient/Population, Intervention/ Indicator, Comparison, Outcome, and (optional) Time element.**

 CENsational Pearl of Wisdom!

P: Population *in the study/disease you are look-ing at (e.g., age, gender, ethnicity, with a certain disorder)*
I: Intervention *or variable of interest (exposure to a disease, risk behavior, prognostic factor, new process)*
C: Comparison—*who/what is measured "against" this group (could be a placebo or "business as usual" as in no disease, absence of risk factor)*
O: Outcome: *(risk of disease, accuracy of a diagnosis, rate of occurrence of adverse outcome)*
T: Time: *The time it takes to demonstrate an out-come (i.e., the time it takes for the intervention to achieve an outcome or how long the pilot will be held)*

35. Answer: A

Cognitive Level: Application

Rationale: **Insurance companies are included in the transmission of protected health information.** It would not be appropriate to give the information to individu-als (such as the ex-wife/husband or friends who call in). EMS personnel would already have the patient's consent because they brought the patient in to the hospital. The Privacy Rule protects all "individually identifiable health information" held or transmitted by a covered entity (that is, hospital) or its business associate, in any form or media (whether electronic, paper, or oral). The hospital may share protected health information (PHI) during the course of treatment, payment, and health care operations.

36. Answer: D

Cognitive Level: Analysis

Rationale: **Paper allows the evidence to breathe, whereas plastic could destroy the evidence with mold and other issues. Applying and initialing the seals ensures the safety of the evidence because the tape is designed to fracture easily to indicate tampering.** When cutting the clothing off a patient, never cut through any cuts, holes, or other marks that may be entrance/exit wounds or contain evidence. It is important these areas be left unaltered. Each piece of evidence should be gath-ered separately to avoid cross contamination, not piled on top of each other.

 CENsational Pearl of Wisdom!

Evidence collection is an important aspect of emer-gency nursing! Every nurse should understand the concept of "Chain of Evidence" as well as an under-standing of basic forensics. At times the ED becomes the crime scene when the patient arrives.

37. Answer: D

Cognitive Level: Analysis

Rationale: **The DNR order is meant to inform health care providers that the patient does not want life-saving techniques performed at the time of cardiac/ respiratory arrest.** It does not allow the nurse to assume that the patient does not want care for his current condi-tion. Care should be provided to this patient following the standards of care for a stroke patient.

38. Answer: A

Cognitive Level: Recall

Rationale: **Think "quality." Qualitative studies involve questions related to human responses, opinions, and motivations of the participants.** Quantitative studies review data. Systematic reviews involve extensive litera-ture search and retrospective studies follow subjects over time.

CENsational Pearl of Wisdom!

Qualitative studies basically report their findings with words and quantitative studies usually involve numbers. Think door to electrocardiogram time, and so on for quantitative studies.

39. Answer: C

Cognitive Level: Recall

Rationale: **This patient is considered involuntary because he no longer has the capacity to make decisions for himself.** If the patient were not a danger to himself or others, this would be an example of informed consent. Implied consent occurs through the actions of conduct of the patient, as in coming to the ED seeking care or cooperating with a procedure. Express consent is expressed verbally or in writing.

40. Answer: A

Cognitive Level: Application

Rationale: **Allowing time for the information to be processed is necessary because the aging process affects the speed with which cognitive and motor processes are performed.** This does not mean that the activities cannot be performed, but rather that they take longer. Family members should not make these decisions unless it is a situation in which the patient cannot capably process the information and make an informed decision. Reading material postoperatively will not assist in making this decision preoperatively.

41. Answer: C

Cognitive Level: Application

Rationale: **A patient is competent to make his/her own decisions and therefore entitled by the ethical principle of autonomy, the right to make decisions regarding a patient's own body.** Autonomy is the right of the patient to retain control over his or her body. Actions that attempt to persuade or coerce the patient into making a choice are violations of this principle, whether the medical provider believes these choices are in that patient's best interest. Beneficence refers to doing all that can be done to benefit the patient in each situation. All recommended procedures and treatments should consider each patient's individual circumstances. Emergency staff members should be trained in the most current and best practices and must recognize that what is good for one patient will not necessarily benefit another.

Nonmaleficence means "to do no harm." This means that we must also consider whether other people or society could be harmed by a decision made, even if it is made for the benefit of an individual patient. Justice recognizes that there should be fairness in all our decisions, including equal distribution of scarce resources and new treatments.

42. Answer: D

Cognitive Level: Recall

Rationale: **Although it is important for the nurse to document this information in a variance or incident report, this is not to be documented in the patient medical record.** The other answers should all be included in the patient record. Staff that are involved in the care of the patient, interventions performed, and physicians should always be included in all charting.

CENsational Pearl of Wisdom!

Please remember how important narrative charting is! Do not simply use checkmarks to denote all care of a patient. The nurse should be painting a picture with the written word, and it is imperative that a true "picture" of the patient and situation can be derived in cases of possible litigation. This is also true for nonlitiginous situations.

43. Answer: A

Cognitive Level: Recall

Rationale: **Displacement is the defense mechanism illustrated by the adage "kicking the cat."** When the person is unable to confront the coworker who caused the issue, he/she might project that anger on a less threatening person or object. See the following CENsational Pearl of Wisdom! to learn more about the other types of defense mechanisms.

CENsational Pearl of Wisdom!

Defense mechanisms *are an unconscious protective measure that allows us to cope with unpleasant emotions. Some common ones include the following:* **Denial** *is when something is too difficult to handle, the person will "refuse to experience it." It is a way to protect oneself from facing and dealing with the unpleasant consequences and pain that accompany acceptance.*

Repression *is similar to denial; however, repression involves completely forgetting the experience altogether. The memory is buried in the subconscious, thereby preventing painful, disturbing, or dangerous thoughts from entering awareness. This is common with child abuse or other traumatic experiences that occurred early on in development.*

Displacement *is the transfer of emotions from the person who is the target of the frustration to someone or something else entirely. Subconsciously, the confrontation is too risky, so the focus is shifted toward a target or situation that is less intimidating or dangerous.*

Projection *occurs when insecurity about oneself causes to "project" feelings onto others; this is done because to recognize that particular quality in one self would cause pain and suffering.*

Regression *is when a person will revert to an earlier level of development where the less demanding behaviors are a way of protecting one from having to confront the actual situation.*

Rationalization *occurs when a person will justify the bad behavior, often placing the blame on others or incidents that caused or provoked the behavior.*

44. Answer: D

Cognitive Level: Analysis

Rationale: **The patient's education level may affect how he learns, but not his motivation.** Consideration of the behavioral, verbal, and nonverbal clues given by the patient enables the nurse to accurately assess the patient's motivation for learning.

45. Answer: C

Cognitive Level: Recall

Rationale: **NIMS integrates emergency preparedness and response into a national framework for incident management.** The Federal Response Plan was created as a guide for an all-hazards approach to domestic incidents and how to group them. The Disaster Relief and Emergency Assistance Act was enacted as statutory authority for most federal disaster response activities and created the Federal Response Plan. The FBI is not involved in emergency preparedness.

 CENsational Pearl of Wisdom!

Incident Command Structures *are based on a three-organization system: incident command, multiagency coordination, and public information*

46. Answer: B

Cognitive Level: Application

Rationale: **Short-term goals are the only ones that the ED nurse will be able to provide in this setting.** There is no long-term, ongoing relationship in the ED setting (typically!). Middle range and tertiary range goals do not exist.

47. Answer: C

Cognitive Level: Analysis

Rationale: **Meeting and documenting the standards of care may not prevent litigation, but these actions will certainly provide support that the standards of care were known and adhered to.** Actions should be documented for all patients, not just for difficult ones. Documentation of nurse-to-patient ratios does not relieve the nurse of the responsibility to provide care within accepted standards. Accepted practice is to document what was done for a patient, not what was *not done*.

48. Answer: B

Cognitive Level: Recall

Rationale: **The plaintiff must prove that the care received was substandard.** It is not necessary to prove intent to cause harm. Mitigating circumstances are issues that would be brought up by the defendant, not the plaintiff. Negligence is by definition an unintentional tort or a civil wrong done without intent by the defendant; therefore, it is not necessary to demonstrate lack of intent.

49. Answer: B

Cognitive Level: Recall

Rationale: **Negligence is the most common unintentional tort involving health care personnel.** Negligence committed by a professional is malpractice, but not all malpractice is negligence. Malpractice is a more restricted, specialized kind of negligence, defined as a violation of professional duty to act with reasonable care and in good faith. Assault and battery are intentional torts.

50. Answer: B

Cognitive Level: Application

Rationale: **If a patient sues a nurse for negligence, the patient must prove that the nurse owed him a specific duty and that the nurse breached this duty.** A breach of duty in this case means that the nurse did not provide care within the accepted standard. A breach is not always willful, as implied in option A. Threatening a patient is assault, more accurately described as a direct invasion of a patient's rights rather than a breach of duty. Confining a patient to a psychiatric unit without a physician's order is false imprisonment, another example of direct invasion of a patient's rights.

51. Answer: D

Cognitive Level: Application

Rationale: **The plaintiff must prove that the injuries sustained were real or actual.** The plaintiff must prove that the defendant owed him a specific duty; that the defendant breached this duty; that the plaintiff was harmed physically, mentally, emotionally, or financially; and that the defendant's breach of duty caused this harm. The plaintiff must also prove foreseeability and damages.

 CENsational Pearl of Wisdom!

The requirements for nursing malpractice include the following elements:

Duty: *There must be a duty owed to the patient. For example, the patient is owed a safe environment, and a nurse has a duty to follow orders and care for the patient.*

Breach of duty: *The specific duty owed to the patient has been breached, meaning that the duty has not been met. In terms of safe environment, the nurse forgets to put the bed rail up and the patient falls. The nurse's failure to maintain the patient's safe environment would constitute a breach of duty.*

Damages: *The breach of duty must have caused injuries that result in damages. The injuries the patient suffered when falling out of bed are the damages that can be claimed. If the patient was not injured, there are no damages.*

Cause: *This is generally the most difficult element to prove in a medical malpractice lawsuit. There must be a direct cause-and-effect link between the breach of duty and the injury. The breach of duty must have caused the injury. In the example, if the nurse had not left the bed railing down, the patient would not have fallen. The nurse's breach of duty caused the injury.*

52. Answer: A

Cognitive Level: Application

Rationale: **Confidentiality between patient and nurse (or physician) should be breached to alleviate a threat to another person.** Medical personnel have a duty to

warn the intended victim (if known) and the authorities. Warning the patient not to commit a felony or weighing the seriousness of the threat is not sufficient grounds for relief from the duty to warn.

53. Answer: C

Cognitive Level: Application

Rationale: **Medical personnel have a duty to warn the intended victim (if known) and the authorities if there is potential for harm to others.** Even though the medical personnel may not know who the victim might be, there is an obligation to tell the authorities about the condition of the patient. The other options do not pose a threat to anyone.

54. Answer: B

Cognitive Level: Analysis

Rationale: **The date of the last menstrual period provides information about the likelihood of a first-trimester pregnancy.** This information may affect medications ordered and radiographic procedures performed. The number of pregnancies and live births is important information, but it has no impact on ordered medications or radiographic procedures. Information about known sexual partners is only important in the presence of a sexually transmitted infection. Sibling health history will not impact this situation.

55. Answer: B

Cognitive Level: Application

Rationale: **The nurse has a duty of care to the patient and to the public and must report the crime to the authorities.** Regardless of the mother's wishes, the child has been harmed and a report to the authorities is necessary. Even though the emergency physician may talk to the mother and the mother may be encouraged to reconsider her wishes, the fact remains that the crime must be reported and evidence must be collected.

56. Answer: A

Cognitive Level: Analysis

Rationale: **A women's shelter can provide many services that are necessary for the mother including safety for herself and her child while keeping her location confidential.** The welfare bureau is a state agency that provides funds for food, shelter, or other necessities for people who need it. Homeless shelters and soup kitchens are voluntary organizations for people in need of shelter and food. They do not necessarily have resources to accommodate patients at risk for abuse.

57. Answer: B

Cognitive Level: Recall

Rationale: **All patients experiencing contractions must be medically screened before transport.** Whether it is obvious that the patient is in labor or not, she must be medically screened and examined before the decision is made to transport to another facility. The emergency department does not have the right to refuse treatment to a patient before medically screening the patient.

58. Answer: A

Cognitive Level: Recall

Rationale: **To ensure that patients are not denied care on the basis of their ability to pay, they must be medically screened and stabilized before their ability to pay is determined.** Failure of a hospital to comply may result in denial of Medicare funding. Only hospitals accepting Medicare funding are required to have some beds available for the indigent. EMTALA does not address payment for services as part of the admission procedure. It only addresses medical screening and stabilization of patients before transport or the determination of ability to pay for services rendered.

59. Answer: D

Cognitive Level: Recall

Rationale: **Statutory law is law made by federal and state legislatures.** Medicare law is an example of a federal statute. Ordinances are laws passed by cities or local jurisdictions such as parking regulations. Common law is the body of law formed by judicial decisions in a courtroom setting. Constitutional law is the supreme law of the land.

CENsational Pearl of Wisdom!

Statutes: *The term "statute" simply refers to a law enacted by a legislative body of a government, whether federal or state. Federal laws (statutes) are enacted by the United States Congress and must be followed by every state in the country. The United States Constitution is the supreme law of the land. No federal or state law may violate it. However, federal laws do not cover all areas of the law, and that is when state (or local) laws will apply.*

Regulations: *State executive agencies carry out state laws through the development and enforcement of regulations (also called rules or administrative laws) and have the effect of law. Someone violating a regulation is, in effect, violating the law that created it. Regulations are designed to increase flexibility and efficiency in the operation of laws. Most regulations are developed and enacted through a rule-making process, which includes public input. State agencies hold open meetings and public hearings, allowing citizens to participate in the creation of regulations.*

Ordinances: *A state may delegate certain powers to other units of government within the state. County and municipal governments enact laws, often called ordinances, via specific powers granted to them by the state. County and municipal ordinances apply to everyone within the county or municipality limits. These ordinances may not violate state or federal laws.*

Common law: *This is considered to be "judge-made" law. It consists of the rules of law that come from the written decisions of judges who hear and decide litigation. Judges are empowered to make these decisions by the constitution and statutes. When a judge decides a case and publishes a written decision, the decision becomes the precedent for future litigation.*

60. Answer: D

Cognitive Level: Analysis

Rationale: **Battery is the nonconsensual, intentional, offensive touching of another person.** Unlike assault, you do not have to warn the victim or make the victim fearful before you hurt for it to count as battery. If a nurse surprises the patient and pushes the patient from behind, that would qualify as battery. Assault and battery occur simultaneously when an individual threatens to harm someone and then physically harms that person. Assault is the intention to cause harm with the ability to carry through with it. It involves making someone fear that you will cause harm. You do not have to actually harm someone to commit assault. Threatening verbally or pretending to hit are both examples of assault that can occur in the health care setting. A breach of duty occurs when care falls below the standards or is omitted. Proximate cause is proof that a breach of duty caused injury to an individual.

61. Answer: C

Cognitive Level: Recall

Rationale: **Involuntary consent applies when an individual refuses treatment but a physician, other official as authorized by law, or law enforcement issues orders for care to be provided for a designated period of time.** When an individual in a life- or limb-threatening situation is unable to provide consent, it is assumed that consent is present to save the limb or life; this is known as implied consent. Informed consent is obtained when a physician/provider has explained a procedure, risk, and alternate treatment options to a patient. Express consent is a voluntary consent for treatment from a competent person.

62. Answer: C

Cognitive Level: Analysis

Rationale: **If the nurse recognizes that the incident is a mandatory reportable incident, even if the physician disagrees, it is the nurse's responsibility to report it to the designated authority.** The nurse shares equally with the physician in this legal responsibility.

 CENsational Pearl of Wisdom!

Anytime the nurse feels uncomfortable about situations such as these, never hesitate to contact the charge nurse, department director, or administrative personnel on call.

63. Answer: A

Cognitive Level: Analysis

Rationale: **Although exact volume and acuity levels can be somewhat unpredictable, the manager should track both over time so that numbers and type of staff are appropriately placed.** Staffing patterns are unit specific and standardization is irrelevant. TJC's standard for integrating emergency services is not directly related to the question.

 CENsational Pearl of Wisdom!

ENA has a position statement on this aspect of care on its website under position statements at www.ena. org. Use position statements to help with issues that arise in emergency departments. They can help outline the issue and provide support for needed changes.

64. Answer: D

Cognitive Level: Analysis

Rationale: **This situation describes a quality improvement process.** This reflects an interdisciplinary approach to process improvement for better patient experience or outcome. It is not intended to generate or validate a scientific knowledge base such as research. The element of data collection is found in research also. In the research process, however, data collection occurs later (after a literature review and after decisions have been made regarding conceptual or theoretical framework and research design). Indicator relevance testing is not a recognized entity in either process.

65. Answer: A

Cognitive Level: Recall

Rationale: **The patient's needs for continuous monitoring, assessment, and interventions vary. The acuity level, complexity of care, and potential needs during the intrahospital transport will determine the combination of personnel needed on the transport team.** The patient's acuity will also dictate the treatment plan during the transport, which may include medications. The patient's weight may add to the overall transport issues as far as manpower is concerned.

66. Answer: A

Cognitive Level: Analysis

Rationale: **Brainstorming is a problem-solving method that rapidly generates a large number of alternatives.** Quality and practicality are unimportant. Some wild and crazy solutions emerge and make the process fun; such unconventional ideas help participants unleash their creativity.

67. Answer: D

Cognitive Level: Recall

Rationale: **The fifth and sixth grade levels are the best for written instructions.** There is a formula that is applied to written papers to help decide which grade level it is written toward. This is called the FRY formula and takes into account length of words and syllables.

68. Answer: B

Cognitive Level: Application

Rationale: **Federal laws allow management to prevent employees from engaging in collective bargaining in patient care areas.** The same laws prohibit managers from preventing union activities during nonworking hours, from withholding desirable assignments from staff engaging in union activities, and from providing special favors to discourage union activity or membership.

69. Answer: C

Cognitive Level: Recall

Rationale: **Announcing topics helps the patient or family member focus on specific areas of the discharge instructions.** For instance, announce the topic of new medications, then activity, and so on. An active voice, specific instructions, and short words or sentences, as well as no jargon is the better way to teach discharge instructions because they will assist with recall for the patient at a later time. Utilizing stories can also help and repetition can help embed the information into the patient's memory.

70. Answer: B

Cognitive Level: Analysis

Rationale: **Optimal customer service includes all staff, at all levels, in all disciplines.** The committee works best when the problem is "owned" by those delivering service to customers as well as those in authority. An all-nurse committee places inappropriate emphasis on nursing. It is evident that nurses do have a great deal of patient contact and, therefore, opportunity to set a customer-friendly tone; however, there are countless factors that are not directly related to nursing, such as billing, medical diagnosis, and housekeeping. Waiting for complaints is passive, and an after-the-damage-is-done strategy, which is limited to monitoring and does not improve goals.

71. Answer: D

Cognitive Level: Recall

Rationale: **Certifications, courses, and licenses are considered credentials.** Experience is one's work history. Educational preparation refers to degrees held as well as academic institutions and programs attended. Personal qualities are subjectively measured and include such things as perceptions of voice, dress, sense of humor, and energy level.

72. Answer: A

Cognitive Level: Analysis

Rationale: **Self-scheduling is the option usually found in shared governance models, which emphasize staff accountability and involvement in operating a**
unit. Management scheduling, or having a designated staff leader for scheduling, places the work of schedule preparation directly on the manager (or designee); it deemphasizes staff maturity and responsibility. A centralized system with computer-generated scheduling would provide little opportunity for staff input and is a poor fit with the decentralized approach underlying the shared governance model.

73. Answer: B

Cognitive Level: Recall

Rationale: **The purpose of nursing research is to generate a scientific knowledge base for validating and improving practice.** Although the professional status of emergency nursing may be incidentally enhanced by research, such enhancement is not the focus or goal. Identification of new problems may be an outcome of nursing research, but most research depends on problem or question identification. Emergency nurses may have opportunities to participate in medication studies and product evaluation programs, but neither represents the purpose of nursing research.

74. Answer: A

Cognitive Level: Application

Rationale: **A study that examines thoughts and perceptions is one that lends itself to a qualitative design. Qualitative research is concerned with understanding human beings and the nature of their transactions with themselves and their surroundings.** The process is not quasi-scientific, rather a well-accepted mode of rigorous, systematic inquiry used in the social sciences. Quantitative research methods analyze data statistically while striving for precision and control over external variables. Experimental research involves doing something to some of the subjects and not doing something to others; in it, subjects are randomly assigned to either group.

75. Answer: D

Cognitive Level: Application

Rationale: **The best choice in this situation is to help the new nurse by performing the procedure with him.** Doing the procedure for him or referring him to an outside resource (book or person) will not enhance the graduate nurse's technical skills to fulfill this patient's needs now. In addition, he may need assistance in physically locating the urethra (beyond a description). Documentation of a procedure should be done only by the nurse completing the procedure.

References

Agency for Healthcare Research and Quality. (2011, July). *Types of health care quality measures.* Rockville, MD: Author. http://www.ahrq.gov/talkingquality/measures/types.html (67)

Agency for Healthcare Research and Quality. (2018, May). *Emergency Severity Index (ESI): A triage tool for emergency departments.* Rockville, MD: Author. http://www.ahrq.gov/professionals/systems/hospital/esi/index.html (7)

Airlift Northwest Medical Control. (n.d.). *Orientation manual.* Retrieved from https://em.uw.edu/sites/em.uw.edu/files/6%20%20ALNW_orientation_June_2011%5B1%5D.pdf (24)

American College of Emergency Physicians. (2012a). Health care system surge capacity recognition, preparedness, and response. Policy statement. *Annals of Emergency Medicine, 59*(3), 240. Retrieved from https://www.acep.org/patient-care/policy-statements/health-care-system-surge-capacity-recognition-preparedness-and-response/ (1)

American Nurses Association. (2012b). *Nursing care and do not resuscitate (DNR) and allow natural death (AND) decisions.* Retrieved from https://www.nursingworld.org/~4ad4a8/globalassets/docs/ana/nursing-care-and-do-not-resuscitate-dnr-and-allow-natural-death-decisions.pdf (36)

American College of Emergency Physicians. (2017). *Boarding of admitted and intensive care patients in the emergency department.* Policy statement. Retrieved from https://www.acep.org/globalassets/new-pdfs/policy-statements/boarding-of-admitted-and-intensive-care-patients-in-the-emergency-department.pdf (25)

American Nurses Association. (2015). *Incivility, bullying, and workplace violence.* Position statement. Retrieved from http://www.nursingworld.org/MainMenuCategories/WorkplaceSafety/Healthy-Nurse/bullyingworkplaceviolence/Incivility-Bullying-and-Workplace-Violence.html (26)

American Nurses Association. (2015). *Violence & bullying.* Practice and policy. Retrieved from https://www. nursingworld.org/practice-policy/work-environment/violence-incivility-bullying/ (43)

American Trauma Society. (n.d.). Retrieved from https://www.amtrauma.org (23)

American Trauma Society. (n.d.). *Trauma center levels explained.* Retrieved from https://www.amtrauma.org/page/traumalevels (22)

Assistant Secretary for Preparedness Response. (2016, November). *The 2017-2022 health care preparedness and response capabilities.* Retrieved from http://www.phe.gov/Preparedness/planning/hpp/reports/Documents/2017-2022-healthcare-pr-capablities.pdf (1)

Baldwin, S. B., et al. (2011). Identification of human trafficking victims in health care settings. *Health and Human Rights, 13*(1). (16–18)

Barr, J., et al. (2013). Clinical practice guidelines for the management of pain, agitation, and delirium in adult patients in the intensive care unit. *Critical Care Medicine, 41*(1), 263–306. (20)

California Hospital Association. (n.d.). *Sample hospital evacuation checklist.* Retrieved from https://www.calhospitalprepare.org/sites/main/files/file-attachments/cha_hospital_activation_of_the_emergency_operations_plan_checklist_final_0.pdf (1)

Campanelli, C. M. (2012). American Geriatrics Society updated beers criteria for potentially inappropriate medication use in older adults: The American Geriatrics Society 2012 Beers Criteria Update Expert Panel. *Journal of the American Geriatrics Society, 60*(4), 616. Retrieved from https://www.ncbi.nlm.nih.gov/pmc/articles/PMC3571677 (20)

Center for Disease Control and Prevention. (2016). *Protecting healthcare personnel.* Retrieved from https://www.cdc.gov/hai/prevent/ppe.html (6)

Centers for Medicare and Medicaid Services. (n.d.). *Emergency Medical Treatment and Labor Act (EMTALA).* Retrieved from http://www.cms.gov/Regulations-and-Guidance/Legislation/EMTALA/index.html (10)

Centers for Medicare and Medicaid Services. (2012, March). *Emergency Medical Treatment & Labor Act (EMTALA).* Retrieved from https://www.cms.gov/Regulations-and-Guidance/Legislation/EMTALA/ (57, 58)

Crime Scene Investigator Network. *Sample handling considerations for biological evidence and DNA extracts.* Retrieved from http://www.crime-scene-investigator.net/sample-handling-considerations-for-biological-evidence-and-DNA-extracts.html (35)

Daly, J., Speedy, S., & Jackson, D. (2017). *Contexts of nursing: An introduction.* Chatswood: Elsevier Health Sciences. (70)

Duke University. (updated 2018, September). *Introduction to evidence-based practice: Types of studies.* Retrieved from https://guides.mclibrary.duke.edu/ebmtutorial/study-types (32, 37, 64, 74)

Edgerton, G. Cultural Awareness International. (2013). *Communicating effectively with non-native English speakers.* Retrieved from https://culturalawareness.com/communicating-effectively-non-native-english-speakers/ (9)

Emergency Nurses Association. (n.d.). *Forensic evidence collection in the emergency care setting.* Position statement. Retrieved from https://www.ena.org/docs/default-source/resource-library/practice-resources/position-statements/forensic-evidence-collection-in-the-emergency-care-setting.pdf?sfvrsn=a1f89eba_4 (35)

Emergency Nurses Association. (n.d.). *Staffing and productivity in the emergency department.* Position statement. Retrieved from https://www.ena.org/docs/default-source/resource-library/practice-resources/position-statements/staffingandproductivityemergencydepartment.pdf?sfvrsn=c57dcf13_6 (63)

Emergency Nurses Association. (2011). *Emergency nursing scope and standards of practice (1st ed.)*. Des Plaines, IL: Author. (12)

Emergency Nurses Association. (2017). Crowding, boarding, and patient throughput. Position statement. Retrieved from https://www.ena.org/docs/default-source/resource-library/practice-resources/position-statements/crowdingboardingandpatientthroughput.pdf?sfvrsn = 5fb4e79f_4 (25)

Emergency Nurses Association. (2017b). *Emergency nursing core curriculum* (7th ed.). St. Louis, MO: W.B. Saunders Company. (15, 27, 59, 67, 68, 72)

Fee, C., et al. (2012). Association of emergency department length of stay with safety-net status. *JAMA, 307*(5), 476–482. doi:10.1001/jama.2012.41 (24)

Fuchsberg, A. L. (2016, January). *What are the elements of a nursing malpractice claim?* Retrieved from https://www.fuchsberg.com/medical-malpractice/2016/01/20/4-elements-nursing-malpractice/ (50, 51)

Gilboy, N., Tanabe, P., Travers, D., & Rosenau, A. M. (2011). Emergency Severity Index (ESI): A triage tool for emergency department care, version 4. *In Implementation handbook 2012 edition*. AHRQ Publication (12-0014). (7, 54)

Gurney, D., et al. (2017). Nursing code of ethics: Provisions and interpretative statements for emergency nurses. *Journal of Emergency Nursing, 43*(6), 497–503. Retrieved from https://www.ena.org/docs/default-source/resource-library/practice-resources/ethics/ethics.pdf?sfvrsn=cb143931_8 (5)

HHS.gov. *Health information privacy*. Retrieved from https://www.hhs.gov/hipaa/for-professionals/faq/index.html (34)

Howard, P., et al. (2010). *Sheehy's emergency nursing principles and practice* (6th ed.). St. Louis, MO: Mosby Elsevier. (21, 29, 31, 62, 65, 73)

Institute for Workplace Health. (2015, April). Primary, secondary and tertiary prevention. *At Work, 80*. Toronto, Ontario, Canada: Institute for Work & Health. Retrieved from https://www.iwh.on.ca/what-researchers-mean-by-primary-secondary-and-tertiary-prevention (4)

J. Otto Lottes Health Sciences Library. (updated 2018, June). *Evidence based nursing practice*. Retrieved from http://libraryguides.missouri.edu/c.php?g=28271&p=174073 (33)

Jennifer, B., et al. (2018). Nursing five rights of delegation. *StatPearls*. Retrieved from https://www.ncbi.nlm.nih.gov/books/NBK519519/ (28)

The Joint Commission. (2008). *Sentinel event alert, issue 40. Behaviors that undermine a culture of safety*. Retrieved from http://www.jointcommission.org/sentinel_event_alert_issue_40_behaviors_that_undermine_a_culture_of_safety (26)

The Joint Commission. (2016, June). Bullying has no place in health care. *Quick Safety, 24*. Retrieved from https://www.jointcommission.org/assets/1/23/Quick_Safety_Issue_24_June_2016.pdf (26)

The Joint Commission. (2018, June). *Quick safety 42: Identifying human trafficking victims*. Retrieved from https://www.jointcommission.org/joint_commission_advisory_on_identifying_human_trafficking_victims_in_health_care/ (16–19)

Ketamin, H. (2014). *Preparation of the critical patient for aeromedical transport*. Retrieved from https://prehospitalmed.com/2014/06/17/preparation-of-the-critical-patient-for-aeromedical-transport/ (24)

Lazarus, J. (2016). Precepting 101: Teaching strategies and tips for success for preceptors. *Journal of Midwifery & Women's Health*, 61(S1), 11-21. (75)

Legg, T. J. (2018, January). *Conversion disorder: What you need to know*. Retrieved from https://www.medicalnewstoday.com/articles/320587.php (30)

Lippincott Solutions. (2015, March). *10 Patient teaching strategies for nurses*. Retrieved from http://lippincott-solutions.lww.com/blog.entry.html/2015/03/05/10_patient_teaching-Hs1L.html (43)

Massachusetts Board of Registration in Nursing. (2018). *Nursing mandatory abuse reporting*. Retrieved from https://www.mass.gov/guides/nursing-mandatory-abuse-reporting#-board-of-registration-in-nursing:-duty-to-report-abuse- (27, 55)

Mental Health America. (n.d.). *Position Statement 22: Involuntary mental health treatment*. Retrieved from http://www.mentalhealthamerica.net/positions/involuntary-treatment (61)

Mercer Community College PowerPoint Presentation. (n.d.). *Short and long term goal setting*. Retrieved from http://www.mccc.edu/ ~ behrensb/documents/Goal-SettinginPhysicalTherapybjb.pdf (46)

MindTools. (2017). *Brainstorming: Generating many radical, creative ideas*. https://www.mindtools.com/brainstm.html (66)

Minh Le Cong, M. L., et al. (2014, June 17). *Preparation of the critical patient for aeromedical transport*. Retrieved from https://prehospitalmed.com/2014/06/17/preparation-of-the-critical-patient-for-aeromedical-transport/ (24)

Moore, B. L., Geller, R. J., & Clark, C. (2015). Hospital preparedness for chemical and radiological disasters. *Emergency Medicine Clinics*, 33(1), 37–49. (6)

The National Domestic Violence Hotline. (n.d.). What is domestic violence? Retrieved from https://www.thehotline.org/is-this-abuse/abuse-defined/ (56)

National Human Trafficking Hotline. Retrieved from https://humantraffickinghotline.org/ (16–19)

National Human Trafficking Resource Center. *Hotline statistics*. Retrieved from https://humantraffickinghotline.org/states (16–19)

National Academy of Science. (2015). Cognitive aging. *An action guide for health care providers*. Retrieved from http://nationalacademies.org/hmd/ ~ /media/Files/Report%20Files/2015/Cognitive_aging/Action%20

Guide%20for%20Health%20Care%20Providers_
V6.pdf (39)

National Conference of State Legislators. (2018). *Mental health professionals' duty to warn*. Retrieved from http://www.ncsl.org/research/health/mental-health-professionals-duty-to-warn.aspx (53)

NursingHomeAbuseGuide.org. (n.d.). *Assault and battery*. Retrieved from http://www.nursinghomeabuse-guide.org/elder-abuse/assault-and-battery/ (60)

Patient Engagement HIT. (n.d.). *Top 4 patient motivation techniques for health improvement*. Retrieved from https://patientengagementhit.com/news/top-4-patient-motivation-techniques-for-health-improvement (43)

Porath, C., et al. (2013). The price of incivility. *Harvard Business Review*, January–February Issue. Retrieved from https://hbr.org/2013/01/the-price-of-incivility (26)

Porth, L. (2012). Preparedness and partnerships: Lessons learned from the Missouri disasters of 2011. *Missouri Hospital Association*. Retrieved from https://www.jointcommission.org/assets/1/6/Joplin_2012_Lessons_Learned.pdf (1)

Reising, D. L. (2012). Make your nursing care malpractice-proof. *American Nurse Today, 7*(1), 24–28. Retrieved from https://www.americannursetoday.com/make-your-nursing-care-malpractice-proof/ (51)

Orientation to your role as "Medical Control" for Airlift Northwest for Medic One and Trauma Docs. (n.d.). Retrieved from https://em.uw.edu/sites/em.uw.edu/files/6%20%20ALNW_orientation_June_2011%5B1%5D.pdf (24)

Short and Long Term Goal Negotiations. (n.d.). Retrieved from http://www.mccc.edu/~behrensb/documents/GoalSettinginPhysicalTherapybjb.pdf (46)

Skerrett, P. J. (2012, September 24). Suicide often not preceded by warnings. *Harvard Health Publishing*. Retrieved from https://www.health.harvard.edu/blog/suicide-often-not-preceded-by-warnings-201209245331 (14)

Springer, G. (2015). When and how to use restraints. *American Nurse Today, 10*(1), 26–27. Retrieved from http://americannursetoday.com/wp-content/uploads/2014/12/ant1-Restraints-1218_RESTRAINT.pdf (2)

St Joseph University. (n.d.). *How the four principles of health care ethics improve patient care*. Retrieved from https://online.sju.edu/graduate/masters-health-administration/resources/articles/four-principles-of-health-care-ethics-improve-patient-care (40)

Stubenrauch, J. M. (2007). Malpractice vs. negligence. *AJN, American Journal of Nursing, 107*(7), 63. Retrieved from https://journals.lww.com/ajnonline/Fulltext/2007/07000/Malpractice_vs__Negligence.28.aspx (49)

United Nations Office on Drugs & Crime, Human Trafficking webpage. (16–19)

United States Department of Labor Occupational Safety and Health Administration. (n.d.). *Critical incident stress guide*. Retrieved from https://www.osha.gov/SLTC/emergencypreparedness/guides/critical.html (8, 9)

University of Ottawa. (n.d.). *Society, the individual and medicine*. Retrieved from https://www.med.uottawa.ca/sim/data/Prevention_e.htm (4)

U.S. Department of Homeland Security. (n.d.). *NIMS—Frequently asked questions*. Retrieved from https://www.fema.gov/pdf/emergency/nims/nimsfaqs.pdf (44)

U.S. Department of Justice. *National best practices for sexual assault kits*. Retrieved from https://www.ncjrs.gov/pdffiles1/nij/250384.pdf (35)

U.S. Department of Justice Office on Violence Against Women. *National training standards for sexual assault medical forensic examiners*. Retrieved from https://www.ncjrs.gov/pdffiles1/ovw/213827.pdf (35)

Whitbourne, S. K. (2011, October). The essential guide to defense mechanisms. *Psychology Today*. Retrieved from https://www.psychologytoday.com/us/blog/fulfillment-any-age/201110/the-essential-guide-defense-mechanisms (41)

White, B., et al. (2013). Impact of emergency department crowding on outcomes of admitted patients. *Annals of Emergency Medicine, 61*(6), 605–611. (24)

Wilson, L. O. The Second Principle. (n.d.). *Three domains of learning—Cognitive, affective, psychomotor*. Retrieved from https://thesecondprinciple.com/instructional-design/threedomainsoflearning/ (13)

Winterton, D. (2018). *Implied consent in a medical malpractice claim*. Retrieved from https://www.legalmatch.com/law-library/article/implied-consent-in-a-medical-malpractice-claim.html (3, 38, 47, 48)

Wolters Kluwer Office Management & HR. (n.d.). *The dos and don'ts of conducting a job interview*. Retrieved from https://www.bizfilings.com/toolkit/research-topics/office-hr/the-dos-and-donts-of-conducting-a-job-interview (71, 56)

Yorg, A. (2018). *8 Common defense mechanisms how we help and hurt our emotional well-being*. Retrieved from https://www.tonyrobbins.com/mind-meaning/8-common-defense-mechanisms/ (42)

Zibulewsky, J. (2001, October). The emergency medical treatment and active labor act (EMTALA): What it is and what it means for physicians. In *Baylor University Medical Center Proceedings* (Vol. 14, No. 4, pp. 339–346). Taylor & Francis. Retrieved from https://www.ncbi.nlm.nih.gov/pmc/articles/PMC1305897/ (10, 11, 57, 58)

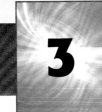

3 Shock

Terry Foster RN, MSN, FAEN, CCRN, CPEN, TCRN, CEN

On the actual Certified Emergency Nurse (CEN) test blueprint, there is not a category marked "Shock." After the last Role Delineation Study (RDS), this category was removed as a separate entity and the content of this topic was redistributed throughout the other categories. For instance, cardiogenic shock was moved into the cardiovascular category. So, the shock states are still on the test, they have just been parceled out among the new category subsets. In this book, it was decided to maintain a chapter on shock for ease of studying this concept. Shock is a hard topic, but with a bit of comprehension of some of the main concepts, it is totally understandable!

1. Which of the following is the common denominator in all forms of shock?
[ ] **A.** Large loss of blood volume
[ ] **B.** Inadequate tissue perfusion
[ ] **C.** Elevated heart rate
[ ] **D.** Inadequate cardiac output

2. Which of the following is the most common form of shock?
[ ] **A.** Hypovolemic
[ ] **B.** Septic
[ ] **C.** Cardiogenic
[ ] **D.** Anaphylactic

3. Which of the following would be an early set of symptoms of toxic shock syndrome?
[ ] **A.** Nausea, vomiting, diarrhea, and fever
[ ] **B.** Hypotension, tachycardia, and cyanosis
[ ] **C.** Scant urine output, hypertension, and rash
[ ] **D.** Disorientation, hypertension, and shivering

4. Which of the following is the main cause of death from a major burn injury during the first 24 hours?
[ ] **A.** Infectious processes
[ ] **B.** Acute Respiratory Distress Syndrome (ARDS)
[ ] **C.** Hypovolemic shock
[ ] **D.** Systemic Inflammatory Response Syndrome (SIRS)

5. During an insertion, a supine, hypovolemic patient has a syncopal episode. Assuring the patient is breathing and has a palpable pulse, the next response should be to:
[ ] **A.** complete the IV insertion and recheck the ABCs.
[ ] **B.** use spirits of ammonia to awaken the patient.
[ ] **C.** abort the IV insertion and move the patient to a cardiac room.
[ ] **D.** obtain a stat ECG and draw cardiac enzymes.

6. Which of the following is the most common pathophysiologic mechanism in anaphylactic shock?
[ ] **A.** Increased intracranial pressure
[ ] **B.** Increased arterial pressure
[ ] **C.** Decreased cardiac output
[ ] **D.** Massive peripheral vasodilation

7. The most common physiologic mechanism in cardiogenic shock is:
[ ] **A.** increased cardiac output.
[ ] **B.** decreased cardiac output.
[ ] **C.** peripheral vasodilation.
[ ] **D.** increased preload.

8. The most common complications of shock include all of the following **EXCEPT**:

[ ] **A.** acute renal failure.

[ ] **B.** disseminated intravascular coagulation (DIC).

[ ] **C.** acute respiratory distress syndrome (ARDS).

[ ] **D.** compartment syndrome.

9. Which of the following diagnostic indicators would be most helpful in the diagnosis of cardiogenic shock?

[ ] **A.** Positive ventilation–perfusion scan

[ ] **B.** Negative Focused Assessment with Sonography for Trauma (FAST) examination

[ ] **C.** Ejection fraction decrease of 20% noted on echocardiogram

[ ] **D.** Hemoglobin decrease of 10 g/dL

10. An elderly patient presents in the ED after a fall down a flight of steps at home. The patient is alert, a cervical spinal injury is ruled out, and the patient is currently being evaluated for further trauma. Vital signs for this patient are as follows:

Blood pressure—88/48 mm Hg
Pulse—64 beats/minute
Respirations—18 breaths/minute
Temperature—98.2° F (36.8° C)
Pulse oximetry—94% on room air

An intravenous fluid bolus of 500 mL has been administered for hypotension. Which of the following current medications that the patient is receiving would explain the slow heart rate?

[ ] **A.** Proton-pump inhibitor

[ ] **B.** Beta-blocker

[ ] **C.** Anticoagulant

[ ] **D.** Antidepressant

11. An unrestrained patient is brought to the emergency department after a motor vehicle crash. He is alert and oriented with the following vital signs:

Blood pressure—88/40 mm Hg
Pulse—42 beats/minute
Respirations—22 breaths/minute
Pulse oximetry—95% on room air
Temperature—99.2° F (37.3° C)

This is most likely due to which of the following types of shock?

[ ] **A.** Hypovolemic

[ ] **B.** Neurogenic

[ ] **C.** Anaphylactic

[ ] **D.** Septic

12. Septic shock in a pediatric patient often has which of the following associated clinical assessment findings?

[ ] **A.** Projectile vomiting

[ ] **B.** Pulmonary edema

[ ] **C.** Petechial rash

[ ] **D.** Jugular venous distension

13. Which of the following is the most common cause of cardiogenic shock?

[ ] **A.** Septal wall rupture

[ ] **B.** Valve dysfunction

[ ] **C.** Infective endocarditis

[ ] **D.** Left ventricular failure

14. Which of the following is the pathophysiologic basis for all forms of cardiogenic shock?

[ ] **A.** Decreased cardiac output

[ ] **B.** Increased cardiac output

[ ] **C.** Decreased preload

[ ] **D.** Mitral regurgitation

15. The pathophysiologic syndrome of shock causes abnormal metabolic changes and an increase in which of the following?

[ ] **A.** Oxygen saturation

[ ] **B.** Glucose

[ ] **C.** Thrombocytes

[ ] **D.** Lactic acid

16. Which of the following are the earliest signs of hypovolemic shock?

[ ] **A.** Tachycardia, restlessness, and thirst

[ ] **B.** Hypoxia, dysrhythmias, and tremors

[ ] **C.** Hypotension, flushed extremities, and anxiety

[ ] **D.** Oliguria, cyanosis, and confusion

17. Which of the following would a patient in septic shock most likely demonstrate?

[ ] **A.** Respiratory acidosis

[ ] **B.** Respiratory alkalosis

[ ] **C.** Metabolic acidosis

[ ] **D.** Metabolic alkalosis

18. Which of the following assessment findings indicates that the compensatory response mechanisms for shock are failing?

[ ] **A.** Cool, clammy skin

[ ] **B.** Pale, moist skin

[ ] **C.** Rapid capillary refill time

[ ] **D.** Mottled, cold skin

19. Which of the following is **NOT** a clinical symptom of cardiogenic shock?
[ ] **A.** Pulmonary edema
[ ] **B.** Jugular venous distension
[ ] **C.** Low central venous pressure
[ ] **D.** Hypotension

20. Which of the following is the primary reason to use vasopressors in the treatment of cardiogenic shock?
[ ] **A.** Increase heart rate
[ ] **B.** Improve tissue perfusion
[ ] **C.** Decrease myocardial contractility
[ ] **D.** Promote vasodilation

21. Which of the following is the first priority when beginning treatment for a patient in septic shock?
[ ] **A.** Oxygen delivery and intravenous access
[ ] **B.** Orthostatic vital signs and temperature
[ ] **C.** Complete blood count and lactic acid levels
[ ] **D.** Intravenous fluid bolus and dopamine infusion

22. Which of the following is **NOT** an initial symptom of anaphylactic shock?
[ ] **A.** Bronchospasm
[ ] **B.** Expiratory wheezing
[ ] **C.** Tachycardia
[ ] **D.** Hyperthermia

23. Which of the following is the antibody/antigen primarily associated with anaphylactic shock?
[ ] **A.** IgM
[ ] **B.** IgG
[ ] **C.** IgA
[ ] **D.** IgE

24. Initial fluid resuscitation for a multiple trauma patient in hypovolemic shock should include which of the following?
[ ] **A.** Crystalloid infusion
[ ] **B.** Colloid infusion
[ ] **C.** Dopamine infusion
[ ] **D.** Hypertonic infusion

25. All of the following are etiologies for hypovolemic shock **EXCEPT**:
[ ] **A.** abdominal trauma.
[ ] **B.** femoral fractures.
[ ] **C.** fatty emboli.
[ ] **D.** dissecting aortic aneurysm.

26. A patient in hypovolemic shock who is concurrently taking a beta-blocker would most likely have which set of basic vital signs?
[ ] **A.** Blood pressure—128/70 mm Hg; pulse: 74 beats/minute
[ ] **B.** Blood pressure—88/50 mm Hg; pulse: 68 beats/minute
[ ] **C.** Blood pressure—84/58 mm Hg; pulse: 130 beats/minute
[ ] **D.** Blood pressure—166/104 mm Hg; pulse: 62 beats/minute

27. After diagnosis and aggressive treatment of septic shock, which of the following are key indicators of continued clinical improvement?
[ ] **A.** Tachycardia and confusion
[ ] **B.** Hypotension with vasopressor support
[ ] **C.** Hypertension and lactic acidosis
[ ] **D.** Normotension and tachycardia

28. Which of the following is **NOT** a normal physiologic compensatory mechanism in hypovolemic shock?
[ ] **A.** Baroreceptors interpret decreased blood flow, which stimulates the pulse to increase.
[ ] **B.** Antidiuretic hormone secretion is increased.
[ ] **C.** Epinephrine secretion stimulates peripheral vasoconstriction.
[ ] **D.** Endotoxin circulation causes hyperthermia.

29. Which of the following is **NOT** an early goal-directed therapy for septic shock?
[ ] **A.** Quick screening for the potential for sepsis
[ ] **B.** Identification of septic symptomology
[ ] **C.** Starting antibiotic therapy before obtaining cultures
[ ] **D.** IV fluid boluses in rapid succession if tolerated

30. The use of intravenous steroids in the patient with septic shock will allow for which of the following effects?
[ ] **A.** Lower blood glucose levels
[ ] **B.** Decrease systemic effects of inflammation
[ ] **C.** Prevent the development of thromboemboli
[ ] **D.** Increase vasoconstriction

31. A multiple trauma patient in hypovolemic shock has received 2 L of intravenous normal saline. He continues to be hypotensive and tachycardic. Which of the following is **NOT** an appropriate action at this time?
[ ] A. Reassess for other potential areas of bleeding.
[ ] B. Start high-dose intravenous vasopressors.
[ ] C. Continue fluid resuscitation while monitoring the patient.
[ ] D. Consider infusing blood products.

32. Which of the following is the leading cause of death in the first 24 hours of a major burn injury?
[ ] A. Hypovolemia
[ ] B. Fluid overload
[ ] C. Infection/sepsis
[ ] D. Multisystem organ failure

33. Which of the following is **NOT** a common complication of shock?
[ ] A. Disseminated intravascular coagulation (DIC)
[ ] B. Multiple pulmonary emboli
[ ] C. Acute respiratory distress syndrome (ARDS)
[ ] D. Acute renal failure (ARF)

34. Which of the following is **NOT** an etiology of cardiogenic shock?
[ ] A. Cardiac tamponade
[ ] B. Hyponatremia
[ ] C. Beta-blocker overdose
[ ] D. Ventricular tachycardia

35. Which of the following is the drug of choice for the treatment of cardiogenic shock?
[ ] A. Dopamine (Intropin)
[ ] B. Dobutamine (Dobutrex)
[ ] C. Nitroglycerin (Trinitrate)
[ ] D. Vasopressin

36. Which of the following statements best describes the pathophysiology behind neurogenic shock? Neurogenic shock is caused by a massive vasodilation from:
[ ] A. suppression of the sympathetic nervous system.
[ ] B. increased intracranial pressure.
[ ] C. the release of histamine.
[ ] D. the systemic inflammatory process.

37. A 60-year-old male is admitted to the emergency department from home for a syncopal episode after having frequent, large amounts of dark red bloody stools this morning. He is 1-week postoperative following a total right hip replacement. He is awake and somewhat confused. His skin is pale and diaphoretic. His vital signs are as follows:

Blood pressure—80/62 mm Hg
Pulse—136 beats/minute
Respirations—26 breaths/minute
Temperature—96.8° F (36° C) (orally)
Pulse oximetry—95% on room air

Which of the following is the priority intervention for this patient?
[ ] A. Prepare for emergency endoscopy with surgery on standby.
[ ] B. Assist with endotracheal intubation and assist respirations as needed.
[ ] C. Draw labs for type and crossmatch and initiate two large-bore intravenous lines.
[ ] D. Discuss end-of-life care wishes with both the patient and family.

38. Assessment of an unrestrained patient from a motor vehicle crash reveals hypotension; warm, dry skin; and bradycardia. Which of the following is the most likely cause?
[ ] A. Cardiogenic shock
[ ] B. Neurogenic shock
[ ] C. Hypovolemic shock
[ ] D. Septic shock

39. Which of the following symptoms would be indicative of the compensatory stage in hypovolemic shock?
[ ] A. Narrowing pulse pressure
[ ] B. Severe hypotension
[ ] C. Increasing lactic acid level
[ ] D. Increasing urine output

40. A patient with pancreatitis is at risk for which of the following two types of shock?
[ ] A. Hypovolemic and Neurogenic
[ ] B. Septic and Anaphylactic
[ ] C. Cardiogenic and Anaphylactic
[ ] D. Hypovolemic and Septic

41. Which of the following is the end result of the activation of the renin–angiotensin–aldosterone system in shock situations?
[ ] **A.** Increased vascular volume
[ ] **B.** Increased urinary output
[ ] **C.** Generalized vasodilation
[ ] **D.** Release of norepinephrine

42. A husband brings his wife to the emergency department for sudden respiratory distress that occurred immediately after eating seafood. She is nonresponsive, her face is flushed, and her lips and tongue have marked swelling. Her blood pressure is 80/42 mm Hg and her pulse is 120 beats/minute.
Which of the following should be administered first?
[ ] **A.** Methylprednisolone (Solu-Medrol)
[ ] **B.** Epinephrine (Adrenalin)
[ ] **C.** Normal saline IV fluid bolus
[ ] **D.** Diphenhydramine (Benadryl)

43. All of the following patient past histories are at increased risk for hypovolemic shock **EXCEPT**:
[ ] **A.** diabetic ketoacidosis.
[ ] **B.** diabetes insipidus.
[ ] **C.** diuretic overuse.
[ ] **D.** digitalis toxicity.

44. The presence of a hemorrhagic shock-like state will initiate which of the following physiologic compensatory mechanisms?
[ ] **A.** Decreased secretion of antidiuretic hormone (ADH)
[ ] **B.** Increased secretion of antidiuretic hormone (ADH)
[ ] **C.** Decreased secretion of epinephrine
[ ] **D.** Decreased secretion of norepinephrine

45. A large pulmonary embolus is most likely to cause which of the following types of shock?
[ ] **A.** Hypovolemic shock
[ ] **B.** Distributive shock
[ ] **C.** Obstructive shock
[ ] **D.** Neurogenic shock

46. On the basis of their predisposition, which of the following patients is most at risk for the development of septic shock?
[ ] **A.** A 40-year-old black male with a history of hypertension
[ ] **B.** A 50-year-old perimenopausal, white female with a history of GERD
[ ] **C.** A 30-year-old white male with a white blood cell count of 1,000 per microliter
[ ] **D.** A 60-year-old Hispanic female on anticoagulants

47. Which of the following symptoms is of most concern in an 84-year-old female regarding responses to potential shock states?
[ ] **A.** Syncopal episodes upon getting out of bed
[ ] **B.** Brief tachycardia upon physical exertion
[ ] **C.** Urine output of 30 mL over the past hour
[ ] **D.** Extremities cool and dry to the touch

48. Which of the following is the first priority emergency intervention for the treatment of all forms of shock?
[ ] **A.** Rapid infusion of intravenous fluids
[ ] **B.** Initiation of vasopressors
[ ] **C.** Administration of high-flow oxygen
[ ] **D.** Airway assessment and maintenance

49. A 5-year-old has been brought to the emergency department by her parents who state she has had persistent vomiting and diarrhea for the past 24 hours. Her general appearance shows she is awake but drowsy. Her color is pale, but her skin is warm and dry. Her weight shows a decrease from her previous weight of 45 lb (20.4 kg) to 42 lb (19 kg). She has no prior medical history. Vital signs are as follows:

Blood pressure—72/64 mm Hg
Pulse—140 beats/minute
Respirations—28 breaths/minute
Pulse oximetry—98% on room air
Temperature—100.4° F (38° C), rectally

Which of the following would be the correct amount of intravenous fluids to infuse as the initial bolus?
[ ] **A.** 190 mL
[ ] **B.** 380 mL
[ ] **C.** 420 mL
[ ] **D.** 840 mL

50. Which of the following is the most common form of distributive shock?
[ ] **A.** Anaphylactic
[ ] **B.** Neurogenic
[ ] **C.** Septic
[ ] **D.** Cardiogenic

51. A patient diagnosed with an acute abdominal aortic dissection is most at risk for which of the following types of shock?
[ ] **A.** Hypovolemic
[ ] **B.** Neurogenic
[ ] **C.** Distributive
[ ] **D.** Cardiogenic

52. Which of the following organs/glands is **NOT** part of the process when the renin–angiotensin–aldosterone system is in operation?
[ ] **A.** Lungs
[ ] **B.** Liver
[ ] **C.** Adrenal gland
[ ] **D.** Thyroid gland

53. Which of the following is **NOT** proper treatment for hypovolemic shock?
[ ] **A.** Placing the patient in Trendelenburg position
[ ] **B.** Oxygen delivery at 100% by non-rebreather mask
[ ] **C.** Administering warmed isotonic solution
[ ] **D.** Covering the patient with warm blankets

54. Which of the following physiologic mechanisms does **NOT** contribute to the development of clinical hypoperfusion in shock?
[ ] **A.** Decreased venous return to the heart
[ ] **B.** Onset of generalized vasodilitation
[ ] **C.** Obstruction of circulating blood volume
[ ] **D.** Increased peripheral vascular resistance

55. Which of the following can lead to the development of an obstructive form of shock?
[ ] **A.** Cardiac dysrhythmia
[ ] **B.** Tension pneumothorax
[ ] **C.** Ectopic pregnancy
[ ] **D.** Bacterial pneumonia

56. A dopamine (Intropin) infusion has been ordered for a patient in cardiogenic shock. Which of the following is **NOT** a precaution for the use of this medication?
[ ] **A.** Close observations for the development of tachydysrhythmias
[ ] **B.** Using a patent central line for drug administration
[ ] **C.** Regular measurements to check for QRS complex prolongation
[ ] **D.** Frequent monitoring of vital signs and urine output

57. A patient in profound hemorrhagic shock is rapidly receiving multiple units of blood through the emergency department's massive transfusion protocol. Which of the following conditions is the most common complication of this treatment?
[ ] **A.** Hyperkalemia
[ ] **B.** Metabolic acidosis
[ ] **C.** Anaphylaxis
[ ] **D.** Acute hemolytic reaction

58. Which of the following patients exhibiting potential shock-like symptoms has the highest triage priority?
[ ] **A.** A 94-year-old female from a nursing home who has cloudy, foul-smelling urine draining from her urinary catheter. She is awake and yelling for the nurse to get out of her kitchen. Vital signs are within normal limits.
[ ] **B.** A 24-year-old man who self-administered his EpiPen 1 hour before arrival after being stung by a wasp. He is alert. Color is flushed. Vital signs are within normal limits except for a pulse rate of 110 beats/minute.
[ ] **C.** A 19-year-old female with a history of vomiting for 6 hours after a night of binge drinking. She is alert. Skin is warm and dry and she is texting on her phone. Vital signs are within normal limits.
[ ] **D.** An 82-year-old male with a long history of smoking is complaining of abdominal and low back pain. He is restless and pale. Vital signs are within normal limits except for blood pressure of 192/108 mm Hg and a pulse rate of 128 beats/minute.

59. Orthostatic vital signs (OSVS) measurements can be an additional assessment tool for the diagnosis of dehydration and/or hypovolemic shock. Which of the following is a true statement regarding this tool?
[ ] **A.** OSVS are not accurate in patients older than 65 or younger than 10.
[ ] **B.** Blood pressure, pulse, and respiratory rate should be assessed with the patient lying flat, sitting, and then standing.
[ ] **C.** Often inaccurate, OSVS should be used in conjunction with history, physical assessment, and other diagnostic findings
[ ] **D.** Do not assess OSVS on patients who are presenting with a chief complaint of syncope or vertigo.

60. Which of the following is **NOT** a late sign or symptom of systemic shock?
[ ] **A.** Cyanosis
[ ] **B.** Anuria
[ ] **C.** Obtunded
[ ] **D.** Tachycardia

61. Which of the following patients is most likely to develop hypovolemic shock?
[ ] A. A 23-year-old female with a urinary tract infection
[ ] B. A 50-year-old female with fibromyalgia
[ ] C. An 80-year-old male with chest pain and dyspnea
[ ] D. A 15-year-old male with diabetic ketoacidosis

62. Which of the following is the primary physiologic reason for hypotension and bradycardia in neurogenic shock?
[ ] A. Third spacing of intracellular fluid
[ ] B. Disruption in sympathetic nervous system
[ ] C. Hypersensitivity to allergen
[ ] D. Left ventricular hypertrophy

63. Which of the following would indicate an improvement in a patient experiencing neurogenic shock associated with a spinal cord injury?
[ ] A. Heart rate of 46 beats/minute
[ ] B. Blood pressure of 90/62 mm Hg
[ ] C. Temperature of 98.6° F (37° C)
[ ] D. Respiratory rate of 28 breaths/minute

64. Which of the following indicates that a family member has understood instructions and education regarding their father's situation with cardiogenic shock?
[ ] A. "I understand that my father needs to get to the cath lab immediately."
[ ] B. "I was told that it is good that his blood pressure is so low."
[ ] C. "We should still be able to go on our planned cruise in 10 days."
[ ] D. "I heard that dad had a problem with too much oxygen getting to his cells?"

65. Which of the following would be a potential cause of septic shock?
[ ] A. Pyelonephritis
[ ] B. Diabetic ketoacidosis
[ ] C. Cardiac tamponade
[ ] D. Tension pneumothorax

66. Which of the following interventions would **NOT** indicate to the ED nurse that obstructive shock symptoms have been mitigated?
[ ] A. Successful pericardiocentesis performed
[ ] B. A 36-week gestation patient turned to the left side
[ ] C. 14 g cathlon inserted into second intercostal space
[ ] D. Bilateral normal saline boluses infusing

67. A slight increase in diastolic blood pressure in early shock is due to an increase in:
[ ] A. stroke volume.
[ ] B. heart rate.
[ ] C. vascular tone.
[ ] D. renal perfusion.

68. Which of the following explains the term "permissive hypotension" as it relates to treating a patient in hypovolemic shock?
[ ] A. Treating hypotension only when the patient is comatose
[ ] B. Treating hypotension to a systolic pressure of 90 mm Hg
[ ] C. Treating hypotension only when it is associated with tachycardia
[ ] D. Treating hypotension with aggressive fluid management

69. Which of the following describes the expected action of the pulse pressure in hypovolemic shock?
[ ] A. Remains unchanged
[ ] B. Widens
[ ] C. Narrows
[ ] D. Is unobtainable

70. Baroreceptors, a collection of sensitive cells that monitor blood pressure and volume, are found in the:
[ ] A. pons and medulla.
[ ] B. aortic arch and carotid arteries.
[ ] C. aorta and renal arteries.
[ ] D. spleen and mesenteric artery.

71. Which of the following findings would most likely indicate obstructive shock rather than hypovolemic shock?
[ ] A. Neck vein distension
[ ] B. Widening pulse pressure
[ ] C. Orthostatic hypotension
[ ] D. Reflex tachycardia

72. Which of the following would indicate a potential shock situation in a 3-year-old pediatric patient?
[ ] A. Blood pressure of 92/60 mm Hg
[ ] B. Pulse rate of 110 beats/minute
[ ] C. Responsive to painful stimuli only
[ ] D. Responsive to verbal stimuli

73. Outcomes for septic shock will be most effective when which of the following guidelines are followed?
[ ] **A.** Withholding antibiotic therapy until cultures are obtained
[ ] **B.** Determining sepsis diagnosis after culture results
[ ] **C.** Early implementation of diuretic therapy
[ ] **D.** Aggressive intravenous fluid management

74. Trendelenburg position in the treatment of shock is contraindicated because of all of the following **EXCEPT**:
[ ] **A.** increased intracranial pressure.
[ ] **B.** increased venous return.
[ ] **C.** increased abdominal organ ischemia.
[ ] **D.** increased diaphragmatic pressure.

75. Treatment of hypovolemic shock is considered successful when which of the following changes are evident?
[ ] **A.** Capillary refill is 4 seconds.
[ ] **B.** Urine output is at least 20 mL/hour for 4 hours.
[ ] **C.** Electrocardiogram changes resolve.
[ ] **D.** Systolic blood pressure is greater than 90 mm Hg.

Answers/Rationales

1. Answer: B

Nursing Process: Analysis

Rationale: **The bottom line, physiologically, in all forms of shock is inadequate tissue perfusion.** A large loss of blood volume is a cause of hypovolemic shock, and inadequate cardiac output is often a cause of cardiogenic shock. Tachycardia is a symptom seen in all forms of shock, except in neurogenic.

 CENsational Pearl of Wisdom!

To really understand shock, you have to get down to the cellular level where the delivery of oxygen occurs. In a shock state, oxygen is not available to the cells to perform all of their functions. When attempting to metabolize carbohydrates, for example, the creation of adenosine triphosphate (ATP), our energy source, is dramatically reduced in an anaerobic environment. When aerobic metabolism is present, each molecule of carbohydrate can generate at least 36 molecules of ATP. When anaerobic metabolism occurs, that amount of ATP goes down to 1! A big difference!!!

2. Answer: A

Nursing Process: Analysis

Rationale: **The most common form of shock is hypovolemic, accounting for more than one-third of all ED visits related to shock.** Septic is the next most common form of shock.

3. Answer: A

Nursing Process: Assessment

Rationale: **Nausea, vomiting, diarrhea, and fever are often the early signs of toxic shock because it often mimics flulike symptoms.** Hypotension, tachycardia, rash, disorientation, and scant urine are often later symptoms seen in toxic shock. Hypertension is not seen in this condition.

 CENsational Pearl of Wisdom!

This is a prime example of reading the test items very closely. The word "early" is the clue in the question. Read every word! Also, delete those items that are known to be wrong immediately. Hypertension would not be a symptom or manifestation of a shock state. So, then the test taker is now down to two options instead of four!

4. Answer: C

Nursing Process: Analysis

Rationale: **The main cause of death from a major burn injury during the first 24 hours is hypovolemic shock.** While losing capillary membrane permeability, the patient begins to third space and the intravascular volume is quickly depleted. Infection is most likely to develop after 24 to 36 hours. ARDS and SIRS are multisystem complications that may develop a few days after the initial injury.

CENsational Pearl of Wisdom!

Hypovolemic shock can occur because of an absolute loss of volume, such as in a ruptured aortic aneurysm or it can happen because of the third spacing concept mentioned. The fluid is there, but it is not able to participate in any of the normal functions. Remember that hypovolemic shock is a loss of preload!

5. Answer: A

Nursing Process: Intervention

Rationale: **In this situation, complete the intravenous needle insertion and recheck the ABCs. After assuring that the ABCs are intact, the most helpful intervention would be to initiate IV fluids; thus, the intravenous line must be started.** The patient is already supine. Another team member could elevate the legs, but the line is imperative. The patient has most likely experienced a vasovagal response. Spirits of ammonia might be an option, but the IV line is the higher priority. The patient does not need to be placed in a different room; and unless the patient manifests other symptomatology that makes the nurse concerned about a cardiac problem, the electrocardiogram and cardiac enzymes would not be necessary.

6. Answer: D

Nursing Process: Analysis

Rationale: **Massive peripheral vasodilation is the most common pathophysiologic mechanism in anaphylactic shock. Histamine and other biochemicals cause an increase in capillary membrane permeability, which results in the massive vasodilation.** This causes the red, flushed skin and tissue swelling. Intracranial pressure is not immediately affected. Arterial pressure is decreased and cardiac output may actually initially be increased because of the body's response to the antigen.

 CENsational Pearl of Wisdom!

Remember that anaphylactic shock is one of the shock states that occur under the heading of "distributive shock." This is a vasodilatory type of shock which helps us remember that vasodilation is the root cause. Other distributive shocks are septic and neurogenic. These are caused by a loss of afterload!

7. Answer: B

Nursing Process: Analysis

Rationale: **The most common physiologic mechanism in cardiogenic shock is decreased cardiac output.** Peripheral vasodilation may occur, but it is not the primary causative mechanism. Depending on the cause, the preload is increased, the afterload is decreased, and myocardial contractility is impaired.

8. Answer: D

Nursing Process: Analysis

Rationale: **Compartment syndrome is NOT a common complication of shock. This is an event that occurs usually due to an orthopedic event such as crush injury, a fracture (the most common cause of compartment syndrome), burns, bites, or frostbite. It can cause grave consequences for the extremity involved. Abdominal compartment syndrome can also occur, but it is not as frequent and is not a complication of shock.** Even though a patient may only be in shock for a short amount of time, serious multisystem complications may develop from this brief period of tissue hypoperfusion such as acute renal failure, disseminated intravascular coagulation, and acute respiratory distress syndrome.

9. Answer: C

Nursing Process: Assessment

Rationale: **An ejection fraction (EF) decrease of 20% would be the best diagnostic indicator in the diagnosis of cardiogenic shock.** An EF of 55% or higher is considered normal. A decreased EF is seen in cardiogenic shock as well as in congestive heart failure and in some cardiomyopathies. A positive V/Q scan is diagnostic for a pulmonary embolus. A negative FAST examination would not be indicated because it is used to identify blood in the abdomen and a hemoglobin decrease to 10 g/dL would be indicative of hemorrhagic shock.

10. Answer: B

Nursing Process: Assessment

Rationale: **Beta-blockers will mute the normal tachycardic response initially seen in hypovolemia.** This is an important consideration to keep in mind because many patients are on these medications, often puzzling the most experienced clinicians. Proton-pump inhibitors, anticoagulants, and antidepressants usually do not affect the heart rate.

11. Answer: B

Nursing Process: Assessment

Rationale: **The hallmark of neurogenic shock is brady-cardia. This occurs because of the loss of sympathetic responses. The parasympathetic system is in control. The vagal response associated with this system is bra-dycardia.** Hypovolemic, anaphylactic, and septic types of shock all have tachycardia as a predominant symptom.

 CENsational Pearl of Wisdom!

The vagus nerve is the largest of the parasympa-thetic nerves and is responsible for 75% of all para-sympathetic activity. When the sympathetic system cannot function, the parasympathetic system takes over. It is also "craniosacral," which means that if the cervical spine is injured, the patient continues to maintain the parasympathetic system but may lose the sympathetic system which is thoracolumbar. Look up the Autonomic Nervous System for a visual of these two components!

12. Answer: C

Nursing Process: Assessment

Rationale: **Sepsis in a pediatric patient is often accom-panied by a petechial rash, usually secondary to an overwhelming infectious process, such as meningococ-cemia.** Projectile vomiting may be a sign of increased in-tracranial pressure. Pulmonary edema and jugular venous distension are associated with cardiogenic shock.

13. Answer: D

Nursing Process: Analysis

Rationale: **Left ventricular failure is the most common cause of cardiogenic shock, often the result of a myo-cardial infarction with the loss of greater than 40% muscle mass.** Septal wall rupture, acute valve dysfunc-tion, and complications from infective endocarditis can also contribute to cardiogenic shock, but left ventricular failure is the hallmark.

 CENsational Pearl of Wisdom!

Potentially lethal dysrhythmias such as ventricular tachycardia and complete heart block can also be etiologies of sudden cardiogenic shock.

14. Answer: A

Nursing Process: Analysis

Rationale: **Decreased cardiac output is the pathophysi-ologic basis for all forms of cardiogenic shock.** This is due to the heart's inability to meet the normal metabolic de-mands. Both the preload and afterload are increased along with the pulmonary artery pressures. However, the overall cardiac output and blood pressure is significantly decreased. Mitral regurgitation can be an etiology of cardiogenic shock, but it is not the overall pathophysiologic basis.

15. Answer: D

Nursing Process: Analysis

Rationale: **The syndrome of shock slows down meta-bolic processes, causing an increase in lactic acid lev-els.** Lactic acid, an end product of anaerobic metabolism, contributes to peripheral vasodilation, hypotension, and decreased organ perfusion. Oxygen saturation may be de-creased as a result of the lactic acid levels. Thrombocytes are generally not affected unless the shock results in dis-seminated intravascular coagulation (DIC).

16. Answer: A

Nursing Process: Assessment

Rationale: **Tachycardia, restlessness, and thirst are often seen early in hypovolemic shock.** Tachycardia is due to increased epinephrine secretion in response to a decreased preload. Restlessness can occur from the epi-nephrine secretion as well as hypoxemia. Thirst is due to decreased extracellular fluid in mucous membranes as it is being shunted back to core circulation. This epineph-rine secretion is due to the compensatory effects of the "fight-or-flight" response. The other manifestations would occur in later phases.

17. Answer: C

Nursing Process: Analysis

Rationale: **The most common acid–base disturbance in septic shock is metabolic acidosis. Without treatment, metabolic acidosis will become progressively worse; steps need to be taken to bring the patient into a com-pensatory mode to recovery.** Treatment of metabolic acidosis is variable depending on the cause, the degree of acidity, and whether it is acute or chronic. In severe metabolic acidosis, intravenous sodium bicarbonate is sometimes used. If the problem is fixed, the body will regulate itself back to a normal pH; however, there are times when sodium bicarbonate is necessary, especially if the pH is at the 7.0 to 7.1 level.

CENsational Pearl of Wisdom!

Remember that when the body is in metabolic acidosis, the respiratory system will come into play to attempt to compensate for the increased acid. Because the respiratory system is in control of the acid component, carbon dioxide, it will attempt to breathe it off causing an increased respiratory rate and depth of breathing.

18. Answer: D

Nursing Process: Assessment

Rationale: **Mottled, cold skin indicates an often irreversible state of shock and is often accompanied by multisystem organ failure.** Cool, clammy, and moist skin are all indicative of shock, but they are also evidence of the compensatory effects working, causing vasoconstrictive reactions throughout the body. A rapid capillary refill time would be a positive normal response.

19. Answer: C

Nursing Process: Assessment

Rationale: **Cardiogenic shock exhibits a high central venous (right atrial) pressure, not low.** Pulmonary edema, jugular venous distension, and hypotension are manifestations of cardiogenic shock, which are all the result of decreased cardiac output.

20. Answer: B

Nursing Process: Intervention

Rationale: **Vasopressors are used in cardiogenic shock to improve tissue perfusion.** Depending on the type, vasopressors are used to increase peripheral vasoconstriction and thereby increase major organ and tissue perfusion. Tachycardia is often a side effect of vasopressors and needs to be monitored closely. They would not be used to decrease contractility or promote vasodilation, which are both negative responses.

CENsational Pearl of Wisdom!

Keep in mind that contractility is synonymous with the word inotropic. On the test, they may use the word, positive- or negative-inotropic response. Chronotropic response is the same as the heart rate.

21. Answer: A

Nursing Process: Intervention

Rationale: **Oxygen delivery and volume replacement are the main priorities in beginning to treat a patient in septic shock. Fluid replacement will allow oxygen and nutrients to perfuse impaired tissues and organs in septic shock.** OSVS and temperatures are often unreliable in assessing for septic shock. A complete blood count (CBC) and lactic acid levels will be performed, but the priorities are oxygenation and intravenous access. Dopamine may be started, but the intravenous access must be present to utilize it or other pressor agents as well as the fluid bolus.

22. Answer: D

Nursing Process: Assessment

Rationale: **Hyperthermia is usually not associated with anaphylactic shock.** Although the skin is flushed and warm, a rise in actual temperature does not occur. Bronchospasm, expiratory wheezing, and tachycardia are all classic signs of anaphylactic shock, along with anxiety, hypotension, and peripheral edema.

CENsational Pearl of Wisdom!

There have been rare cases of extreme heat-related events associated with strenuous activity causing anaphylaxis. When patients have a repeat attack of anaphylaxis after an initial positive response and with no further exposure to the offending allergen, it is known as biphasic anaphylaxis.

23. Answer: D

Nursing Process: Analysis

Rationale: **The mechanism of anaphylaxis is mediated primarily by antibodies—specifically those of the immunoglobulin E (IgE) class**. These antibodies recognize the offending antigen and bind to it. The IgE antibodies also bind to specialized receptor molecules on mast cells and basophils, causing these cells to release their stores of inflammatory chemicals such as histamine, serotonin, and leukotrienes, which have a number of effects, including constriction of the smooth muscles, which leads to breathing difficulty; dilation of blood vessels, causing skin flushing and hives; and an increase in vascular permeability, resulting in edema and hypotension. IgM is an immunoglobulin that helps protect the body from new bacterial invasions. IgG is an antibody that responds to organisms that have invaded the body before. They have a "memory." IgA antibodies are located in mucous membranes found in the lungs, intestines, stomach, and sinus areas and work in the immune system of these mucous membranes. They are present in saliva, blood, and tears.

24. Answer: A

Nursing Process: Intervention

Rationale: **Two large-bore IVs with infusion of 2 L of normal saline or lactated ringer's is the standard treatment for a multiple trauma patient in hypovolemic shock. Either is accepted now.** Colloid infusions can be acceptable, but they are not the first-line fluid of choice. Dopamine may be utilized for renal perfusion after initial fluid resuscitation measures are completed. Hypertonic fluids such as 3% and 5% saline have been suggested, but further trials and studies need to be completed.

25. Answer: C

Nursing Process: Analysis

Rationale: **Hypovolemic shock may often be seen in internal bleeding from abdominal trauma, femoral fractures, and dissecting aortic aneurysm.** The chest, abdomen, pelvis, and femur areas can accommodate several units of blood and should be assessed for in occult bleeding. Fatty emboli are not associated with hypovolemic shock.

26. Answer: B

Nursing Process: Assessment

Rationale: **Beta-blocker medications will mute the normal tachycardic response to hypovolemic shock. A blood pressure of 88/50 with a pulse of 68 demonstrates this effect of beta-blocker activity in a shock situation.** This can often be a missed assessment point when hypotension is present, but tachycardia is absent, giving the clinician a false sense of reassurance. Owing to the beta-blocker, the body is not able to compensate by increasing the heart rate, which can compound the shock state. A blood pressure of 128/70 and a pulse rate of 74 are normal vital signs. A blood pressure of 84/58 with a heart rate of 130 would be a normal variation that would be experienced by a patient not on beta-blocker medications. A blood pressure of 166/104 with a heart rate of 62 would not represent a shock state because this patient is not hypotensive or tachycardic.

27. Answer: D

Nursing Process: Evaluation

Rationale: **Normotension and tachycardia are signs of clinical improvement in a patient with septic shock.**

The elevated heart rate is in response to the infection and is being tolerated as evidence by the normal blood pressure. Confusion, hypotension while receiving vasopressor support, hypertension, and the presence of lactic acidosis would not be indicators of positive improvements for the patient.

28. Answer: D

Nursing Process: Analysis

Rationale: **Endotoxin circulation is associated with septic shock, not hypovolemic shock.** In hypovolemic shock, the body compensates for the shock state by increasing the heart rate through sympathetic stimulation, one of which occurs through the baroreceptor response, secreting antidiuretic hormone for water and sodium uptake to keep fluid within the body, and epinephrine secretion to facilitate peripheral vasoconstriction.

 CENsational Pearl of Wisdom!

Baroreceptors are located in the aortic arch and the carotid bodies and respond to changes in vascular tone that is impacted by the blood pressure. When these are stimulated, they activate the sympathetic nervous system and contribute to the aldosterone cascade that also helps maintain body water and assists with vasoconstriction in an effort to increase the blood pressure. When the body is in shock, it does everything it can to hold water in so it can increase its intravascular volume and blood return to the right side of the heart.

29. Answer: C

Nursing Process: Intervention

Rationale: **Although treatment should not be delayed, cultures should be quickly obtained before starting antibiotic therapy.** Quick screening and identification of symptoms are crucial in the initial diagnosis of sepsis. Once the potential for sepsis is identified, fluid boluses are indicated if concurrent hypotension is present.

 CENsational Pearl of Wisdom!

Antibiotic therapy is extremely important in the care of the patient with sepsis. Every hour of delay in starting antibiotics can increase the mortality rate by 8%!

30. Answer: B

Nursing Process: Intervention

Rationale: **The use of steroids in septic shock is primarily to decrease the systemic effects of inflammation.** Although their use may be controversial in other situations, the anti-inflammatory effects of the steroids, in conjunction with other forms of aggressive treatment, are standard in the treatment of septic shock. Steroid administration will not lower blood glucose (on the contrary, steroids will increase blood glucose levels), prevent thromboembolic disease, or increase the likelihood of vasoconstriction.

31. Answer: B

Nursing Process: Intervention

Rationale: **High-dose vasopressors are not indicated in the treatment of hypovolemic shock.** This patient may require more fluids and/or blood products. The patient may continue to be symptomatic because of occult bleeding sites not yet identified.

32. Answer: A

Nursing Process: Analysis

Rationale: **The leading cause of death during the first 24 hours after a major burn injury is hypovolemia. As a result of the burn injury, third spacing begins to occur causing a dramatic decrease in intravascular volume and perfusion.** After 24 to 48 hours, infection, sepsis, and major organ failure are more likely to be contributing factors in the cause of death.

33. Answer: B

Nursing Process: Evaluation

Rationale: **Multiple pulmonary emboli are not common complications of shock.** Disseminated intravascular coagulation (DIC), acute respiratory distress syndrome (ARDS), and acute renal failure (ARF) are all common complications of shock and are the result of prolonged impaired perfusion.

34. Answer: B

Nursing Process: Analysis

Rationale: **Hyponatremia is not a known factor in the development of cardiogenic shock.** Cardiac tamponade (blood in the pericardial space) impairs the myocardial ability to pump, leading to a shock state. A beta-blocker overdose and dysrhythmias such as ventricular tachycardia will dramatically suppress cardiac output and predispose the patient to shock.

 CENsational Pearl of Wisdom!

Cardiac tamponade is a cause of obstructive shock. Beck's triad, explaining the three symptoms of cardiac tamponade, is always on the CEN examination. The triad includes muffled heart sounds, hypotension, and distended neck veins.

35. Answer: B

Nursing Process: Intervention

Rationale: **Dobutamine is a potent vasopressor but has less of a tendency to increase the heart rate as opposed to dopamine.** Tachycardia is a dangerous side effect of dopamine, and can worsen cardiogenic shock because of the increased myocardial demands. Therefore, dobutamine is the preferred drug for cardiogenic shock. Vasopressin is used to treat hypotension in patients who are suffering from a vasodilatory type of shock. It is used for these patients after there is no response from fluid boluses and catecholamine infusions. Nitroglycerin is a nitrate utilized in the treatment of renal failure and angina and congestive heart failure with a myocardial infarction. Nitroglycerin would bring blood pressures down because of its vasodilatory effects. It would be contraindicated in hypotension.

36. Answer: A

Nursing Process: Analysis

Rationale: **Neurogenic shock is caused by a massive vasodilation from impaired function of the sympathetic nervous system. Without the sympathetic nervous system, the vasculature responds only to the parasympathetic nervous system and, therefore, vasodilates.** In neurogenic shock, the intracranial pressure is unaffected. Although both are forms of distributive shock, the vasodilation from histamine release occurs in anaphylactic shock and vasodilation in the inflammatory processes occurs in septic shock.

 CENsational Pearl of Wisdom!

The sympathetic nervous system (SNS) and parasympathetic nervous system (PNS) work opposite of each other. In general, the SNS makes body systems work faster and harder and also allows for vasoconstriction. The PNS is the relaxation system that causes vasodilation and also causes slower responses such as bradycardia. The one system that is "backwards" is the gastrointestinal system. The SNS relaxes the GI system, whereas the PNS causes cramping and increased peristalsis. The PNS causes pupillary constriction and the SNS causes pupillary dilation.

37. Answer: C

Nursing Process: Intervention

Rationale: **This patient is obviously bleeding and is in apparent profound hypovolemic shock. The number one priority for this patient is two large-bore intravenous (IV) lines and lab studies including a type and crossmatch. Labs should be drawn as the IV lines are initiated.** Intubation and end-of-life issues are not currently applicable in this situation. Endoscopy may be indicated once the patient is stabilized.

CENsational Pearl of Wisdom!

When patients are hypovolemic, be sure to start large-bore intravenous lines. They should be at least 18 g or above. For the patient in profound shock, if it can be done, place 16 or 14 g. The patient will not know the difference! And remember to infuse normal saline if blood products are in the patient's future!

38. Answer: B

Nursing Process: Assessment

Rationale: **Bradycardia is the hallmark symptom of neurogenic shock.** Spinal trauma, from a motor vehicle crash, may cause an interruption in the sympathetic nervous system integrity. Although the patient may be hypotensive, the skin is often warm and dry in neurogenic shock. Hypovolemic, septic, and cardiogenic shock would most likely have tachycardia, hypotension, and cool, moist skin.

39. Answer: D

Nursing Process: Evaluation

Rationale: **Increasing urine output indicates that renal perfusion is maintained and is a sign of compensated hypovolemic shock.** A narrowing pulse pressure, severe hypotension, and increased lactic acid levels are indicative of uncompensated forms of shock.

CENsational Pearl of Wisdom!

Watching the urine output is the best way to keep informed regarding the perfusion of the "gut." The work of the kidneys reflects the perfusion status. It has been said in the past, "The kidneys are the window to the viscera." Old adage, but true!

40. Answer: D

Nursing Process: Analysis

Rationale: **A patient with pancreatitis is especially prone to both hypovolemic and septic shock. Severe dehydration from vomiting and diarrhea is often seen in pancreatitis, leading to hypovolemia. Pancreatitis can also be hemorrhagic. When this type is present, there is a risk of hypovolemic shock. The inflammatory process associated with pancreatitis and exacerbated by the hypovolemia can lead to sepsis.** Patients with pancreatitis are not at high risk for cardiogenic, neurogenic, or anaphylactic shock (unless they were to react to antibiotics given for septic shock!).

41. Answer: A

Nursing Process: Analysis

Rationale: **The renin–angiotensin–aldosterone system is activated when decreased extracellular fluid and hypotension is present. The end result is the reabsorption of sodium and water in the body, which causes an increase in vascular volume.** In shock, the body needs to reserve as much water as it can and keep it in the intravascular system. It also causes vasoconstriction from the release of aldosterone in the process. It does not release norepinephrine. Urinary output is reduced and therefore concentrated. If fluid is retained in the body, the urinary output would decrease.

CENsational Pearl of Wisdom!

When the renin–angiotensin–aldosterone system is activated, the kidneys release renin, which then causes the secretion of angiotensinogen. The angiotensinogen initiates the release of angiotensin I, which is converted to angiotensin II. This occurs in the lungs. Remember this! The angiotensin II then causes the release of aldosterone, which does the good part of producing the end product of sodium and water reabsorption. It also causes vasoconstriction to try to increase the blood pressure. This system is very important! Hint-Hint.

42. Answer: B

Nursing Process: Intervention

Rationale: **Epinephrine (Adrenalin) is the drug of choice for anaphylaxis and impending anaphylactic shock.** This is often followed by IV fluids, an antihistamine such as diphenhydramine (Benadryl), and a steroid dose such as methylprednisolone (Solu-Medrol). Return of symptoms can occur later, which is known as biphasic anaphylaxis.

43. Answer: D

Nursing Process: Analysis

Rationale: **Digitalis toxicity is not a contributing factor in hypovolemic shock.** Diabetic ketoacidosis, diabetes insipidus (lack of antidiuretic hormone), and diuretic overuse all can contribute to the development of severe dehydration and hypovolemic shock.

44. Answer: B

Nursing Process: Analysis

Rationale: **A hemorrhagic shock state will cause an increased secretion of antidiuretic hormone (ADH).** ADH helps restore lost fluid volume by increasing the uptake of sodium and water. There will be a decreased urine output, which is the desired compensatory effect in shock. Epinephrine and norepinephrine are released because of the sympathetic nervous system stimulation to compensate for the shock state.

45. Answer: C

Nursing Process: Analysis

Rationale: **A large pulmonary embolus can obstruct outflow of blood from the heart and lungs, thereby causing an obstructive form of shock.** Other causes of obstructive shock include cardiac tamponade and a gravid uterus lying on the inferior vena cava.

46. Answer: C

Nursing Process: Analysis

Rationale: **Immunosuppressed patients are at significant risk for the development of septic shock.** Steroids, chemotherapy, radiation therapy, HIV positive status, splenectomy, and stress contribute to immunosuppression. Hypertension, gastroesophageal reflux disease, and anticoagulant therapy do not predispose patients to sepsis.

47. Answer: A

Nursing Process: Assessment

Rationale: **Syncopal episodes in an elderly patient can be life-threatening.** Elderly patients may have unique symptoms of shock, so the patient would need to be quickly assessed for orthostatic hypotension, cardiac dysrhythmias, or hypovolemia from dehydration as the cause for the syncope. All of these can make the elderly patient at risk for falls, which can contribute to other catastrophic events for this age group. Tachycardia after exertion and urine output of 30 mL/hour are normal parameters. Cool extremities that are dry to touch would not raise a red flag for this patient.

 CENsational Pearl of Wisdom!

Also, remember that the elderly patient, like the pediatric patient, can decompensate very quickly!

48. Answer: D

Nursing Process: Intervention

Rationale: **Airway assessment and maintenance is always the number one priority in the care of a patient in shock.** Administration of intravenous fluids, oxygen, or vasopressors will not do any good in the treatment of shock if the airway is not assessed and maintained. If the patient does not have a patent airway, no other interventions will matter.

49. Answer: B

Nursing Process: Intervention

Rationale: **The standard intravenous fluid dose for pediatric patients is 20 mL/kg. Since this child now weighs 19 kg, multiply 19 times the 20 ml.** The correct bolus dose is 380 ml. The amount used for fluid resuscitation in a neonate is 10 mL/kg and may be used in children with cardiac histories. This child had no prior medical history. When calculating the dosage for the bolus, be sure to change the pounds to kilograms. This is the most common mistake that is made.

 CENsational Pearl of Wisdom!

Pediatric boluses should be given over 5 to 20 minutes and repeated as necessary while monitoring the child.

50. Answer: C

Nursing Process: Analysis

Rationale: **Septic shock is the most common form of distributive shock.** Distributive shock is caused by a vasodilation that occurs with a subsequent loss of afterload. Anaphylactic and neurogenic shock are forms of distributive shock, but they are not as common. Cardiogenic shock is not a form of distributive shock. Cardiogenic shock occurs due to the loss of the pumping ability of the heart.

51. Answer: A

Nursing Process: Analysis

Rationale: **Hypovolemic shock is the type of shock most often associated with dissecting aortic aneurysms.** As the intravascular blood volume decreases from the dissection, the hypovolemic shock progresses until the aorta can be repaired. Many complications can ensue from this brief, catastrophic hypovolemic state when the actual rupture occurs.

52. Answer: D

Nursing Process: Analysis

Rationale: **The thyroid gland is not involved in the process of the renin–angiotensin–aldosterone system.** At the forefront is the renal system that causes the release of renin. Angiotensin I is converted to angiotensin II in the lungs. Aldosterone is released from the adrenal glands. The liver is involved in the secretion of angiotensinogen.

 CENsational Pearl of Wisdom!

The sequence of events in the renin–angiotensin–aldosterone cascade is Renin → Angiotensinogen → Angiotensin I → Angiotensin II → Aldosterone.

53. Answer: A

Nursing Process: Intervention

Rationale: **Trendelenburg position is not recommended in the treatment of hypovolemic shock anymore. This position has been proven to have negative effects on a patient in shock. The proper position now is "shock" position or "modified Trendelenburg," which is to keep the body flat and elevate the feet/legs.** Providing oxygen via a non-rebreather mask at high flow to maintain the pulse oximetry reading between 94% and 98% is necessary. It is important to be concerned about hyperoxia; however, in the early stages of care, it is acceptable and recommended to provide the high-flow oxygen for a period of time. Keeping the patient warm is also important because hypothermia can cause many complications including acidosis and coagulopathies. Administration of warmed isotonic fluids is important for the patient. The intravenous lines will also be necessary for possible blood products.

 CENsational Pearl of Wisdom!

Modified Trendelenburg is the position of choice now. It can be difficult especially with lower extremity injuries.

54. Answer: D

Nursing Process: Analysis

Rationale: **Peripheral vascular resistance is decreased in clinical hypoperfusion, not increased.** Other factors that do contribute to the development of symptoms include decreased venous return to the heart, vasodilitation causing distributive types of shock, and an obstruction of circulating blood volume.

55. Answer: B

Nursing Process: Analysis

Rationale: **A tension pneumothorax is a major factor in the development of obstructive shock.** The tension pneumothorax causes a gradual compression on the mediastinum, including the heart and great vessels, which obstructs the venous return and impairs contractility. A cardiac dysrhythmia may lead to cardiogenic shock. Ectopic pregnancies are associated with hypovolemic shock. Bacterial pneumonia can progress to septic shock.

56. Answer: C

Nursing Process: Evaluation

Rationale: **Dopamine (Intropin) does not affect prolongation of the QRS complex.** Dopamine can cause tachydysrhythmias, requires a central IV line for administration and frequent monitoring of vital signs and urine output. Although dopamine can be used for cardiogenic shock, dobutamine (Dobutrex) is the preferred drug because it has less of a tendency to cause tachydysrhythmias.

 CENsational Pearl of Wisdom!

Infusion through a central line is preferred for dopamine; however, a large access peripheral line can be used if a central line is not available.

57. Answer: A

Nursing Process: Evaluation

Rationale: **After massive transfusions, hyperkalemia is of great concern because of the potential for dysrhythmias and muscular irritability. Hyperkalemia can occur because of the breakdown of cells as blood is stored. Each unit of blood given can increase the patient's potassium level. Consider this if the patient is already hyperkalemic before blood administration.** Metabolic acidosis, anaphylaxis, and hemolytic reactions are of concern, but are less frequently a complication.

CENsational Pearl of Wisdom!

Always reassess a patient after any intervention for a shock-like state. The ever-changing hemodynamics need to be assessed often.

58. Answer: D

Nursing Process: Assessment

Rationale: **The restless 82-year-old male with low back and abdominal pain, history of heavy smoking and hypertension, and tachycardia needs to be immediately assessed for an abdominal aortic aneurysm, which would place him at great risk for hypovolemic shock. His past history of heavy smoking places him at risk for these conditions and he is at the highest risk at this time.** The 24-year-old with the wasp sting is stable at this time and already has epinephrine on board. The 94-year-old is at risk for sepsis but is stable at this time. It would be important to determine her normal mentation to determine if today's confusion is new or old. The 19-year-old female with a history of vomiting is also stable.

59. Answer: C

Nursing Process: Assessment

Rationale: **OSVS are an unreliable method for assessing for fluid loss or hypovolemic shock and should be used only in conjunction with history, assessment, and other diagnostic indicators. Patients can falsely compensate while sitting, thus masking the true effects of hypovolemia.** Even though this test does carry some concern for its validity, it remains an accepted test and can provide objective data for the potential diagnosis of bleeding or dehydration. It can be performed on patients of any age. Only blood pressure and pulse rate are measured for this test. It can be performed on those with syncope, but these patients should be closely monitored during the test.

CENsational Pearl of Wisdom!

OSVS have been traditionally performed in the lying, sitting, and standing positions with changes such as a decrease in blood pressure or an increase in heart rate creating a positive report of this test. The Emergency Nurses Association has released a "Clinical Practice Guideline" recommending that these vital signs be performed lying, standing at 1 minute, and standing at 3 minutes. Criteria for changes in this manner of testing are drop in systolic pressure of 10 mm Hg, drop in diastolic pressure of 20 mm Hg, or increase in pulse rate of 20 beats/minute.

One of the best times to utilize OSVS is in those patients who present to the ED several days after a traumatic event with vague symptoms of abdominal pain or shortness of breath. OSVS can be positive and point the care provider in the direction of a ruptured spleen that has tamponaded off in the early stages and is now actively bleeding.

60. Answer: D

Nursing Process: Assessment

Rationale: **Tachycardia is often an early sign in shock because of the initial release of epinephrine and the attempt in the cardiovascular system to compensate for a decreased volume.** Cyanosis, anuria, and obtunded mental status are all late signs of shock.

61. Answer: D

Nursing Process: Analysis

Rationale: **Diabetic ketoacidosis, especially in a young patient, often presents after prolonged vomiting, diarrhea, and decreased oral intake, and may be accompanied by an infection and hypovolemic shock.** The patient with the urinary tract infection may be at risk for sepsis. The patient with chest pain and dyspnea could develop cardiogenic shock. The patient with fibromyalgia is not at risk for a shock state. The question asked was relative to hypovolemic shock.

62. Answer: B

Nursing Process: Assessment

Rationale: **Neurogenic shock occurs when there is a disruption in the sympathetic nervous system, allowing the parasympathetic nervous system to take over, which causes hypotension and bradycardia.** No other form of shock causes these connected symptoms. Third spacing of intracellular fluid leads to hypovolemia. Left ventricular hypertrophy may be a contributing factor for cardiogenic shock. A hypersensitivity reaction would involve anaphylactic shock.

63. Answer: C

Nursing Process: Evaluation

Rationale: **Patients with neurogenic shock associated with spinal cord injuries have difficulty maintaining their** temperature control. This is known as poikilothermia. A normalized temperature would be a positive turn for a patient with this type of shock. A heart rate of 46 beats/minute would be part of the symptomatology for neurogenic shock as would the hypotension and the rapid breathing.

64. Answer: A

Nursing Process: Evaluation

Rationale: **According to the SHOCK trial, the best possible treatment for cardiogenic shock is immediate percutaneous coronary intervention (PCI or coronary artery bypass graft (CABG). These dramatically reduce the mortality rate.** It is best to provide this option within 90 minutes, but it can be performed as much as 12 hours later with good results. Thinking that the patient will be well enough to travel in 10 days is not realistic on the part of the adult child. Low blood pressures do not help perfuse the patient's body and the problem is inadequate oxygenation of the cells, not too much oxygen.

 CENsational Pearl of Wisdom!

It is generally a good idea to always anticipate the worst thing that could happen to a patient. That way, you are never surprised. Always err on the side of caution. Think of the worst and hope for the best!

65. Answer: A

Nursing Process: Analysis

Rationale: **Pyelonephritis is an infectious disease and, therefore, would be the disease process most likely to cause septic shock.** Diabetic ketoacidosis would most likely cause a hypovolemic type of shock because of its dehydration properties. Cardiac tamponade and tension pneumothorax are both causes of obstructive shock.

66. Answer: D

Nursing Process: Evaluation

Rationale: **Normal saline boluses would not treat an obstructive shock patient. This would be indicated in situations involving hemorrhagic or hypovolemic shock.** A patient would receive a pericardiocentesis to treat a cardiac tamponade which causes obstructive shock. A pregnant patient would need to be turned to her left side to keep the gravid uterus off of the inferior vena cava, thus preventing or treating hypotension associated with obstructive shock. A needle decompression would be used to treat a tension pneumothorax, which would also cause obstructive shock.

67. Answer: C

Nursing Process: Analysis

Rationale: **Increased vascular tone in early shock will cause a slight increase in the diastolic pressure.** In early shock, the heart rate and the stroke volume will increase but is not the causative factor in the change in diastolic pressure. Renal perfusion will actually decrease at a later time.

68. Answer: B

Nursing Process: Intervention

Rationale: **Treating the hypotension to maintain a systolic pressure of 90 mm Hg is a form of permissive hypotension. As long as the MAP remains approximately 65, the patient is being perfused.** Aggressive measures such as copious fluid management may actually cause the injured area to bleed more and can cause more issues such as hypothermia, as well as diluting clotting factors and hemoglobin which is the oxygen-carrying capacity. Maintaining a systolic blood pressure of 90 mm Hg is carefully managed until definitive care can be provided. It is not appropriate to wait to treat hypotension until tachycardia or unconsciousness occurs. The patient may be taking beta-blockers, which would not allow tachycardia to occur, and hypotension should be treated before the patient has a decreased mentation.

69. Answer: C

Nursing Process: Analysis

Rationale: **The pulse pressure in hypovolemic shock becomes narrower as the shock progresses.** Pulse pressure is the difference between the systolic and diastolic measurements of the blood pressure. This change in pulse pressure is an indication that the cardiac output is declining and peripheral vascular resistance is increasing.

 CENsational Pearl of Wisdom!

The pulse pressure will widen in increased intracranial pressure.

70. Answer: B

Nursing Process: Analysis

Rationale: **Baroreceptors are located in the aortic arch and carotid arteries.** In a shock-like state, these sensitive cells can detect even the slightest decrease in pressure or volume and quickly send messages to the medulla. The medulla sets into motion a series of compensatory mechanisms for the body to address the shock. Responses to this include the release of epinephrine, which increases heart rate and peripheral vasoconstriction in an effort to increase the blood pressure.

71. Answer: A

Nursing Process: Analysis

Rationale: **Neck vein distension is often seen in conditions that cause obstructive shock.** These include cardiac tamponade, tension pneumothorax, and pulmonary embolism. A widening pulse pressure is seen in increased intracranial pressure. Orthostatic hypotension can be seen in dehydration, hypovolemic shock, vasodilator therapy, and diuretic overuse. Reflex tachycardia can occur when there is a sudden change in blood volume, with orthostatic hypotension being one of the major causes.

CENsational Pearl of Wisdom!

Reflex tachycardia can also be seen with nitroglycerin use because of the vasodilation that occurs. The sympathetic nervous system responds with tachycardia because it senses that there is not enough blood flow in the widened vascular system.

72. Answer: C

Nursing Process: Assessment

Rationale: **A child who is responsive to painful stimuli only or demonstrates lethargy is a potential candidate for the diagnosis of shock.** A blood pressure of 92/60 in a 3-year-old is not hypotensive. The pulse rate of 110 beats/minute is also not indicative of gross tachycardia in this patient. Responding to verbal stimuli would be a good response.

CENsational Pearl of Wisdom!

Remember that hypotension is one of the last signs in children. They have much better vascular tone than do adults and therefore are able to maintain their blood pressure for a much longer period of time.

73. Answer: D

Nursing Process: Evaluation

Rationale: **Aggressive fluid management is a major factor in the effective treatment of septic shock.** Although

initial blood cultures can be obtained while initiating treatment, antibiotics should never be held for any period of time to obtain cultures. Sepsis can be readily identified before any culture results are obtained. Diuretics would be counterproductive in a shock state.

74. Answer: B

Nursing Process: Intervention

Rationale: **Trendelenburg position's only benefit is that it increases venous return. It is not recommended for patients in shock.** The negative effects are an increase in intracranial pressure, increased abdominal organ ischemia, and increased diaphragmatic pressure causing a decrease in tidal volume and an eventual decrease in respirations and oxygen perfusion.

75. Answer: D

Nursing Process: Evaluation

Rationale: **The treatment of hypovolemic shock is considered effective when the systolic blood pressure is at least 90 mm Hg.** This is in conjunction with assessments of heart rate, capillary refill of 2 seconds or less, and a urine output of at least 30 mL/hour. ECG changes, with the exception of heart rate, generally do not occur in hypovolemic shock.

References

American Academy of Allergy, Asthma and Immunology. (2015). *Life-threatening allergic reactions are triggered by heat and exertion.* Retrieved from https://www.aaaai.org/global/latest-research-summaries/New-Research-from-JACI-In-Practice/life-threatening-allergic-reaction (22)

Dolan, C. (2016). *Biphasic anaphylaxis—what you need to know.* Allergy Lifestyle. Retrieved from https://www.allergylifestyle.com/biphasic-reaction (22)

Drugs.com. (2017, March 31). *Vasopressin dosage.* Retrieved from https://www.drugs.com/dosage/vasopressin.html (35)

Emergency Nurses Association. (2017). Emergency nursing core curriculum (7th ed.). St. Louis, MI: Elsevier. (8, 16, 37, 47, 50, 55, 59, 60, 66)

Emergency Nurses Association. (2018). Emergency nursing pediatric course: provider manual (5th ed.). Des Plaines, IL: Emergency Nurses Association. (12, 49, 72)

Emergency Nurses Association Clinical Practice Guidelines. (2015). *Orthostatic vital signs.* Retrieved from https://www.ena.org/docs/default-source/resource-library/practice-resources/cpg/orthostaticvitalsign-scpg.pdf?sfvrsn=c73c24a6_12 (59)

Gurney, D. (2014). Trauma nursing core course: provider manual (7th ed.). Des Plaines, IL: Emergency Nurses Association. (2, 4, 5, 10, 11, 25, 31–33, 38, 39, 52, 53, 57, 69, 75)

Hammond, B. A., et al. (2013). Sheehy's manual of emergency care (7th ed.). St. Louis, MO: Elsevier. (3, 5, 22, 29, 41, 42, 46, 48, 58, 61, 63, 65)

Hannon, R. A., et al. (2016). Porth pathophysiology: concepts of altered health states. Philadelphia, PA: Wolters & Kluwer. (1, 6, 7, 14, 15, 17, 23, 27, 28, 36, 44, 54, 62, 67, 70)

John, U. (2018, September 12). *Hemorrhagic shock treatment and management.* Medscape. Retrieved from https://emedicine.medscape.com/article/432650-treatment (24)

Joseph, M. (2016, January 18). *Blood pressure assessment in the hypovolemic shock patient.* EMS1. Retrieved from https://www.ems1.com/ems-products/Ambulance-Disposable-Supplies/articles/479223-Blood-pressure-assessment-in-the-hypovolemic-shock-patient/ (69)

Kollef, M. (2017). The Washington manual of critical care. Philadelphia, PA: Wolters & Kluwer. (18, 26, 29, 30, 51, 68, 73)

Medscape. (2018). *Dopamine Rx.* Retrieved from https://reference.medscape.com/drug/intropin-dopamine-342435#11 (56)

Medscape. (2018). *Nitroglycerin IV.* Retrieved from https://reference.medscape.com/drug/glyceryl-trinitrate-iv-iv-nitroglycerin-nitroglycerin-iv-342278 (35)

Parillo, P. E., et al. (2018). Critical care medicine. Philadelphia, PA: Elsevier. (2, 9, 13, 17, 19, 20, 40, 45, 56)

Phillip, L. (2017, March). *Overview of the autonomic nervous system.* Merck Manual. Retrieved from https://www.merckmanuals.com/professional/neurologic-disorders/autonomic-nervous-system/overview-of-the-autonomic-nervous-system (11)

Richard, F. (2018, February 15). *The importance of the vagus nerve.* Very Well Health. Retrieved from https://www.verywellhealth.com/the-importance-of-the-vagus-nerve-1746123 (5, 11)

Walls, R. (2013). Rosen's emergency medicine: concepts & clinical practice (8th ed.). Philadelphia, PA: Elsevier. (21, 34, 35, 43, 71, 74)

WebMD. (2018). *What is an immunoglobulin test?* Retrieved from https://www.webmd.com/a-to-z-guides/immunoglobulin-test#1 (23)

Xiushui, R. (Mike). (2017, January 11). *Cardiogenic shock treatment and management.* Medscape. Retrieved from https://emedicine.medscape.com/article/152191-treatment (64)

4 Environmental Emergencies

Joan Somes, PhD, RN-BC, CEN, CPEN, FAEN, NRP

Environmental emergencies cover a broad spectrum of topics and information. Patients may present with concerns ranging from snake bites to sunstroke. Although rapidly carrying out the traditional steps of airway, breathing, circulation, and disability (neurologic findings), as well as supporting them, are important first steps, often it is the fine details in the history and a thorough head-to-toe survey that will provide clues to definitive care. On the Certified Emergency Nurse test, environmental issues are combined with toxicology and communicable diseases, totaling 15 items. To be sure that this content is completely covered, this book also contains a chapter on toxicology (Chapter 5) and information related to communicable diseases in the medical emergencies chapter (Chapter 7).

1. While obtaining the history from a patient who presents with multiple puncture wounds on his arm, the patient states he was ". . .fishing in the river and was bitten by a big, ugly fish with whiskers!" One of the punctures seems to have a long spine (very thin, long bone) poking out from it. Which type of aquatic creature does the emergency nurse suspect caused this injury?
[ ] **A.** Shark
[ ] **B.** Jellyfish
[ ] **C.** Catfish
[ ] **D.** Fire coral

2. Which of the following would be appropriate treatment for a patient who has been stung by a catfish?
[ ] **A.** Soak the area in hot water (temperature: 110° F to 115° F [43° C to 46° C]) for 60 to 90 minutes, and then explore the wound in surgery to remove the spine.
[ ] **B.** Pull out the spine, soak the area in sea or salt-water solution for 30 minutes, and apply vinegar to the area.
[ ] **C.** Administer diphenhydramine orally, remove the spine, cleanse with soap and water, and apply an ice pack to the area.
[ ] **D.** Neutralize the nematocysts, and apply shaving cream, paste of flour, talc, or baking soda to the area and shave it.

3. Soft-tissue radiologic examinations may be most useful after:
[ ] **A.** a tiger shark bite.
[ ] **B.** exposure to a Portuguese Man of War.
[ ] **C.** tangling with an octopus.
[ ] **D.** an attack by a sting ray.

4. A patient presents with swelling of his or her lips, face, and mouth; generalized hives and itching; as well as tachycardia, hypotension, and generalized weakness. The history reveals that the patient was at the beach when the symptoms started. Which of the following is the most likely etiology for these symptoms?
[ ] **A.** A venom-specific reaction
[ ] **B.** Anaphylactic reaction to venom
[ ] **C.** Overexposure to the sun
[ ] **D.** Extracellular fluid dehydration

5. The most commonly needed type of care related to aquatic creature injury will be related to:
[ ] **A.** anaphylaxis and hypotension.
[ ] **B.** paralysis and muscle weakness.
[ ] **C.** infection and tissue necrosis.
[ ] **D.** vomiting and bloody diarrhea.

6. Which of the following is the most correct statement related to aquatic organisms and risks posed to rescuers?
[ ] **A.** There is little risk to rescuers and health care providers.
[ ] **B.** There is no potential risk if the animal is dead.
[ ] **C.** There is high risk if stinger protection is not used.
[ ] **D.** There is low risk if alcohol is used to neutralize toxins.

7. Which of the following statements regarding injury prevention education related to aquatic organisms is correct?
[ ] **A.** It is safe to pick up dead aquatic creatures with bare hands.
[ ] **B.** Wearing stinger suits and gloves are important when snorkeling.
[ ] **C.** Aquatic envenomation is easy to avoid if one is simply careful.
[ ] **D.** Staying out of the water and on the beach will eliminate chance of envenomation.

8. A patient states that he "tangled with a jellyfish earlier in the day while on vacation." He complains of severe pain where the jellyfish tentacles struck him. Which action will provide the most pain relief?
[ ] **A.** Soak the area in warm water for 45 minutes.
[ ] **B.** Have the patient rub the area to dislodge nematocysts.
[ ] **C.** Soak the area in a solution of acetic acid 5%.
[ ] **D.** Administer intravenous diphenhydramine (Benadryl).

9. Which of the following aquatic creatures releases a heat-susceptible toxin, which is deactivated by soaking the area in 110° F to 115° F (43° C to 46° C) water for 60 to 90 minutes?
[ ] **A.** Jelly fish
[ ] **B.** Fire coral
[ ] **C.** Portuguese Man of War
[ ] **D.** Sting ray

10. The venom of aquatic organisms will most likely cause:
[ ] **A.** weakness.
[ ] **B.** hemolysis.
[ ] **C.** hypertension.
[ ] **D.** bradycardia.

11. A child is brought to the emergency department in the early afternoon with a fresh raccoon bite. The raccoon ran away. There are several puncture wounds and a crushing laceration of the child's hand. Which of the following infectious agents is of highest concern?
[ ] **A.** Staphylococcus
[ ] **B.** Pasteurella
[ ] **C.** Rabies
[ ] **D.** Clostridium

12. A parent presents with their infant requesting a "rabies shot" because they saw a bat flying in the child's bedroom. The emergency nurse would anticipate:
[ ] **A.** reassuring the parent that unless a wound is found there is no risk of rabies.
[ ] **B.** administering Rabies Immune Globulin and first dose of Rabies vaccine.
[ ] **C.** setting up appointments for the series of rabies injections twice a day for 21 days.
[ ] **D.** initiating prophylactic intravenous antibiotics as soon as possible.

13. A patient presents after being bitten by a snake that he describes as having red, yellow, and black bands on the body and a black head. He states that several tiny punctures and scratch marks are seen at the site he was bitten. The nurse should monitor for:
[ ] **A.** pain, swelling, bullae at site, and hypotension.
[ ] **B.** paresthesias, dysesthesias, and respiratory distress.
[ ] **C.** localized tissue edema, redness, and necrosis.
[ ] **D.** rapid onset of coagulopathy and bleeding.

14. Administration of snake bite anti-venom is:
[ ] **A.** risky due to the possibility of adverse reaction.
[ ] **B.** dependent on identification of the type of snake.
[ ] **C.** most effective if given within 6 hours of a bite.
[ ] **D.** indicated in both Viperidae and Elapidae snake bites.

15. Which type of snake bite would require obtaining laboratory studies that includes coagulation studies, blood type, and creatinine kinase level, as well as performing serial measurements on the leg where the bite occurred?
[ ] **A.** Rattle snake
[ ] **B.** Coral snake
[ ] **C.** Sea snake
[ ] **D.** Bull snake

16. Which of the following statements made by a patient treated for snake bite would indicate that he or she understands proper preventative care?
[ ] **A.** "I need to have additional anti-venom injections in 3, 7, and 14 days."
[ ] **B.** "The anti-venom you gave me will keep the wound from getting infected."
[ ] **C.** "It is OK to pick up snakes as long as I grab them right behind the eyes."
[ ] **D.** "I should always wear boots or high-top shoes when hiking in the woods."

17. Which of the following would be proper treatment for a victim of a snake bite?
[ ] **A.** Applying a proximal tourniquet
[ ] **B.** Utilizing ice on the extremity
[ ] **C.** Administering a tetanus injection
[ ] **D.** Soaking the area in warm water

18. Hymenoptera is an insect that leaves a venom-filled stinger in the victim. This venom frequently causes anaphylaxis. Which of the following is the most likely to pose this risk to a sensitized patient?
[ ] **A.** Mosquito
[ ] **B.** Sand flea
[ ] **C.** Spider
[ ] **D.** Fire ant

19. A patient presents with redness, swelling, fever, and pain in an arm that was stung by several wasps 3 days previously. This patient is most likely experiencing which of the following?
[ ] **A.** Infectious cellulitis of the area and needs an oral antibiotic
[ ] **B.** A delayed reaction to the wasp venom and needs anti-venom
[ ] **C.** Continued IgE-mediated reaction and needs antihistamine
[ ] **D.** Non-wasp bite-related and needs further investigation

20. Which of the following is the most frequently reported vector-borne illness in the United States?
[ ] **A.** Tick-borne Ehrlichiosis
[ ] **B.** Rocky Mountain Spotted Fever
[ ] **C.** Lyme disease
[ ] **D.** Colorado tick fever

21. A patient diagnosed with Lyme's disease presents with nausea and vomiting. Which stage of the disease is this patient experiencing?
[ ] **A.** Stage 1
[ ] **B.** Stage 2
[ ] **C.** Stage 3
[ ] **D.** Stage 4

22. A patient presents with concerns they may have contracted a tick-related illness. Which of the following pieces of information obtained from the patient would help to reduce the likelihood of tick-borne illnesses?
[ ] **A.** A tick engorged to the size of a pea was found on the patient.
[ ] **B.** The patient has been camping in a wooded, grassy area.
[ ] **C.** The tick was found crawling around on the patient's leg.
[ ] **D.** The patient has not been outside, but his dog goes to the park.

23. Rocky Mountain Spotted Fever (RMSF) typically presents with a history of the patient having visited:
[ ] **A.** the Rocky Mountains in Nevada.
[ ] **B.** the grassy plains in Missouri.
[ ] **C.** the rocky seashore in Oregon.
[ ] **D.** the glacier fields in Montana.

24. A patient presents with a high fever, chills, severe headache, confusion, nausea, and vomiting. You also notice a red, nonitchy rash on the patient's wrists, palms, ankles, and feet. Which question answered in the affirmative might pinpoint the source of these symptoms best?
[ ] **A.** "Have you been around someone else with these symptoms?"
[ ] **B.** "Have you taken any new medications or used new soaps lately?"
[ ] **C.** "Have you been out walking in an area that is grassy or wooded?"
[ ] **D.** "Have you been wading in a weedy pond that has ducks lately?"

25. Which of the following statements made by a patient being discharged with a tick bite indicates the need for further instructions?
[ ] **A.** "I need to get antibiotics every time I find a tick walking on me."
[ ] **B.** "When I go walking I will wear my pants tucked into my socks."
[ ] **C.** "To remove a tick—grab the head with tweezers and twist it off."
[ ] **D.** "I will use tick repellant when walking in areas with known ticks."

26. An 8-year-old child is being evaluated for sudden onset of weakness and frequent falling. On examination, the child appears to have an acute ascending, flaccid paralysis that started 1 day before and is worsening. It is determined that the child has been restless and irritable, complaining of paresthesias, myalgias, and fatigue over the last several days. The child spent last week at camp and the mother said they pulled several ticks off the child when he came home. Which of the following is the highest possibility?

[ ] **A.** Second stage of Lyme's disease
[ ] **B.** Onset of human tick paralysis
[ ] **C.** Closed head injury
[ ] **D.** Guillain-Barré syndrome

27. A patient states he was cleaning out an old shed when he felt a sharp pain in his left hand. He then suddenly developed an aching pain in this hand, with severe abdominal pain and nausea. Based on this information, which of the following would have most likely bitten this patient? Vital signs are as follows:

Blood pressure—180/112 mm Hg
Pulse—138 beats/minute
Respirations—16 breaths/minute
Pulse oximetry—97% on room air
Temperature—98.8°F (37.1°C)

[ ] **A.** Brown recluse spider
[ ] **B.** Copperhead snake
[ ] **C.** Black widow spider
[ ] **D.** Brown nose bat

28. A patient presents with a small area of blackened tissue on his hand that started with itching and swelling 2 days before. Purplish blisters with adjacent purpura are seen in the area. Which of the following provides the best information for diagnosis?

[ ] **A.** He was piling wood when a brown recluse spider bit his hand.
[ ] **B.** While cleaning an outhouse, he was bitten by a black widow spider.
[ ] **C.** A rabid bat bit him while sleeping in a small one-room cabin.
[ ] **D.** When walking in a grassy wooded area, he was bitten by a deer tick.

29. Neurotoxin released by the black widow spider can lead to:

[ ] **A.** hypotension and tachycardia.
[ ] **B.** urticaria and necrosis.
[ ] **C.** tingling and muscle fasciculation.
[ ] **D.** hemolysis and renal failure.

30. Anticipated therapy for a black widow spider bite would include which of the following?

[ ] **A.** Immediate debridement of area
[ ] **B.** Administration of corticosteroids
[ ] **C.** Immediate intravenous antibiotics
[ ] **D.** Anti-venom after skin testing

31. Which of the following pathophysiologic events occurs with frostbite-associated tissue damage?

[ ] **A.** Vasodilatory capillary leak
[ ] **B.** Sludging-related thrombosis
[ ] **C.** Cardiopulmonary ice crystals
[ ] **D.** Decreased vessel permeability

32. Which of the following is a true statement regarding superficial frostbite?

[ ] **A.** Water-filled blisters occur.
[ ] **B.** The skin is usually necrotic.
[ ] **C.** There is no sensation in the area.
[ ] **D.** Skin is hard and nonpliable.

33. Which of the following would be proper care for frostbitten feet?

[ ] **A.** Rewarming should occur when there is no further chance of refreezing.
[ ] **B.** The feet should rest on the bottom of a basin filled with hot water.
[ ] **C.** A hair dryer can be used if hot water is not available immediately.
[ ] **D.** Warming should occur in 15- to 30-minute increments for 5 to 6 hours.

34. Which of the following statements made by a patient being discharged with frostbite would indicate a positive understanding?

[ ] **A.** "I will stop using my aspirin and ibuprofen."
[ ] **B.** "I will continue to wear tightly fitting stockings."
[ ] **C.** "I will drink more coffee to help healing."
[ ] **D.** "I will keep my feet elevated to heart level."

35. A patient was found outside on a cold, rainy night. The patient is unresponsive, naked, and with skin that is cold to the touch. There are no signs of shivering, and the cardiac rhythm is slow and irregular. The 12-lead electrocardiogram (ECG) shows an extra positive deflection between the QRS complex and ST segment. The emergency nurse would suspect which of the following core temperatures and level of hypothermia?

[ ] **A.** 93° F to 95° F (35° C to 36° C), mild hypothermia

[ ] **B.** 86° F to 93° F (30° C to 34° C), moderate hypothermia

[ ] **C.** 83° F to 85° F (28° C to 29° C), severe hypothermia

[ ] **D.** Less than 83° F (27° C), profound hypothermia

36. A severely hypothermic patient in cardiac arrest is brought to the emergency department with CPR in progress. The cardiac monitor shows ventricular fibrillation. In addition to continuing compressions and ventilations, which of the following should the team perform?

[ ] **A.** Rewarm the patient before attempting emergency drugs or defibrillation.

[ ] **B.** Administer 2 mg intravenous epinephrine before defibrillation and rewarming.

[ ] **C.** Defibrillate the patient once, then aggressively rewarm before further shocks.

[ ] **D.** Rapidly push 500 mg amiodarone (Cordarone) intravenously while rewarming.

37. Which of the following types of medications would predispose a patient found lying unresponsive on the bathroom floor to be hypothermic?

[ ] **A.** Phenothiazines

[ ] **B.** Beta-blockers

[ ] **C.** Opioids

[ ] **D.** Stool softeners

38. A shivering patient brought to the emergency department by EMS has a core temperature of 90° F (32° C). Rewarming would be most easily and effectively carried out by which of the following methods?

[ ] **A.** Wrapping in a reflective blanket

[ ] **B.** Forced-air warming blanket

[ ] **C.** Warmed intravenous fluid bolus

[ ] **D.** Extracorporeal Membrane Oxygenation (ECMO)

39. During the process of rewarming and resuscitation, it is important to monitor for "after drop." Which of the following events can occur during this process?

[ ] **A.** Blood pH drops into acidotic state due to return of circulation

[ ] **B.** Drop in BP when cool blood from extremities reaches the core

[ ] **C.** Potassium level drops due to reactivation of cellular activity

[ ] **D.** Bradycardia recurs due to increased peripheral circulation

40. A patient presents with complaints of a deep throbbing pain in his joints, especially his shoulders which has been progressively worsening over the past 2 hours. He also offers complaints of being extremely tired and is noted to have a mottled-looking skin rash with pitting edema of the extremities. Which of the following would best describe his recent activity?

[ ] **A.** Hiking in the woods

[ ] **B.** Mountain climbing

[ ] **C.** Cave exploring

[ ] **D.** Diving in a deep lake

41. Decompression sickness is caused by which of the following?

[ ] **A.** Oxygen floating through the blood

[ ] **B.** Nitrogen bubbles sequestering in the joints

[ ] **C.** Carbon monoxide gathering in the tissues

[ ] **D.** Hydrogen atoms under the diaphragm

42. A patient presents with shortness of breath, confusion, and bleeding from the ears. Friends state he was diving on a wreck when he surfaced rapidly after he had accidently jabbed his hand with a knife while prying something loose from the wreckage. Bleeding is controlled at the site. Which of the following is the first priority for this patient's care? Vital signs are as follows:

Blood pressure—96/64 mm Hg
Pulse—110 beats/minute
Respiratory rate—36 breaths/minute
Pulse oximetry—90% on room air
Temperature—98.4° F (36.8° C)

[ ] **A.** Clean and suture the laceration.

[ ] **B.** Arrange for hyperbaric chamber.

[ ] **C.** Assist with a needle decompression.

[ ] **D.** Rapidly give 2 liters IV crystalloids.

43. On a warm, humid, summer day, the local school marching band has been practicing dress rehearsal formations for several hours. Eight of the students began complaining of dizziness and nausea. On arrival at the emergency department, all students are conscious with complaints of increased thirst, dizziness, nausea, and headaches. Active vomiting is present in four of them. They are pale and diaphoretic. What is the most likely cause of these symptoms?

[ ] **A.** Heat cramps
[ ] **B.** Heat exhaustion
[ ] **C.** Heat stroke
[ ] **D.** Heat hysteria

44. Which of the following would be most concerning regarding a patient diagnosed with heat stroke?

[ ] **A.** Persistent lack of shivering
[ ] **B.** Pink/reddish-colored urine
[ ] **C.** Sinus tachycardia on the monitor
[ ] **D.** Presence of a Lichtenberg Figure

45. Which of the following is the safest and most effective way to cool a patient with heat exhaustion?

[ ] **A.** Covering the lower trunk with ice packs
[ ] **B.** Gastric lavage with 2 L of iced saline
[ ] **C.** Utilizing fans on the patient with sprayed water
[ ] **D.** Immersing the patient into a tub of cold water

46. A group of nursing friends are attending a nursing conference in a mountainous area. On arrival, several of the group become irritable and are complaining of persistent headache, nausea, and extreme fatigue. There is a planned event that afternoon to the summit of one of the near mountains. Which of the following would be the best recommendation for those feeling ill?

[ ] **A.** Take 1,000 mg acetaminophen, increase fluids, and attend the trip.
[ ] **B.** Drink two large glasses of nonalcoholic fluids, rest, and decline the trip.
[ ] **C.** Increase noncaffeinated fluids, eat some protein, and attend the trip.
[ ] **D.** Eat and drink normally, go on the trip, but decline the hike.

47. Which of the following is the primary cause of death in most submersion injuries?

[ ] **A.** Aspiration
[ ] **B.** Bradycardia
[ ] **C.** Hypothermia
[ ] **D.** Hypoxia

48. Research related to drowning outcome predictions has shown which of the following situations has the highest potential for survival?

[ ] **A.** Submersion for only 5 to 10 minutes or less
[ ] **B.** Resuscitation continued for 25 minutes or greater
[ ] **C.** Circulation and breathing returned at the scene
[ ] **D.** Patient required ventilation, but no compressions

49. Circulation has been restored and assisted ventilations continue in a patient rescued from a pond. Continued care will initially focus on treating which of the following disorders?

[ ] **A.** Respiratory alkalosis and hypercarbia
[ ] **B.** Hypocarbia and cellular hypoxemia
[ ] **C.** Pulmonary infection and aspiration
[ ] **D.** Cerebral edema and hypothermia

50. A patient found submerged in a cold stream has been carried into the emergency department by the family. The clothing is soaking wet. The patient mumbles when shaken, is breathing 6 breaths/minute, and has wet lung sounds. The pulse rate is 58 beats/minute and weak, skin is cool, and capillary refill is 3 seconds. Which of the following best describes priority of care for this patient?

[ ] **A.** Warm to 96° F (35.6° C), intubate and apply positive end-expiratory pressure.
[ ] **B.** Warm, suction fluids/debris from lungs during bronchoscopy and give diuretics.
[ ] **C.** Immobilize neck and place on Continuous Positive Airway Pressure (CPAP).
[ ] **D.** Administer atropine and a vasopressor and place in postural drainage position.

51. A family presents to the emergency department with complaints of severe itching, especially at night. All have linear red papules, visible threadlike burrows, and excoriations at the wrists, ankles, armpits, and between their fingers and toes. Which of the following statements indicates clear understanding of the diagnosis and appropriate follow up?

[ ] **A.** "This is due to tick bites. I will wear long sleeves and pants tucked into my socks when outside."
[ ] **B.** "This is due to allergies. I won't include strawberries or peanuts in the meals I make for my family."
[ ] **C.** "This is due to scabies. I will launder our bed linens in hot water and dry using the hottest drier cycle."
[ ] **D.** "This is due to lice. I will soak all our combs, brushes, and hair barrettes in a 50% bleach water solution."

52. History elicits that a patient was found in a burning shed. There is black soot on the face and upper chest. Both arms and hands have blistered and peeling skin. Which of the following is the highest life-threat concern?
[ ] A. Hypothermia due to significant skin loss
[ ] B. Hypovolemia due to fluid loss from burns
[ ] C. Electrolyte imbalance from fluid shifts
[ ] D. Swelling of the upper airway tissues

53. Which of the following would be a correct assumption regarding stocking type burns on the feet or both hands on a child?
[ ] A. This is normal as children are curious.
[ ] B. This will require admission to a burn unit.
[ ] C. This should raise suspicion for maltreatment.
[ ] D. This will be treated using sulfa ointment.

54. A store clerk was stocking cleaning supplies when the box cutter sliced open several bottles of the cleaner. The fluid splashed over the clerk's hands, arms, and legs. The cleaner contains hydrofluoric acid. Which of the following orders would the emergency nurse expect to be prescribed for this patient?
[ ] A. Flush area with a prepared solution of calcium gluconate.
[ ] B. Irrigate area with 1 liter warmed saline and report pH.
[ ] C. Wash area with mixture of sodium bicarbonate and ringers lactate.
[ ] D. Apply thin layer of water-based ointment (Bacitracin) to the area.

55. Which of the following is a priority risk to consider when caring for a patient presenting with a chemical burn?
[ ] A. Not having the proper agent needed to neutralize the chemical
[ ] B. Creating a hazardous gas when applying water to area
[ ] C. Exposing the caregivers to the chemical during treatment
[ ] D. Hypokalemia when chemical is absorbed into bloodstream

56. A little league player collapses after a light pole he was standing next to was hit by lightning. Which of the following actions would be an appropriate measure after maintaining scene safety?
[ ] A. Check immediately for long-bone fractures that need immobilization.
[ ] B. Worry about cervical spine injury when attempting to resuscitate.
[ ] C. Immediately tilt the head back opening the airway to ventilate.
[ ] D. Begin chest compressions assuming ventricular fibrillation is present.

57. A patient presents to the emergency department after being "knocked flat" while he was playing golf. His only complaint is that he "feels weird." During assessment, a reddened fern-shaped pattern across his back is noted. He denies any pain to the area. Based on this presentation which of the following would be appropriate actions?
[ ] A. Look for entrance and exit wounds
[ ] B. Intubate the patient to protect his airway
[ ] C. Check the lactate level on the patient
[ ] D. Monitor cardiac rhythm and urine color

58. A patient was removed from a burning house. Which of the following would be a priority test?
[ ] A. Pulse oximetry
[ ] B. 12-Lead ECG
[ ] C. Carboxyhemoglobin
[ ] D. Urine myoglobin

59. A patient is brought to the emergency department with burns sustained when he fell backward into a fire pit. The palms of his hands have linear charred markings and are leathery to palpation. His lower back and upper posterior thighs have reddened, blistered areas and his nylon shorts are melted into his skin. When the shorts are pulled away, the underlying skin is patchy white or charred-looking. The patient complains of pain to his back and thighs, but not his buttocks or hands. Which of the following would be the suspected depth of burn associated with his hands and buttocks?
[ ] A. Superficial epidermal—first degree
[ ] B. Superficial partial thickness—second degree
[ ] C. Deep partial thickness—second degree
[ ] D. Full thickness—third degree

60. An adult patient with significant deep partial-thickness burns is being stabilized and the calculated amount of warmed fluid has been administered. Which of the following is the best indicator that the correct amount of fluid has been administered?
[ ] A. The respiratory rate is 32 breaths/minute.
[ ] B. The mean arterial pressure is 45 mm Hg.
[ ] C. The urine output is 58 mL/hour.
[ ] D. The pulse rate is 136 beats/minute.

61. Several members of an extended family visiting the area for a family reunion present with similar symptoms that began approximately 4 hours before. They complain of nausea, vomiting, trouble swallowing, crampy diarrhea, and generalized weakness. The nurse notes slurred speech, and when asked about the constant eye rubbing, the presence of blurred vision is discovered. It also appears that eyelids are drooping slightly on several of the patients. Based on these symptoms and characteristics of the group, which of the following questions would assist in helping to diagnosis this disease process?

[ ] **A.** "Have all of you eaten some of the same food?"
[ ] **B.** "Were all of you playing in the hotel pool area?"
[ ] **C.** "Have any of you been licked by the same dog?"
[ ] **D.** "Did any of you drink the same home-made juice?"

62. Which of the following would confirm a diagnosis of food poisoning?

[ ] **A.** Stool positive for blood
[ ] **B.** Altered serum electrolytes
[ ] **C.** Normal white blood cell count
[ ] **D.** Sample of food ingested

63. A day care provider brings three of her own children to the emergency department for evaluation of a 2-day history of abdominal pain, bloating, gas, and greasy diarrhea that floats in the toilet. Several other children from the day care have similar symptoms. Many of the children have gluten, soy, and milk allergies/intolerances, so typically they do not eat the same foods. Which of the following is the most likely source of these symptoms?

[ ] **A.** Day care's Golden Retriever
[ ] **B.** Gelatin snack served daily
[ ] **C.** Local community splash pad
[ ] **D.** Local park's drinking fountain

64. Which of the following would be an appropriate response in guiding someone who is traveling to a location where the water is not guaranteed to be safe to drink?

[ ] **A.** "Use over-the-counter loperamide (Imodium) if diarrhea occurs."
[ ] **B.** "Boil all drinking water for at least 5 minutes before use."
[ ] **C.** "Avoid raw fruits, vegetables, and salads while in the country."
[ ] **D.** "Take preventative antiparasitic medications as prescribed."

65. A 2-year-old child is brought to the emergency department for evaluation of a reddened circle about an inch in diameter with an intermittent ridge line around most of the circumference on the left arm. The parents are concerned regarding the potential of ringworm as the family dog was recently treated for this. Which of the following should the emergency nurse expect if ringworm is present?

[ ] **A.** A black light shined on the area that fluoresces is proof of ringworm.
[ ] **B.** A social worker may be needed to investigate this type of injury.
[ ] **C.** Clippings or scrapings showing bacteria will prove ringworm.
[ ] **D.** The area will turn purple if swabbed with a Betadine/peroxide mixture.

66. Four employees at the local gardening center were unloading a truck when the forklift pierced a box of insecticide causing it to spill over all of them. Within minutes, all have classic symptoms of exposure. Which of the following symptoms would be expected with this contamination?

[ ] **A.** Uncontrollable tearing and salivation
[ ] **B.** Stuffy nose and constipation
[ ] **C.** Hot, dry skin and anxiety
[ ] **D.** Flushed skin and dilated pupils

67. A tanker truck involved in a crash has several containers of cyanide that are leaking. Which of the following would the emergency department need to obtain in preparation for potential patients?

[ ] **A.** Atropine and pralidoxime (2-PAM)
[ ] **B.** Benzodiazepines
[ ] **C.** Hydroxocobalamin
[ ] **D.** 0.5% bleach solution

68. A plumber presents after a mishap while unblocking a drain. Prior attempts involved lye and toilet bowl cleaner. A sudden eruption from the drain pipe totally drenched the plumber. On arrival to the emergency department, his clothing is still dripping with the contents of the attempts and the standing water in the pipe. Which of the following would be the first step in caring for this patient?

[ ] **A.** Assist the patient in removing his shirt and pants.
[ ] **B.** Douse the patient with 0.5% hypochlorite mixture.
[ ] **C.** Assist the patient in showering for 30 minutes in hot water.
[ ] **D.** Obtain and don personal protective equipment.

69. During a breach at a local nuclear energy plant, a radioactive was released. No explosion or radioactive dust cloud was created. Which of the following is the most important question to ask each patient as they present for treatment?
[ ] **A.** "How far from the plant were you?"
[ ] **B.** "Were you inside or outside a building?"
[ ] **C.** "What symptoms are you having?"
[ ] **D.** "Are you wearing the same clothing?"

70. Symptoms of acute radiation poisoning include which of the following?
[ ] **A.** Vomiting, watery diarrhea, and fever occurring within hours
[ ] **B.** Immediate painful blistering and sloughing of all exposed skin
[ ] **C.** Muscle cramping, prolonged seizures, and respiratory distress
[ ] **D.** Pulmonary edema, uncontrollable coughing, and tearing of eyes

71. A critical tool needed during assessment of an event involving radiation release would be a/an:
[ ] **A.** cardiac monitor.
[ ] **B.** capnography detector.
[ ] **C.** Geiger counter.
[ ] **D.** glucose meter.

72. A 55-year-old patient was lighting the barbeque grill when it flashed over. He presents with redness and blistering of his chest, abdomen, and entire right arm and hand. Using the rule of 9's, what percentage of body surface area is involved to be used to calculate fluid volume replacement?
[ ] **A.** 7%
[ ] **B.** 17%
[ ] **C.** 27%
[ ] **D.** 37%

73. A behavioral health patient sticks a pilfered paper clip into the electrical wall socket in the bathroom. The staff hears a snap, sees a flash, the patient stiffens and falls to floor unresponsive, and the lights go out in the bathroom. In addition to thinking "Stabilize the ABC's," which of the following should be considered?
[ ] **A.** Percent body surface area burned
[ ] **B.** Are burns superficial or deep dermal
[ ] **C.** Immediate carboxyhemoglobin level
[ ] **D.** Look for an entrance and exit wound.

74. Multiple hospital staff report to the emergency department with sudden onset of severe abdominal cramping and diarrhea. Upon assessment, it is determined that all ate the "cafeteria special," meat and gravy over noodles, earlier in the shift. All are normothermic with no vomiting. What is the anticipated action for these patients?
[ ] **A.** Initiate intravenous (IV) fluids and give IV ondansetron (Zofran).
[ ] **B.** Encourage increased oral fluids and rest.
[ ] **C.** Determine blood type anticipating bloody diarrhea.
[ ] **D.** Administer intravenous antibiotics and admit.

75. Patients involved in environmental emergencies present to the emergency department with a variety issues, causative factors, symptoms, and complaints. Which of the following is the priority action when providing care for an unstable victim of an unknown environmental problem?
[ ] **A.** Assess to ensure airway is intact.
[ ] **B.** Check ventilations for adequacy.
[ ] **C.** Palpate skin for capillary refill.
[ ] **D.** Don personal protective equipment.

Answers/Rationales

1. Answer: C

Nursing Process: Analysis

Rationale: **Identifying the type of aquatic creature causing the injury will be important to determine which type of treatment is most effective. Aquatic organisms with spines/whiskers (including the catfish) cause multiple puncture wounds, release a toxin from their spines, and often leave small pieces of the spine/whiskers broken off in the wounds.** Each of the other aquatic organisms has a different method of protecting itself and affecting their victim.

(Clue on test taking—Read the questions very carefully. If you read this question with an eye for detail, you will notice that the patient was fishing in the lake. The other three options would not be found in the lake!)

 CENsational Pearl of Wisdom!

With the increasing number of people participating in ocean-related activities such as skin diving, snorkeling, and beach vacations, there have been an increased number of aquatic organism injuries. One does not need to go in the water to come into contact with aquatic creatures that cause injury. Additionally, now with the ease and speed of air travel, it is possible for nurses nowhere near an ocean to encounter sea water-based organism-related injuries as patients may wait until they return home to seek medical attention. Treatment will vary depending on the type of organism, thus being able to identify the causative agent will be important for correct therapy.

2. Answer: A

Nursing Process: Intervention

Rationale: **Initially soaking the area in hot water (110° F to 115° F [43° C to 46° C]) will deactivate the venom. Surgical removal under magnification followed by vigorous irrigation with warm saline is recommended to find and wash away all broken spine pieces.** The wound is usually left open to allow for drainage and less risk of overwhelming infection. Option D would be appropriate for fish with stingers. Options C and D are incorrect answers.

 CENsational Pearl of Wisdom!

Aquatic Animal	Cause of Injury	Also Known As (AKA)	Treatment
Biters	Wound is usually torn skin, avulsion, or deep puncture	Sharks, barracuda, octopus, moray eels, sea snakes, killer whales	Radiograph for broken teeth/bones, foreign bodies, etc. Clean and irrigate wound Generally wound is left open Antibiotics and tetanus immunization
Stingers	Nematocysts embed in skin and release venom	Jellyfish, hydrozoans, Portuguese Man of War, fire coral, sea wasps, anemones	Remove any remaining parts Prevent nematocyst activation by rinsing in salt water/saline Soak in vinegar Apply shaving cream or baking soda paste Shave area
Spiny creatures	Puncture and release a toxin	Sting rays, scorpion fish, lion fish, sea urchins, catfish	Soak in hot water (110°–115° F [43°–46° C]) for 60–90 min to deactivate venom Look for and remove puncturing part

3. Answer: D

Nursing Process: Intervention

Rationale: **Sting rays often leave part of the stinging barb in the victim and either a soft-tissue radiograph** or ultrasound is needed to determine if there is a foreign body in the wound. Although a shark bite may involve bony portions of the body, an radiograph may not be necessary based on size and location of the wound. Portuguese Man of War and octopi do not leave radiopaque bony fragments. They leave nematocysts that are not radiopaque, so will not show up on radiograph.

CENsational Pearl of Wisdom!

Nematocysts are small, specialized cells found in the tentacles of jellyfish and other coelenterates designed to protect themselves or paralyze prey. Each cell contains a tiny venomous barb, which when stimulated, is released into the victim, injecting a poisonous liquid. This poison subdues smaller fish, but only leads to local irritation in people when they brush against a jellyfish or even a detached piece of jellyfish.

An old wives' tale is to urinate on the area, but actually any fluid that is not at the salinity of ocean water will actually stimulate any nematocysts that are still stuck to the skin leading to more barbs being stimulated.

4. Answer: B

Nursing Process: Analysis

Rationale: **Although hypotension and tachycardia are also signs of venom reactions, this patient is presenting with classic anaphylaxis symptoms—hives, itching, and swelling of the face, mouth, and lips.** Venom-related reactions are typically weakness and paralysis. Treatment should be aimed at the histamine reaction and circulatory collapse and should be treated as such with epinephrine, diphenhydramine (Benadryl), and H_2-blockers such as famotidine (Pepcid) and fluids. Overexposure to the sun would cause more heat exhaustion or heat stroke-like symptoms, including an increased temperature. The hives, itching, and swelling would not be caused by the sun exposure nor would they be associated with dehydration although the tachycardia, hypotension, and generalized weakness could be manifestations of this process.

5. Answer: C

Nursing Process: Intervention

Rationale: **Injuries caused by aquatic organisms often take place in water that is contaminated and are puncture wounds (which are traditionally the wound most likely to become infected) that do not drain well. They may also have small bits of foreign body parts in them (especially if exposed to a spiny creature). Any injected venom is also irritating to the tissue; thus necrosis, infection, and ulceration are much more common.**

Anaphylaxis, hypotension, muscle weakness, and paralysis are concerns, but are not the most common problems. Vomiting and diarrhea are not usually associated with envenomation by aquatic creatures.

CENsational Pearl of Wisdom!

Neutralizing toxins in wounds caused by aquatic creatures is recommended, but, more importantly, a thorough cleansing/irrigating of the wound(s) along with prophylactic antibiotics, as well as allowing the injury to heal by secondary intention, is recommended. Also ensure the patient is updated on tetanus immunization.

6. Answer: C

Nursing Process: Analysis

Rationale: **Rescuers and care providers must take precautions with proper PPEs to prevent accidental exposure to retained nematocysts or tentacles containing venom. Forceps or hemostats should be utilized to remove stingers or barbs to prevent being stuck.** Even dead organisms will release toxins, and alcohol typically does not neutralize venom.

7. Answer: B

Nursing Process: Analysis

Rationale: **Appropriate protection, such as footwear, gloves, and even some kind of skin covering to prevent injury, is recommended when in the water, as is shuffling one's feet when walking in the sand near the water. Accidentally brushing against, or stepping on unseen aquatic organisms, and reaching into small holes where an aquatic organism is hiding are the most common ways people are injured in the water by marine creatures.** Often the creatures bury themselves in the sand or are so well camouflaged that they are not easily seen and so are accidentally stepped on. "Water's edge" injuries are just as common when aquatic creatures wash up on the beach. Venom from dead marine creatures is just as toxic.

8. Answer: C

Nursing Process: Intervention

Rationale: **Jellyfish and other coelenterates have stingers containing toxin. Acetic acid 5% (vinegar) will inactivate the venom.** Immediately rinsing with salt water, soaking in vinegar, and then shaving the area will remove the nematocysts and decrease the pain. Rubbing the affected area or pouring fresh water over it will activate the nematocysts that contain the toxin. Itching is handled with topical steroids, anesthetics, or antihistamines after nematocysts are removed and the area is cleaned.

9. Answer: D

Nursing Process: Analysis

Rationale: **Sting rays, catfish, angel fish, sea urchins, scorpion fish, and lion fish have spinous processes or whiskers that release toxin when they puncture the skin of the victim. This venom is deactivated by soaking the area in hot (110° F to 115° F [43° C to 46° C]) water for 60 to 90 minutes.** Venom from stinging marine creatures—fire coral, jellyfish, and Portuguese Man of War—is deactivated by acetic acid 5% (vinegar).

10. Answer: A

Nursing Process: Assessment

Rationale: **Envenomation by marine creatures results in muscle weakness, paresthesias, hypotension, tachycardia, seizures, and cardiac arrest.** Venom may also cause anaphylaxis.

11. Answer: C

Nursing Process: Analysis

Rationale: **Wild animals, especially bats, and also skunks and raccoon, are the most common source of rabies. Raccoons tend to be nocturnal, so it is unusual behavior for it to be out during daylight, making the bite even more suspicious.** Staphylococcus is most commonly associated with human bites, Pasteurella with cat bites, and Clostridium is not related to bites but is typically food that is bitten and ingested.

12. Answer: B

Nursing Process: Intervention

Rationale: **Because the bite of a rabid bat is so small, difficult to find, generally unfelt during sleep, and the high risk that the bat could have rabies, the recommendation is that if a bat is seen in a room where someone was sleeping, they should receive the rabies series. Initial treatment is with Rabies Immune Globulin (RIG) and the first dose of Rabies vaccine if the patient has not been vaccinated previously.** Antibiotics will not help. Rabies vaccine is no longer administered twice a day for 21 days and there is a high risk for this patient per the CDC as this is a child. Other high-risk patients include someone found altered due to alcohol or drugs, the elderly, or sound sleepers.

CENsational Pearl of Wisdom!

Initially treating someone for rabies is carried out with Rabies Immune Globulin (RIG) and the first dose of Rabies vaccine if the patient has not been vaccinated previously. Twenty units/kg of RIG is administered as much as possible around the wound if a bite site can be identified. The rest is given IM at a distant site on the body. The patient will also need either human diploid cell vaccine (HCDC) or rabies vaccine adsorbed (RVA) 1 mL on days 0, 3, 7, and 14, or only on days 0 and 3 if previously immunized.

13. Answer: B

Nursing Process: Assessment

Rationale: **A red, yellow, and black banded snake that leaves punctures and scratch marks is classically a coral snake (Elapidae). The venom of a coral snake can cause paresthesias, dysesthesias (abnormal sensation), and neuromuscular blockade leading to respiratory distress. Some patients will only experience mild swelling and paresthesias at the bite site. Symptoms may take up to 13 hours to present.** There are other harmless snakes with similar coloring; thus, it is important to know the types of snakes in your area. The other three options are more typical with a pit viper bite.

CENsational Pearl of Wisdom!

Although venomous snakes are found in almost all 50 of the United States, only about 10 to 15 deaths occur per year. The two most common types of venomous snakes are Viperidae (pit vipers and vipers, AKA rattle snakes, timber snakes, cottonmouths, copperheads, and water moccasins) and Elapidae (coral and sea snakes). It is said that about 20% of pit viper bites (recognized by fang or puncture marks) are considered "dry" with no venom released. Typically, Viperidae venom causes pain, swelling, bruising, bullae, and local tissue damage; along with coagulopathy, hemorrhage, hypotension, shock, and death. Elapidae (coral snake) venom causes neurologic symptoms, including paresthesias, dysesthesias, and neurologic blockade that can lead to respiratory distress and arrest, although typically the reaction is mostly localized. Anaphylactic reaction to either venom is also common.

14. Answer: C

Nursing Process: Intervention

Rationale: **Snake anti-venom crotaline polyvalent immune fab (CroFab) is primarily intended for pit viper envenomations and should be administered within 4 to 6 hours of the bite.** It should be used only if the patient is experiencing symptoms because the drug is expensive and up to 50% of pit viper bites do not inject venom. Adverse reactions are rare with these newer versions of anti-venom, but can occur, especially, if the patient has received anti-venom in the past. The manufacturer recommends being ready to treat anaphylaxis, but notes it is rarely necessary. CroFab is not indicated for coral snake bites.

 CENsational Pearl of Wisdom!

Although it is not necessary to skin test for CroFab®, it is best to start the administration of the intravenous drip at a slow pace for at least 20 to 30 minutes. The rate can then be increased.

15. Answer: A

Nursing Process: Analysis

Rationale: **Crotaline snakes (pit vipers), of which rattle snakes are one type, have a toxin that contains an enzyme and protein that causes swelling, cellular tissue damage, and coagulopathy that can lead to hemorrhage, shock, and death. As a result of the swelling and cellular disruption in the limb where the bite occurred, compartment syndrome is a frequent consequence. Monitoring for bleeding issues as well as compartment syndrome will be important.** Coral and sea snake venom causes nervous system disruption. Bull snakes are harmless.

16. Answer: D

Nursing Process: Evaluation

Rationale: **Most snake bites occur on the ankle and lower leg when a hiker accidentally disrupts a snake's nap. Understanding that wearing boots or high-top shoes will provide protection is a positive indicator for discharge instructions.** Anti-venom does not protect from an infection—a common problem with snake bites. Rabies vaccine is given on days 0, 3, 7, and 14. Snake anti-venom is given immediately and until symptoms are gone. Picking up a venomous snake is just asking for trouble, because this will irritate it and will positively make the hiker a new victim!

17. Answer: C

Nursing Process: Intervention

Rationale: **Any open wound is a risk for tetanus, so ensuring the patient's tetanus status is current is the best answer in this case.** Tourniquets are not helpful and should be avoided. Ice is not advised. Applying heat will speed the spread of venom and is not recommended.

18. Answer: D

Nursing Process: Analysis

Rationale: **Hymenoptera is the most common venomous insect and include bees, wasps, hornets, and fire ants. Forty to fifty deaths per year are attributed to anaphylaxis caused by hymenoptera stings.** Although there are biting spiders that produce venom, they are not hymenoptera; neither are sand fleas or mosquitoes—even though their bites can be miserable.

 CENsational Pearl of Wisdom!

People allergic to bee stings (one of the hymenoptera) should not take bee pollen to counteract local allergens. There have been documented cases of anaphylaxis as the result of this home remedy because of the pollen containing bee saliva, which seems to set off the allergic reaction.

19. Answer: A

Nursing Process: Analysis

Rationale: **These findings and story fit better with an infectious process because any opening in the skin can become infected, including wasp bites. The stinger may be acting as a foreign body.** Some infected wasp bites have been cultured with interesting pathogens because of where they often procure the food they eat. The story also fits better with infection than reaction, because even delayed IgE-mediated reactions typically occur within 24 hours of exposure. There is no anti-venom for wasp bites.

20. Answer: C

Nursing Process: Analysis

Rationale: **The CDC reports a dramatic increase in the number of cases of Lyme disease (now the most common vector and sixth most reported infectious disease) and has now been found in an increasing number of states in the United States.** This disease was originally thought to be only in limited areas of this country. Additionally, because the symptoms are often so vague, has stages, can have life-altering consequences, and is so easily treated, it is important to obtain a history related to possible exposure and be aware of the stages of Lyme disease.

21. Answer: B

Nursing Process: Assessment

Rationale: **Dissemination of the disease occurs during Stage 2 of Lyme's disease. During Stage 2, symptoms of Stage 1 cease and the patient may actually think they are cured. They may develop nausea, vomiting, and a diffuse rash (rather than the bull's-eye rash seen in Stage 1). This typically occurs 4 to 10 weeks after the tick bite.** Stage 1 of Lyme's disease usually presents 3 to 30 days after the tick bite with flu-like symptoms (fever, chills, fatigue, body aches, headache, and the "classic" bull's-eye rash anywhere on the body). Stage 1 symptoms go away on their own, with or without treatment. Patients who do not complete therapy will progress to Stage 2 where often symptoms are not recognized as Lyme disease. The patient then progresses to Stage 3 (weeks to years after the bite) when symptoms can include joint pain, cardiac rhythm disturbances, neurologic problems (Bell's palsy, meningitis, and impaired cognition), return of rash, or hepatitis. There is no Stage 4.

 CENsational Pearl of Wisdom!

Stage 2 of Lyme disease can include signs of arthritis, general rash, poor motor coordination, malaise, fatigue, Bell's palsy, and A-V blocks.

22. Answer: C

Nursing Process: Analysis

Rationale: **The general consensus is that a tick must be latched onto the victim, feeding by sucking blood, and potentially instilling saliva into the victim for any of the disease organisms carried by ticks to be transmitted. It would not be crawling around the body.** In fact, most sources say the tick must have been eating long enough to become engorged to infect the patient (Lyme's disease transmission is thought to take up to half a day). Finding an engorged tick puts the patient at risk and obtaining a history of the patient or the dog being in a grassy or wooded area places both at risk. Pets are a good vehicle for ticks to be brought inside and transferred to humans. A close "tick check" is always in order.

23. Answer: B

Nursing Process: Assessment

Rationale: **Despite the name "Rocky Mountain Spotted Fever," ticks, which bear the name of the disease, are**

found in grassy or wooded areas and typically not in rocky or icy places, or the seashore. This tick-borne disease is found in all areas of the country, but Arkansas, Missouri, North Carolina, Oklahoma, and Tennessee account for over 60% of reported cases.

24. Answer: C

Nursing Process: Assessment

Rationale: **These symptoms are consistent with Rocky Mountain Spotted Fever (RMSF)—one of the tick-borne diseases. Ticks that spread this disease hang out in grassy or wooded areas. RMSF is considered deadly if not treated early with doxycycline.** The other questions will not obtain information related to risk of a tick causing the symptoms. The pond may have a parasite that causes cercarial dermatitis, which has this distribution of a rash, but no fever and is not treated with antibiotics. This would be an odd distribution for allergic reaction to medication and particularly for soap as one would expect the soap to come in contact with other parts of the body.

25. Answer: A

Nursing Process: Evaluation

Rationale: **A walking tick has not latched on, sucked blood, or transmitted a tick-borne disease to the patient. Additionally, most patients with a tick exposure will not be prophylactically treated, but the provider will treat based on disease risk in area and type of disease risk.** It is appropriate to tuck pants legs into socks to keep ticks and other insects off of the ankle areas. Removing ticks can be accomplished by using tweezers, and a twisting motion and tick repellant would be correct.

 CENsational Pearl of Wisdom!

Be sure to instruct patients about preventing tick-borne illnesses. They can do this best by wearing light-colored clothing, long pants tucked into socks, and long-sleeved shirts. Tick bites are prone to infection because of retained mouth parts, so teach the patient to watch for signs of infection and always remember to check on tetanus status.

26. Answer: B

Nursing Process: Analysis

Rationale: **A rare but deadly tick-related disease is tick paralysis. It is most typically seen in pets and small** children and is often confused with Guillain-Barré disease because of the ascending paralysis that leads to respiratory muscle paralysis and death. The same ticks that cause Lyme disease and other tick-related diseases can produce this toxin. Lyme disease does not typically cause early neurologic symptoms. The ticks should lead one to suspect tick paralysis rather than Guillain-Barré, and the symptoms of paresthesias and myalgias are not consistent with a head injury.

 CENsational Pearl of Wisdom!

In the show Emergency! Dr. Joe Early cured a case of tick paralysis in a young boy brought to the ED with these symptoms after ruling out polio. Emergency nurse Dixie McCall did the careful search and found the tick in the child's hair.

The symptoms are related to a salivary toxin in the tick, not an infectious agent. Symptoms usually occur 2 to 7 days after the tick attachment. Removal of the tick will lead to resolution of the symptoms.

27. Answer: C

Nursing Process: Analysis

Rationale: **Black widow spiders flourish in old sheds, barns, garages, outhouses, and other dark secluded spaces. Symptoms of a bite include a sharp pinprick sensation followed by an aching pain. Other symptoms include acute abdominal pain, nausea, vomiting, hypertension, and tachycardia. Black widow venom is a neurotoxin that can take effect in as little as 30 minutes.** Copperhead snake bites cause respiratory symptoms and severe pain at the site, bat bites carry a high risk for rabies that take time to develop, and brown recluse spider bites cause a necrotic bite area that can require skin grafting.

28. Answer: A

Nursing Process: Analysis

Rationale: **Brown recluse spiders like wood piles and other storage areas. The bite is often painless, until the toxin starts to cause itchy vesicles, bullae, and swelling in 1 to 3 hours. Hemorrhage into the area creates a painful purpuric area, which progresses into a necrotic ulcer.** None of the other bites will cause a wound or symptoms such as these.

29. Answer: C

Nursing Process: Assessment

Rationale: **Black widow spider neurotoxin causes nausea and weakness as well as hypertension and** tachycardia. Other symptoms include muscle fasciculations, spasm, tingling, altered mental status, and potentially seizures. Renal failure from hemolysis can occur with brown recluse bites. Brown recluse bites, not black widow, can demonstrate urticaria and a necrotic wound.

 CENsational Pearl of Wisdom!

Even if you do not know the answer to this question, careful reading can help you! The stem states that it is a neurotoxin causing the symptoms. The only option that would match a neurotoxin would be the tingling and muscle fasciculation.

30. Answer: D

Nursing Process: Intervention

Rationale: **Black widow spider anti-venom is available, although in short supply. Its biggest risk is anaphylaxis, so skin testing is recommended. Symptoms can usually be treated with opioids and benzodiazepines.** Steroids have been shown to be of little use, antibiotics are not indicated unless the wound becomes infected, and there typically is no area to debride as there might be in a brown recluse bite.

31. Answer: B

Nursing Process: Analysis

Rationale: **When frostbite occurs, the blood becomes "slushy" while surrounding tissues develop ice crystals. The slowed, and often stopped, blood flow forms clots or thromboses, which lead to further impaired cellular perfusion, ischemia, and cellular death.** Although the vessels remain vasoconstricted, they become more permeable leading to edema of the tissue and further sludging. Ice crystals typically are found in peripheral areas (ears, feet, fingers, nose, and cheeks), but not in central areas.

 CENsational Pearl of Wisdom!

Always remember to avoid rubbing frostbitten areas or allowing the victim to walk on frozen feet. This will cause increased damage to the tissues. Blankets should not be used directly on skin because they can cause tissue damage and sloughing.

32. Answer: A

Nursing Process: Assessment

Rationale: **Both superficial and deep frostbite can cause blisters; however, superficial blisters are water-filled**

and deep are hemorrhagic. Deep frostbite is usually identified as having cyanotic, necrotic coloration with anesthesia to the affected area. The skin is hard, cool to the touch, and nonpliable. Superficial frostbite tissue is pale and edematous, with tingling and a burning sensation.

33. Answer: A

Nursing Process: Intervention

Rationale: **Frostbitten areas should be rewarmed only when there is no chance for refreezing.** Areas of the frostbitten area should not be against basins or other objects as this can increase chances of cellular damage from ice crystals puncturing the cellular walls. Water baths should be used to thaw-frozen areas. Never use dry heat. Rapid, not slow rewarming is recommended.

34. Answer: D

Nursing Process: Evaluation

Rationale: **Patients who have had frostbite will need to be on bed rest with their feet at heart level to promote circulation to and from the feet.** The toes need padding between them and a loose dressing applied to prevent any pressure to the areas that were frostbitten. Aspirin or ibuprofen is often used to improve blood flow, which was sludgy from clot formation. Caffeine causes vasoconstriction, as does smoking, so both should be discouraged.

 CENsational Pearl of Wisdom!

There are now facilities using fibrinolytics to bust the tiny clots found in frostbitten patients. Some are using the intravenous approach, others intra-digital injections. Both methods report improved outcomes.

35. Answer: B

Nursing Process: Analysis

Rationale: **This patient is demonstrating symptoms of moderate hypothermia, especially taking into consideration where they were found. An Osborne or J-wave, an extra notching after the QRS complex, is often associated with moderate hypothermia, as is atrial fibrillation.** Mildly hypothermic patients still shiver, are usually responsive, and are initially tachycardic. Severely hypothermic patients are either in ventricular fibrillation or a very slow atrial fibrillation or other slow rhythm with no spontaneous respirations. In profound hypothermia, the patient will display either pulseless electrical activity (PEA) or asystole and will appear dead with a flat electroencephalogram (if available). This is usually an irreversible stage.

 CENsational Pearl of Wisdom!

Paradoxical undressing: *This is a theory that as the patient's temperature drops through the moderate hypothermic stage into severe hypothermia, loss of vascular tone occurs. This causes peripheral vasodilation and the feeling that they are flushed and hot. Thus, many times hypothermic patients are found with their clothing removed. Obviously, this cools them even further and faster.*

Cold diuresis: *Another finding with hypothermic patients is that vasoconstriction during the mild hypothermic state leads fluids to shunt to the core. The kidneys are not able to concentrate the urine and interpret this as fluid overload, so cold diuresis occurs. During the process of resuscitation, one must replace volume, but balance replacement against the pulmonary edema that often occurs as the result of increased vascular permeability occurring during severe hypothermic stages.*

36. Answer: C

Nursing Process: Intervention

Rationale: **The 2015 American Heart Association (AHA) recommends immediate defibrillation (rather than wasting time to check the temperature first), start chest compressions and ventilations, gives a 1-mg dose of epinephrine, and initiate rewarming if hypothermia is suspected.** Evidence related to the use of defibrillation and medications in a severely hypothermic cardiac arrest is mostly theoretical; however, repeated defibrillations do not seem to be successful until the body is warmed to 86° F (30° C). Studies have shown a standard dose of epinephrine may lead to return of spontaneous circulation. Larger doses of epinephrine have caused poorer outcomes and antiarrhythmics have not been effective until the body is warmed. (Also, the dose noted is incorrect!) There is also a theoretical concern of medicines accumulating and not being metabolized in a severely hypothermic patient, so repeated doses are not recommended.

37. Answer: A

Nursing Process: Analysis

Rationale: **Phenothiazines, barbiturates, and neuromuscular-blocking agents decrease a person's ability to shiver, which is the body's method of creating heat.** This predisposes them to hypothermia. None of the other options decrease the ability to shiver.

CENsational Pearl of Wisdom!

Other factors that predispose a patient to hypothermia include being very young and very old because pediatric and geriatric patients tend to have less body fat to keep them warm. Pediatric patients also do not shiver effectively. Alcohol, trauma, diabetes, and shock also can lead to hypothermia. Patients found lying on a tile or concrete floor or on the ground will leech their body heat into that cooler mass and they will quickly become hypothermic.

38. Answer: A

Nursing Process: Intervention

Rationale: **This patient is only mildly hypothermic as they are still shivering and creating their own heat. Passive rewarming with the use of a reflective blanket similar to those used by athletes will help reflect that heat back toward the patient and is the easiest, yet still effective way to warm the patient.** Forced warm air blankets can actually cause vasodilation in the extremities, mobilizing the colder blood in the periphery leading to further cooling in the core. Warmed IV fluid boluses are listed as part of plan for the moderately hypothermic patient but they do not transfer much heat to the person; thus, other internal warming methods (warm water lavage of thoracic cavity, etc.) are recommended. ECMO (Extracorporeal Membrane Oxygenation) is recommended for severe hypothermia.

39. Answer: B

Nursing Process: Analysis

Rationale: **Rewarming shock (afterdrop) occurs when colder blood from the extremities reaches the core during the warming process.** Hypotension and dysrhythmias may be prevented by warming the trunk first and then the extremities once the core temperature has risen. Metabolism is slowed during hypothermia and arterial blood gas (ABG) results often do not reflect actual pH because of the blood being warmed in the blood gas analyzer. Potassium levels typically go up with hypothermia and atrial fibrillation or ventricular fibrillation are common rewarming rhythms.

40. Answer: D

Nursing Process: Analysis

Rationale: **Dives to depths of 30 feet or deeper, length of time breathing compressed air from a tank, and rate of ascent to the surface are the three components that can lead to decompression sickness (the bends). This can include pain in the joints, skin, peripheral nerves, or spinal cord. Patients may also have pitting edema, itching,** mottled skin rash, and excessive fatigue. In more severe cases, the patient may have respiratory distress, nervous system involvement, and signs of shock. None of the other activities would set the patient up for this disease process.

41. Answer: B

Nursing Process: Analysis

Rationale: **Decompression sickness occurs when nitrogen, which dissolves in the tissues during the dive, expands during ascent to the surface. The expanding nitrogen bubbles put pressure on the various body parts causing symptoms. This classically occurs if the patient ascends too quickly and without allowing the nitrogen bubbles to be reabsorbed.** Typically, oxygen is utilized by the body, so it does not dissolve into the tissues like nitrogen, which is not utilized. There should be no carbon monoxide involved, and hydrogen gas collecting under the diaphragm would be a different issue.

42. Answer: B

Nursing Process: Intervention

Rationale: **This patient is showing signs of severe Decompression Sickness (DCS) and will need to be placed in a decompression (hyperbaric) chamber to decrease the size of the nitrogen gas bubbles and eliminate them.** It is important to assess for a pneumothorax/tension pneumothorax and treat shock; but hypotension, respiratory distress, and neurologic symptoms are consistent with DCS type II, which requires a hyperbaric chamber. Suturing the laceration can be accomplished later because bleeding is controlled at this time.

CENsational Pearl of Wisdom!

The number of hyperbaric chambers in the United States able to handle a patient suffering Decompression Sickness seems to be limited based on a survey done in 2016. Of the 361 chambers in the United States that handle hyperbaric oxygen (HBO) situations, only 43 responded that they were able to handle high-acuity patients emergently. This is important information to have on hand for those nurses who work in areas that have locations such as lakes, rivers, or water-filled mining pits with depths greater than 30 feet deep. Early identification of patients who might need these services is of great value so that calls can be expedited!

43. Answer: B

Nursing Process: Analysis

Rationale: **Altered mental status associated with nausea, vomiting, and sweating because of extreme heat is typical of heat exhaustion.** The students have been creating body heat as they march; they are in uniforms that do not allow efficient cooling via passive loss of heat; high humidity makes sweating less efficient and if practicing marching formations, there will be no shade; thus, there are multiple reasons for students to develop this syndrome. Heat cramps could also develop, but symptoms for this would be muscle cramping that usually occurs in the shoulders, thighs, and abdominal wall. In heat stroke, typically the patient can be confused, ataxic, and anxious or unresponsive with hot, flushed, and dry skin, rather than actively sweating. Heat hysteria is not a documented heat-related condition.

 CENsational Pearl of Wisdom!

For those patients exercising in the heat, some diaphoresis can occur. Classic or nonexertional heat stroke does present with hot, dry skin. Be aware though that just because diaphoresis is present, it does not mean it is not heat stroke!

44. Answer: B

Nursing Process: Analysis

Rationale: **One of the consequences of heat exhaustion is the breakdown of skeletal muscle tissue leading to rhabdomyolysis, which presents as pinkish to dark red-colored urine.** This occurs because of the release of myoglobin into the plasma. "Rhabdo" can lead to renal failure if sufficient fluids are not flushed through the kidneys. One of the challenges when cooling a hyperthermic patient is preventing shivering because this actually creates heat. Sinus tachycardia is expected. A Lichtenberg Figure is associated with a lightning strike at the point of entry. This transient discoloration lasts for only a few hours.

 CENsational Pearl of Wisdom!

Alert! Rhabdomyolysis is an important disease process that nurses should understand. It can occur for many reasons, including heat-related events such as heat stroke or heat exhaustion. Other causes are sports-related muscle injuries, status asthmaticus, status epilepticus, infections, illicit drug use such as LSD and cocaine, statins, and crush injuries (to name a few). One of the most common patients seen in the ED at risk for this is the elderly patient who has fallen, is unable to get up, and is found hours later.

One of the classic signs for this is a positive urine dipstick for blood, but no red blood cells are seen microscopically. CK (creatinine kinase) is elevated in this disease process and can be extremely high.

45. Answer: C

Nursing Process: Intervention

Rationale: **Wet skin with fans on is one of the most effective and efficient ways to cool someone with heat exhaustion.** Ice packs can be used in areas of superficial arteries such as the groin and ankles, but covering the entire lower torso with ice and immersion tend to cause shivering that is counter-effective. Gastric lavage is an extreme measure and would only be used in critical situations. Replacing fluids and electrolytes, either orally or intravenously, is also indicated. Replacing fluids only is a major mistake in caring for these individuals.

46. Answer: B

Nursing Process: Intervention

Rationale: **At 4,900 feet, oxygen does not attach to hemoglobin as readily, leading to symptoms of tissue hypoxia which can include headache, fatigue, nausea, weakness, irritability, and dehydration. Acute mountain sickness, the milder form of altitude sickness, typically improves with rest, fluids, and time as the body acclimates to the altitude and the patient feels better within a day or two.** Ascending higher into the mountains will increase symptoms and may progress to high-altitude cerebral edema (HACE) or high-altitude pulmonary edema (HAPE). Activities such as hiking will increase symptoms and risk. Going on the trip higher into the mountain is ill-advised.

 CENsational Pearl of Wisdom!

Both HAPE and HACE can be fatal. HAPE is a noncardiac version of pulmonary edema. Gradual ascent to high altitudes can help with acclimation and the ultimate treatment may be rapid descent to lower altitudes. For those individuals who are arriving by air to high altitudes, altitude sickness can begin the minute the doors to the airplane open. Checking pulse oximetry upon arriving can be eye opening!! Oxygen is one of the most important treatments for these maladies.

47. Answer: D

Nursing Process: Analysis

Rationale: **Although all are components of and may contribute to submersion-related deaths, it is hypoxia that leads to cerebral edema and brain death, which is the primary cause of the patient's death.** Aspiration (often just a small amount of fluid) tends to initiate a cascade of events, leading to laryngospasm, pulmonary injury, and shunting that leads to further hypoxia. Bradycardia is the result of hypoxia and hypothermia will depend on the situation. A significant number of submersion deaths are related to small amounts of water (children falling into pails of water); thus, hypothermia is not part of the equation. A few drowning-related deaths do not take on water into the lungs because of intense laryngospasm that causes hypoxia and death.

48. Answer: C

Nursing Process: Assessment

Rationale: **Obtaining a history of what happened immediately upon finding the patient is an extremely important factor in determining how long to attempt resuscitation. The need for compressions and ventilations is not an indication of poor prognosis if the patient recovers a pulse and spontaneous respirations within a short time—typically before transport.** Data indicate that if resuscitation (compressions and/or ventilations) has to continue 25 minutes after removal from the water, the patient has a poor chance of survival. There are anecdotal cases of successful resuscitation cases after 10 minutes of submersion; but studies have shown even with immediate Basic Life Support (BLS) and Advanced Cardiac Life Support (ACLS) chances of recovery drop from 90% if less than 5 minutes of submersion to 44% after 5 to 10 minutes of submersion and to 12% after 10 minutes of submersion despite resuscitative attempts unless the water was very cold. Then the patient must be warmed before terminating efforts. Death is not always immediate, but often delayed and due to multisystem organ failure or brain insult.

49. Answer: D

Nursing Process: Intervention

Rationale: **Typically, most submersion patients are hypothermic and will develop cerebral edema secondary to hypoxia. Treatment will need to focus on rewarming the patient and ensuring the brain is receiving enough oxygen by correcting pulmonary and circulation issues.** The patient will show metabolic acidosis on ABG report because of altered metabolism, and although they may initially have had hypercarbia, this should correct to normal with return of circulation. Signs of extreme hypocarbia (less than 10 mm Hg) would indicate poor circulation or that the patient is being overly ventilated (less than 34 mm Hg). $ETCO_2$ levels should range from 35 to 45 mm Hg. Not all patients aspirate or develop pneumonia, and a "monitor for development" attitude is generally recommended. Ensuring the patient's tissues are adequately oxygenated and ventilated is the focus.

50. Answer: A

Nursing Process: Intervention

Rationale: **Warming and ensuring adequate ventilation and oxygenation is the priority. These actions will improve lung sounds, heart rate, and blood pressure.** Deep suctioning and diuretics, atropine, or vasopressors have not been found to be helpful. Unless history indicates the need to protect the neck, this action has been found to be unnecessary in most submersion injuries. The respiratory rate is not fast enough to use Continuous Positive Airway Pressure (CPAP).

51. Answer: C

Nursing Process: Evaluation

Rationale: **This family has scabies based on location of itching, burrows, and excoriations. Often found in bed lines and clothing, high heat will kill scabies and their eggs. Placing nonwashable items in sealed plastic bags for 1 to 2 weeks may also kill scabies.** A pediculicide that is applied to the skin may be ordered. Lice and their nits are found in the hair, tick bites can be anywhere and do not typically have burrows, and allergic reactions to food typically do not appear in this distribution.

52. Answer: D

Nursing Process: Analysis

Rationale: **Soot on the patient's face and chest and being found in an enclosed space implies possible inhalation issues associated with breathing in of the soot and possibly heat from the fire. Both can lead to airway compromise—swelling of the upper airway and surfactant damage leading to hypoxia.** Once the airway is managed, the care will need to switch to fluid volume replacement and keeping the patient warm. Fluid shifts that affect electrolytes will occur and need to be addressed in the next 24 hours, but is not the priority issue.

 CENsational Pearl of Wisdom!

Be concerned about airway compromise in patients who were in small places with the smoke and fire. Look for sooty sputum, stridor, burns to the face, and singed nasal hair and eyebrows. Hoarseness, voice changes, and/or agitation associated with signs of facial burns listed earlier should raise a red flag for the nurse to be prepared to intubate the patient. Waiting could create a situation in which the airway closes completely and there is no chance to successfully place an endotracheal tube. Remember!!! Infants have teeny tiny tracheas! It does not take much to completely occlude their airways!!

53. Answer: C

Nursing Process: Analysis

Rationale: **Burns on both the hands or both the feet, in a stocking pattern, or resembling a hot item should be suspicious for maltreatment and child protection should be contacted.** Obtaining a consistent story as to how the injuries occurred may rule out intentional cause, but suspicion needs to occur. Not all children will require admission to the burn unit; however, follow up with a burn center is recommended. Burns are no longer always treated with sulfa-based ointments. Water-based ointments such as bacitracin may be used, especially on the face, ears, neck, and buttocks.

54. Answer: A

Nursing Process: Intervention

Rationale: **The fluoride ion in hydrofluoric acid binds with calcium ions and will continue to "burn" until neutralized with calcium gluconate.** While waiting for the calcium gluconate, flushing with water will help dilute the pollution, but 1 liter will not be sufficient. The patient should be put in a running stream of water. Other chemicals will not help, and the wound should not be covered with an ointment until the area has been completely treated with calcium chloride. Often a paste of calcium chloride is applied so it will continue to help treat this type of burn that is due to a localized hypocalcemia and will neutralize the fluoride ions found in this product.

 CENsational Pearl of Wisdom!

A dermal burn from hydrofluoric acid can actually cause a systemic hypocalcemia because of the binding of the fluoride and available calcium ions. This may need to be treated with intravenous calcium. Consider the manifestations of hypocalcemia, including Trousseau's sign (carpopedal spasm with inflation of blood pressure cuff) and Chvostek's sign (facial twitching when facial nerve is tapped).

55. Answer: C

Nursing Process: Analysis

Rationale: **Chemicals on patients are easily transferred to caregivers during interventions unless precautions— wearing personal protective equipment (PPE)—are taken.** Neutralizing the agent is rarely indicated as dilution with large amounts of water is usually recommended for almost all chemical exposures. Sufficient water typically does not lead to issues with gas formation; however, part of PPE includes wearing a mask to eliminate this problem. Wearing PPEs would be the priority in dealing with chemical concerns. Electrolyte changes would generally not be a concern.

56. Answer: B

Nursing Process: Intervention

Rationale: **An ever-present concern with electrical energy is muscle spasm caused when electricity courses through the body. Energy from the lighting can travel from the pole through the ground to the player and cause spasm of the heart, neck, and other muscles of the body. Due to this a jaw-thrust maneuver, which would protect the C-spine should be utilized to open this airway.** Before starting chest compressions, one should check for a pulse and respiratory effort and not assume ventricular fibrillation. Attending to the airway would take precedence over long bone fractures or other injuries sustained.

 CENsational Pearl of Wisdom!

Although both asystole and ventricular fibrillation can occur with a lightning strike, asystole is more common. It is thought that if ventricular fibrillation does occur, it is the result of continued hypoxia after the initial asystole converted to a sinus rhythm with subsequent deterioration to this dysrhythmia.

57. Answer: D

Nursing Process: Intervention

Rationale: **Cardiac dysrhythmias and muscle contractions, leading to release of myoglobin which turns urine a pink to reddish color, are two consequences of lightening injury.** Rhabdomyolysis is the outcome of this released myoglobin and can be a precursor to acute renal failure. The fern-shaped pattern is called a Lichtenberg Figure and is present for a short period of time after a lightning strike. Being "knocked flat" in conjunction with the transient hyperpigmentation on the back are good indications the patient may have sustained a lightning strike. There will be no entrance or exit wounds and the airway is generally not affected if the patient remains conscious. A lactate level would not be necessary.

58. Answer: C

Nursing Process: Intervention

Rationale: **Incomplete combustion in a fire releases carbon monoxide (CO), which is measured with a** carboxyhemoglobin (HbCO) test. High levels of CO require placement of high-flow oxygen and extremely high levels may require transfer to a hyperbaric chamber as CO leads to hypoxia and neurologic sequelae. Pulse oximetry is inaccurate in the presence of carbon monoxide poisoning as the pulse oximetry reads that something is attached to the hemoglobin molecule but does not differentiate between oxygen and carbon monoxide. An abnormal 12 lead will not diagnose the problem (abnormalities may be seen due to cardiac cellular hypoxia). Urine myoglobin will take time to appear.

59. Answer: D

Nursing Process: Assessment

Rationale: **The patient's hands and buttocks are full thickness—often called third degree—burns because they are charred or patchy white in color and painless because nerve endings have been destroyed.** Superficial epidermal (first degree) burns are red and painful. Superficial partial thickness and deep partial thickness (second degree) are usually blistered and painful. The patient may not realize some areas do not have pain because of the pain in the areas with more superficial burns.

60. Answer: C

Nursing Process: Evaluation

Rationale: **Adequate fluid resuscitation is evidenced by urine output of at least 50 mL/hour. Watching urine output is considered to be the best way to monitor fluid resuscitation now.** Concern for rhabdomyolysis would increase the desired urine output to at least 100 mL/hour; however, for the adult patient an output of 50 mL or more per hour is considered adequate. The respiratory rate and pulse rate would not indicate adequate fluid resuscitation. The mean arterial pressure reading of 45 mm Hg would be present with a blood pressure of 74/30 mm Hg, which would not be a desired endpoint for fluid resuscitation.

61. Answer: A

Nursing Process: Analysis

Rationale: **These patients all have symptoms (trouble swallowing, thick speech, visual problems, drooping eyelids, and generalized weakness) consistent with botulism, spread by ingesting the same contaminated food.** All developing symptoms at the same time is a significant clue. Diseases implied by the other questions would not include symptoms described. Legionnaires typically presents with respiratory symptoms after being in a humid area, or an area where clouds of water are spewed. Rabies involves exposure to an animal with

rabies saliva. Symptoms would include tingling at bite site, flu-like symptoms, confusion, agitation, and excessive salivation. Nonpasteurized juices often contain *Escherichia coli*, but other foodborne illnesses including *Staphylococcus aureus*, *Clostridium perfringens*, *Bacillus cereus*, campylobacter, Listeria, salmonella, and norovirus can cause abdominal pain, vomiting, fevers, and diarrhea, including bloody diarrhea.

 CENsational Pearl of Wisdom!

Be suspicious any time a group of people present with similar symptoms! Consider exposure to the same bacteria or virus. Be aware of warnings posted by the local Department of Health or the CDC. Reporting multiple victims with similar symptoms may assist in controlling an outbreak. This author had to treat an entire family when a dog in the early stage of rabies was at the same family reunion and licked ice cream cones they all were eating!

62. Answer: D

Nursing Process: Analysis

Rationale: **Food poisoning involves the ingestion of a toxin, typically created by Staphylococcus *aureus*, *Clostridium perfringens*, or *Bacillus cereus* and is characterized by vomiting within 2 to 6 hours of ingesting the toxin. A sample of the toxin in the food ingested is required to make the diagnosis.** Many people present stating they have "food poisoning" when, in fact, they have gastroenteritis or an infectious diarrhea. Blood tests will show how the person is responding to the illness, but will not confirm the actual toxin ingested. Stool specimens would assist in the diagnosis only if the patient is infected with a bacterial, viral, parasitic, or protozoan agent. Blood in the stool alone would not diagnose these patients.

63. Answer: C

Nursing Process: Analysis

Rationale: **Abdominal pain, bloating, gas, and greasy diarrhea that floats is consistent with Giardia, which most frequently is found in backcountry streams and lakes, but also can be found in municipal swimming pools, splash pads, and whirlpools.** Most municipal well water is treated to prevent this; however, home wells may be contaminated. Even if the water to make gelatin is contaminated, boiling it to make the gelatin will kill Giardia. Dogs can, in theory, transmit a gastrointestinal illness to people, but dog stool would have to be ingested by the children. Giardia can also be transmitted to humans if they have been in pools or bodies of water, but in this scenario the dog was not in contact with the splash pad.

64. Answer: C

Nursing Process: Intervention

Rationale: **Uncooked fruits, vegetables, and salad materials in developing nations, as well in the United States, are at risk of being contaminated by *E. coli* and other bacteria during the growing process and can lead to gastrointestinal illness (vomiting, diarrhea, fever, and potential life-threatening renal failure) if ingested.** Washing does not always eliminate the bacterium, which is often incorporated into the structure of these foods. It is not recommended to use an anti-diarrheal as this can slow the digestive system and prolong exposure to the bacteria. Boiling water for 1 minute will kill *E. coli* and other bacteria. Antiparasitic agents will not help to fight against a bacterial infection.

 CENsational Pearl of Wisdom!

Acids in the stomach actually kill most E. coli encountered; therefore, taking medications that decrease acids in the stomach such as omeprazole (Prilosec) or pantoprazole (Protonix), and so on, may increase the risk of developing an E. coli infection.

65. Answer: B

Nursing Process: Intervention

Rationale: **The description of this "ring" actually fits more closely with a description of a human bite rather than ringworm and is therefore suspicious for abuse. Ringworm presents as small red, round patches that have a crusted appearance.** Not all ringworm fluoresces under a black light. If this is ringworm, the clippings/scrapings will show the fungus (scrapings are placed in a drop of potassium hydroxide [KOH] to diagnose) and will not turn purple if swabbed with Betadine and hydrogen peroxide. Ringworm is a fungus not a bacteria. (This is an actual case in which the child was bitten by another child at the day care.)

66. Answer: A

Nursing Process: Analysis

Rationale: **Insecticides cause the toxidrome associated with a cholinergic crisis. SLUDGE (Salivation, Lacrimation, Urination, Diarrhea, Gastrointestinal distress, and Emesis) is one mnemonic to help remember the symptoms associated with a cholinergic problem.** Pupils

will be pinpoint and treatment continues until symptoms abate and pupils dilate. All other symptoms listed are consistent with anticholinergic agents.

 CENsational Pearl of Wisdom!

Toxidromes are constellations of symptoms that pinpoint a specific agent. Cholinergics are wet! Anticholinergics are dry! Another mnemonic for this is MUDDLES that stands for miosis, increased urination, defecation, diaphoresis, lacrimation, excitation, and salivation. Anticholinergics cause hot, dry, flushed skin and mental status changes. A mnemonic for this process is "mad as a hatter, blind as a bat, red as a beet, hot as hades, dry as a bone."

67. Answer: C

Nursing Process: Intervention

Rationale: **One antidote for cyanide poisoning is hydroxocobalamin. Most medical facilities have only one to two cyanide kits, so in the process of prepping for victim arrivals, obtaining more kits would be an appropriate measure.** Atropine and pralidoxime (2-PAM) are used for cholinergic crises such as might be seen with Sarin gas or other nerve agents as well as insecticides. Seizures are typically not part of symptoms associated with cyanide; therefore, benzodiazepines would not be needed and bleach is not used to treat this problem.

68. Answer: D

Nursing Process: Intervention

Rationale: **Protecting oneself and avoiding contamination by donning personal protective equipment (PPE) before helping the patient is a priority.** If the patient is able to follow directions, direct him to remove his clothing and shower, but do not assist until protected from injury. More bleach (hypochlorite) will not help this situation.

69. Answer: B

Nursing Process: Assessment

Rationale: **Protection from radiation consists of distance, shielding, and exposure time. Patients inside buildings are more likely to be adequately protected. If they were outside, but there was a wall or structure between the patient and the blast, the risk is decreased.** The farther away from the explosion and the shorter the exposure time, the less risk exists for the patient. Clothing is most likely not contaminated, unless the patient was involved in a dust cloud or an explosion. Lack of immediate symptoms may not indicate exposure as they may not occur for several days.

70. Answer: A

Nursing Process: Assessment

Rationale: **Radiation sickness affects the gastrointestinal tract, blood production, and the cardiovascular/neurologic systems. Sloughing of the gastrointestinal tract with vomiting, cramps, and diarrhea can occur within a few hours of exposure.** Blood cell counts may be affected for weeks if the patient survives. The cardiovascular/neurologic system effects also include confusion and nervousness. Blistering and sloughing of skin is more consistent with exposure to a vesicant agent such as mustard gas. Cramping and seizures are consistent with nerve agents. Pulmonary edema, coughing, and tearing are associated with agents such phosgene or anhydrous ammonia.

71. Answer: C

Nursing Process: Assessment

Rationale: **A Geiger counter will provide evidence of radioactive materials on their body and clothing, which could cause a threat to the care providers.** The knowledge of where to find and how to operate a Geiger counter will be important in an event involving radiation release. Adequate decontamination can be detected as well. The rest of the items are helpful in assessing and monitoring a patient, but do not provide information related to radiation.

72. Answer: C

Nursing Process: Assessment

Rationale: **Using the rule of 9's for an adult, the correct answer is 27% total body surface area (TBSA) burned.** This number is reached by adding 18% for the chest/abdomen and 9% for the hand and arm. The back would be an additional 18%, each leg is 18%, the head is 9%, and the perineal area 1%. The other numbers are incorrect.

CENsational Pearl of Wisdom!

Other burn charts are available (Lund and Browder), which are more accurate, but initial calculation using the rule of 9's is fast and helps to get treatment started. A really rough "guesstimate" uses the patient's palm considering it to equal 1% of the total body surface area. This works well, especially with smaller burns. Until recently, the Parkland formula of 2 to 4 mL × %TBSA burned × weight in kilogram was used to calculate fluid required. Recently, the American Burn Association refined this formula to also look at urine output during resuscitation with a goal of 0.5 mL/kg/hour for adults and 0.5 to 1 mL/kg/hour for children.

73. Answer: D

Nursing Process: Assessment

Rationale: **Because the patient was holding the paperclip, there is good probability that the electricity was conducted through the patient to something wet or metal. Electrical burns often follow blood vessels or nerve pathways through the body leaving an area of char along the route inside the body. Finding the entrance and exit helps to determine the extent of the burn route.** It will not be possible to determine percent of body surface burned or degree at this time. A carbon monoxide level is not indicated.

CENsational Pearl of Wisdom!

Treatment of electrical injury that has traveled through the body will include ABC's; volume replacement must be sufficient to provide a clear urine output of at least 30 to 50 mL/hour, and the patient should be monitored for cardiac dysrhythmias and compartment syndrome. Consider that the patient may be in ventricular fibrillation—the most common dysrhythmia for electrical burns!

74. Answer: B

Nursing Process: Assessment

Rationale: **The "cafeteria special" probably contained *Clostridium perfringens* toxin that developed due to improper storage. Treatment is to replace fluids orally, unless the patient is unable to keep up with volume replacement.** Meat and gravy are a common medium for this toxin, as are hospitals or similar cafeterias. Most patients do not require IV fluids and there is no reason to give ondansetron (Zofran). Typically, diarrhea does not become bloody, and this is not a bacterium that requires antibiotics, but a toxin that needs to run its course.

75. Answer: D

Nursing Process: Intervention

Rationale: **Because many environmental emergencies include toxins, poisons, and other hazardous substances, it is important for emergency nurses to know what they are dealing with. Donning the appropriate PPE before coming into contact with the patient is a major priority. A health care provider that becomes a victim in the process of caring for patients is unable to provide care.** Some may argue that an across-the-room assessment could potentially ensure the airway is intact and ventilations are adequate; however, most of the emergency nurses do not tend to run to treat the ambulatory stable person. It is the patient in trouble that emergency nurses run to help without thinking, end up contaminated, and become a victim themselves. Minimally, an "across-the-room" history will help to determine if it is safe to come into contact with a patient.

References

American Heart Association. (2013). ACLS for experienced providers. Dallas, TX: American Heart Association. (31, 32, 35–39, 47–50, 56, 57, 66, 67, 69, 70, 73)

Balentine, J. R. (2016). *Rocky Mountain Spotted Fever.* Medicinenet.com. Retrieved July 2018, from https://www.medicinenet.com/rocky_mountain_spotted_fever_rmsf/article.htm#where_do_most_cases_of_rmsf_occur_in_the_us (24)

Centers for Disease Control and Prevention. *Lyme disease home page on web site.* Retrieved July 2018, from https://www.cdc.gov/lyme/index.html (20–26, 51)

Centers for Disease Control and Prevention. *Ringworm information for healthcare professionals web site.* Retrieved July 2018, from https://www.cdc.gov/fungal/diseases/ringworm/health-professionals.html (65)

Centers for Disease Control and Prevention. *What causes food poisoning food borne illnesses and germs web site.* Retrieved July 2018, from https://www.cdc.gov/foodsafety/foodborne-germs.html (62–64, 74)

Centers for Disease Control and Prevention. *Why CDC is worried about Lyme disease.* CDC web site on Lyme disease. Retrieved July 2018, from https://www.cdc.gov/lyme/why-is-cdc-concerned-about-lyme-disease.html (20, 23, 25)

Cooper, M. A. (2017). *Lightening injuries treatment and management.* Medscape. Retrieved from https://emedicine.medscape.com/article/770642-treatment (56)

Emergency Nurses Association. (2012). Emergency nursing pediatric course: provider manual (4th ed.). Des Plaines, IL: Emergency Nurses Association. (52)

Emergency Nurses Association. (2014). Trauma nursing core course (7th ed.). Des Plaines, IL: Emergency Nurses Association. (32, 33, 52–55, 58–60, 66, 69, 70–73, 75)

Emergency Nurses Association. (2018). Emergency nursing core curriculum (7th ed.). St. Louis, MO: Elsevier. (1–20, 23, 27–34, 37, 40–47, 50–54, 58–61, 66–71, 75)

Hammond, B., et al. (2013). Sheehy's manual of emergency care (7th ed.). St. Louis, MO: Mosby Elsevier. (52)

Mayo Clinic. (2018). *E. coli.* Retrieved from https://www.mayoclinic.org/diseases-conditions/e-coli/symptoms-causes/syc-20372058 (64)

Mayo Clinic Patient Care and Information. (2018). *Frostbite.* Retrieved July 2018, from https://www.mayoclinic.org/diseases-conditions/frostbite/symptoms-causes/syc-20372656 (31–34)

Michel, S., et al. (2018). *83 Implementation of a remote frostbite protocol in the use of thrombolytics with improved salvage rate journal of burn care and research.* Retrieved https://academic.oup.com/jbcr/article-abstract/39/suppl_1/S46/4965378?redirectedFrom=fulltext (34)

Muscal, E. (2017). *Rhabdomyolysis.* Medscape. Retrieved from https://emedicine.medscape.com/article/1007814-workup#c7 (44)

5 Toxicology and Substance Abuse

Bill Light, MSN, RN, CEN, CPEN, TCRN

Toxicology is an especially tough subject! Many of us struggle with this topic, so do not feel bad if you do too! Toxicology is mixed in the blueprint with Environmental Emergencies and Communicable Diseases. There are 15 questions total on these three aspects of emergency nursing. It is hard to determine for sure how these will be divided up. This is why this book has separate chapters on each of these topics. The rationales in these questions are in depth to help you understand the pathophysiology behind them, which should help if you get to a question that stumps you. If you get stuck on the test, just take your time and walk yourself through the background information and you should be able to work around to the correct answer. Good luck!

1. A patient presents to the emergency department after overdosing on an alpha-adrenergic antagonist medication. Which of the following assessment findings would the emergency nurse likely uncover?
[ ] **A.** Warm, flushed skin
[ ] **B.** Decreased respirations
[ ] **C.** Elevated blood pressure
[ ] **D.** Increased serum glucose

2. A patient presents with an ingestion of an unknown substance. The emergency nurse notes the patient to have bradycardia, diminished bowel sounds, miosis, and cool, dry skin. Which of the following agents did the patient most likely ingest?
[ ] **A.** Opioid
[ ] **B.** Anticholinergic
[ ] **C.** Sedative-hypnotic
[ ] **D.** Sympathomimetic

3. A patient arrives in the emergency department after a toxic ingestion of carbidopa/levodopa (Sinemet). Which of the following sets of symptoms would the emergency nurse most likely observe in this patient on initial assessment?
[ ] **A.** Tachycardia, miosis, flushed skin
[ ] **B.** Dry mouth, absent bowel sounds, fever
[ ] **C.** Increased urine output, hypertension, confusion
[ ] **D.** Hallucinations, bradycardia, cool/clammy skin

4. The emergency nurse should prepare to administer which of the following medications to a patient with symptoms of organophosphate overdose?
[ ] **A.** Glucagon (GlucaGen)
[ ] **B.** Flumazenil (Romazicon)
[ ] **C.** Physostigmine (Antilirium)
[ ] **D.** Atropine sulfate (Atropine)

5. The emergency nurse suspects that an inebriated patient in the emergency department has ingested methanol after which of the following odors is noted on the patient's breath?
[ ] **A.** Bitter almond
[ ] **B.** Moth balls
[ ] **C.** Formalin
[ ] **D.** Garlic

6. Emergency Medical Services personnel arrive in the emergency department with a patient with a depressed mental status and slowed respirations. They state that no pill bottles or needles were found at the scene, but they did find a white powdery substance and a pipe that the patient appeared to have been smoking. Which of the following additional symptoms should the emergency nurse anticipate assessing?
[ ] **A.** Tachycardia
[ ] **B.** Hot, dry skin
[ ] **C.** Hypertension
[ ] **D.** Pinpoint pupils

7. A child is brought to the emergency department after ingesting oleander. The nurse should monitor the patient for:

[ ] **A.** drooling.
[ ] **B.** dysarthria.
[ ] **C.** bradycardia.
[ ] **D.** constipation.

8. Which of the following is the appropriate antidote for an ingestion of acetaminophen (Tylenol)?

[ ] **A.** Succimer (Chemet)
[ ] **B.** Deferoxamine mesylate (Desferal)
[ ] **C.** Romazicon (flumazenil)
[ ] **D.** N-Acetylcysteine (Mucomyst)

9. Which of the following symptoms are considered among the first symptoms of iron toxicity?

[ ] **A.** Fever over 101° F (38.3° C)
[ ] **B.** Fecal impactions
[ ] **C.** Coagulopathies
[ ] **D.** Diarrhea

10. When assessing a patient with a suspected overdose of warfarin (Coumadin), the emergency nurse would anticipate which of the following?

[ ] **A.** Purpura to skin
[ ] **B.** Pain to posterior calf
[ ] **C.** Elevated partial thromboplastin time (PTT)
[ ] **D.** Decreased international normalized ratio (INR)

11. Tricyclic antidepressant overdoses have three main toxic features. These features are cardiotoxicity, adrenergic blocking, and:

[ ] **A.** anticoagulation.
[ ] **B.** anticholinergic effects.
[ ] **C.** sympathomimetic effects.
[ ] **D.** central nervous system excitation.

12. After chewing rhubarb leaves, a 3-year-old is brought to the emergency department. The emergency nurse should assess for which of the following conditions?

[ ] **A.** Lethargy
[ ] **B.** Dysphagia
[ ] **C.** Bradycardia
[ ] **D.** Hypertension

13. A patient presents to the emergency department after overdosing on levothyroxine (Synthroid). Among other symptoms, the patient has a core body temperature of 106.4° F (41.3° C). In addition to active external cooling methods, which of the following interventions would be optimal in this situation?

[ ] **A.** Give acetaminophen (Tylenol) orally.
[ ] **B.** Provide acetylsalicylic acid (Aspirin) rectally.
[ ] **C.** Administer ketorolac (Toradol) intravenously.
[ ] **D.** Instill Lugol iodine solution via nasogastric tube.

14. Which of the following would be most likely noted by the emergency nurse in a patient with a known benzodiazepine overdose?

[ ] **A.** Miosis
[ ] **B.** Diarrhea
[ ] **C.** Bradypnea
[ ] **D.** Hyperthermia

15. Borborygmus would be associated with which of the following toxic overdoses?

[ ] **A.** Cocaine
[ ] **B.** Tincture of opium
[ ] **C.** Donepezil (Aricept)
[ ] **D.** Alprazolam (Xanax)

16. A 15-year-old presents to the emergency department with tachycardia; dry, flushed skin; confusion; and restlessness. The patient's friends say that they were all at a party and ate some "stinkweed." Recognizing this as jimson weed, which of the following interventions is **NOT** indicated in this scenario?

[ ] **A.** Providing a cooling blanket
[ ] **B.** Administering physostigmine
[ ] **C.** Performing endotracheal intubation
[ ] **D.** Administering IV crystalloid solution

17. On assessment of a patient with a suspected single-drug intentional overdose, the emergency nurse notes dilated pupils; hypoactive bowel sounds; and hot, dry, and flushed skin. Which of the following medications would be the most likely source of the overdose based on the symptoms present?

[ ] **A.** Alprazolam (Xanax)
[ ] **B.** Amitriptyline (Elavil)
[ ] **C.** Methylphenidate (Ritalin)
[ ] **D.** Morphine sulfate (Roxanol)

18. Following interventions for a pure beta$_2$-cholinergic antagonist overdose, which of the following assessments would indicate treatment was successful?

[ ] **A.** Increased heart rate

[ ] **B.** Decreased respiratory rate

[ ] **C.** Increased moisture to skin

[ ] **D.** Decreased diastolic blood pressure

19. Which of the following beta$_2$-adrenergic effects would the emergency nurse anticipate finding in an overdose of a medication in this class?

[ ] **A.** Increased sweating

[ ] **B.** Decreased heart rate

[ ] **C.** Increased tidal volume

[ ] **D.** Decreased blood sugar

20. A patient is brought to the emergency department after a suspected overdose. The patient has altered perceptions of reality, shallow respirations, dysarthria, and ataxia. The emergency nurse suspects which of the following to be the causative substance?

[ ] **A.** Phencyclidine (PCP)

[ ] **B.** Cannabis (Marijuana)

[ ] **C.** Gamma-hydroxybutyrate (GHB)

[ ] **D.** Lysergic acid diethylamide (LSD)

21. A patient with a history of alcohol abuse comes to the emergency department 12 hours after last drinking complaining of nausea and palpitations. The patient is tremulous and reports feeling anxious. Which medication can the nurse anticipate being the first ordered in this scenario?

[ ] **A.** Thiamine (vitamin B$_1$)

[ ] **B.** Lorazepam (Ativan)

[ ] **C.** Phenytoin (Dilantin)

[ ] **D.** Haloperidol (Haldol)

22. The following rhythm strip is seen on the monitor of a patient who just arrived in the emergency department with a possible ingestion.

Which of the following medications most likely caused this rhythm change?

[ ] **A.** Hydroxyzine (Vistaril)

[ ] **B.** Nifedipine (Procardia)

[ ] **C.** Nortriptyline (Aventyl)

[ ] **D.** Ephedrine (Primatene)

23. Two hours after taking an overdose of acetaminophen (Tylenol), a patient arrives in the emergency department. Based on the nomogram for acute ingestion, when can the emergency nurse expect to draw a blood acetaminophen level?

[ ] **A.** Immediately

[ ] **B.** In 1 hour

[ ] **C.** In 2 hours

[ ] **D.** In 4 hours

24. The emergency nurse knows that erethism, associated with mercury toxicity, primarily affects which of the following systems?

[ ] **A.** Neurologic

[ ] **B.** Genitourinary

[ ] **C.** Cardiovascular

[ ] **D.** Gastrointestinal

25. A child is brought to the emergency department after ingestion of prenatal vitamins. The child is noted to have symptoms consistent with an iron toxicity greater than 20 mg/kg and chelation therapy with deferoxamine (Desferal) is administered by continuous intravenous infusion. Which of the following symptoms would indicate the infusion should be discontinued?

[ ] **A.** Hypotension

[ ] **B.** Hematochezia

[ ] **C.** Return of yellow urine

[ ] **D.** Resolution of abdominal pain

26. A patient is brought to the emergency department 15 minutes after ingesting a full bottle of the tricyclic antidepressant amitriptyline (Elavil). Which of the following interventions would **NOT** be utilized in this scenario?

[ ] **A.** Gastric lavage

[ ] **B.** Syrup of ipecac

[ ] **C.** Activated charcoal

[ ] **D.** Electrocardiogram (ECG)

27. Ingestion of the leaves of which of the following plants would be associated with buccal lesions and throat irritation?

[ ] **A.** Coca

[ ] **B.** Cannabis

[ ] **C.** Potato plants

[ ] **D.** Philodendron

28. During the past 3 hours, several adult patients have presented to the emergency department with similar symptoms, which include vomiting, severe diarrhea, and abdominal cramps. Each patient reports eating at the same restaurant the previous night with no other commonalities identified. Based on this information, the triage nurse suspects that these patients were exposed to which type of food poisoning?
[ ] **A.** Botulism
[ ] **B.** Listeriosis
[ ] **C.** Salmonella
[ ] **D.** Staphylococcal

29. Urine alkalization is most likely to be considered in patients who overdose on which of the following types of medications?
[ ] **A.** Sulfonylureas
[ ] **B.** Cephalosporins
[ ] **C.** Calcium channel blockers
[ ] **D.** Phosphodiesterase inhibitors

30. A patient with a long history of benzodiazepine use is brought to the emergency department for a reported overdose of approximately 35 tablets of lorazepam (Ativan). The patient is unresponsive and mildly cyanotic with the following vital signs:

Blood pressure—88/64 mm Hg
Respirations—7 breaths/minute, shallow and regular
Heart rate—52 beats/minute, strong and regular
Pulse oximetry—86% on room air

The emergency nurse considers the following interventions. Which one would be the highest priority in this situation?
[ ] **A.** Infuse 20 mL/kg isotonic crystalloid bolus.
[ ] **B.** Administer flumazenil (Romazicon) IV push.
[ ] **C.** Deliver ventilations at 14 breaths/minute.
[ ] **D.** Initiate chest compressions at 100/minute.

31. Which of the following medications is most commonly used to treat anticholinergic delirium?
[ ] **A.** Naloxone (Narcan)
[ ] **B.** Lithium
[ ] **C.** Physostigmine (Antilirium)
[ ] **D.** Atropine

32. A chronic alcoholic patient presents to the ED with ethanol intoxication. Which of the following laboratory results is most consistent with this scenario?
[ ] **A.** Hyperkalemia
[ ] **B.** Hyponatremia
[ ] **C.** Hyperglycemia
[ ] **D.** Hypomagnesemia

33. A patient presents to the triage desk and complains of arthritis pain and tinnitus. The patient has been taking nonprescription medications for pain relief. Based on the chief complaints, the emergency nurse should ask about the use of which of the following medications?
[ ] **A.** Naproxen (Aleve)
[ ] **B.** Ibuprofen (Motrin)
[ ] **C.** Acetaminophen (Tylenol)
[ ] **D.** Acetylsalicylic acid (Aspirin)

34. While administering dimercaprol (British anti-Lewisite) to a patient, the emergency nurse knows which of the following is optimal regarding administration?
[ ] **A.** Intramuscular injection
[ ] **B.** Oral dose with 16 ounces of water
[ ] **C.** Intravenous infusion over 60 minutes
[ ] **D.** Rapid intravenous infusion over 5 minutes

35. A nondiabetic patient arrives in the emergency department after an intentional overdose of the biguanide antihyperglycemic agent metformin (Glucophage). The emergency nurse would anticipate which of the following finding if a toxic amount was taken?
[ ] **A.** Bradycardia
[ ] **B.** Hypoglycemia
[ ] **C.** Metabolic acidosis
[ ] **D.** Fruity odor to breath

36. A patient who is actively hallucinating is brought to the emergency department by friends. They say that the patient used either D-lysergic acid diethylamide (LSD) or phencyclidine (PCP) at a concert. During triage, which assessment finding indicates that the patient may have ingested PCP?
[ ] **A.** Paranoia
[ ] **B.** Nystagmus
[ ] **C.** Dilated pupils
[ ] **D.** Altered mood

37. For a patient with a suspected cholinergic agent exposure, which of the following symptoms would the emergency nurse consider the highest priority?
[ ] **A.** Diaphoresis
[ ] **B.** Tachycardia
[ ] **C.** Flushed skin
[ ] **D.** Constricted pupils

38. After an ingestion, a patient develops acute blindness and emergency treatment is provided. Ingestion of which of the following would most likely be associated with this scenario?
[ ] **A.** Hydraulic brake fluid
[ ] **B.** Camping stove fuel
[ ] **C.** Skin cleanser
[ ] **D.** Mouthwash

39. A patient presents to the emergency department with a recent history of overuse of oral antacids. The emergency nurse would anticipate which of the following laboratory findings?
[ ] **A.** Hyperkalemia and hypercalcemia
[ ] **B.** Hypocalcemia and hypomagnesemia
[ ] **C.** Hypercalcemia and hypophosphatemia
[ ] **D.** Hypermagnesemia and hyperphosphatemia

40. A patient is treated for a cholinergic exposure. Which of the following manifestations would indicate successful treatment?
[ ] **A.** Miosis
[ ] **B.** Dry skin
[ ] **C.** Tachycardia
[ ] **D.** Hypotension

41. A patient is being treated for an intentional overdose of metformin (Glucophage). Which of the following would indicate that treatment has been successfully completed?
[ ] **A.** Venous pH of 7.29
[ ] **B.** Blood glucose level of 60 mg/dL
[ ] **C.** Lactate level of 1.1 mmol/L
[ ] **D.** Urine output of 3.5 mL/kg/hour

42. The emergency nurse expects a patient with hypotension, widened QRS complex tachycardia, dry, hot skin, respiratory depression, and decreased level of consciousness to have most likely overdosed on which of the following substances?
[ ] **A.** Lorazepam (Ativan)
[ ] **B.** Amitriptyline (Elavil)
[ ] **C.** Carbidopa/levodopa (Sinemet)
[ ] **D.** Benzoylmethylecgonine (cocaine)

43. Signs and symptoms of cyanide exposure are best demonstrated by which of the following?
[ ] **A.** Hallucinations, hypotension, tachycardia
[ ] **B.** Bradycardia, odor of bitter almonds, pH 7.62
[ ] **C.** Bradypnea, decreased mental status, SpO$_2$ 97%
[ ] **D.** Cyanosis, elevated serum lactate level, tachypnea

44. The emergency nurse may anticipate intravenous thiamine to be given for which of the following purposes?
[ ] **A.** Treatment of Addison's crisis
[ ] **B.** Management of pernicious anemia
[ ] **C.** Prevention of Wernicke's encephalopathy
[ ] **D.** Reducing the international normalized ratio (INR)

45. During initial care of a patient with acute lead toxicity, the emergency nurse knows that which of the following findings is most associated with this exposure?
[ ] **A.** Serum pH 7.48
[ ] **B.** Hemoglobin 8.2 g/dL
[ ] **C.** Heart rate 36 beats/minute
[ ] **D.** Respirations 10 breaths/minute

46. A comatose adult with a suspected barbiturate overdose is brought to the emergency department. If gastric lavage is ordered, which of the following would indicate correct performance of the intervention?
[ ] **A.** Instill 300 mL of fluid.
[ ] **B.** Insert an 18 French gastric tube.
[ ] **C.** Administer activated charcoal before lavage.
[ ] **D.** Place patient in a right lateral Trendelenburg position.

47. The classic triad of symptoms associated with an opiate overdose is respiratory depression, central nervous system depression, and:
[ ] **A.** miosis.
[ ] **B.** diuresis.
[ ] **C.** tachycardia.
[ ] **D.** hyperthermia.

48. A patient with a cocaine overdose presents to the emergency department with a temperature of 105.1° F (40.6° C). The emergency nurse anticipates which of the following interventions to be optimal in this situation?
[ ] **A.** Insertion of rectal ibuprofen (Advil)
[ ] **B.** Application of ice packs to the groin and axilla
[ ] **C.** Administration of oral acetaminophen (Tylenol)
[ ] **D.** Initiation of intravenous Dantrolene (dantrolene sodium)

49. While caring for a patient with carbon monoxide poisoning, which of the following is the most likely cause of the patient's confusion?
[ ] **A.** Airway obstruction
[ ] **B.** Impaired gas exchange
[ ] **C.** Oxygen delivery failure
[ ] **D.** Arrested cellular metabolism

50. During the treatment of a patient who drank antifreeze, which of the following would be an expected outcome?
[ ] **A.** Declining serum methanol level
[ ] **B.** Increasing serum ethanol level
[ ] **C.** Rising potassium level
[ ] **D.** Decreasing serum calcium level

51. A patient who ingested the tricyclic antidepressant doxepin (Sinequan) is brought to the emergency department. In addition to supportive measures, the nurse administers sodium bicarbonate IV push. Monitoring for which of the following would best indicate treatment had its intended effect?
[ ] **A.** Acid–base status
[ ] **B.** Neurologic status
[ ] **C.** Respiratory status
[ ] **D.** Cardiovascular status

52. The emergency nurse administered activated charcoal with sorbitol to a patient. Which of the following would be cause for concern?
[ ] **A.** Absent bowel sounds
[ ] **B.** Three episodes of diarrhea
[ ] **C.** Mean arterial pressure of 83 mm Hg
[ ] **D.** Passage of copious dark stool

53. Which of the following would the emergency nurse expect to find in a patient with a known amphetamine overdose?
[ ] **A.** Hypotension
[ ] **B.** Tachycardia
[ ] **C.** Hot, dry skin
[ ] **D.** Constricted pupils

54. Which of the following interventions is most likely to be effective in a patient who overdoses on a beta-adrenergic blocker?
[ ] **A.** Glucagon
[ ] **B.** Epinephrine
[ ] **C.** Calcium gluconate
[ ] **D.** Digoxin immune fab

55. After ingesting 10 mg of the antihypertensive drug clonidine (Catapres) in a suicide attempt, a patient is brought to the emergency department with a decreased level of consciousness. Following steps to secure the airway and obtain vascular access, the emergency nurse should anticipate administering:
[ ] **A.** naloxone.
[ ] **B.** calcium chloride.
[ ] **C.** magnesium sulfate.
[ ] **D.** sodium bicarbonate.

56. For which of the following exposures would charcoal hemoperfusion be indicated?
[ ] **A.** Methanol
[ ] **B.** Digitalis (Digoxin)
[ ] **C.** Amitriptyline (Elavil)
[ ] **D.** Coumadin (warfarin)

57. An unresponsive patient is brought to the emergency department after a possible overdose. If the emergency nurse wants to determine whether the patient ingested an opioid rather than a sedative, which of the following would help make this determination?
[ ] **A.** Bradycardia
[ ] **B.** Hypertension
[ ] **C.** Constricted pupils
[ ] **D.** Absent bowel sounds

58. A patient, after ingesting nightshade, is treated with physostigmine. Which of the following would indicate this treatment had its intended effect?
[ ] **A.** Pupils dilate
[ ] **B.** Heart rate increases
[ ] **C.** Blood pressure rises
[ ] **D.** Hallucinations subside

59. Which of the following laboratory values is most consistent for a patient with an untreated acute salicylate overdose?
[ ] **A.** A serum pH of 7.49
[ ] **B.** A serum glucose of 150 mg/dL
[ ] **C.** A serum potassium of 2.9 mEq/L
[ ] **D.** A serum creatinine level of 9.9 mg/dL

60. When giving activated charcoal in small intermittent doses, the best explanation of the rationale for this method is that small doses:
[ ] **A.** increase the binding of toxins.
[ ] **B.** decrease the likelihood of bowel obstruction.
[ ] **C.** lessen the onset of electrolyte disturbances.
[ ] **D.** reduce the incidence of vomiting and aspiration.

61. When evaluating the effectiveness of treatment for organophosphate poisoning, the emergency nurse should prepare to administer additional antidote if a patient continues to display which of the following signs or symptoms?
[ ] **A.** Tachycardia
[ ] **B.** Hot, dry skin
[ ] **C.** Pinpoint pupils
[ ] **D.** Dry mucous membranes

62. The following electrocardiogram is associated with which of the following overdoses?

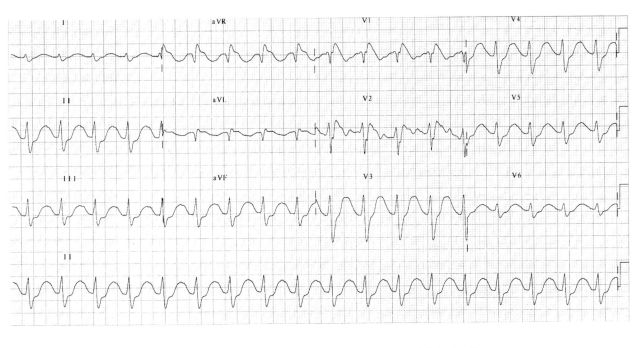

[ ] **A.** Doxepin (Sinequan)

[ ] **B.** Diltiazem (Cardizem)

[ ] **C.** Propranolol (Inderal)

[ ] **D.** Carvedilol (Coreg)

63. A patient is brought to the emergency department after a possible cocaine overdose. Which of the following would the emergency nurse expect to note?

[ ] **A.** Miosis

[ ] **B.** Sudation

[ ] **C.** Catatonia

[ ] **D.** Borborygmus

64. A patient is unintentionally exposed to a large quantity of insecticide and brought to the emergency department for treatment. Which of the following sets of symptoms would be the most likely seen on assessment when the patient arrives?

[ ] **A.** Urination, elevated serum pH, diarrhea

[ ] **B.** Lacrimation, respiratory crackles, miosis

[ ] **C.** Bradycardia, muscle cramping, dry cough

[ ] **D.** Absent bowel sounds, drooling, defecation

65. Dimercaprol (British anti-Lewisite) is prescribed for a patient in the emergency department. The emergency nurse suspects the patient has which of the following presenting complaints?

[ ] **A.** Exposure to anthrax

[ ] **B.** Ingestion of mercury

[ ] **C.** Inhalation of cyanide gas

[ ] **D.** Consumption of ethylene glycol

66. A patient presents with an opioid overdose. Which of the following symptoms would be most likely uncovered by the emergency nurse?

[ ] **A.** Diarrhea, dilated pupils, tachypnea

[ ] **B.** Confusion, cool extremities, miosis

[ ] **C.** Bradypnea, diaphoresis, thready pulses

[ ] **D.** Bradycardia, hot and dry skin, hyperthermia

67. A child is brought to the emergency department after accidentally dousing himself in lamp oil while attempting to drink it. After immediate decontamination, the emergency nurse knows that interventions for which system is the next highest priority?

[ ] **A.** Pulmonary
[ ] **B.** Neurologic
[ ] **C.** Cardiovascular
[ ] **D.** Gastrointestinal

68. Treatment is undertaken for a calcium channel blocker overdose. The emergency nurse knows that treatment has been effective if the patient's:

[ ] **A.** heart rate decreases.
[ ] **B.** temperature decreases.
[ ] **C.** serum glucose increases.
[ ] **D.** blood pressure increases.

69. Which of the following substances is considered a sympathomimetic?

[ ] **A.** Phencyclidine (PCP)
[ ] **B.** Fentanyl (Sublimaze)
[ ] **C.** Physostigmine (Antilirium)
[ ] **D.** Gamma-hydroxybutyric acid (GHB)

70. Which of the following findings is associated with successful treatment for a flunitrazepam (Rohypnol) overdose?

[ ] **A.** Decrease in agitation
[ ] **B.** Increase in heart rate
[ ] **C.** Decrease in serum pH
[ ] **D.** Increase in blood pressure

71. A patient with an unknown single-drug overdose presents to the emergency department and is given a dose of naloxone (Narcan) to determine whether opioids are present. Which of the following findings would indicate opioids were the substance ingested?

[ ] **A.** Drying of skin
[ ] **B.** Dilated pupils
[ ] **C.** Decreased heart rate
[ ] **D.** Assisted ventilation

72. Which of the following medications should the emergency nurse be prepared to administer to a patient with a toxic acetaminophen (Tylenol) level?

[ ] **A.** Succimer (Chemet)
[ ] **B.** Flumazenil (Romazicon)
[ ] **C.** Deferoxamine (Desferal)
[ ] **D.** Acetylcysteine (Acetadote)

73. A patient is treated with deferoxamine (Desferal) following a drug toxicity. Which of the following would be the most likely agent involved in this situation?

[ ] **A.** Prenatal vitamins
[ ] **B.** Methamphetamine
[ ] **C.** Nortriptyline (Aventyl)
[ ] **D.** Nitroprusside (Nipride)

74. Which of the following interventions would be the highest priority for an unresponsive patient with an overdose of the sulfonylurea agent glipizide?

[ ] **A.** 20 mL/kg IV bolus of isotonic crystalloid
[ ] **B.** Octreotide (Sandostatin) 80 mg IV bolus
[ ] **C.** 25 g IV push of dextrose in 50 mL water
[ ] **D.** 15 g of oral glucose solution (Glutose 15)

75. A patient with an acute cyanide ingestion is brought to the emergency department by a private vehicle. Which of the following interventions takes the highest priority?

[ ] **A.** Administer cyanide antidote.
[ ] **B.** Perform gastric lavage.
[ ] **C.** Give activated charcoal.
[ ] **D.** Manage seizure activity.

Answers/Rationales

1. Answer: A

Nursing Process: Assessment

Rationale: **Warm and flushed skin is the most likely of the findings to be uncovered.** Alpha-adrenergic antagonists would result in vasodilation (warm and flushed skin, hypotension), glycogenesis (decreased blood glucose), and dry skin. Alpha receptors of the sympathetic system do not affect the respiratory drive, which are controlled by the beta$_2$ receptors, and this would make bradypnea an unlikely finding. Because vasodilation is a result of alpha-adrenergic antagonists, a finding of hypotension, rather than hypertension, would be more likely. And, finally, because this medication would cause glycogenesis, it is more likely for the patient to present with hypoglycemia as opposed to hyperglycemia.

 CENsational Pearl of Wisdom!

Remember to keep it simple! Many (if not most) questions on the examination will fall back to the basics. Remember, in Toxicology the basics are the toxidromes. Take the time to really learn them. I promise it will be time VERY well spent!

2. Answer: A

Nursing Process: Assessment

Rationale: **The opioid toxidrome includes bradycardia, constricted pupils (miosis), hypotension, hypothermia, diminished bowel sounds, bradypnea, and no change in diaphoresis; therefore, opioid would be the most likely choice in this scenario.** Anticholinergics and sympathomimetics are known to have tachycardia, rather than bradycardia, mydriasis (dilated pupils) rather than miosis, and increased body temperature. Sedative-hypnotics are known to cause bradycardia, diminished bowel sounds, and cool, dry skin, but are not associated with miosis.

3. Answer: B

Nursing Process: Assessment

Rationale: **Dry mouth, absent bowel sounds, and fever are all symptoms consistent with toxicity from this medication.** Carbidopa/levodopa (Sinemet) is a Parkinsonian drug and produces symptoms from the anticholinergic toxidrome. These symptoms often include tachycardia, dilated pupils (mydriasis), hypertension, hyperthermia, decreased or absent bowel sounds, and inhibition of diaphoresis. Although tachycardia and flushed skin may be seen, mydriasis, rather than miosis, would be expected in this situation. Hypertension and confusion (due to body temperatures over 41° C [105.8° F] causing denaturing of neurotransmitters and creating psychosis) may be expected; however, the blockade of muscarine binding sites inhibits fluid mobilization and would more likely decrease, rather than increase, urine production. The patient may have hallucinations, and would likely have tachycardia, rather than bradycardia, and hot and dry skin, rather than cool and clammy skin.

 CENsational Pearl of Wisdom!

Many times the same basic content will be referenced in the questions in different ways. Notice how often the concept of toxidrome symptoms comes up. That is not a cheat, it is reality. Think about your practice and how often you see a patient and begin planning care around the symptoms displayed or the symptoms associated with the chief complaint. The examination is no different. So, again, I emphasize, understand the basics and do not try to memorize all the individual drug effects; learn their class and the majority of the work is done!

4. Answer: D

Nursing Process: Intervention

Rationale: **The antidote is an anticholinergic agent such as atropine, which is given in large doses.** Organophosphate poisoning leads to cholinergic overstimulation. Physostigmine is a cholinergic agent and will worsen symptoms. Flumazenil reverses the sedative effects of benzodiazepines. Glucagon is the antidote for beta-adrenergic blockers.

 CENsational Pearl of Wisdom!

Organophosphate poisoning is a cholinergic crisis that can happen with products such as bug spray. Think "wet" with cholinergic situations because all body fluids that can be secreted are in this situation. A good mnemonic to use for this is MUDDLES. This stands for Miosis, and then increased Urination, Defecation, Diaphoresis, Lacrimation, Excitation, and Salivation. This happens with biochemical substances such as Sarin gas as well.

5. Answer: C

Nursing Process: Assessment

Rationale: **Formalin is a characteristic breath odor in methanol poisoning because formic acid is a metabolite of methanol.** Several poisons may be indicated by the presence of associated breath odors. Bitter almond, for example, is characteristic of cyanide. The odor of moth balls is characteristic of camphor and naphthalene. Garlic is characteristic of arsenic, organophosphates, phosphorous, selenium, and thallium.

 CENsational Pearl of Wisdom!

Another important key is to make a short list of exceptional findings or special cases. Know the basics of the toxidromes, and then tack on to that the handful of special findings such as, in this case, characteristic odors.

6. Answer: D

Nursing Process: Assessment

Rationale: **This patient shows signs of a possible opioid overdose, which includes the depressed mental state and decreased respiratory rate. Opioids, except for meperidine, cause pinpoint pupils. Other signs of opioid toxicity include bradycardia, hypotension, flushed cool skin, bradypnea, and decreased bowel sounds.** Hypertension and tachycardia would not be anticipated in opioid overdose. Hot, dry skin is seen with an anticholinergic overdose, because the lack of diaphoresis in this specific toxicity leads to hyperthermia but would not be seen in opioid overdose.

7. Answer: C

Nursing Process: Assessment

Rationale: **Oleander is a plant that can produce cardiac glycoside effects. Symptoms of toxicity are similar to those of digoxin toxicity and include dysrhythmias (especially bradycardia), hyperkalemia, anorexia, nausea, vomiting, altered mental status, and visual disturbances.** Dysarthria, drooling, and constipation are not associated with oleander toxicity.

 CENsational Pearl of Wisdom!

After you have mastered the core content, such as toxidromes in this case, try to learn examples of drugs or plants that produce these effects. Questions will often change it up by giving you a specific substance and

you need to be able to determine the basic toxidrome it falls within. Other plants that cause digitalis-like symptoms are foxglove and lily of the valley.

8. Answer: D

Nursing Process: Intervention

Rationale: **The antidote for acetaminophen toxicity is N-acetylcysteine, which enhances conversion of toxic metabolites to nontoxic metabolites by providing the substance glutathione that works to clean up the metabolite NAPQI, which causes the liver damage. There are both oral and intravenous preparations of N-acetylcysteine. Mucomyst is the oral form and Acetadote is the intravenous form.** Deferoxamine mesylate is the antidote for iron intoxication. Succimer is an antidote for lead poisoning, and flumazenil reverses the sedative effects of benzodiazepines.

9. Answer: D

Nursing Process: Assessment

Rationale: **The first phase of iron toxicity occurs within 0 to 2 hours after exposure and includes nausea, vomiting, abdominal pain, hematemesis, hematochezia (blood in the stool), and hypotension. Diarrhea, rather than constipation, would be associated with the first phase of iron toxicity.** Fevers are not directly associated with iron toxicity, although they may be noted during the secondary phase because of dehydration. Coagulopathies are more associated with the acidosis of phase three of iron toxicity and not expected in the early phases.

 CENsational Pearl of Wisdom!

The second phase of toxicity occurs within 2 and 48 hours of ingestion and is commonly a resolution of symptoms and perceived improvement in the condition, although the patient may have symptoms of dehydration that may include mild fevers. The third phase often takes 48 to 96 hours to appear and includes symptoms of metabolic acidosis, coagulopathies, hemorrhage, hypovolemic shock, hepatic failure, and renal failure.

Some questions rely on simple recall of facts, while others, like this one, ask you to know not just what happens, but when it happens in the progression of toxicity. Remember, the goal is not to know everything before you enter the examination, but rather not to be thrown off or surprised by questions. Do not be sent into a tailspin during your examination. Take it slow. Learn the basics. Then challenge yourself to sharpen the knowledge you are gaining.

10. Answer: A

Nursing Process: Assessment

Rationale: **Purpura to the skin would be an expected finding in this patient because of the effect of warfarin (Coumadin) in inhibiting the recycling of vitamin K to its usable form.** This reduction in functional vitamin K causes a reduction in vitamin K–dependent reactions that form the clotting factor of the extrinsic cascade: factor VII. It also has a negative impact on nonspecific clotting factors of the common clotting pathway (factors II, IX, and X). The overall toxicity effect of this is a reduction in clotting ability and increased likelihood of bleeding episodes. Because this patient is likely to have bleeding episodes, pain to the posterior calf, a symptom often associated with deep vein thrombosis, is not likely to be seen. Factor VII is measured by the laboratory tests, prothrombin time (PT) and international normalized ratio (INR), rather than the partial thromboplastin time (PTT) test that measures the intrinsic factors (factors VIII, IX, XI, and XII); therefore, an elevation in PTT is not a likely finding in this situation. Because warfarin (Coumadin) inhibits the creation of factor VII, an elevated INR would be anticipated rather than a decreased result.

CENsational Pearl of Wisdom!

PHEW That explanation was a bit intense! Sorry, I think my nerd showed a little on that one. In this review I do not want to dumb anything down and insult you, but I also know that not everyone appreciates the level of detail of pathophysiology that was presented there. I choose to see the best in you. I set the bar as high as I can and encourage you to reach for it. I know you will not always immediately get it, and that is perfectly okay. Just absorb as much as you can and challenge yourself to learn a little more each time. This is how we learn. We try-fail-adapt-overcome! Do not lose heart, you can do this. Remember what I told you earlier? You are AWESOME!

11. Answer: B

Nursing Process: Assessment

Rationale: **The three effects associated with tricyclic antidepressant overdoses are cardiotoxicity (prolonged PR interval, widened QRS, prolonged QT interval, heart blocks, and asystole), adrenergic blocking leading to hypotension, and anticholinergic effects (dry skin and mouth with a depressed level of consciousness).** There are no anticoagulation or sympathomimetic effects and the central nervous system is depressed rather than excited.

12. Answer: B

Nursing Process: Assessment

Rationale: **Dysphagia would be the most likely symptom in this scenario because rhubarb leaves contain oxalic acid, a toxin that irritates the mouth and throat.** The acid may cause edema of the mouth and throat, dysphagia, and increased salivation. Systemic effects include hypocalcemia with calcium oxalate crystals in the urine. Lethargy may occur after ingestion of several plants, especially of the amygdalin-glycoside-cyanide category such as seeds of apples, pears, or apricots, but is not associated with ingestion of rhubarb leaves. Bradycardia is more often found after ingestion of plants that contain cardiac glycosides such as oleander, foxglove, or lily of the valley. Hypertension occurs after ingestion of plants that contain anticholinergic agents such as jimson weed rather than with rhubarb.

13. Answer: A

Nursing Process: Intervention

Rationale: **Acetaminophen is the ideal choice because it will lower the set point without additional negative side effects.** Hyperpyrexia caused by toxicity of thyroid hormone leads to uncontrolled hyperthermia and cellular breakdown, including clotting factor destruction. This is an acute life-threatening condition and must be addressed early. Thyroid hormone stimulates the hypothalamus' temperature-regulating center known as the set point and, when the set point is high, prevents the body's thermoregulatory function from cooling the body down. Antipyretic medications will directly lower this set point and allow the body to assist in dropping the emergent temperature. Because the high temperature can destroy clotting factors, it is advised not to use nonsteroidal anti-inflammatory drugs (NSAIDs) to correct the fever because they may increase the risk of coagulopathies. In addition, salicylates, such as aspirin, can have detrimental effects of clotting ability and also create active metabolites that directly stimulate thyroid release from binding sites. Administering Lugol iodine solution is not incorrect, per se, but it will, at best, only decrease the further release of thyroid, and not do anything to actively stop the life-threatening problems harming the patient. Iodine solution must be given at least 1 hour after antithyroid medications such as methimazole or propylthiouracil (PTU). Therefore, reducing the temperature would be a higher priority.

CENsational Pearl of Wisdom!

Remember, not all high body temperatures are created equal! Patients can be hot due to inability to cool themselves (hyperpyrexia) or overproduction/

overexposure to heat (hyperthermia). Hyperpyrexia, when the set point is high, may be seen with metabolism-induced fevers (illness or inflammation cause set point to rise), increased hormones (hyperthyroidism or pregnancy hormone), or control malfunction (increased intracranial pressure or brain injury disrupts the hypothalamus' ability to dissipate heat normally). Hyperthermia, when heat overcomes the ability to cool, may be seen with high external temperatures (heat stroke) or high internal production of heat (sympathomimetic toxicity). Although the problem (high body temperature) is the same for each of these, the treatment is dramatically different. Understanding the cause of the patient's high body temperature is key to treatment.

14. Answer: C

Nursing Process: Assessment

Rationale: **Benzodiazepines are within the sedative-hypnotic toxidrome and have symptoms of bradycardia, hypotension, hypothermia, decreased bowel motility, and bradypnea.** Constipation, rather than diarrhea, would be associated with benzodiazepine overdose. A decrease in body temperature, rather than hyperthermia, would be anticipated in this situation. Sedative-hypnotics are not normally associated with changes to pupil size.

15. Answer: C

Nursing Process: Assessment

Rationale: **Donepezil (Aricept) is an example of a cholinergic medication and would be associated with increased bowel motility and diarrhea in a toxic overdose.** Borborygmus is the sound of air or fluid moving through the intestines and is commonly known as bowel sounds. Bowel motility, which would lead to increased borborygmus, is primarily governed by neurotransmitters of the parasympathetic nervous system. Cocaine, a member of the sympathomimetic toxidrome, has minimal effect on the gastrointestinal tract, although it may cause a decrease in motility. Opium, the namesake of the opioid class of medications, would cause a decrease in borborygmus. Alprazolam (Xanax) is a benzodiazepine and is associated with a decrease in bowel motility.

16. Answer: C

Nursing Process: Intervention

Rationale: **Jimson weed is not known to cause airway compromise; therefore, endotracheal intubation is not** normally indicated in these patients. Jimson weed is known to elicit anticholinergic properties when consumed. These symptoms may include tachycardia, dry skin, hyperthermia, psychosis and hallucinations, vasoconstriction, mydriasis (dilating pupils), increased blood sugar, and tachypnea. Cooling measures, such as cooling blankets or cool cloths and cooled IV fluids, may be used to treat hyperthermia. Physostigmine is an acetylcholinesterase inhibitor and can, therefore, reverse the peripheral and central manifestations of anticholinergic excess; however, this medication can cause bradycardia and asystole along with other side effects. It must be given very slowly!

 CENsational Pearl of Wisdom!

Anticholinergic manifestations that can be found with medications such as tricyclics can be remembered with the help of a mnemonic: blind as a bat, red as a beet, dry as a bone, mad as a hatter, hotter than Hades. This helps remind us of dilated pupils (blind as a bat), flushed skin (red as a beet), dry mucous membranes and urinary retention (dry as a bone), anxiety or other psychiatric symptoms (mad as a hatter), and hyperthermia (hotter than Hades). Remember that anticholinergics are "dry" and cholinergic issues are "wet."

17. Answer: B

Nursing Process: Analysis

Rationale: **Based on this information and findings of this patient, the only medication that fits all criteria for this toxidrome is amitriptyline (Elavil).** The four medications listed are from the toxidromes of sedatives (alprazolam), anticholinergics (amitriptyline), sympathomimetics (methylphenidate), and opioids (morphine sulfate). The symptoms for anticholinergics include tachycardia, dilated pupils (mydriasis), hypertension, hyperthermia, decreased bowel sounds, tachypnea, and dry skin. The symptoms for opioids include bradycardia, constricted pupils (miosis), hypotension, hypothermia, decreased bowel sounds, bradypnea, and no effect on diaphoresis. The symptoms for sedatives include bradycardia, hypotension, hypothermia, decreased bowel sounds, bradypnea, and no effect on diaphoresis or pupil size. The symptoms for sympathomimetics include tachycardia, dilated pupils (mydriasis), hypertension, hyperthermia, tachypnea, and diaphoresis, and bowel sounds may be hypoactive or hyperactive.

CENsational Pearl of Wisdom!

Remember, analysis questions always require you to bring a little extra to the table! There is nearly always some interpretation that you must do with the information in the question to understand what the answer choices are really indicating. This example, in my opinion, is one of the most straightforward in the analysis style. Here, the question presents you with symptoms you recognize as part of a specific toxidrome. You are then provided with specific medications that you must identify as existing within one of the toxidromes as well. After that, it a simple enough task, to choose the correct choice with a matching toxidrome.

18. Answer: B

Nursing Process: Evaluation

Rationale: **If treatment was successful, decreased respiratory rate would be an expected outcome.** A beta$_2$-cholinergic antagonist, such as ipratropium (Atrovent), would block muscarine receptor sites of acetylcholine and result in unopposed sympathetic stimulation of the beta$_2$-adrenergic receptors primarily in the lungs. Symptoms of the overdose would include tachypnea and bronchodilation if the medication is selective, as was the case in this scenario. In this scenario, we are not looking at the overdose, but rather at a resolution of the overdose symptoms. Increased heart rate would not be expected, both because a decrease in sympathetic stimulation should occur and because with a pure beta$_2$ agent the beta$_1$ receptors of the heart are not likely to be affected. Moisture to the skin and changes in diastolic blood pressure are associated with alpha-receptor activity rather than beta$_2$ receptors and unlikely to be confirmation of successful treatment in this scenario.

CENsational Pearl of Wisdom!

Here is our first example of an evaluation-style question. These can be tricky if you do not understand the intention. In assessment questions, you are tasked to identify the problem on the basis of the assessment of the patient. After that, intervention questions ask you what do you do to fix identified problems. Evaluation questions make you determine whether your intervention worked. So, the question may present a patient with a specific problem, but asks you something like "what indicates treatment was successful?" Be careful not to answer on the basis of symptoms of the condition presented, because if the treatment was successful, the patient will not have that anymore; instead, the patient will have symptoms opposite to that of the problem presented. Just read carefully and be sure to answer the question they asked you, not the question you WANTED them to ask you.

19. Answer: C

Nursing Process: Assessment

Rationale: **Because beta$_2$ receptors are associated with lung function, the most likely symptom to be anticipated would be increased tidal volume.** Adrenergic effects refer to the compensatory responses of the sympathetic system; commonly referred to as the flight-or-fight response. These effects are generated through specific receptor sites throughout the body and include alpha receptors and beta receptors. The beta receptors are differentiated into beta$_1$, beta$_2$, and beta$_3$. The beta$_1$ receptors are almost entirely located in the heart and focus on stimulation of cardiac output such as increasing heart rate, contractility, and automaticity. The beta$_2$ receptors are almost, but not completely, located in the lungs and focus on increasing pulmonary function such as increased respiratory rate and bronchodilation, which increases tidal volume. The beta$_3$ receptors are not completely understood, but have been found in the gallbladder, urinary bladder, and brown adipose tissue and appear to be associated with lipolysis (breakdown of fat for energy), thermogenesis, and bladder relaxation. Although increased sweating would be an adrenergic effect, it is not regulated by the beta$_2$ receptors. Both decreased heart rate and decreased blood sugar are associated with the cholinergic (parasympathetic) system and would not be likely responses in this situation.

CENsational Pearl of Wisdom!

Just a little extra pathophysiology to help your understanding of the adrenergic system. Remember to take from these rationales what you need or can handle and then leave the rest for another time. Learning is a lifelong process and will not be completed in a single sitting.

20. Answer: C

Nursing Process: Analysis

Rationale: **Gamma-hydroxybutyrate (GHB) is a sedative/hypnotic which induces hallucinations and euphoria as well as more commonly associated sedation effects such as respiratory depression.** Phencyclidine (PCP), cannabis (marijuana), and lysergic acid diethylamide (LSD) produce hallucinations and coordination impairment but act as stimulants, rather than as depressants on the respiratory drive.

21. Answer: B

Nursing Process: Analysis

Rationale: **Benzodiazepines such as lorazepam are first-line therapy for the treatment of acute withdrawal syndrome and the prevention and treatment of seizure activity and delirium tremens.** Placebo-controlled trials have demonstrated that phenytoin is ineffective for the secondary prevention of alcohol withdrawal seizures. In addition, phenytoin use has been attributed to respiratory depression in high doses or when combined with alcohol. For the treatment of Wernicke's encephalopathy and thiamine deficiency, the administration of thiamine is recommended; however, this would not be a first-line therapy. Haloperidol has also been used to control the psychiatric symptoms of alcohol withdrawal, including combativeness, delirium, and anxiousness. However, it has been shown to be significantly less effective than benzodiazepines in preventing delirium and can cause torsades de pointes because of prolongation of the QT interval.

 CENsational Pearl of Wisdom!

Remember, certain words and phrases carry specific meaning on the examination. When you encounter words such as priority, primary, *or* initial *interventions, it should lead you to think "Which will actively stop the dying process." This is usually based on stopping the symptoms that are truly harming the patient. In the given example, we see that all four medications are appropriate for this patient, but only Ativan stopped the immediate life-threatening complication. I hope this helps!*

22. Answer: B

Nursing Process: Assessment

Rationale: **This rhythm strip demonstrates both a first-degree heart block and bradycardia. Calcium**

channel blockers such as nifedipine (Procardia) **are known to cause heart blocks and bradycardia.** Hydroxyzine (Vistaril) is an antihistamine drug and will cause tachycardia rather than bradycardia. Nortriptyline (Acentyl) is a tricyclic antidepressant and leads to several toxic cardiac effects including tachycardic dysrhythmias and arrest, but is not traditionally associated with heart blocks and bradycardia. Ephedrine (Primatene) is a sympathomimetic and would cause an increased, rather than a decreased, heart rate and is not associated with heart blocks.

 CENsational Pearl of Wisdom!

Remember that basic rhythm interpretation is fair game on the examination! Remember the five or so basic rhythms you need to know when you go to an ACLS or PALS course? Those are the same ones you need to know for this examination most of the time. Occasionally there will be a tougher rhythm that is very specific to an individual drug or condition, but such cases are the exceptions.

23. Answer: C

Nursing Process: Intervention

Rationale: **Based on the nomogram for acute ingestion, serum acetaminophen levels should be drawn 4 hours after ingestion. Because the ingestion occurred 2 hours before arrival, the level should be drawn 2 hours after arrival to reach the 4-hour level.** Levels drawn sooner or later would not reflect the peak acetaminophen level. An acetaminophen level greater than 150 g/mL 4 hours after ingestion indicates toxicity.

24. Answer: A

Nursing Process: Assessment

Rationale: **Erethism, also known as Mad Hatter Disease, is a neurologic complication of mercury toxicity.** Symptoms associated with erethism include irritability, excitability, excessive shyness, and insomnia. Although acute or chronic symptoms of mercury toxicity may include other symptoms, the classic triad is tremors, gingivitis, and erethism. Erethism is not associated with the genitourinary, cardiovascular, or gastrointestinal systems.

CENsational Pearl of Wisdom!

Okay, I admit it! This was just me sneaking in a fun fact. Not sure it is the more relevant piece of information for the examination, but I did not know it and when I stumbled across it while researching this chapter, I wanted to share it. If you did not know it, do not feel bad; neither did I! But now you know that mercury poisoning causes neurologic manifestations! Just in case!

25. Answer: C

Nursing Process: Evaluation

Rationale: **Indication for discontinuation of deferoxamine therapy in iron toxicity is when urine color normalizes.** The chelation process of deferoxamine on iron leads to a pink or orange-red urine. Therefore, once urine returns to a clear yellow color, the therapy is considered complete. Hypotension and hematochezia are symptoms of phase one of iron toxicity and would not be indicative of successful treatment. Likewise, resolution of abdominal pain is an expected event during the second phase of iron toxicity and would, therefore, not be a good indicator of completion of chelation therapy.

CENsational Pearl of Wisdom!

Iron toxicity often presents in three phases, each with its own set of symptoms. The first phase, often presenting within 0 to 2 hours of ingestion/exposure, is associated with hypotension, hematemesis (bloody emesis), hematochezia (bloody stool), and abdominal pain. The second phase, often presenting between 2 and 48 hours after ingestion, is associated with a resolution of gastrointestinal symptoms. The third phase, often seen approximately 48 to 96 hours after ingestion, is associated with metabolic acidosis, coagulopathy, hemorrhage, shock, and hepatic and renal failure. Some report this second phase as "in between phase one and two." Just remember there is a period of time where the patient seems to be "Okay."

26. Answer: B

Nursing Process: Intervention

Rationale: **Syrup of ipecac is contraindicated in tricyclic antidepressant overdose. Because rapid deterioration**

with cardiovascular collapse and seizures can occur, inducing emesis may lead to airway compromise from aspiration. Gastric lavage could be ordered with endotracheal intubation with proper cuff inflation and mechanical ventilation. Administration of activated charcoal may be delayed. A baseline ECG may be ordered. The patient should be placed on a cardiac monitor because dysrhythmias and cardiac conduction delays are common.

27. Answer: D

Nursing Process: Assessment

Rationale: **Oxalic acid is a skin irritant contained in the leaves of several plants including dieffenbachia, philodendron, and rhubarb. Oxalic acid can cause blisters and ulcerations to the mucous membranes of the mouth and throat when chewed. This irritation can lead to throat swelling, dysphagia, and respiratory distress.** Leaves of the coca plant will cause numbness and anesthesia to the mouth when chewed, but then lead to stimulant effects as they are absorbed in the body. Cannabis leaves contain nearly 500 active chemicals including tetrahydrocannabinol (THC) and have little effect on the buccal cavity when chewed, but they are associated with alterations in perception, increased appetite, and anxiety and several other mood-associated effects. Leaves of some potato plants have an anticholinergic effect including hyperthermia and hallucinations, dry skin, mental excitation, and tachycardia.

CENsational Pearl of Wisdom!

Although it is not always the most common situation we see in our practice, it is far from uncommon for patients to present with ingestions of nonpharmacologic agents such as plants or solutions. There is no chance that we will know every possible toxic substance out there, but see if you can add a few of them to your repertoire here and there.

28. Answer: C

Nursing Process: Analysis

Rationale: **Signs of Salmonella poisoning appear from 12 to 24 hours after the ingestion of contaminated food.** Common foods contaminated with Salmonella include milk, custards and other egg dishes, salad dressings, sandwich fillings, polluted shellfish, and poultry. Staphylococcal symptoms appear suddenly 1 to 6 hours after exposure and include headache and fever. Listeriosis occurs 3 to 21 days after exposure, and, in addition to diarrhea, fever, and headache, it may result in pneumonia, meningitis, and endocarditis. Botulism does not usually cause diarrhea. The symptoms of botulism include bilateral facial weakness, dysphagia, eyelid ptosis (drooping), blurry vision, and paralysis as well as gastrointestional manifestations.

29. Answer: A

Nursing Process: Intervention

Rationale: **Alkalization of urine is considered effective for overdoses involving phenobarbital, sulfonylureas, formaldehyde, and salicylates.** Weak acids may become iontrapped and excreted in the urine when urine pH is increased with controlled administration of alkalizing agents. Alkalinizing the urine does not promote excretion of cephalosporins, calcium channel blockers, or phosphodiesterase inhibitors.

30. Answer: C

Nursing Process: Analysis

Rationale: **Because of the phenomenon explained here, respiratory depression and arrest is the highest priority with an acute benzodiazepine overdose. Of the options presented, mechanical ventilations would be the highest priority because they are both immediate and therapeutic, that is to say, the action directly stops the dying process in the patient.** Benzodiazepines, such as lorazepam (Ativan), act as agonists for the *gamma*-aminobutyric acid (GABA) receptor site and decrease neuronal excitability. The primary effect of benzodiazepines is antianxiety and hypnotic effects; however, in higher doses, this increased resistance to nerve impulse conduction translates into a higher threshold of resistance to muscle firing as well. Therefore, benzodiazepines also are used to inhibit seizure activity by making muscles less able to contract because of an increased resistance threshold. In a toxic overdose setting, the antianxiety and hypnotic properties are not the primary concern, but rather the inhibition of muscle firing; specifically, in voluntary skeletal muscles, but with limited effect on vascular and cardiac smooth muscles. Flumazenil (Romazicon) is the antagonist for benzodiazepines and would act to reverse the effects of the drug within 1 to 3 minutes; however, there are multiple problems with choosing this as the first intervention in this situation. The obvious problem is that flumazenil would take 1 to 3 minutes to work, during which time the patient is still hypoventilated and hypoperfused; not optimal. Also, this patient is described as having chronic benzodiazepine use, which would impart tolerance

to the medication. Flumazenil is contraindicated in patients with chronic benzodiazepine use because of an increased risk of rebound sedation as well as of intractable seizure activity following rapid administration of the reversal agent. In chronic tolerance cases, the recommended weaning of benzodiazepines with flumazenil is over the course of weeks to months and not recommended for rapid reversals. Chest compressions and intravenous fluid boluses are not incorrect in this situation, but they do not serve to correct the primary life-threatening problem, which is respiratory depression; therefore, they would not take precedence over ventilations.

 CENsational Pearl of Wisdom!

Do not hate me for that one! I know it was probably frustrating. Let me explain a bit about why this type of question is so important and why it is an analysis-style question rather than intervention. Many times on the examination, you will be presented with four good choices! They are sometimes all appropriate in the given situation. The question becomes not which one will I do, but which one will I do first *to best provide therapeutic and immediate life-saving interventions. As explained, there are multiple choices that are valid and if you stop at the first choice that is appropriate, you will get the question incorrect. When you see a question that has multiple "good" answers, ask yourself what is the crisis in this situation. That is, what is actually harming the patient and what will best correct that. It may be best because it is most readily available, targets the specific cause of harm in the patient, or does not create secondary complications. They are not always easy, but they will show up both on the examination and in your emergency department!*

31. Answer: C

Nursing Process: Intervention

Rationale: **Physostigmine acts by interfering with the metabolism of acetylcholine; therefore, increasing the cholinergic effects of acetylcholine in the body and reversing anticholinergic delirium.** Remember that physostigmine must be given slowly because of the side effects! Naloxone is used in opiate overdose. Lithium is not used as an antidote in any scenario. Atropine is used in beta-adrenergic blocker, calcium channel blocker, and organophosphate and physostigmine poisonings.

32. Answer: D

Nursing Process: Assessment

Rationale: **The most common cause of hypomagnesemia is alcoholism and is commonly associated with poor dietary intake, diarrhea-induced hypophosphatemia that drives down magnesium levels, and metabolic acidosis and magnesiuric effects which both lead to low levels of serum magnesium.** Potassium levels are usually not elevated with chronic alcoholism. Alcohol is a known diuretic and is more likely to cause hypernatremia as opposed to hyponatremia. Because of liver damage and lack of glycogen stores, chronic alcoholics are more likely to be hypoglycemic than hyperglycemic.

33. Answer: D

Nursing Process: Assessment

Rationale: **Tinnitus is the most common central nervous system sign of mild salicylate toxicity. Patients taking medications that contain salicylates at doses prescribed for arthritis may develop mild toxicity (salicylism).** Ibuprofen usually causes GI upset and blurred vision. Acetaminophen toxicity causes liver failure. Naproxen may cause GI bleeding without other GI symptoms and may also mask infection.

34. Answer: A

Nursing Process: Intervention

Rationale: **The only route that dimercaprol may be safely administered is via the intramuscular route.** Dimercaprol (British anti-Lewisite) is a chelating agent used to treat toxicity with select heavy metals including arsenic, lead, gold, and mercury. This medication is only effective in parenteral routes and is not effective orally. Dimercaprol is contraindicated in iron, selenium, silver, uranium, and cadmium toxicities because of the toxic complex that dimercaprol forms with these metals. Owing to the toxic interaction with iron, dimercaprol is contraindicated via the intravenous route, either slow or rapid infusion, because it chelates heme molecules in the red blood cells leading to life-threatening anemias in some cases.

35. Answer: C

Nursing Process: Assessment

Rationale: **Metabolic acidosis would be a more likely finding in this situation.** The antidiabetic medication class of biguanide, of which metformin is a member, acts more prominently by inhibiting liver glucose production rather than, as other antidiabetic medications do, decreasing cellular resistance of insulin. Therefore, biguanides only drop blood sugar to the euglycemic threshold of the body and are not commonly associated with hypoglycemic emergencies. They do, however, inhibit liver breakdown of lactate molecules and can lead to metabolic lactic acidosis in overdoses. Hypoglycemia is rarely seen with biguanide overdose. Bradycardia would not be a direct consequence of biguanide overdose, although dysrhythmias may be seen secondary to the acidotic state. Ketones on the breath, which have a fruity odor, would be a consequence of diabetic ketoacidosis and not from the use of biguanide medications. In this scenario, the patient is specifically stated as not being diabetic, so ketones on the breath are unlikely.

36. Answer: B

Nursing Process: Assessment

Rationale: **Nystagmus would be the most compelling symptom presented to indicate PCP was ingested rather than LSD.** Phencyclidine is an anesthetic with severe psychological effects. It blocks the reuptake of dopamine and directly affects the midbrain and thalamus. Bidirectional nystagmus and ataxia are common physical findings of PCP use. Dilated pupils are evidence of LSD ingestion. Paranoia and altered mood occur with both PCP and LSD ingestion.

37. Answer: A

Nursing Process: Analysis

Rationale: **Diaphoresis would be the most concerning symptom in this situation because it indicates the level of toxicity of the cholinergic agent as well as having a primary impact on gas exchange through fluid production in the lungs.** Cholinergic agents lead to symptoms of the parasympathetic system, which include vasodilation, decreased serum glucose, decreased cardiac function (including bradycardia, conduction blocks, and decreased contractility), bradypnea, and bronchoconstriction. However, because of the relative strength imbalance between the adrenergic (sympathetic) receptors and the cholinergic (parasympathetic) receptors in the $beta_1$ and $beta_2$ sites, lability in heart rate and respirations are often seen. In addition, with cholinergic toxicity, the effects of the muscarinic and nicotinic pathways, which have primary control over fluid mobilization in the body, we find that excessive fluid production from all fluid-producing cells often occurs. Tachycardia in this situation would be a sympathetic reflex as part of compensation and not directly life threatening. Flushed skin would indicate vasodilation, which may have a secondary impact on vascular resistance and blood pressure; but it would be a circulatory concern and would not take priority over the airway obstruction of fluid production. Constricted pupils would be a symptom of parasympathetic stimulation and expected in this situation, although they do not pose an immediate life-threatening concern.

CENsational Pearl of Wisdom!

Remember that cholinergic crises are "wet." All bodily fluids are sent into overdrive!

38. Answer: B

Nursing Process: Analysis

Rationale: **Visual disturbances and blindness are associated with toxicity of methanol. Methanol is found in several chemicals including windshield washer fluid, canned fuels, and alternative automobile fuel.** Ethylene glycol, another alternative alcohol, leads to acidosis and renal failure. Ethylene glycol is often found in solvents and as an antifreeze agent in automotive fluids such as hydraulic brake fluid. Isopropanol, the least toxic of the alternate alcohols, metabolizes quickly into acetone and, although toxic and able to cause profound central nervous system and respiratory depression, is lost in respiratory expressions rapidly and can be managed with supportive care. Isopropanol is found in disinfectants and skin cleansers. Ethanol is safe for human consumption and is nontoxic in moderate doses. Ethanol, much like isopropanol, can be an effective solvent and is used in certain cleansers and tinctures. Owing to ethanol's nontoxic nature, it is often found in products intended for internal use, such as mouthwash. If ingested in small amounts, it is unlikely to cause harm.

CENsational Pearl of Wisdom!

Another place to find methanol is moonshine!

39. Answer: C

Nursing Process: Analysis

Rationale: **The most likely findings would be hypercalcemia and hypophosphatemia.** Oral antacids are comprised of one of four primary active ingredients: aluminum hydroxide, magnesium hydroxide, sodium bicarbonate, and calcium carbonate. In most liquid antacids, such as Mylanta or Maalox, the active ingredient is aluminum hydroxide, which acts by deactivating the gastric enzyme pepsin and by increasing the mucosal lining of the stomach; but it has a side effect of binding to phosphates in the gastrointestinal tract and causing hypophosphatemia. The other common liquid antacid is milk of magnesium, which contains magnesium hydroxide. Magnesium hydroxide works by binding in stomach acid to produce

magnesium chloride, thereby reducing acid directly but also producing a biologically available magnesium compound in the process. The side effects of magnesium hydroxide are diarrhea and hypermagnesemia. One of the solid antacids containing sodium bicarbonate is Alka-Seltzer or baking soda and it acts by binding to gastric hydrochloric acid to reduce pH; but it has a side effect of producing sodium, which can be freely absorbed to elevate serum sodium levels. The most common oral antacid is calcium carbonate, such as in Tums, and this most potent usable antacid completely neutralizes available stomach acids. However, approximately one-third of the calcium gets absorbed into the bloodstream, causing elevations in serum calcium, and binds to phosphate ions, causing hypophosphatemia. Therefore, regardless of the agent used, the following effects are common (number of agents that cause each is listed in parenthesis): metabolic alkalosis (4), hypercalcemia (2), hypophosphatemia (2), hypernatremia (1), hypermagnesemia (1) or hypomagnesemia (1), and hypokalemia (3).

It is unlikely for this patient to have hyperkalemia because magnesium, calcium, and sodium bicarbonate all have a reducing effect on serum potassium levels. Hypercalcemia, rather than hypocalcemia, is a common effect. Although hypermagnesemia is possible, none of the agents are known to cause hyperphosphatemia but rather cause hypophosphatemia.

CENsational Pearl of Wisdom!

This was a fun fact for you. We all know the basics of antacids, but did you know how they each work? I cannot say I had a comprehensive understanding of them myself before I researched them extensively so do not feel a bit of shame if you did not either. Again, my goal is to raise the bar for you and push you to take your understanding to a new level.

40. Answer: B

Nursing Process: Evaluation

Rationale: **Drying of the skin would be an indication that the cholinergic toxicity effect has been resolved.** This toxidrome often causes lability, as either elevated or decreased heart rate, respirations, and blood pressure, and is not known to directly change body temperature. Miosis is a symptom of cholinergic exposure; therefore, its presence would not indicate successful treatment. Tachycardia and hypotension may be symptoms of cholinergic crisis; however, the treatment of cholinergic exposure would not intentionally create an abnormally high heart rate or an abnormally low blood pressure. Tachycardia and hypotension in this case would indicate that patient was overtreated and a new problem, potentially anticholinergic crisis, was created.

41. Answer: C

Nursing Process: Evaluation

Rationale: **A lactate level of 1.1 mmol/L would be in the standard reference range and indicate the lactic acidosis caused by the toxicity has been resolved.** Remember that biguanide antihyperglycemic agents, including metformin (Glucophage), act by inhibiting liver glucose production rather than, as other antidiabetic medications do, by decreasing cellular resistance of insulin. Therefore, biguanides only drop blood sugar to the euglycemic threshold of the body and are not commonly associated with hypoglycemic emergencies. They do, however, inhibit liver breakdown of lactate molecules and lead to metabolic lactic acidosis in overdoses. A venous pH of 7.29 would indicate an acidotic state and would not indicate successful treatment in this situation. Because biguanide overdose is not normally associated with hypoglycemia, a blood glucose level of 60 mg/dL would not necessarily indicate successful treatment. Although increased urine output may be present in a patient who is hyperglycemic, which is likely in a patient who has access to antidiabetic medications, it would be indicative of the condition of hyperglycemia, rather than the toxic effects of metformin (Glucophage) and would not be associated with effective treatment of the toxicity.

42. Answer: B

Nursing Process: Assessment

Rationale: **Patients with toxicity from tricyclic antidepressants may present with cardiotoxicity (wide-complex tachydysrhythmias), anticholinergic effects (hyperthermia, dry skin, tachycardia), and anti-adrenergic effects (vasodilation, hypotension). Tricyclic antidepressants** (modernly referred to as cyclic antidepressants) have three primary effects that lead to unique symptoms in toxic exposures. The first two effects are due to an inhibition of norepinephrine and serotonin reuptake, which, in therapeutic levels, increases synaptic firing and stimulates elevations in mood, memory, and alertness. At toxic levels, serotonin inhibits norepinephrine release from adrenergic nerves leading to beta$_2$-adrenergic blockade as well as generates increased levels of nitrous oxide from endothelial cells, which leads to alpha-adrenergic antagonist effects including severe vasodilation and hypotension. The second mechanism seen in toxic tricyclic exposure is a reduction of sodium fast channels in cardiac myocytes, leading to delayed cardiac conduction and widening of QRS complexes. The third mechanism of action during toxicity is the blockade of

cholinergic and histaminergic receptors, which manifests as the anticholinergic effects of lack of fluid mobilization (dry skin, dry mouth, and prevention of thermodissipation effects of diaphoresis).

 CENsational Pearl of Wisdom!

Have you seen the secret yet? The key to understanding toxicology is not in memorizing every possible presentation for every individual agent. It is knowing the toxidromes and the key features to each one. It is with this knowledge that Poison Centers are able to so effectively identify the probable toxic agents and recommend treatment. Trust yourself! Know the core content of the toxidromes and apply the presenting symptoms to that.

43. Answer: C

Nursing Process: Analysis

Rationale: **Bradypnea, decreased mental status, and normal pulse oximetry would be expected in this situation.** Cyanide affects the body primarily by attaching to metalloenzymes found inside cells and inactivating them by preventing cytochrome oxidase. This blockade of a primary enzymatic reaction within cells prevents mitochondria from performing oxidative phosphorylation and prevents it from performing aerobic cellular respiration. This essential process forces affected cells into anaerobic metabolism and dramatically increases lactic acid production at the cellular level. It is this key feature that creates a set of very specific symptoms including hypotension, bradycardic dysrhythmias, respiratory depression/arrest, decreased mental status, seizure, and metabolic acidosis, but maintains an adequate serum oxygen level (because oxygen is carried by hemoglobin and stored on myoglobin but cannot be used by cells). It is the relatively normal oxygen levels which create the clinical confusion, because they produce normal oxygen saturations and normal skin color (noncyanotic) while the patient has all the other signs or hypoxia. Tachycardia, serum alkalosis, and cyanosis would not be expected in cyanide exposure.

44. Answer: C

Nursing Process: Intervention

Rationale: **Thiamine deficiency is known to contribute to Wernicke's encephalopathy and Korsakoff's syndrome; therefore, administration of thiamine is an expected treatment for both of these conditions.** Addison's crisis is caused by insufficient adrenal hormones and is treated with intravenous hydrocortisone (Solu-Cortef) or another corticosteroid. Pernicious anemia is caused by a deficiency of vitamin B_{12} and is treated with subcutaneous vitamin B_{12} injections, not thiamine which is vitamin B_1. Elevated international normalized ratio (INR) is treated with infusions of fresh frozen plasma and cryoprecipitate as well as vitamin K.

45. Answer: B

Nursing Process: Assessment

Rationale: **A mild anemia, such as a hemoglobin level of 8.2 g/dL, may be likely with lead toxicity.** Common symptoms of acute lead toxicity include neurologic changes (mood lability, tremors, concentration impairment, memory loss), renal failure, anemia, and gastrointestinal upset (diarrhea, vomiting, nausea, and anorexia). Metabolic acidosis, rather than alkalosis, would be expected because of renal failure and an increase in positive ions in the blood. Lead toxicity tends to create a stressed state in the body due to gastrointestinal losses and renal failure; therefore, tachycardia, rather than bradycardia, and tachypnea, rather than bradypnea, would be more likely.

46. Answer: A

Nursing Process: Intervention

Rationale: **An adult receiving gastric lavage should have 200 to 300 mL of fluid instilled at a time.** The fluid should then be removed by gravity or gentle suction. Larger amounts may cause the pyloric sphincter to open and force the toxins into the small intestine. Smaller amounts may not distend the stomach enough to open the rugae and be able to clear the pill fragments out of these folds. The patient should be placed in the left lateral Trendelenburg position. A large-bore gastric tube (22 to 36 French) should be used, with the average size for an adult being 32 to 36 French. Activated charcoal should be instilled after lavage has been completed; otherwise, it would be washed out during the lavage process.

47. Answer: A

Nursing Process: Assessment

Rationale: **The classic triad of symptoms associated with an opiate overdose is respiratory depression, central nervous system depression, and miosis (constricted pupils).** Alterations in urinary output, including diuresis, are not associated with opiate overdoses. Bradycardia, as opposed to tachycardia, and hypothermia, as opposed to hyperthermia, are associated with opiate overdoses.

48. Answer: B

Nursing Process: Intervention

Rationale: **Active external cooling methods, such as application of ice packs, are much more likely to be**

effective than pharmacologic interventions which focus on reduction of the set point. Hyperthermia in sympathomimetic overdoses is driven primarily by excessive thermogenesis because of increased activity and muscle firing rather than through hyperpyrexia and endocrine activity. Administration of ibuprofen or acetaminophen is unlikely to be effective in reducing the temperature of this patient. Dantrolene sodium, a postsynaptic muscle inhibitor, may be effective in blocking further temperature generation by inhibiting muscle firing, although it will do little to reduce the current temperature and, therefore, would not take precedence over active cooling measures in this patient.

 CENsational Pearl of Wisdom!

Dantrolene, which works on the skeletal muscles, can have some serious hepatotoxic side effects and is not usually the first line of defense for disease processes such as that listed in question 48. The most common reason to use this medication is in a situation of malignant hyperthermia that is most often seen during surgery. However, be aware that the use of Succinylcholine (Anectine) can also cause malignant hyperthermia!

49. Answer: C

Nursing Process: Analysis

Rationale: **The primary toxic effect of carbon monoxide (CO) is competitive binding to hemoglobin, which prevents the carrying and delivery of oxygen to cells; therefore, the primary cause of confusion would be oxygen delivery failure.** Carbon monoxide has no direct impact on airway patency or gas exchange in the lung fields. Although there is some evidence that carbon monoxide may bind to cardiac myoglobin and have increased cardiovascular metabolism impairment, the toxicity much more directly retarding cellular metabolism is cyanide.

 CENsational Pearl of Wisdom!

Once you have the pathophysiology of a toxicity in your grasp, you find that questions become a lot more straightforward. Take it slow and add what you can each time you get the opportunity. Ask questions when you see new or unfamiliar cases in your practice. Examples will always help you solidify your understanding!

50. Answer: B

Nursing Process: Evaluation

Rationale: **The most likely outcome in this situation would be rising ethanol levels. The dehydrogenase sites are saturated when ethanol levels are 100 mg/dL or above; therefore, increasing serum ethanol levels would be an expected outcome of therapy.** Antifreeze contains ethylene glycol which, when metabolized by the liver, produces toxic metabolites. Medical therapy for ethylene glycol ingestion includes blocking the metabolism of the drug by saturating alcohol dehydrogenase sites with ethanol to prevent the production of toxic metabolites as well as administration of sodium bicarbonate for acidosis. Ethylene glycol, rather than methanol, is a more common ingredient in antifreeze, so declining methanol levels would be less likely associated with this treatment; however, because treatment involves binding to the dehydrogenase sites, the levels of the alternate alcohol (ethylene glycol or methanol) should remain the same if treatment is successful. Ethylene glycol toxicity leads to hypocalcemia and hyperkalemia through chelation of calcium by oxalates and metabolic acidosis, respectively. Therefore, treatment of this toxicity should lead to increasing calcium levels and decreasing potassium levels.

51. Answer: D

Nursing Process: Evaluation

Rationale: **The primary effect of administering sodium bicarbonate is to reverse QRS prolongation and hypotension. The actual mechanism of action is not well understood, but it may inhibit binding of tricyclic antidepressants to the myocardial sodium channels.** The toxic effects of tricyclic antidepressants include cardiotoxicity (prolongation of conduction leading to dysrhythmias and arrest), adrenergic blockade (alpha-receptor blockades leading to hypotension), and anticholinergic stimulation (including dry, flushed skin, hyperthermia, tachycardia). Management of tricyclic antidepressant overdose is focused on reversing cardiotoxicity. Seizures may occur, but administration of benzodiazepines, rather than sodium bicarbonate, will suppress this symptom. The administration of sodium bicarbonate does not directly affect respiratory status. Acid–base status should also be monitored, but effectiveness is based on cardiac response.

52. Answer: A

Nursing Process: Evaluation

Rationale: **A contraindication to the administration of sorbitol is a bowel ileus because increasing lumen pressures proximal to a bowel obstruction** exacerbates the risk of bowel perforation; therefore, absent bowel sounds would be a cause for concern in this situation. Sorbitol is a cathartic agent that may be added to activated charcoal to increase elimination of charcoal-bound toxins from the gastrointestinal tract. Sorbitol is a sugar-alcohol and is known to stimulate bowel motility by increasing intra-intestinal osmolality and drawing extra-intestinal fluids into the large intestine. Episodes of diarrhea would be an expected outcome of sorbitol administration and not concerning with only the three episodes noted. Loss of fluid through the gastrointestinal tract is a concern and could lead to hypotension; however, a mean arterial pressure of 83 mm Hg (potentially 110/70) is a normotensive value and not cause for alarm. The goal of activated charcoal with sorbitol is to bind toxins with charcoal and increase their elimination in the stool; therefore, copious dark stool would be expected if this treatment was successful.

53. Answer: B

Nursing Process: Assessment

Rationale: **Amphetamines are central nervous system stimulants that cause sympathetic stimulation, including hypertension, tachycardia, vasoconstriction, and hyperthermia.** Hot, dry skin is seen with anticholinergic agents such as jimsonweed and tricyclic antidepressants. Pupils are dilated, not constricted, with amphetamine overdose.

54. Answer: A

Nursing Process: Intervention

Rationale: **Glucagon would be the most beneficial intervention because its primary activity on cells is to stimulate the production of cAMP; therefore, it will bypass the blockade applied by the beta-adrenergic blocking agent.** Beta-adrenergic blockers decrease heart rate (negative chronotrope) and decrease systolic blood pressure (negative inotrope) by indirectly reducing the production of cyclic adenosine monophosphate (cAMP), which inhibits the influx of calcium into muscle cells via the L-type calcium channels. Epinephrine would be less effective in this situation because the effect of the beta-adrenergic blocker is to specifically counter the function of catecholamines such as epinephrine. Calcium gluconate, although effective in calcium channel blocker overdose, would not overcome the cAMP reduction which allows calcium to use the calcium channel to enter the cells and would therefore be less effective on a beta-adrenergic blocker overdose. The digoxin immune fab is a specifically engineered molecule that binds to digoxin and renders it functionally inert but would have no effect on beta-adrenergic blocker overdoses.

55. Answer: A

Nursing Process: Intervention

Rationale: **Clonidine may stimulate the production of an opioid-like substance in high doses; therefore, the priority intervention of reversing the life-threatening depressant effects of opioids would be anticipated.** Clonidine is an imidazoline antihypertensive agent that stimulates alpha-adrenergic receptors in the central nervous system. Investigational uses include detoxification of opioid dependence. Calcium chloride, magnesium sulfate, and sodium bicarbonate would be neither indicated nor offer life-saving effect.

56. Answer: B

Nursing Process: Intervention

Rationale: Charcoal hemoperfusion is an extracorporeal technique by which blood is filtered through activated charcoal to remove toxins. **Unfortunately, this process only works on a limited number of substances including digitalis, paraquat, phenobarbital, Tegretol, and theophylline.** Methanol, amitriptyline, and Coumadin do not respond to charcoal hemoperfusion therapies. Charcoal hemoperfusion is different than hemodialysis. Alcohol ingestions can be treated with hemodialysis.

CENsational Pearl of Wisdom!

There are several very important interventions, just as hemoperfusion, which have quite limited applications. Just because they are not universal does not mean they do not provide a valuable therapy. Knowing the limitations of an intervention can often be key!

57. Answer: C

Nursing Process: Assessment

Rationale: **Constricted pupils would be a good assessment finding to help determine the likely ingestion was a narcotic and help the nurse provide definitive treatment promptly.** The toxidrome for opioids and sedative-hypnotics are nearly identical in that they both cause bradycardia, hypotension, hypothermia, decreased bowel sounds, bradypnea, and have no change in skin moisture. However, the difference between these two classes of medication is that opioids are known to cause constricted pupils, whereas sedative-hypnotics do not normally change pupil size. Bradycardia and absent bowel sounds are common with both types of ingestion and would not specifically assist with determining definitive treatment. Hypertension is not associated with either class of medication and would, therefore, not be anticipated.

58. Answer: D

Nursing Process: Evaluation

Rationale: **Resolution of hallucinations would indicate a reversal of the anticholinergic effects and, therefore, successful treatment.** Nightshade is known to have anticholinergic properties that may include tachycardia, dry skin, hyperthermia, psychosis and hallucinations, vasoconstriction, mydriasis (dilating pupils), increased blood sugar, and tachypnea. Physostigmine is a cholinergic agent which can be used to counter the effects of anticholinergic toxicity. Increased heart rate, elevated blood pressure, and dilated pupils are all signs of an anticholinergic effect and these effects, therefore, would not indicate success in treatment.

59. Answer: C

Nursing Process: Analysis

Rationale: **Salicylates create a direct stimulation of the $beta_2$-adrenergic receptors, leading to respiratory alkalosis which, in turn, drives calcium and potassium losses in the urine as carbon dioxide is lost in the respiratory drive.** Salicylates, such as Aspirin, are metabolized into salicylic acid and lead to, in overdoses, a profound metabolic acidosis. The acidosis is exacerbated through three primary mechanisms: loss of bicarbonate, inability to excrete phosphoric and sulfuric acids, and stimulation of gluconeogenesis and ketoacid production. Low serum pH, rather than elevated, would be consistent in this untreated situation. Hypoglycemia due to metabolism stimulation as oxidative phosphorylation is uncoupled by salicylate metabolites is more likely than elevated serum glucose. Although renal insufficiency may be seen, it is generally mild and would certainly not be anticipated to raise serum creatinine as high as 9.9 mg/dL.

60. Answer: D

Nursing Process: Intervention

Rationale: **Large quantities of activated charcoal, when given in a short period of time, are known to distend the stomach wall and stimulate gastric contraction and regurgitation. By giving smaller intermittent doses, this risk decreases. It is also easier for the patient to take in smaller doses.** Giving smaller intermittent doses of activated charcoal does not reduce the risk of developing a bowel obstruction nor does it increase the binding ability of the charcoal. Activated charcoal is not associated with electrolyte disturbances regardless of the rate at which it is administered.

CENsational Pearl of Wisdom!

Do not forget the basics. It is not always the flashy interventions or therapies that show up on the examination. Remembering your basic nursing interventions is vital for all certified emergency nurses!

61. Answer: C

Nursing Process: Evaluation

Rationale: **If the nurse notes constricted pupils, adequate anticholinergic intervention has not been reached and subsequent dose(s) should be administered.** Organophosphate agents act as cholinergic agonists and lead to symptoms which include vasodilation, decreased serum glucose, fluid production such as diaphoresis and bronchorrhea, constricted pupils, bradycardia, and bradypnea. Atropine, the antidote for organophosphate poisoning, is an anticholinergic agent and would counter the cholinergic (parasympathetic) symptoms of the exposure. Tachycardia; hot, dry skin; and dry mucous membranes would all be expected findings of the successful treatment with the anticholinergic medication.

62. Answer: A

Nursing Process: Analysis

Rationale: **Doxepin (Sinequan) is a tricyclic antidepressant (TCA) and its toxicity is associated with these changes.** Tricyclic antidepressants block voltage-gated sodium channels causing electrocardiogram changes such as prolonged PR interval, widened QRS complexes, and prolonged QT intervals. Diltiazem (Cardizem) is a calcium channel blocker and is associated with heart blocks and bradycardia which is not depicted in this strip. Propranolol (Inderal) and Carvedilol (Coreg) are a beta-adrenergic blockers and, similar to calcium channel blockers, leads to bradycardia and heart blocks.

CENsational Pearl of Wisdom!

Remember earlier I said there could be rhythms based on very specific conditions or toxicities? Here it is! TCAs have a specific pathophysiologic effect on sodium channels and create a very unique rhythm. Can you think of a few other examples? Like hyperkalemia? Hypomagnesemia?

63. Answer: B

Nursing Process: Analysis

Rationale: **Sudation is another term for diaphoresis and would be the most likely symptom of those listened.** Cocaine acts as a sympathomimetic agent and leads to stimulation of the adrenergic receptor sites. Symptoms may include vasoconstriction, hypertension, increased serum blood sugar, diaphoresis, dilation of the pupils, central nervous system stimulation or excitation, tachycardia, tachypnea, and decreased bowel motility. Miosis, constriction of the pupils, is not associated with cocaine toxicity. Catatonia, a state of stupor or psychomotor immobility, is not an expected effect of sympathomimetic overdose. Borborygmus, or bowel sounds, would not be an expected finding but rather a lack of bowel sounds would be more likely noted in this case.

CENsational Pearl of Wisdom!

Remember your diagnostic terms and anatomy and physiology definitions. Find ways to keep look-alike/sound-alike terms clear. For instance, do you have trouble with miosis and mydriasis? Try this: Miosis is the smaller word; the smaller word makes the smaller pupils—Miosis is pupillary constriction. Mydriasis is the larger word; the larger word makes the larger pupils. Or the "D" in mydriasis stands for "dilation." Mydriasis is pupillary dilation.

64. Answer: B

Nursing Process: Assessment

Rationale: **Lacrimation (tearing), respiratory crackles (due to stimulation of bronchial secretions), and miosis would all be symptoms consistent with this toxidrome.** Insecticides commonly work by stimulating muscarinic and nicotinic pathways of the parasympathetic nervous system and, therefore, are associated with symptoms of the cholinergic toxidrome. The cholinergic toxidrome includes constricted pupils (miosis), increased bowel motility, and increased fluid production. This toxidrome causes lability in heart rate, blood pressure, and respiration, which is to say it may produce high or low findings in each. Although urination and diarrhea would be expected findings, acidosis, rather than elevated serum pH, would be more likely due to gas exchange obstruction from fluid production in lungs and lactic acid production due to cellular hypoperfusion. Bradycardia may be typical in cholinergic exposures but muscle weakness, rather than cramping, and moist, rattling cough, rather than dry cough would be more likely in this scenario. And, finally, although drooling and defecation would be expected symptoms, increased bowel motility, rather than absent bowel sounds, would be a more anticipated symptom.

65. Answer: B

Nursing Process: Analysis

Rationale: **Dimercaprol (British anti-Lewisite) is a chelating agent used to treat heavy metal exposures including arsenic, lead, gold, and mercury.** Anthrax is a bacterial infection treated with long-course antibiotics such as ciprofloxacin or doxycycline and supportive care. Cyanide exposures are treated with hydroxocobalamin or with the classic cyanide kit which includes amyl nitrite, sodium nitrite, and sodium thiosulfate. Ethylene glycol is treated with ethanol to prevent liver metabolism of the alternate alcohol into toxic metabolites while treatments such as dialysis is implemented.

    CENsational Pearl of Wisdom!

Cyanide treatment with amyl nitrite, sodium nitrite, and sodium thiosulfate consists of causing a low level of methemoglobinemia—which is not a good thing—but better than cyanide poisoning! Cyanide likes methemoglobin much better and will bind with it to create cyanomethemoglobin. The sodium thiosulfate then creates thiocyanate and it is then excreted in the urine. Utilizing hydroxycobalamin creates cyanocobalamin, which is then excreted also through the renal system. Some significant side effects can occur when using hydroxycobalamin including hypertension, urine discoloration, and anaphylaxis and an inability to use with hemodialysis. It should also not be administered in the same line with medications such as diazepam (Valium), dopamine, or dobutamine.

Another important note is that patients with smoke inhalation should not receive the sodium nitrite unless the carboxyhemoglobin level is verified as under 10%. Otherwise, it can extend the effects of the CO, which would decrease the oxygen-carrying capacity of the patient's blood.

66. Answer: B

Nursing Process: Assessment

Rationale: **Symptoms of opioid toxicity include bradycardia, constricted pupils (miosis), hypotension, decreased body temperature, decreased bowel sounds,** **bradypnea, and decreased mental status.** Diarrhea, dilated pupils, tachypnea, diaphoresis, thready pulses (associated with vasoconstriction), hot and dry skin, and hyperthermia would not be associated with a patient who overdosed on an opioid substance.

67. Answer: A

Nursing Process: Intervention

Rationale: **Pulmonary complications would be the highest priority for interventions after decontamination stopped continued exposure.** Petroleum distillates, such as kerosene, lighter fluid, lamp oil, turpentine, and certain pesticides, pose a direct threat through ingestion, aspiration, and absorption through skin. The most life-threatening complications normally occur from aspiration and pulmonary problems. In this situation, the child potentially drank and then was subsequently exposed to the petroleum distillate through skin absorption. Complications to neurologic and cardiovascular systems would be possible but would result secondary to respiratory insufficiencies. The gastrointestinal tract may be altered, and problems may arise from exposure, but would not take priority over the pulmonary system.

68. Answer: D

Nursing Process: Evaluation

Rationale: **An increase in the patient's blood pressure is an indication of successful treatment.** Signs of calcium channel overdoses include hypotension (due to negative inotropic effects), bradycardia/heart blocks (due to negative chronotropic effects), decreased or altered level of consciousness (in response to both hypotension and bradycardia), nausea, vomiting, and hyperglycemia (resulting from pancreatic L-type calcium channel blockage and resultant insulin resistance in the cells). A decrease in the patient's heart rate and an increase in the patient's serum glucose levels all indicate that treatment is not working. The patient's temperature does not usually change with either the overdose of calcium channel blockers or the treatment for it.

69. Answer: A

Nursing Process: Assessment

Rationale: **The example of a sympathomimetic is phencyclidine (PCP).** The sympathomimetic class of medications are substances commonly referred to as "uppers" and include street drugs such as methamphetamine or cocaine, psychedelic agents such as phencyclidine (PCP) or D-lysergic acid diethylamide (LSD), and prescription medications such as albuterol, dopamine, or amitriptyline. Fentanyl is in the opioid class, physostigmine belongs to the cholinergic class, and gamma-hydroxybutyric acid (GHB) falls into the sedative-hypnotic toxidrome as a barbiturate.

70. Answer: D

Nursing Process: Evaluation

Rationale: **An increase in blood pressure would indicate successful treatment.** Symptoms of flunitrazepam (Rohypnol) overdose include CNS depression (amnesia, confusion, unconsciousness) and hypotension. Because CNS depression is a side effect of this drug, a decrease in agitation is not an indication of successful treatment. Depressed respiratory effort coupled with hypotension is likely to cause an acidosis with a low serum pH; therefore, a reduction in serum pH would not indicate effective treatment. Bradycardia is not a significant finding in this overdose; therefore, elevation in the heart rate is not associated with successful treatment.

71. Answer: B

Nursing Process: Evaluation

Rationale: **Reversal of opioid toxicity would likely cause the heart rate to increase, pupil size to increase, blood pressure to rise, bowel sounds to increase, and respirations to increase.** Moisture to the skin is not normally affected by opioids and would, therefore, not be expected to change when an opioid reversal agent is administered. Bradycardia is a symptom of opioid toxicity; therefore, naloxone administration would not cause further bradycardia and not prove that opioids were the cause. Requiring assisted ventilations would be indicated if the patient became bradypneic or otherwise had interruption of ventilations; therefore, this would not be expected if opioid toxicity were removed following administration of naloxone (Narcan).

 CENsational Pearl of Wisdom!

Remember that if Naloxone (Narcan) is going to work, it will occur within the first few minutes of administration. The patient will often awaken agitated and may require some strong arms to keep the person in the bed! The effects of Naloxone (Narcan) will last for about 20 to 90 minutes, after which the patient may require redosing.

72. Answer: D

Nursing Process: Intervention

Rationale: **It takes up to 24 hours for acetaminophen (Tylenol) to accumulate in the liver and cause liver damage; therefore, acetylcysteine (Mucomyst or Acetadote) can be given up to 24 hours after ingestion and still be effective.** Although acetylcysteine (Mucomyst or Acetadote) should be given earlier, such as 2 or 4 hours after ingestion, it is still effective up to 24 hours later. Acetylcysteine (Mucomyst) should not be given with charcoal, because charcoal will absorb acetylcysteine (Mucomyst) and prevent it from being absorbed into the body where it can effectively reduce acetaminophen (Tylenol) levels. Acetylcysteine (Mucomyst or Acetadote) should be given before liver enzymes elevate to prevent liver damage. Succimer (Chemet) is the chelating agent for lead poisoning. Flumazenil (Romazicon) is used to reverse the effects of benzodiazepines and Deferoxamine (Desferal) is the antidote for iron toxicity.

73. Answer: A

Nursing Process: Intervention

Rationale: **Deferoxamine (Desferal) is the antidote for iron. Prenatal vitamins are a common source of elemental iron.** Methamphetamine, tricyclic antidepressants such as nortriptyline, and nitroprusside are not treated with deferoxamine.

74. Answer: C

Nursing Process: Intervention

Rationale: **The highest priority intervention for this patient would be to restore serum glucose with a bolus of IV dextrose solution.** Sulfonylureas act by blocking potassium channels in pancreatic beta cells which results in additional insulin release. This excess insulin in the system can lead to life-threatening hypoglycemia in overdoses. Oral glucose would also meet this need, but it is contraindicated in a comatose patient because of the risk for aspiration. In addition, the 15 g of dextrose would be much slower to reach the cells and would, therefore, not take precedence over IV dextrose. Intravenous fluid bolusing would be helpful in a patient with hyperglycemia and subsequent volume depletion, but it would not be a result from a patient overdosing on a sulfonylurea medication. Octreotide would be a reversal agent for sulfonylurea overdose because it would stop the pancreas from secreting insulin; however, the immediate crisis in this situation is not the medication, but rather the hypoglycemic shock it has caused.

 CENsational Pearl of Wisdom!

Another example of multiple "good" choices, but understanding the situation and underlying pathophysiology helps you see which one is the priority in this situation. Be sure to read all of the question and take everything into account when reading the stem of the question! The answers lie within!

75. Answer: A

Nursing Process: Intervention

Rationale: **The cyanide antidote should be administered before decontaminating the GI tract or managing seizure activity.** Because cyanide is rapidly absorbed and causes cellular hypoxia, reversing the hypoxia takes priority. One method of treating cyanide is administering the classic cyanide kit which contains an amyl nitrite inhaler or ampule that can be broken and placed in the oxygen mask and sodium nitrite, both of which create methemoglobin and attract cyanide away from the respiratory enzyme cytochrome oxidase. Sodium thiosulfate is also used; it forms nontoxic thiocyanate and removes the cyanide from the body. Performing gastric lavage, giving activated charcoal, and managing seizures are not incorrect, but do not reverse the immediate life-threatening symptom of cellular hypoxia.

 CENsational Pearl of Wisdom!

Amyl nitrite and sodium nitrite both do the same thing! Utilize the amyl nitrite first, which then buys the emergency nurse time to start an intravenous line. Once the line is established, remove the amyl nitrite before administering the sodium nitrite. A low level of methemoglobinemia is desired. The reversal agent for methemoglobinemia is methylene blue. This is why this medication is also found in the cyanide kit. Symptoms of methemoglobinemia are presence of cyanosis with no respiratory distress or relief with administration of oxygen and blood draw that looks like chocolate.

References

Adal, A. (2018, January 6). *Heavy metal toxicity.* Medscape. Retrieved from https://emedicine.medscape.com/article/814960-overview (24, 34, 45, 65)

Benzer, T. I. (2015, December 29). *Gamma-hydroxybutyrate toxicity.* Medscape. Retrieved from https://emedicine.medscape.com/article/820531-overview (20, 70)

Björnsson, E. (2017). Hepatotoxicity by drugs: The most common implicated agents. *International Journal of Molecular Sciences, 17,* 224. Retrieved from ijms-17-00224-v2.pdf (48)

Buggs, A. M. (2017, October 18). *Emergent management of lead toxicity.* Medscape. Retrieved from https://emedicine.medscape.com/article/815399-overview (45)

Cohen, B., et al. (2013, December). Efficacy of urine alkalinization by oral administration of sodium bicarbonate: A prospective open-label trial. *The American Journal of Emergency Medicine, 31*(12), 1703–1706. doi:10.1016/j.ajem.2013. (8, 29, 31)

Cooper, J. S. (2015, December 29). *Sedative-hypnotic toxicity.* Medscape. Retrieved from https://emedicine.medscape.com/article/818430-overview (14, 20, 21, 30, 57, 70)

D'Orazio, J. L. (2018, May 30). *Hallucinogen toxicity.* Medscape. Retrieved from https://emedicine.medscape.com/article/814848-overview (36)

Emergency Nurses Association. (2017). Emergency nursing core curriculum (7th ed.). Chicago, IL: Elsevier Saunders. (1, 3, 11, 15, 19, 21, 24–26, 28, 34, 37, 40, 43, 46, 47, 51, 52, 56, 60, 63, 66, 67, 73)

Farrell, S. E. (2018, January 22). *Acetaminophen toxicity.* Medscape. Retrieved from https://emedicine.medscape.com/article/820200-overview (8, 23, 72)

Gresham, C. (2018, June 13). *Benzodiazepine toxicity.* Medscape. Retrieved from https://emedicine.medscape.com/article/813255-overview (14, 21, 30, 57)

Inna, L. (2018). *Cyanide toxicity treatment and toxicity.* Medscape. Retrieved from https://emedicine.medscape.com/article/814287-treatment#d (11)

Kathuria, P., et al. (2018, April 3). *Lead toxicity.* Medscape. Retrieved from https://emedicine.medscape.com/article/1174752-overview (45)

Katz, K. D. (2017, September 5). *Organophosphate toxicity.* Medscape. Retrieved from https://emedicine.medscape.com/article/167726-overview (4, 61)

Kearney, J. F. (2015, December 29). *Oxalate poisoning.* Medscape. Retrieved from https://emedicine.medscape.com/article/817016-overview (12, 27)

Keyes, D. C. (2017, December 5). *Ethylene glycol toxicity.* Medscape. Retrieved from https://emedicine.medscape.com/article/814701-overview (50)

Kolecki, P. (2018, July 17). *Sympathomimetic toxicity.* Medscape. Retrieved from https://emedicine.medscape.com/article/818583-overview (48, 53, 63, 69)

Korabathina, K., et al. (2017, January 30). *Methanol toxicity.* Medscape. Retrieved from https://emedicine.medscape.com/article/1174890-overview (5, 38)

Korosh Sharain, A. M. (2015, December). Chronic alcoholism and the danger of profound hypomagnesemia. *The American Journal of Medicine, 128*(12), e17–e18. doi:10.1016/j.amjmed.2015.06.051. (32)

Lafferty, K. A. (2017, January 14). *Barbiturate toxicity.* Medscape. Retrieved from https://emedicine.medscape.com/article/813155-overview (21, 29, 46, 69)

Levine, M. D., et al. (2017, December 17). *Alcohol toxicity.* Medscape. Retrieved from https://emedicine.medscape.com/article/812411-overview (5, 21, 32, 38, 44, 50)

Leybell, I., et al. (2018, January 2). *Cyanide toxicity.* Medscape. Retrieved from https://emedicine.medscape .com/article/814287-overview (43, 75)

Madhusmita, M. (2018, February). *Thyroid storm treatment and management.* Retrieved from https://emedicine .medscape.com/article/925147-treatment#d7 (13)

Medscape. *Acetylcystine.* Retrieved from https://reference .medscape.com/drug/acetadote-cetylev-antidote-acetylcysteine-antidote-343740#11 (8)

Olson, D. A. (2017, August 13). *Mercury toxicity.* Medscape. Retrieved from https://emedicine.medscape.com/ article/1175560-overview (24)

Olson, K. R. (2018, January 19). *Warfarin and superwarfarin toxicity.* Medscape. Retrieved from https://emedicine .medscape.com/article/821038-overview (10)

Patel, V., et al. (2017, January 4). *Digitalis toxicity.* Medscape. Retrieved from https://emedicine.medscape .com/article/154336-overview (7)

Ramnarine, M., et al. (2017, October 27). *Anticholinergic toxicity.* Medscape. Retrieved from https://emedicine .medscape.com/article/812644-overview (3, 16, 31, 58)

Rega, P. P. (2015, December 29). *LSD toxicity.* Medscape . Retrieved from https://emedicine.medscape.com/ article/1011615-overview (36)

Richards, J. R. (2017, December 26). *Methamphetamine toxicity.* Medscape. Retrieved from https://emedicine .medscape.com/article/820918-overview (48, 53, 63, 69)

Riley, D. (2017, December 15). *Clonidine toxicity.* Medscape. Retrieved from https://emedicine.medscape.com/ article/819776-overview (55)

Rosenbloom, M. (2017, December 26). *Vitamin toxicity.* Medscape. Retrieved from https://emedicine.medscape .com/article/819426-overview (25, 73)

Sharma, A. (2018, January 18). *Beta-blocker toxicity.* Medscape. Retrieved from https://emedicine.medscape .com/article/813342-overview (54)

Silverthorn, D. U. (2016). Human physiology: An integrated approach (7th ed.). Austin, TX: Pearson. (13, 15, 18, 19, 22, 30, 39, 44, 45, 48–50, 52, 54, 55, 59, 62, 64, 67, 74)

Spanierman, C. S. (2018, January 5). *Iron toxicity.* Medscape. Retrieved from https://emedicine.medscape .com/article/815213-overview (9, 25, 73)

Stephens, E. (2017, October 6). *Opioid toxicity.* Medscape. Retrieved from https://emedicine.medscape.com/ article/815784-overview (2, 6, 47, 55, 57, 66, 71)

Su, M., et al. (2017, April 27). *Anticholinergic poisoning.* UpToDate. Retrieved from https://www.uptodate.com/ contents/anticholinergic-poisoning (3, 16, 31, 58)

ToxTidbits. (2016, June). *The Maryland Poison Center's Monthly Update: Physostigmine for anticholinergic toxicity.* Retrieved from http://mdpoison.com/media/SOP/mdpoisoncom/ToxTidbits/2016/June%20 2016%20ToxTidbits.pdf (16)

Tsai, V., et al. (2017, December 12). *Tricyclic antidepressant toxicity.* Medscape. Retrieved from https://emedicine. medscape.com/article/819204-overview (11, 42, 51, 62)

Waseem, M., et al. (2017, December 20). *Salicylate toxicity.* Medscape. Retrieved from https://emedicine.medscape .com/article/1009987-overview (33, 59)

West, P. L. (2015, April 20). *Phencyclidine toxicity.* Medscape. Retrieved from https://emedicine.medscape .com/article/816348-overview (36)

Wolf, Y. (2017, August 24). *Rapid Review: Anticholinergic Toxidrome.* RoshReview. Retrieved from: https://www .roshreview.com/blog/rapid-review-anticholinergic-toxidrome/ (16)

Zimmermann, B. B. (2013). Sheehy's manual of emergency care (7th ed.). St. Louis, MO: Elsevier. (1–4, 9–11, 14–19, 21, 24–28, 31, 34–37, 40, 43–48, 51, 52, 56–58, 60–61, 63–67, 73)

6 Neurologic Emergencies

Cathy C. Fox, RN, CEN, CPEN, TCRN, FAEN

On the Certified Emergency Nurse (CEN) test, neurologic emergencies are included in the blueprint under "Neurological Emergencies." This portion of the actual test will comprise 16 questions spread across the spectrum of illnesses and injuries that affect this system. To prepare for the test effectively, this chapter will focus on potential test items related to the neurologic system.

Each of the following neurologic questions will be utilized as both a testing tool *and* as a teaching tool in the answer pages! Rationales for each correct answer and untrue answers are part of the teaching process. Additional information has been supplied in various areas to include some "CENsational Pearls of Wisdom!" to assist you as you prepare for the CEN examination.

1. A patient is brought into the emergency department after a spinal cord injury. He is unable to move below the level of the injury. An indwelling urinary catheter is inserted because:
[ ] **A.** the bladder is areflexic.
[ ] **B.** the patient is unable to ambulate.
[ ] **C.** voluntary reflex bladder emptying occurs.
[ ] **D.** hematuria may be present.

2. A patient arrives via EMS in full tonic-clonic seizures. His airway is patent and suction is at the bedside. The patients' phenytoin (Dilantin) level is 3 µg/mL. Normal is 10 to 20 µg/mL. The emergency nurse is ready to infuse phenytoin (Dilantin) 1 g (1,000 mg) via intravenous (IV) line. The emergency nurse should infuse this medication in:
[ ] **A.** Dextrose 5% in water as quickly as possible.
[ ] **B.** 3% normal saline at 75 mL/minute.
[ ] **C.** 0.9% normal saline at 50 mL/minute.
[ ] **D.** lactated ringer's solution at 100 mL/minute

3. A patient presents to the emergency department complaining of pain in her jaw. The emergency nurse notes facial drooping to the corner of the mouth on the left side. Which of the following cranial nerves (CN) is affected?
[ ] **A.** Cranial nerve VI (Abducens)
[ ] **B.** Cranial nerve VIII (Acoustic)
[ ] **C.** Cranial nerve V (Trigeminal)
[ ] **D.** Cranial nerve III (Oculomotor)

4. A provider has just asked the patient "How many fingers do you see?" This question is assessing which of the following cranial nerves?
[ ] **A.** Cranial nerve II (Optic)
[ ] **B.** Cranial nerve III (Oculomotor)
[ ] **C.** Cranial nerve IV (Trochlear)
[ ] **D.** Cranial nerve VI (Abducens)

5. During a neurologic examination, the patient is unable to raise his eyebrows or close his eyes tightly against resistance. Which of the following cranial nerves might be damaged?
[ ] **A.** Cranial nerve II (Optic)
[ ] **B.** Cranial nerve V (Trigeminal)
[ ] **C.** Cranial nerve VII (Facial)
[ ] **D.** Cranial nerve XII (Hypoglossal)

6. An 8-month-old presents with a hematoma on his head. According to developmental milestones, which of the following is the most likely explanation for the hematoma?
[ ] **A.** He fell off a slide while playing.
[ ] **B.** He fell while pulling up to a standing position.
[ ] **C.** He climbed out of his crib.
[ ] **D.** He bumped into a coffee table while walking.

7. A 13-year-old presents with a laceration to the occiput after a fall with numbness and tingling to the extremities. Which of the following is the priority nursing intervention?
[ ] **A.** Assess the airway while maintaining cervical spine immobilization.
[ ] **B.** Insert two large-bore IVs and administer a normal saline bolus.
[ ] **C.** Apply a pressure dressing and obtain a type and crossmatch.
[ ] **D.** Place the patient on a cardiac monitor and pulse oximetry.

8. A 4-month-old presents with decreased feeding and increased somnolence. He has had two episodes of vomiting in the last 3 hours. Vital signs are as follows:

Blood pressure—108/38 mm Hg
Pulse—66 beats/minute
Respirations—30 breaths/minute
Temperature—97.0° F (36.1° C)

Which of the following is the most likely cause of these symptoms?
[ ] **A.** Dehydration
[ ] **B.** Increased intracranial pressure
[ ] **C.** Autonomic dysreflexia
[ ] **D.** Increased intra-abdominal pressure

9. A 5-week-old is brought in by his parents for concern of fever and being inconsolable at home. Upon assessment, the emergency nurse notes that the infant is irritable, exhibits a high-pitched cry, has areas of purpura on his extremities, and has a rectal temperature of 102.0° F (38.9° C). Which of the following are these signs and symptoms most consistent with?
[ ] **A.** Henoch-Schönlein purpura
[ ] **B.** Meningococcemia
[ ] **C.** Idiopathic thrombocytopenic purpura
[ ] **D.** Kawasaki disease

10. A patient presents to the triage desk 20 hours after a motorcycle crash without a helmet. The emergency nurse notes bruising to the mastoid process and periorbital ecchymosis. Which of the following types of head injury is most likely?
[ ] **A.** Epidural hematoma
[ ] **B.** Subdural hematoma
[ ] **C.** Depressed skull fracture
[ ] **D.** Basilar skull fracture

11. Which of the following patients is most at risk for a diagnosis of encephalitis?
[ ] **A.** A 16-year-old with nuchal rigidity and a headache. He has not had a tetanus immunization since his childhood immunizations.
[ ] **B.** A 4-year-old with nuchal rigidity and a headache. She is behind in her immunization schedule and is recovering from chicken pox.
[ ] **C.** An 8-year-old with a recent history of a viral illness and has been being medicated with aspirin for fever control.
[ ] **D.** A 9-year-old with a recent history of a viral illness diagnosed as measles. No medication has been used in this child.

12. A young adult presents to the emergency department complaining of numbness and paresthesia of her hands and feet, as well as lower leg muscle weakness. She works as a child care provider and had a recent viral illness. Which of the following disease processes is the highest probability for this patient?
[ ] **A.** Myasthenia gravis
[ ] **B.** Guillain-Barré syndrome
[ ] **C.** Botulism poisoning
[ ] **D.** Organophosphate poisoning

13. Four patients with the complaint of headache present to the triage desk within minutes of each other. Which of the following statements made by these patients would indicate the most emergent situation?
[ ] **A.** "I have a throbbing headache that's been coming on for several days. Can you turn off the lights?"
[ ] **B.** "This terrible headache hit me so quick while I was watching TV. It's getting worse and now I'm throwing up."
[ ] **C.** "I have a really bad headache and my neck hurts. I've been so stressed lately."
[ ] **D.** "I tripped over a rug and have a laceration on my head. It bled a lot and sure hurts."

14. Which of the following are typical signs of increased intracranial pressure?
[ ] **A.** Decreased pulse rate and decreased respiratory rate
[ ] **B.** Numbness of fingers and decreased temperature
[ ] **C.** Increased pulse rate and decreased blood pressure
[ ] **D.** Decreased mentation and increased respiratory rate

15. A patient suffered a thoracic-level spinal injury from a diving accident. To initiate cardiopulmonary resuscitation (CPR) at the poolside, which of the following measures would be most important?

[ ] **A.** Hyperextend the neck to clear the airway before mouth-to-mouth resuscitation.

[ ] **B.** Administer CPR in a prone position.

[ ] **C.** Do not administer CPR after a head injury.

[ ] **D.** Elevate the mandible with a jaw thrust to assess airway with the head in a neutral position.

16. A paraplegic patient presents to the emergency department complaining of a headache. He is noted to be flushed and is sweating profusely. Which of the following should be the first action for this patient?

[ ] **A.** Apply compression stockings.

[ ] **B.** Lower his head to increase cerebral circulation.

[ ] **C.** Massage lower extremities to cause vasodilation.

[ ] **D.** Assess for a blocked urinary catheter.

17. Which of the following would be the first intervention when assisting a patient experiencing a tonic-clonic seizure?

[ ] **A.** Place a tongue blade between the patient's teeth.

[ ] **B.** Restrain the patient from all movements to avoid injury.

[ ] **C.** Turn the patient onto their side and observe them.

[ ] **D.** Protect the patient from hitting their arms against close objects.

18. Which of the following would be the primary nursing goal when caring for a 4-year-old with meningitis?

[ ] **A.** Increase stimulation opportunities to prevent coma.

[ ] **B.** Provide an opportunity for therapeutic play.

[ ] **C.** Reduce the pain related to nuchal rigidity.

[ ] **D.** Place a urinary catheter to monitor urine output.

19. A 1-year-old girl has experienced a febrile seizure. Which of the following statements made by the parents would indicate that they understood the discharge instructions regarding temperature control?

[ ] **A.** "We will use alcohol baths if her temperature gets too high."

[ ] **B.** "We will keep her temperature down with tepid sponge baths and acetaminophen (Tylenol)."

[ ] **C.** "We will give her the phenobarbital when the temperature is above 101° F (38.3° C)."

[ ] **D.** "We will use ice baths if her temperature goes up and we cannot get it to come down."

20. A patient presents with a known history of migraine headaches. The emergency nurse prepares for which of the following treatment regimens?

[ ] **A.** IV fluid bolus, antiemetic, and Morphine

[ ] **B.** IV fluid bolus, hydromorphone (Dilaudid), and antiemetic

[ ] **C.** Antihistamine, antiemetic, and IV fluid bolus

[ ] **D.** Antihistamine, Nitroglycerin sublingual, and IV fluid bolus

21. When asking health history questions about the child admitted with Reye's syndrome, which of the following would be considered a common finding?

[ ] **A.** Parental administration of acetaminophen for fever

[ ] **B.** Recent streptococcal infection

[ ] **C.** Recent sickle cell crisis

[ ] **D.** Recent influenza illness with aspirin administration

22. An infant with a high-pitched cry, irritability, and fever is being prepped for a lumbar puncture (LP). Which of the following is an appropriate position for this patient during this procedure?

[ ] **A.** Lateral with knees to chest and chin to chest

[ ] **B.** Lateral with legs extended and arms above the head

[ ] **C.** Placing the patient in the prone position

[ ] **D.** Placing the patient in the supine position

23. A patient with suspected bacterial meningitis had a lumbar puncture (LP) with cerebral spinal fluid (CSF) sent to the laboratory for evaluation. The emergency nurse would suspect which of the following laboratory values?

[ ] **A.** Increased WBC, increased protein, and decreased glucose

[ ] **B.** Increased WBC, increased protein, and increased glucose

[ ] **C.** Decreased WBC, decreased protein, and increased glucose

[ ] **D.** Decreased WBC, decreased protein, and decreased glucose

24. A patient presents with hemiplegia that started 1 hour before arrival. A computed tomography (CT) scan of the head is negative and the physician has ordered administration of tissue plasminogen activator (TPA/Activase). The emergency nurse knows that which of the following is the maximum dose of TPA?

[ ] **A.** 80 mg

[ ] **B.** 90 mg

[ ] **C.** 120 mg

[ ] **D.** No maximum, because the dosage is based on weight.

25. Receptive aphasia results from damage to which area of the brain?
[ ] **A.** Parietal lobe
[ ] **B.** Occipital lobe
[ ] **C.** Temporal lobe
[ ] **D.** Frontal lobe

26. During neurosurgical evaluation of an unresponsive patient, the physician evaluates the oculocephalic reflex (doll's eye phenomenon). When the head is rotated to the left, the patient's eyes also move to the left. What does this finding indicate?
[ ] **A.** No abnormality
[ ] **B.** Damage to Cranial Nerve I (Olfactory)
[ ] **C.** Damage to the fovea
[ ] **D.** A lesion on the brain stem

27. Which of the following would be the primary intervention for a patient complaining of headache and neck pain and does not recall events leading up to his arrival in the emergency department? On arrival, the patient has a Glasgow Coma Scale of 14. A hematoma is palpated from the occipital to the frontal skull areas.
[ ] **A.** Perform a complete head-to-toe assessment.
[ ] **B.** Apply cervical immobilization.
[ ] **C.** Administer opioid analgesics for complaints of pain.
[ ] **D.** Obtain a specimen to determine blood alcohol level.

28. Thirty minutes after a patient is admitted to the emergency department, the emergency nurse performs a repeat neurologic examination. The patient does not follow commands, but after several attempts by the nurse to apply noxious stimuli, he opens his eyes and moves the nurse's hand. The patient utters a one-word response to the nurse. Which of the following is the correct Glasgow Coma Scale for this patient?
[ ] **A.** 5
[ ] **B.** 7
[ ] **C.** 10
[ ] **D.** 12

29. Which of the following signs and symptoms would indicate the presence of a spinal cord injury?
[ ] **A.** Hypertension with tachycardia
[ ] **B.** Numbness and tingling in the extremities
[ ] **C.** Cloudy cerebrospinal fluid (CSF)
[ ] **D.** Presence of exophthalmos

30. Which of the following conditions indicates an ovoid-shaped pupil?
[ ] **A.** Traumatic orbital injury
[ ] **B.** Intracranial hypertension
[ ] **C.** History of cataract surgery
[ ] **D.** Pontine hemorrhage

31. A patient receiving pharmacologic medications for combativeness associated with a head injury responds to noxious stimuli only. Which of the following scores on the Ramsay Score for Sedation (RASS) would be documented?
[ ] **A.** 1
[ ] **B.** 3
[ ] **C.** 5
[ ] **D.** 15

32. In an adult patient with head injuries, which of the following medications can be administered before sedating the patient with succinylcholine (Anectine)?
[ ] **A.** Atropine
[ ] **B.** Ketamine (Ketalar)
[ ] **C.** Lidocaine (Xylocaine)
[ ] **D.** Meperidine (Demerol)

33. Which of the following assessment findings would be associated with a patient with an intracranial pressure (ICP) reading of 35 mm Hg?
[ ] **A.** Narrowed pulse pressure
[ ] **B.** Hypothermia
[ ] **C.** Cheyne-Stokes respirations
[ ] **D.** Kussmaul's respirations

34. Which of the following interventions will decrease elevated intracranial pressure (ICP)?
[ ] **A.** Frequent suctioning of the airway
[ ] **B.** Administering morphine for pain
[ ] **C.** Maintaining the patient in trendelenburg position
[ ] **D.** Administering mannitol (Osmitrol)

35. Which of the following is **NOT** an early symptom of multiple sclerosis (MS)?
[ ] **A.** Diplopia
[ ] **B.** Scotomas
[ ] **C.** Weakness
[ ] **D.** Paralysis

36. A patient is brought to the emergency department by ambulance with a chief complaint of lethargy. Two days before the patient was in a high-speed motor vehicle accident and refused care. Since that time, she has complained of headaches and drowsiness. Her friend states that it has now become difficult to wake her up. Assessment reveals a right pupil that is fixed and dilated with papilledema present. The Glasgow Coma Scale score is 8. Which of the following types of injury does this patient exhibit?
[ ] **A.** Subdural hematoma
[ ] **B.** Epidural hematoma
[ ] **C.** Diffuse axonal injury
[ ] **D.** Postconcussion syndrome

37. Which of the following areas of the brain controls the respiratory and cardiac systems?
[ ] **A.** Medulla
[ ] **B.** Frontal lobe
[ ] **C.** Diencephalon
[ ] **D.** Hypothalamus

38. Which of the following is a potential complication when utilizing succinylcholine (Anectine) for rapid sequence intubation (RSI) in a patient diagnosed with Guillan-Barre?
[ ] **A.** Hypernatremia
[ ] **B.** Hyperkalemia
[ ] **C.** Hypokalemia
[ ] **D.** Hyponatremia

39. Which of the following head injuries results in a collection of blood between the skull and the dura mater?
[ ] **A.** Subdural hematoma
[ ] **B.** Subarachnoid hemorrhage
[ ] **C.** Epidural hematoma
[ ] **D.** Contusion

40. A mother brings her 1-year-old child, who fell down the stairs 2 hours ago, to the emergency department. The child is dirty and wearing clothing that is inappropriate for the cold weather. The child cries when the head and neck are palpated. Bruises at various stages of healing are noted on the buttocks and back. As the physician enters the room, the child begins seizing. This child should be evaluated for which of the following conditions?
[ ] **A.** Coagulation disorder
[ ] **B.** Meningitis
[ ] **C.** Subdural hematoma
[ ] **D.** Leukemia

41. A patient with a diagnosis of ischemic stroke is being prepped for the initiation of tissue plasminogen activator (TPA).. The patient is on the cardiac monitor. Oxygen has been applied at 2 L/nasal cannula. Labetalol (Normodyne) 5 mg intravenous was administered. A light, warm blanket has been applied. Which of the following would indicate that proper interventions have been completed that allow for the administration of this medication?
[ ] **A.** Pulse rate of 120 beats/minute
[ ] **B.** Blood pressure of 168/98 mm Hg
[ ] **C.** Pulse oximetry reading of 94%
[ ] **D.** Temperature of 98.6° F (37° C)

42. Which of the following would be an ominous sign in a 1-year-old child with a possible neck injury?
[ ] **A.** Heart rate of 60 beats/minute
[ ] **B.** Respiratory rate of 30 breaths/minute
[ ] **C.** Capillary refill time of 3 seconds
[ ] **D.** Positive Babinski's reflex

43. While caring for a patient with a ventriculostomy, the emergency nurse notices that the intracranial pressure (ICP) reading is 30 mm Hg. The emergency nurse assesses the patient and the ICP monitor and determines that the drain is open. Which of the following would be the appropriate immediate intervention for this patient?
[ ] **A.** Move the head from a rotated position to the midline.
[ ] **B.** Lower the head of the bed to the Trendelenburg position.
[ ] **C.** Close the stopcock on the ventriculostomy.
[ ] **D.** Elevate the head of the bed to high Fowler's position.

44. A patient involved in a 20-foot fall sustains a fracture with spinal cord transection at the level of C_6. This injury will result in which of the following findings?
[ ] **A.** Quadriplegia with diaphragmatic breathing and gross arm movements
[ ] **B.** Quadriplegia with total loss of respiratory function
[ ] **C.** Paraplegia with variable loss of intercostal and abdominal muscle use
[ ] **D.** Paraplegia with loss of bowel and bladder function

45. All of the following can be used for blood pressure control for the cerebral vascular accident (CVA) patient **EXCEPT**:
[ ] **A.** Nicardipine (Cardene)
[ ] **B.** Nitroprusside (Nipride)
[ ] **C.** Labetalol (Normodyne)
[ ] **D.** Cardizem (Diltiazem)

46. Which of the following statements made by a patient being discharged with a new prescription for phenytoin (Dilantin) indicates that the patient understands their instructions?
[ ] **A.** "I know that if I miss a routine dose I cannot easily make it up."
[ ] **B.** "I am glad to know that I won't have to have routine lab tests."
[ ] **C.** "I am aware that if I stop taking this medication I am at risk for status epilepticus."
[ ] **D.** "It's good that I don't have to worry about a bunch of adverse effects from this drug."

47. Which of the following would be the priority action if an ischemic stroke patient receiving tissue plasminogen activator (TPA) infusion begins to vomit bright red blood?
[ ] **A.** Notify the physician.
[ ] **B.** Place a nasogastric tube.
[ ] **C.** Decrease the infusion.
[ ] **D.** Stop the infusion.

48. Which of the following is **NOT** a clinical manifestation of Parkinson's disease?
[ ] **A.** Shuffling gait
[ ] **B.** Bradykinesia
[ ] **C.** Rigidity
[ ] **D.** Alopecia

49. Which of the following medications is commonly used to treat the symptoms of Parkinson's disease?
[ ] **A.** Pramipexole (Mirapex)
[ ] **B.** Reserpine (Serpalan)
[ ] **C.** Haloperidol (Haldol)
[ ] **D.** Valproic acid (Depakote)

50. The National Institutes for Health Stroke Scale (NIHSS) can be linked to outcomes. Which of the following indicates the meaning of the higher scoring?
[ ] **A.** Better outcome
[ ] **B.** Better orientation
[ ] **C.** Increased risk factors
[ ] **D.** Poorer outcome

51. A 28-year-old woman comes to the emergency department with blurred vision and drooping of the right eyelid. She also complains of intermittent episodes of muscle weakness and states that at times her neck does not feel strong enough to support her head. She tires when eating and takes frequent breaks during a meal. Several times, she has had to close her mouth using her hand because "the muscles in my face feel so weak." Which of the following is the probable diagnosis for this patient?
[ ] **A.** Myasthenia gravis
[ ] **B.** Bell's palsy
[ ] **C.** Trigeminal neuralgia
[ ] **D.** Glioblastoma

52. Which of the following tests is frequently used to diagnose myasthenia gravis?
[ ] **A.** Lumbar puncture
[ ] **B.** Tensilon test
[ ] **C.** Allen's test
[ ] **D.** Magnetic resonance imaging (MRI)

53. Which of the following medications is **NOT** used to reduce the spasticity or pain associated with multiple sclerosis (MS)?
[ ] **A.** Diazepam (Valium)
[ ] **B.** Baclofen (Lioresal)
[ ] **C.** Gabapentin (Neurontin)
[ ] **D.** Cyclophosphamide (Cytoxan)

54. Alzheimer's disease is characterized by profound impairment of cognitive functions. Which of the following is the cause of this disorder?
[ ] **A.** Destruction of motor cells in the pyramidal tracts
[ ] **B.** Metabolic disorder involving the adrenal glands
[ ] **C.** Cerebral atrophy and cellular degeneration
[ ] **D.** Degeneration of the basal ganglia

55. An emergency nurse is caring for a patient who has suffered a closed head injury and has elevated intracranial pressure (ICP). Which of the following guidelines should the nurse follow when maintaining the patency of the endotracheal tube?
[ ] **A.** Suction every 2 hours
[ ] **B.** Instill normal saline before suctioning
[ ] **C.** Lower the head of the bed before suctioning
[ ] **D.** Suction only when necessary

56. A patient with complaints of seeing "zigzagging lines" in her visual field after waking this morning presents to the emergency department. She now complains of a right temporal headache accompanied by nausea and photosensitivity. Based on these symptoms, the patient is evaluated for which of the following conditions?
[ ] **A.** Sinusitis
[ ] **B.** Meningitis
[ ] **C.** Migraine headache
[ ] **D.** Trigeminal neuralgia

57. Which of the following medications is utilized as preventative treatment for migraine headache?
[ ] **A.** Propranolol (Inderal)
[ ] **B.** Ondansetron (Zofran)
[ ] **C.** Codeine
[ ] **D.** Diphenhydramine (Benadryl)

58. A patient is prescribed ergotamine (Cafergot) for treatment of her headache. This medication has a cumulative effect that increases the risk of drug overdose. Clinical manifestations of ergotamine overdose (ergotism) include which of the following symptoms?
[ ] **A.** Diplopia
[ ] **B.** Hypotension
[ ] **C.** Numbness
[ ] **D.** Ataxic gait

59. A patient arrives by ambulance for evaluation of seizure activity after falling on the ground while engaged in an argument with his employer. He is screaming and violently flinging his extremities. No evidence of incontinence or tongue biting is present. Prehospital providers state that this episode has lasted for 40 minutes. Based on this information, this patient is most likely to be diagnosed with which of the following conditions?

[ ] **A.** Pseudoseizures
[ ] **B.** Absence (petit mal) seizures
[ ] **C.** Tonic-clonic (grand mal) seizures
[ ] **D.** Focal seizures

60. Temporary periods of cerebral ischemia may result in symptoms associated with which of the following conditions?

[ ] **A.** Transient ischemic attacks (TIAs)
[ ] **B.** Hypercapneic encephalopathy
[ ] **C.** Disequilibrium syndrome
[ ] **D.** Transtentorial herniation

61. Which of the following medications is used to treat an acute cerebrovascular accident (stroke)?

[ ] **A.** Tissue Plasminogen Activator (TPA)
[ ] **B.** Tenecteplase (TNK)
[ ] **C.** Reteplase (Retevase)
[ ] **D.** Streptokinase (Streptase)

62. Which of the following responses from a new emergency nurse on an orientation test would indicate knowledge of the neurologic problem related to difficulty in transforming sound into patterns of understandable speech?

[ ] **A.** Receptive aphasia
[ ] **B.** Dysphagia
[ ] **C.** Expressive aphasia
[ ] **D.** Apraxia

63. The emergency nurse is discharging a patient with a probable diagnosis of Alzheimer's versus dementia. Which of the following statements made by the family indicates an understanding of the explanations provided to them?

[ ] **A.** "We understand that hallucinations and delusions are not as common as with other forms of dementia."
[ ] **B.** "We know that he is losing his mental abilities and this will interfere with his daily activities and social interactions."
[ ] **C.** "We are glad to know that there are medications out there that we will discuss with his doctor that will cure him."
[ ] **D.** "We understand that this disease called Alzheimer's is not very common for dementia patients."

64. Which of the following is one of the most malignant and rapidly growing forms of brain tumor?

[ ] **A.** Astrocytoma
[ ] **B.** Meningioma
[ ] **C.** Neuroma
[ ] **D.** Glioblastoma

65. Children below the age of 8 years are most likely to injure which portion of the vertebral column?

[ ] **A.** C_6 to C_7
[ ] **B.** C_1 to C_3
[ ] **C.** C_5 to C_6
[ ] **D.** C_7 exclusively

66. Which of the following is an important anatomical consideration for an infant regarding the potential of hypovolemia related to head and neck trauma?

[ ] **A.** Open suture lines
[ ] **B.** Lax neck muscles
[ ] **C.** Large head
[ ] **D.** Short trachea

67. Clinical symptoms of autonomic dysreflexia include headache, profuse sweating, piloerection (gooseflesh), hypertension, and bradycardia. This syndrome occurs in patients with injuries at or above which of the following levels?

[ ] **A.** S_5
[ ] **B.** L_1
[ ] **C.** T_6
[ ] **D.** T_{12}

68. A patient is being treated in the emergency department after a high-speed motor vehicle crash. He is complaining of pain to his lower thoracic spine area and is paralyzed from the waist down. He is noted to have hypotension. Computed tomography (CT) demonstrates a fracture at T_9. Which of the following is the most probable reason for his hypotension?

[ ] **A.** Neurogenic shock
[ ] **B.** Hypovolemic shock
[ ] **C.** Septic shock
[ ] **D.** Spinal shock

69. Which of the following is the most common manifestation of central cord syndrome?

[ ] **A.** Quadriplegia
[ ] **B.** Priapism
[ ] **C.** Upper extremity paralysis
[ ] **D.** Poikilothermia

70. Which of the following types of medications would be prescribed for a patient diagnosed with temporal arteritis?
[ ] **A.** Steroids
[ ] **B.** Anticonvulsants
[ ] **C.** Muscle relaxants
[ ] **D.** Antihistamines

71. Which of the following symptoms is associated with a cluster headache?
[ ] **A.** Tearing
[ ] **B.** Fever
[ ] **C.** Aphasia
[ ] **D.** Epistaxis

72. A patient presents to the triage desk and states, "This is the worst headache of my life." The patient is well known by the staff with a past history of migraine headaches and hypertension. He is vomiting on arrival. He requests to have the lights off in his room, and on assessment, the emergency nurse notes that his speech is abnormal. The patient is rubbing the back of his neck and he states that it "just hurts so much when I move my head down." All of the following make this person high risk for a catastrophic event **EXCEPT**:
[ ] **A.** intensity of the headache.
[ ] **B.** pain to the posterior neck area.
[ ] **C.** history of migraine headaches.
[ ] **D.** speech abnormalities.

73. When evaluating parameters, which of the following would have the most negative impact on a patient with a closed head injury?
[ ] **A.** Blood pressure—90/42 mm Hg
[ ] **B.** Cerebral perfusion pressure—85 mm Hg
[ ] **C.** Urine output—48 mL in 1 hour
[ ] **D.** Serum osmolality—280 mOsm

74. A patient with a ventriculostomy in place is noted to have an increasing intracranial pressure. Which of the following corrections would help remedy this situation?
[ ] **A.** Turn the head to the right.
[ ] **B.** Place the patient supine.
[ ] **C.** Remove C-Collar on neck.
[ ] **D.** Increase activity in the room.

75. Which of the following is the earliest indicator of change in a patient's neurologic status?
[ ] **A.** Pupillary reaction
[ ] **B.** Motor response
[ ] **C.** Capillary refill
[ ] **D.** Level of consciousness (LOC)

Answers/Rationales

1. Answer: A

Nursing Process: Intervention
Rationale: **After a spinal cord injury, the bladder will lose nerve innervation to sense when the bladder is full. The bladder becomes areflexic, which is why many spinal cord injured patients require straight catherization or an indwelling urinary catheter.** A patient who is unable to ambulate may still be able to urinate. Voluntary reflex bladder emptying may occur at the time of the initial injury to the spinal column, especially if the bladder is full upon injury or trauma but is not a reason to insert a urinary catheter. Hematuria is not always present in a spinal column injury patient and may indicate a urologic injury.

2. Answer: C

Nursing Process: Intervention
Rationale: **Phenytoin (Dilantin) must be mixed in normal saline and administered via an intravenous pump at no greater than 50 mg/minute. It can also be mixed in lactated ringer's solution, but the rate of the infusion is too fast in this option.**

If phenytoin (Dilantin) is mixed in dextrose, it will crystalize and render the medication and fluid unable to administer. Never give phenytoin (Dilantin) rapid IV push because it can drop the blood pressure, increase drowsiness, and may cause cardiac dysrhythmias. It would be inappropriate to mix 3% normal saline as this would not routinely be given unless there was an issue with possible head injury or severe hyponatremia and it is not an appropriate diluent for Phenytoin (Dilantin).

 CENsational Pearl of Wisdom!

Administering phenytoin (Dilantin) often requires a slower rate than the recommended 50-mg/minute because of the pain that it causes the patient. Remember to check with the patient as they may not offer that it is extremely painful. Fosphenytoin (Cerebyx) can be given faster—at 150 mg/minute, and is not venous irritating/painful, so, it is a good alternative for the phenytoin (Dilantin). Both medications must be monitored for hypotension and cardiac dysrhythmias.

3. Answer: C

Nursing Process: Analysis

Rationale: **Cranial nerve V (Trigeminal) deals with facial, cheek, and chin movement.** Cranial nerve III (Oculomotor) constricts the pupil and is responsible for helping with eyeball movement. Cranial nerve VI (Abducens) rotates the eyeball outward, and cranial nerve VIII (Acoustic) deals with hearing and balance.

 CENsational Pearl of Wisdom!

Cranial Nerves Mnemonic and Functions			
On	I	Olfactory	Smell
Old	II	Optic	Visual acuity, count fingers, and dark vs. light
Olympus	III	Oculomotor	Constricts pupil, opens eyelid, extraocular eye movements (EOMs)
Towering	IV	Trochlear	Look down and outward (EOMs)
Tops	V	Trigeminal	Forehead, cheek, and chin movement and sensation, jaw movement
A	VI	Abducens	Rotates eyeball outward (EOMs)
Fin	VII	Facial	Smile, closes the eyelid, raising eyebrows, facial movement, tears, and saliva production
And	VIII	Acoustic (vestibulocochlear)	Hearing and balance
German	IX	Glossopharyngeal	Swallow and gag reflex
Viewed	X	Vagus	Swallowing, parasympathetic responses of heart, lungs, and abdominal viscera
Some	XI	Spinal accessory	Shoulder shrug and head turning
Hops	XII	Hypoglossal	Tongue movement, speech, and swallowing

4. Answer: A

Nursing Process: Assessment

Rationale: **Cranial nerve II, the Optic nerve, assesses visual acuity, dark versus light, and the counting of fingers.** Cranial nerve III, Oculomotor, gives the eye the ability to constrict the pupils, move the eyeball, and open the eyelid. Cranial nerve IV, Trochlear, allows the eye to look downward and outward and cranial nerve VI, Abducens, assists the eyeball to rotate outward.

 CENsational Pearl of Wisdom!

The cranial nerves that move the eyeball are CN III, CN IV, and CN VI (Oculomotor, Trochlear, and Abducens). These nerves are responsible for the muscles that innervate the globe. A mnemonic to help remember this is: "3,4,6 makes my eyes do tricks!" PS—Remember this one! You might need to recall it for the test!

5. Answer: C

Nursing Process: Assessment

Rationale: **The Facial nerve, CN VII, controls facial expression and taste in the anterior two-thirds of the tongue. This nerve has five branches and the temporal branch allows the patient to raise their eyebrows and close their eyes.** The other branches are the zygomatic, buccal, mandibular, and cervical. CN II, the Optic nerve, allows the patient to have vision, perceive light, and constrict the pupil. CN V, the Trigeminal nerve, controls jaw movement and facial sensation. CN XII, the Hypoglossal nerve, controls tongue movement.

 CENsational Pearl of Wisdom!

Cranial nerves V (Trigeminal) and VII (Facial) should be assessed when dealing with trigeminal neuralgia and Bell's palsy, CVA, or possible TIA.

(continued)

Bell's palsy is usually manifested by unilateral facial paralysis, inability to close one eye or move facial muscles, drooling, and pain behind the ear. The extremities are not affected. Trigeminal neuralgia is manifested as sudden, severe pains associated with one of the branches of CN V. At times, a "tic" or muscle spasm accompanies the pain. Usually a computed tomography (CT) is performed to rule out stroke.

6. Answer: B

Nursing Process: Analysis

Rationale: **Developmental milestones for 7 to 12 months old include pulling themselves up to a standing position and then cruising along a stationary item depending on emerging or advanced skill level.** An 8-month-old cannot climb a slide and does not possess the fine motor dexterity to climb out of a crib unassisted or walk independently.

7. Answer: A

Nursing Process: Intervention

Rationale: **Assessment of the pediatric trauma patient should always begin with inspecting the airway and maintaining cervical spine stabilization. With a presentation of numbness and tingling in the extremities, the patient is at great risk for spinal cord injury.** Although intravenous access may be important, there is nothing to indicate that this patient is in need of a normal saline bolus nor is it the first priority for this patient. The dressing may also be necessary, but again there is nothing that indicates the bleeding is uncontrolled requiring blood replacement. The cardiac monitor and pulse oximetry are good care options, but the airway and cervical spine issues are the highest priority.

8. Answer: B

Nursing Process: Analysis

Rationale: **Increased intracranial pressure produces observable signs and symptoms depending on the stage of increased pressure. Early signs include headache, nausea and vomiting, altered level of consciousness, and drowsiness.** Late signs include increased systolic blood pressure, bradycardia, widening pulse pressures, and dilated nonreactive pupils. Hypothermia, bradycardia, and a widened pulse pressure are indicative of increased intracranial pressure. Two episodes of vomiting in 3 hours should not cause these symptoms. Autonomic dysreflexia is a hypertensive emergency and occurs in patients who have a history of spinal cord injuries. There is no indication in the stem of the question to indicate increased intra-abdominal pressure.

 CENsational Pearl of Wisdom!

Neurologic Signs of Early versus Late Intracranial Pressure (ICP)

Early Signs of Increased ICP
- *Restlessness or altered level of consciousness*
- *Nausea and vomiting (can be with or without nausea)*
- *Headache*
- *Amnesia*
- *Behavioral changes that progress to confusion drowsiness, or impaired judgment*

Cushing's Triad = Very LATE Sign of Increased ICP
- *Increased systolic BP with widening pulse pressure*
- *Profound bradycardia*
- *Abnormal respirations*

Other Late Signs of Increased ICP
- *Dilated nonreactive pupils*
- *Unresponsiveness*
- *Abnormal posturing (flexion, extension, or flaccidity)*

Herniation
- *Increasing ICP causes herniation ("shift") of brain tissue*
- *Etiology can be many, that is, tumor, bleeding, and swelling*
- *All other signs and symptoms of herniation are usually present to some degree*
- *Altered level of consciousness (LOC), posturing, and vital sign changes*
- *Uncal herniation—dilated pupils unilaterally or bilaterally*
- *Central herniation—bilateral constricted pupils*

9. Answer: B

Nursing Process: Analysis

Rationale: **Meningococcemia is a potentially life- or limb-threatening clinical entity in which the organism *Neisseria meningitidis* gains access to the bloodstream. It is characterized by rapid onset of petechiae and purpuric lesions and is spread by oral or nasal droplets. Additional signs and symptoms include irritability, fever/temperature instability, bleeding from puncture sites, tachycardia, poor perfusion, hypotension, gangrene, and tissue necrosis (late).** Henoch-Schönlein purpura (HSP) is a disease of the skin, mucous membranes, and sometimes other organs that most commonly affects children following an infectious process such as a throat infection. Palpable purpura (small, raised areas of bleeding underneath the skin), joint pain, and abdominal pain can occur. Chronic kidney disease can follow this disease process. Idiopathic thrombocytopenic purpura (ITP) is a disorder affecting both children and adults that can lead to easy or excessive bruising and bleeding. The bleeding results from unusually low levels of platelets and the cells that help blood clot. Children often develop ITP after a viral infection and usually recover fully without treatment. In adults, the disorder is often long term. Depending on the level of platelets, manifestations can range from minimal to potentially fatal with internal bleeding. Kawasaki disease affects children and includes fever, rash, swelling of the hands and feet, irritation and redness of the whites of the eyes, and swollen lymph glands in the neck with irritation and inflammation of the mouth, lips, and throat. The effects of Kawasaki disease are rarely serious. The acute phase of the condition commonly lasts 10 to 14 days or more. Most children recover fully. In some cases, Kawasaki disease can lead to long-term heart complications.

10. Answer: D

Nursing Process: Assessment

Rationale: **Battle's sign (mastoid bruising) and raccoon eyes (periorbital ecchymosis) are signs of a basilar skull fracture and indicates that blood may be leaking into the periorbital and mastoid spaces. These signs do not usually present until 12 to 24 hours after the initial injury to the base of the skull.** Epidural hematoma is usually caused by an arterial bleed between the skull and the dura mater because of laceration of the middle meningeal artery with a direct blow to the head. Unconsciousness followed by a lucid period and then rapid change to a decreased level of consciousness are landmark signs of this problem. Subdural hematomas occur more frequently and are characterized by bleeding in the subdural space between the dura mater and arachnoid. Classic presentation results in a venous bleed with loss of consciousness, fixed and dilated pupils with immediate surgical intervention often required. A depressed skull fracture would be indicated by a depression in the integrity of the skull with soft tissue injury.

 CENsational Pearl of Wisdom!

This is an excellent example of reading the question very closely for small clues. The major clue here is that the patient arrived "20 hours after a motorcycle crash without a helmet." That points to the answer of basilar skull fracture with the presenting manifestations.

11. Answer: D

Nursing Process: Analysis

Rationale: **Acute encephalitis (inflammation of the brain parenchyma) can be caused by bacterial, viral, or parasitic infections and can be seen in children with systemic infectious childhood illnesses such as measles.** It occurs more often in children less than 10 years of age. Children who take aspirin with a viral illness are at increased risk of presenting with Reye's syndrome. Reye's syndrome is rarely seen today because education of the risk of using aspirin products during viral illnesses has been greatly appreciated. Any child with fever and nuchal rigidity should be placed on droplet precautions until a diagnostic lumbar puncture (LP) can be completed to rule out meningitis. Immunization history is not relevant in these situations.

12. Answer: B

Nursing Process: Assessment

Rationale: **Guillain-Barré syndrome is an acute idiopathic poly-neuropathic disorder affecting the motor component of the peripheral nerves. It affects people between the age of 16 and 30 years of age and over 50% of those affected have had a recent viral illness.** Classic presentation is ascending, bilateral weakness progressing from the extremities upward and inward. Myasthenia gravis is a chronic autoimmune disorder caused by a defect in neuromuscular transmission occurring more frequently in women also between the ages of 20 and 30 years of age. Ocular dysfunction is the most common initial symptom ptosis (eyelid drooping), diplopia with sustained directional gaze, and difficulty keeping the eye closed. Botulism poisoning presents after ingestion, inhalation, or wound contamination with botulism toxin. Patient presentation includes symmetrical descending flaccid paralysis with ptosis and blurred vision, which then progresses to flaccid paralysis and respiratory distress. Organophosphate poisoning is an acetylcholinesterase inhibitor disrupting and blocking the effects of acetylcholinesterase. Presentation includes skeletal muscle twitching, cramping, flaccid paralysis, tachycardia, pinpoint pupils (miosis), diaphoresis, hypersecretion of the salivary glands, lacrimal glands, sweat, and bronchial glands, nausea, vomiting, and diarrhea.

 CENsational Pearl of Wisdom!

Organophosphate poisoning occurs with bug sprays and also with sarin gas. This is a cholinergic crisis that is "wet." A mnemonic to help remember the manifestations of this process are:

(continued)

SLUDGEM

Salivation and increased secretions

Lacrimation

Urinary incontinence

Defecation incontinence (diarrhea)

Gastroesophageal effects (nausea, vomiting, and diarrhea)

Miosis (pinpoint pupils)

13. Answer: B

Nursing Process: Analysis

Rationale: **The timing of onset of symptoms with progressing severity of symptoms should be considered higher acuity. A patient with sudden onset of headache and vomiting should be considered high priority as this may be indicative of pathophysiologic events such as herniation or subarachnoid hemorrhage.** A throbbing headache with photophobia is indicative of a classic migraine. A bad headache in the occipital/neck area may also be indicative of a migraine or a tension type of headache. Head lacerations usually bleed quite a bit because of the vascularity of the head. This option indicated that the bleeding had stopped at this time.

CENsational Pearl of Wisdom!

From a triage standpoint, always consider a sudden onset—especially one that is like a "thunderbolt"— and pain of highest intensity, to be a possibility for grave consequences.

14. Answer: A

Nursing Process: Assessment

Rationale: **Cushing's triad/response is a late sign of increased intracranial pressure and includes: reflex bradycardia, high systolic or widened pulse pressure and breathing abnormalities, which can result in a decreased respiratory effort.** Numbness of the fingers and decreased temperature are not associated with increased intracranial pressure. A decreased level of consciousness (mentation) would occur in increased intracranial pressure but not the increased respiratory rate.

CENsational Pearl of Wisdom!

The response to increase in blood pressure when intracranial pressure is increasing occurs

automatically to maintain cerebral perfusion pressure (CPP). It is a response to the formula, CPP = MAP − ICP. MAP is mean arterial pressure and ICP is intracranial pressure. The body must maintain a cerebral perfusion pressure of at least 60 mm Hg in order to perfuse the brain. The blood pressure increases to maintain the CPP when intracranial pressure is increased.

15. Answer: D

Nursing Process: Intervention

Rationale: **Initiating CPR starts with opening the airway. Jaw thrust is the most effective way to open the airway in a patient with a suspected spinal cord injury.** CPR cannot be effectively administered in a prone position, and many patients with a catastrophic head injury in association with a spinal injury who present in cardiopulmonary arrest may require CPR. Cervical spine injury should be considered until proven otherwise thus hyperextending the neck would not be recommended.

16. Answer: D

Nursing Process: Intervention

Rationale: **This patient is demonstrating manifestations of autonomic dysreflexia. This is the sudden onset of an abnormal sympathetic nervous system response to a noxious stimuli such as a full bladder, full rectum, or pressure on an ulcer. The symptoms include bradycardia, hypertension, headache, flushing, and excessive sweating.** Emergency treatment involves raising the head of the bed and loosening any constricting clothing. If compression stockings are present on the patient, they should be removed to encourage venous pooling. The most important intervention for this response is to resolve the offending stimulus. Assess for G-I or G-U-related situations. Often irrigation of a urinary catheter or unkinking the tubing may relieve the sympathetic response. Enemas or removal of an impaction may be necessary. Antihypertensives can be given, but the hypertension will not resolve until the stimulus has been removed.

17. Answer: C

Nursing Process: Intervention

Rationale: **The most important measure to take when assisting a person who is actively seizing is to ensure airway patency and prevent further injury. The patient should be rolled onto their side to facilitate drainage of secretions from the airway. The extremities and head should be protected from injury, but the**

patient should be turned first. Motor activity should be monitored and length of time of the seizure activity should be noted. Placing a tongue blade or mouth block may cause more injury. Restraining the patient is not appropriate.

 CENsational Pearl of Wisdom!

Many times, there seems to be two appropriate answers for the question. Always choose the one that has to do with airway!

18. Answer: C

Nursing Process: Analysis

Rationale: **In addition to treating infection and minimizing exposures, pain management is a high priority. Minimizing pain contributes to reducing increased metabolism, glucose utilization, and intracranial pressure.** You would not want to increase stimulation to the child because this will increase metabolic demands and glucose needs. Measuring urine output is important but a urinary catheter should not be placed unless it is absolutely necessary due to the potential of introducing another focus of infection.

19. Answer: B

Nursing Process: Evaluation

Rationale: **Between 25% and 30% of children who have suffered a febrile seizure may have reoccurrences. Keeping the temperature from increasing rapidly may contribute to the prevention of febrile seizures. Tepid sponge bath, administering antipyretics, and increasing fluid intake during febrile illnesses are key to preventing febrile seizures.** An ice bath is too cool to bring the temperature down and the temperature should be brought down slowly by using tepid water between 60° F and 100° F (16° C to 38° C). Alcohol baths was an accepted form of temperature control in years past, but it was then realized that the alcohol could be absorbed through the skin, causing alcohol poisoning. Phenobarbital does not affect temperature.

20. Answer: C

Nursing Process: Intervention

Rationale: **Over 23 million patients suffer from migraine headaches. Current treatment standards for patients with migraine headaches include providing** hydration (oral or intravenous), antiemetics (ondansetron hydrochloride [Zofran]), and/or antihistamines (intravenous diphenhydramine or Benadryl), and NSAIDS [Ibuprofen, Motrin]). Narcotic analgesics should be avoided because of the possibility of a rebound headache and addiction. Nitroglycerin sublingual should be avoided because of the vasodilatory affect, which can increase the intensity of the headache.

21. Answer: D

Nursing Process: Assessment

Rationale: **The characteristic presentation of a child with Reye's syndrome is use of salicylates during a viral illness, followed by mental status change and evidence of fatty deposits in the liver.** Sickle cell crisis is often triggered by stress, illness, extreme changes in temperature (cold weather), or infection, but is not associated with Reye's syndrome. Acetaminophen (Tylenol) use or bacterial streptococcal infection has not been linked to Reye's syndrome. Influenza-like illnesses or viral conditions should be treated with antipyretics such as acetaminophen or Tylenol.

 CENsational Pearl of Wisdom!

Early manifestations of Reye's syndrome are lethargy and vomiting, which is associated with encephalopathy. These symptoms usually occur within the first 2 days of the illness.

22. Answer: A

Nursing Process: Intervention

Rationale: **Optimal positioning for a lumbar puncture in an infant is sitting upright or on their side with knees flexed and chin to chest.** Older children or adults may be sitting on the side of the bed, leaning over a bedside table. A prone position is not appropriate and the supine position would not provide access to the spinal area. The child or infant would have to be in a curled position in order to access the proper location for needle insertion.

 CENsational Pearl of Wisdom!

Remember that all children and infants should be monitored very closely during this procedure because of the positioning. Watch respirations and pulse oximetry.

23. Answer: A

Nursing Process: Analysis

Rationale: **Characteristics of CSF with bacterial meningitis include elevated WBC, elevated protein, decreased glucose, and positive gram stain with turbid or cloudy CSF.** Bacterial meningitis can be fatal in 50% of patients. Common agents include *Streptococcus pneumoniae*, *Neisseria meningitidis*, *Haemophilus influenzae*, or group B *streptococci*, and *Listeria monocytogenes*.

 CENsational Pearl of Wisdom!

Type of Meningitis	CSF Pressure	Protein	Glucose	WBC
Bacterial	↑ Elevated	↑ Elevated	↓ Decreased	↑ Increased (>1,000 cells/μL)
Viral	Normal (may be mildly increased)	↓ Decreased	Normal	↑ Increased (10–1,000 cells/μL)

24. Answer: B

Nursing Process: Intervention

Rationale: **TPA is administered as a weight-based dose of 0.9 mg/kg, but with a maximum dose of 90 mg in the patient presenting with a stroke.** TPA is the only thrombolytic approved for use in stroke patients.

 CENsational Pearl of Wisdom!

Be cautious with computer-generated ordering and medication screens. Near misses have occurred because of wrong orders being "clicked" and pharmacy errors regarding placing a "stop" on the dose at 90 mg!

25. Answer: C

Nursing Process: Analysis

Rationale: **The temporal lobe contains the auditory association area. If this area is damaged in the dominant hemisphere, the patient hears words but does not know their meaning.** It is also associated with memory.

Damage to the parietal lobe affects the patient's ability to identify special relationships with the environment. This has to do with sensory information that is obtained through the sense of touch. It also is a focus for the sensation of pain. When damaged, the occipital lobe affects visual associations; therefore, the patient can visualize objects but cannot identify them. The frontal lobe acts as the center for the ability to reason and express the spoken word, to understand right from wrong, cognition, and socialization skills.

26. Answer: D

Nursing Process: Assessment

Rationale: **Evaluation of brain stem function can be done in an unconscious patient by testing the oculocephalic reflex. When the patient's head is rotated, the eyes should move in a direction opposite to the head movement. Brain stem damage is indicated if the eyes move in the same direction as head movement.** Cranial nerve I is the olfactory nerve; damage to this nerve results in the inability to identify odors. The fovea is the center of the retina's macula, the area of greatest visual acuity.

Evaluation of this reflex is contraindicated in a patient with suspected cervical spine injury or who has not had the cervical spine cleared.

Assessment Technique for the Oculocephalic Reflex

1. Briskly rotate the head from side to side, or
2. Briskly flex and extend the neck.

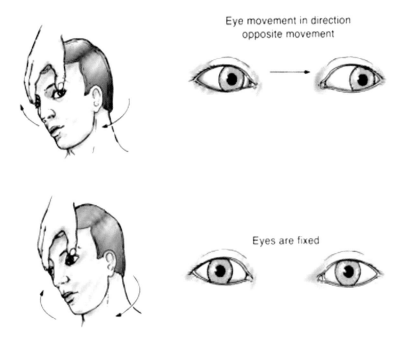

Findings

- When the head is rotated, the eyes should move in the direction opposite to the head movement *(top)*. (If the head is rotated to the left, the eyes appear to move to the right.) Alternative method: When the neck is flexed, the eyes appear to look upward; when the neck is extended, the eyes look downward.
- When the doll's eye reflex is absent, the eyes do not move in the sockets and thus follow the direction of passive rotation. Loss of the oculocephalic reflex in the comatose patient indicates a lesion at the pontine–midbrain level of the brainstem.

Reprinted with permission from Hickey, J. (2013). Clinical practice of neurological & neurosurgical nursing (7th ed.). Philadelphia, PA: Wolters Kluwer Health.

27. Answer: B

Nursing Process: Intervention

Rationale: **Immobilization of the head and neck reduces the risk of further damage to the cervical spine. This patient arrived with a large hematoma to his head, which indicates some type of trauma. All patients with suspected head and neck trauma should be immobilized until all seven cervical vertebrae are cleared by radiograph visualization or computed tomography (CT).** A complete head-to-toe assessment (secondary survey) should be performed after CT (computed tomography) scan or radiologic examination. Airway, breathing, and circulation are assessed as the cervical spine is immobilized, and the patient is evaluated for potential life-threatening injuries (primary survey).

Administering opioid analgesics to a patient with altered mental status or head injuries is not a primary intervention because opioids can increase respiratory depression and hypotension in patients with head injury. Obtaining a specimen for blood alcohol level helps determine the amount of alcohol the patient has consumed and its possible relationship with the patient's level of consciousness. Although this is useful information, it is not a primary intervention.

28. Answer: C

Nursing Process: Evaluation

Rationale: **This patient is given 5 points for purposeful movement to pain (motor), 3 points for inappropriate words (verbal), and 2 points for eye opening in** response to painful stimuli. **The total score is 10.** Remember! The lowest score on a Glasgow Coma Scale is 3—not 0! Highest potential scoring is 15.

 CENsational Pearl of Wisdom!

Eye Opening	
Spontaneous	4
To speech	3
To pain	2
None	1
Verbal Response	
Oriented	5
Confused	4
Inappropriate words	3
Moans	2
None	1
Motor Response	
Follows commands	6
Localizes pain	5
Withdrawals	4
Decorticate (flexion)	3
Decerebrate (extension)	2
None	1

Reprinted with permission from Leonard, L. S. (2017). The Washington manual of emergency medicine (1st ed.). Philadelphia, PA: Wolters Kluwer Health.

29. Answer: B

Nursing Process: Assessment

Rationale: **A patient with possible spinal cord injury typically complains of numbness and tingling in the extremities or an inability to detect sensation.** Bradycardia and hypotension would be expected with spinal cord injury not hypertension and tachycardia. Cloudy CSF is associated with bacterial infections such as meningitis. Exophthalmos is an abnormal protrusion of the eyeball associated with orbital tumors, thyroid disorders, and orbital cellulitis.

30. Answer: B

Nursing Process: Assessment

Rationale: **An ovoid pupil is the midpoint between a normally round pupil and a fully dilated and fixed pupil and is a sign of increased intracranial pressure.** Traumatic orbital injury results in a jagged-appearing pupil or a tear-drop–shaped pupil as with a globe rupture.

A keyhole-shaped pupil is common in patients who have had an iridectomy as part of cataract surgery. A pontine hemorrhage causes the pupils to be pinpoint.

31. Answer: C

Nursing Process: Evaluation

Rationale: **The modified Ramsay Score for Sedation (RASS) measures the level of sedation achieved with pharmacologic agents. A Ramsay score of 5 suggests that the patient responds only to noxious stimuli.** A patient who is anxious, agitated, or restless has a Ramsay score of 1. A patient who is cooperative, tranquil, and oriented has a score of 2. A patient who responds to voice and verbal commands has a Ramsay score of 3. A patient who responds to gentle shaking scores a 4. A patient who shows no response to noxious stimuli is considered a 6 on the scale. The scale ranges from 1 to 6 only.

32. Answer: C

Nursing Process: Intervention

Rationale: **Succinylcholine is a neuromuscular-blocking agent that can increase intracranial pressure (ICP) in a patient with head injuries. Administering 1 mg/kg of lidocaine provides ICP control.** Atropine is the premedication of choice for children receiving succinylcholine because it decreases the bradycardia that occurs with succinylcholine administration. Ketamine and meperidine are contraindicated in a patient with head injuries because they increase ICP.

 CENsational Pearl of Wisdom!

There is some controversy regarding the use of lidocaine as a pretreatment because of inconsistent studies. It is an accepted practice.

33. Answer: C

Nursing Process: Assessment

Rationale: **Normal ICP should be less than 0 to 20 mm Hg. Widening pulse pressure, hyperthermia, and Cheyne-Stokes respirations are signs of increased ICP.** Kussmaul's respirations are associated with diabetic ketoacidosis.

 CENsational Pearl of Wisdom!

Different books may provide different numbers on normal values such as intracranial pressure readings. One book may document it as 0 to 20, whereas another will state 0 to 15. They are usually close together and neither are necessarily incorrect.

34. Answer: D

Nursing Process: Intervention

Rationale: **Mannitol is an osmotic diuretic that decreases intracranial pressure (ICP).** Suctioning the patient's airway should be minimized to prevent increased ICP. Morphine should be used cautiously in a patient with a head injury or increased ICP because the drug's respiratory depressant effects are considerably enhanced in these situations. A patient with a head injury should have his head elevated 30 degrees to promote venous drainage. Placing a patient in trendelenburg position obstructs venous return from the brain and increases ICP.

35. Answer: D

Nursing Process: Assessment

Rationale: **Paralysis is a late symptom of multiple sclerosis (MS).** The earliest clinical signs of MS may be vague, such as weakness, numbness, or tingling in limbs; visual blurring; or urinary changes. Motor symptoms initially present as weakness and then progress to paralysis. Diplopia (double vision) or scotoma (area of depressed vision in the visual field) may also present early in the disease.

CENsational Pearl of Wisdom!

Multiple sclerosis is a disease process that affects the myelin sheath of the central nervous system. Guillain-Barré syndrome affects the myelin sheath of the peripheral nervous system.

36. Answer: A

Nursing Process: Analysis

Rationale: **A subdural hematoma, occurring between the dura mater and the arachnoid layer of the meninges, is bleeding that causes direct pressure to the surface of the brain. Signs and symptoms appear within 48 hours (acute) and can be delayed as long as several months (chronic).** Symptoms of an epidural hematoma include a history of momentary loss of consciousness followed by a lucid period after which the patient's mental status deteriorates rapidly due to the presence of bleeding from the middle meningeal artery. The clinical manifestations of a diffuse axonal injury are immediate and prolonged coma with decorticate or decerebrate posturing. Manifestations of postconcussion syndrome include headache, dizziness, irritability, poor judgment, and insomnia.

CENsational Pearl of Wisdom!

When patients arrive in the ED with a headache, always ask if they have fallen and hit their head within the past 2 to 3 months. The term "chronic subdural hematoma" occurs at later dates as the vessels bleed a little at a time. Two patients who are at increased risk for this are the geriatric patient and the alcoholic because of their smaller brain mass (atrophy occurs with both of these) and their tendency to fall. Those on blood thinners are at even higher risk. Think of these things when assessing patients at either the triage area or as the primary nurse.

37. Answer: A

Nursing Process: Analysis

Rationale: **The medulla controls the arterioles, the blood pressure, and the rate and depth of respirations. Severe injury to this area generally results in death.** The medulla also controls yawning, coughing, vomiting, and hiccoughing. The frontal lobe of the cerebrum controls personality, judgment, thought, and logic. The diencephalon contains the thalamus, which is the sensory pathway between the spinal cord and the cortex of the brain. The hypothalamus regulates body temperature, appetite, and sleep.

38. Answer: B

Nursing Process: Analysis

Rationale: **Hyperkalemia can occur if succinylcholine (Anectine) is used for the induction of rapid sequence intubation in the patient with Guillain-Barre and in the later stages of those with spinal cord injuries, burns, and strokes.** The uptake of acetylcholine at the neuromuscular junction is increased in these disease processes as well as the medication, succinylcholine. This allows for the release of potassium and can cause a fatal hyperkalemia. Those patients who have disease processes that lend toward increased potassium levels can also be at risk, such as renal failure, large crush injuries, or even digitalis toxicity. Sodium is not affected by this medication and disease processes.

39. Answer: C

Nursing Process: Analysis

Rationale: **An epidural hematoma results from blood collecting between the skull and the dura mater.** A subdural hematoma is commonly caused by trauma or violent shaking (shaken baby syndrome) and results in a collection of venous blood between the dura mater and the arachnoid mater. A subarachnoid hemorrhage is a collection of blood between the pia mater and the arachnoid membrane. A contusion is a bruise on the surface of the brain.

40. Answer: C

Nursing Process: Assessment

Rationale: **This child has classic signs of a traumatic head injury such as subdural hematoma, which is caused by venous bleeding between the dura and the arachnoid layers. This injury is frequently associated with child abuse.** A patient with a history of coagulation or hematologic disorders may present with ecchymosis, petechiae (in platelet disorders), or purpura. Meningitis is associated with lethargy, irritability, fever, seizures, and headache. Petechiae and purpura are present in meningococcemia.

 CENsational Pearl of Wisdom!

When assessing any patient, the history, psychological findings, and patient's overall appearance must also be considered to determine whether the signs and symptoms are consistent with the patient/caregivers history. Remember that we need to focus on the "chief complaint," but we also must look at our patients holistically!

41. Answer: B

Nursing Process: Evaluation

Rationale: **According to the stroke guidelines for care, a systolic blood pressure above 180 mm Hg requires treatment before the initiation of TPA. Labetalol (Normodyne) was given before with a blood pressure now of 168/98 mm Hg, which demonstrates that the Labetalol (Normodyne) was successful in lowering the systolic pressure below 185 mm Hg.** A systolic blood pressure that remains above 185 mm Hg is a contraindication to TPA initiation. Acceptable pressures are systolic below 185 mm Hg and diastolic below 110 mm Hg. Uncontrolled hypertension increases the risk of intracranial bleeding. Tachycardia would not necessarily contraindicate the administration unless it was associated with bleeding/hypovolemia. The pulse oximetry reading and temperature are not included in the criteria, although it is recommended to supplement for SaO_2 below 94%. Hyperthermia can increase the morbidity rate, but in this scenario, the temperature is normal and a light, warm blanket was applied for patient comfort.

 CENsational Pearl of Wisdom!

Other exclusion criteria are head trauma, previous recent stroke or intracranial bleed, and laboratory tests that indicate bleeding potential (platelets, international normalized ratio [INR], protime). Other considerations include resolving symptoms, recent surgery, recent gastrointestinal hemorrhage, recent myocardial infarction, and seizure at onset of event.

42. Answer: A

Nursing Process: Assessment

Rationale: **The normal heart rate for a 1-year-old child ranges from 90 to 120 beats/minute. Bradycardia is a sign of increasing intracranial pressure.** Normally, respirations for a child of this age range from 20 to 30 breaths/minute. Capillary refill time less than or equal to 3 seconds is a normal finding. For children below the age of 2, a positive Babinski's reflex is a normal finding.

43. Answer: A

Nursing Process: Intervention

Rationale: **A rotated head position will prevent venous outflow via the jugular veins and contribute to increased intracranial pressure (ICP). The head of the bed should be maintained at 30 degrees, and hyperextension, flexion, and rotation of the head should be avoided.** Placing the patient in Trendelenburg position by lowering the head of the bed would increase the pressure on the brain. Closing the stopcock on the ventriculostomy causes the ICP to rise because there is no longer an outlet for the cerebrospinal fluid (CSF).

44. Answer: A

Nursing Process: Assessment

Rationale: **A patient with an injury at C_6 will have quadriplegia with diaphragmatic breathing and gross motor arm movements. The patient may also suffer from hypotension and an atonic bladder.** An injury at level C_2 results in total loss of respiratory function and movement from the shoulders down. Paraplegia with loss of portions of intercostal and abdominal muscles is indicative of injury at T_1 to L_2. An injury below L_2 results in mixed motor sensory loss and bowel and bladder dysfunction.

45. Answer: D

Nursing Process: Intervention

Rationale: **Cardizem is typically used to treat tachycardia, such as that associated with atrial fibrillation with a rapid ventricular rate.** Nicardipine (Cardene), nitroprusside (Nipride) and labetalol (Normodyne) are all agents used to reduce blood pressure in ischemic stroke.

46. Answer: C

Nursing Process: Evaluation

Rationale: **One of the most common causes of seizures in a patient taking phenytoin (Dilantin) is discontinuation of the medication.** Because of the slow absorption of phenytoin from the GI tract, daily drug routines can be easily adjusted when a dose is missed. The patient also needs to be made aware of possible adverse effects of his medications. Phenytoin is metabolized in the liver, and both the inactive metabolites and unchanged drug are excreted in the urine. Because phenytoin has many hematopoietic adverse effects, blood work (including complete blood count, liver, and renal function studies) should be obtained on a regular basis. Serum levels should also be monitored because serum concentrations increase disproportionately to dosing regimens.

47. Answer: D

Nursing Process: Intervention

Rationale: **Tissue plasminogen activator (TPA) is a fibrinolytic medication that decreases the patient's ability to clot. The infusion should be stopped immediately.** While a patient is receiving TPA, all invasive procedures should be avoided because of the increased risk of bleeding; therefore, a nasogastric tube should not be placed. The physician should be notified, but the priority is to stop the infusion.

 CENsational Pearl of Wisdom!

When administering TPA, a bolus of 10% of the total dose is given IV push and then the infusion is provided over 1 hour.

48. Answer: D

Nursing Process: Assessment

Rationale: **Alopecia (hair loss) is not a manifestation of Parkinson's disease.** The symptom that typically characterizes this disease is a faint tremor that slowly progresses in intensity. As the patient's muscle tone becomes more rigid, the gait takes on a shuffling appearance. The patient's face is masklike, and his/her speech is slow and monotone. Movements are slow (bradykinesia). It is common for the patient to develop dysphagia and drooling. The patient's judgment becomes impaired even though actual intelligence remains unaffected.

49. Answer: A

Nursing Process: Intervention

Rationale: **Pramipexole (Mirapex) is a dopamine agonist. It activates dopamine receptors, which mimic or copy the function of dopamine in the brain.** Reserpine (Serpalan) is used for hypertension, some psychiatric disorders, and tardive dyskinesia. Haloperidol (Haldol) is used in the treatment of schizophrenia. Valproic acid (Depakote) is an antiseizure medication that can cause tremors.

 CENsational Pearl of Wisdom!

The use of dopamine-blocking drugs has been linked to pharmacologically induced parkinsonism. Dopamine and acetylcholine are neurotransmitters that act on the input nuclei to the basal ganglia. When dopamine (an inhibitor) is reduced, acetylcholine (an excitatory neurotransmitter) becomes predominant and precipitates tremor.

50. Answer: D

Nursing Process: Analysis

Rationale: **The higher the score, the more deficits are present, which indicates a worse outcome for the patient. A score of 0 would indicate no deficits present for a patient with a normal examination.** The NIHSS assesses the patient's level of consciousness, orientation, response to commands, gaze, visual fields, facial movement, motor function, limb ataxia, sensation, language, articulation, and extinction.

51. Answer: A

Nursing Process: Analysis

Rationale: **The primary symptom of myasthenia gravis is weakness of voluntary muscles, especially those of the face. This weakness may temporarily improve with short periods of rest.** Myasthenia gravis affects two to three times more women than men until age 40. This disease may result from a defect at the myoneural junction. Bell's palsy is an inflammatory reaction involving the facial nerve presenting as ipsilateral facial paresis. This patient also has blurred vision and difficulty eating, which would not indicate Bell's palsy. Trigeminal neuralgia is characterized by sudden episodes of ipsilateral facial pain. Glioblastomas are intracranial tumors that present with symptoms of increased intracranial pressure and focal deficits.

52. Answer: B

Nursing Process: Analysis

Rationale: **In the Tensilon test, edrophonium (Tensilon) is administered by intravenous infusion to a patient exhibiting signs of muscle weakness. Significant improvement, lasting approximately 4 to 5 minutes, in the patient's muscle tone indicates a positive diagnosis for myasthenia gravis.** A lumbar puncture (LP) is frequently performed to assist in diagnosing meningitis. An Allen's test is performed to evaluate the circulatory function of the ulnar artery before obtaining arterial blood gases (ABG) to verify collateral circulation before accessing the radial artery. An MRI is effective in detecting degenerative central nervous system diseases, malignant tumors, and oxygen-deprived tissue, but none of these findings are associated with myasthenia gravis.

53. Answer: D

Nursing Process: Intervention

Rationale: **Cytoxan is a chemotherapeutic agent used to slow growth of cancer cells and interfere with their spread throughout the body.** Diazepam, baclofen, and gabapentin are associated with the medical management of patients with multiple sclerosis (MS). Diazepam and baclofen are primarily effective in decreasing the spasms and stiffness associated with the disease, whereas gabapentin relieves pain as well as spasticity.

54. Answer: C

Nursing Process: Evaluation

Rationale: **Alzheimer's disease is a neurologic and degenerative disorder resulting from cerebral atrophy and cellular degeneration. Predominating symptoms are mental status changes, increased anxiety, forgetfulness, and eventually, the inability to recognize significant others and perform activities of daily living.** Destruction of motor cells in the anterior gray horns and pyramidal tracts can result in the symptoms associated with amyotrophic lateral sclerosis. Metabolic disorders may cause altered cognitive function but can be reversed by correction of the underlying problem. Degeneration of the basal ganglia is usually associated with Parkinson's disease.

55. Answer: D

Nursing Process: Intervention

Rationale: **Suctioning should occur only when necessary and should be done quickly with less than 10 seconds at a time.** Suctioning will cause coughing, which increases both intrathoracic and intracranial pressure. Suctioning should not occur every 2 hours but should be performed in case of elevated peak pressures or visible secretions accompanied by respiratory assessments that support the need. The instillation of normal saline before suctioning increases ventilator-associated pneumonia. Lowering the head of the bed will elevate the ICP. The head of the bed should be maintained at 30 degrees.

56. Answer: C

Nursing Process: Assessment

Rationale: **This patient is experiencing a migraine headache. Vision changes such as "zig-zag lines," a unilateral headache, nausea, and photosensitivity are common manifestations of this type of headache.** Sinusitis is described as pain or pressure over the maxillary or frontal sinus areas. The pain can be reproduced by palpation. Meningitis presents with symptoms of fever, headache, severe neck discomfort, and irritability. Typically, there's an altered level of consciousness. Trigeminal neuralgia is characterized by ipsilateral facial pain from the side of the mouth to the ear, eye, or nostril on the same side.

 CENsational Pearl of Wisdom!

Migraines are more prevalent in women than men, and there can be a familial tendency. Migraines are divided into three phases: aura (vision disturbances, confusion, paresthesia), which precedes the headache and lasts from 15 to 30 minutes; headache, characterized by a throbbing pain that usually begins as unilateral and can progress to bilateral accompanied by nausea or vomiting; and postheadache, noted by scalp tenderness and muscular aching of the neck.

57. Answer: A

Nursing Process: Intervention

Rationale: **Propranolol (Inderal), a beta-blocker, is one of the most commonly prescribed drugs for the prevention of migraines.** Ondansetron (Zofran) is an antiemetic used to control the nausea and vomiting associated with a migraine headache. Codeine can be given for the pain of a full-blown migraine. Diphenhydramine (Benadryl) is useful in treating cluster headaches and can be used in the treatment of migraine headaches, but not the prevention.

58. Answer: C

Nursing Process: Assessment

Rationale: **Symptoms of ergotamine overdose occur in response to intense vasoconstriction, which can produce signs and symptoms of peripheral vascular ischemia. In addition to numbness and tingling of fingers and toes, the patient may experience muscle pain and weakness, gangrene, and hypertension as well as dysrhythmias and myocardial infarction.** Diplopia and ataxia are not associated with ergotamine tartrate overdose.

59. Answer: A

Nursing Process: Assessment

Rationale: **Emotional upset usually precedes a pseudoseizure, which generally lasts longer than a true seizure.** In a true seizure, the patient may scream at the onset of the event but repetitive, consistent movement of the extremities is ongoing. Absence, or petit mal, seizures are manifested by an absence of consciousness for 5 to 10 seconds. Tonic-clonic (grand mal) seizures present with the following pattern: aura, cry, loss of consciousness, fall, tonic-clonic movement, and incontinence. Focal seizures involve one area of the body (which varies from patient to patient) and are not associated with an altered mental state.

CENsational Pearl of Wisdom!

Remember that patients do not have to have a loss of consciousness in order to manifest a seizure!

60. Answer: A

Nursing Process: Analysis

Rationale: **Transient ischemic attacks (TIAs) are temporary episodes of neurologic dysfunction in response to brief episodes of cerebral ischemia. Most commonly, a TIA presents as weakness of the lower face and upper and lower extremities (either right or left sided) as well as dysphagia, which may occur multiple times during the day.** Between each attack, neurologic findings are normal. Hypercapneic encephalopathy is seen in patients with problems associated with chronic respiratory acidosis. Disequilibrium syndrome is an acute complication of peritoneal dialysis or hemodialysis. Transtentorial herniation occurs as a result of downward pressure from edema in the parietal or frontal lobes.

61. Answer: A

Nursing Process: Intervention

Rationale: **Thrombolytics are part of a drug therapy that dissolves clots by fibrinolysis. Tissue plasminogen activator (Activase) is the only approved thrombolytic for use in acute ischemic stroke. Studies are in progress regarding the use of Tenecteplase (TNK) in acute stroke but are not approved at this time.**

CENsational Pearl of Wisdom!

Thrombolytics are utilized within the 3-hour time period as recognized by the American Heart Association and for a select group of individuals within a 4.5-hour time period. Also remember that thrombolytic therapy should be started within 60 minutes of arrival to the ED (door to needle).

62. Answer: C

Nursing Process: Evaluation

Rationale: **The new emergency nurse would provide the correct response if she/he stated that expressive aphasia is represented by the inability to speak words even though the patient is able to comprehend the spoken word. This is indicative of stroke syndromes on the left side of the brain (right-sided hemiplegia).** Receptive aphasia is an impaired ability to understand spoken words. Dysphagia refers to difficulty in swallowing, which occurs when injury affects the vertebrobasilar region. Apraxia is the inability to perform a learned movement, such as using a comb, brushing one's teeth, or waving goodbye.

63. Answer: B

Nursing Process: Evaluation

Rationale: **Alzheimer's disease is a type of dementia. Generally, dementia is defined as a decline in thinking, reasoning, and/or remembering. People with Alzheimer's disease have difficulty carrying out daily tasks they have performed routinely and independently throughout their lives and they can have difficulty with social interactions.** Alzheimer's disease accounts for 60% to 80% of all cases of dementia. This terminal, progressive brain disorder has no known cause or cure. Hallucinations and delusions can occur later in the disease process for these patients.

64. Answer: D

Nursing Process: Analysis

Rationale: **The glioblastoma and medulloblastoma are two of the most malignant and rapidly growing brain tumors. They are difficult to excise and can cause death within months.** An astrocytoma is a slower growing form of glioma. A meningioma is benign and frequently encapsulated. A neuroma is an extremely slow growing tumor that arises from any of the cranial nerves.

65. Answer: B

Nursing Process: Analysis

Rationale: **When a young child is placed in a safety restraint seat facing the front of the car, the risk of cervical fracture at the C_1 to C_3 level increases because of the fulcrum effect as the child's head whips forward in an accident.** For several reasons, a child's cervical spine is more susceptible to injury than an adult. The other options are more common injuries in older children and adults.

CENsational Pearl of Wisdom!

Spinal Anatomical and Physiologic Changes in Children

- *The vertebral bodies of children are wedged anteriorly and tend to slide forward with flexion.*
- *The neck ligaments of children are more lax.*
- *The neck muscles of children are weaker.*
- *The upper cervical spine facets of children are flatter.*

SCIWORA stands for Spinal Cord Injury Without Radiographic Abnormality that is found in children only. This is under some regrouping at this time since with magnetic resonance imaging (MRI) we can actually determine some of these injuries. If you see it on the test, the answer is usually that an MRI is necessary to identify this disorder. The child may complain of neurologic deficits that were present but are now absent. The child must be "packaged" and sent to a facility that can provide MRI imaging. Do not discount children's complaints of these deficits!

66. Answer: A

Nursing Process: Assessment

Rationale: **An infant's open suture lines can allow for a greater amount of bleeding into the head and can actually bleed significantly enough to cause hypovolemia with hypotension and a shock state.** The lax neck muscles, large head, and short trachea do not impact the potential for blood loss in an infant.

 CENsational Pearl of Wisdom!

A child with a subdural hematoma exhibits bulging fontanels because the sutures separate as intracranial pressure (ICP) increases. Always check fontanels when assessing an infant.

67. Answer: C

Nursing Process: Assessment

Rationale: **Autonomic dysreflexia is associated with spinal cord injuries at or above the T_6 level.**

 CENsational Pearl of Wisdom!

Autonomic dysreflexia occurs in the postacute phase when reflex activity has returned. A massive vasoconstriction creates a dangerous hypertensive situation.

68. Answer: B

Nursing Process: Analysis

Rationale: **Neurogenic shock occurs with fractures at T_6 or above. This patient's most likely cause of shock is hypovolemic, which must be discovered thorough examination and testing for etiologies within the chest and abdomen. Because of his paralysis from the T_9 fracture, he will not be able to feel discomfort in either of these areas. It is therefore important to recognize these principles and not assume that the hypotension derives from the lower thoracic spinal area.** Septic shock would not appear this early and is associated with infectious disease processes. Spinal shock revolves around a temporary cessation of feeling and motor power below the level of the lesion. This can happen immediately after the event or may appear several days later. This also impacts bowel and bladder functions. Hypotension is not a part of spinal shock.

 CENsational Pearl of Wisdom!

Remember that with neurogenic shock, hypotension will be present with bradycardia—not tachycardia!

69. Answer: C

Nursing Process: Assessment

Rationale: **Central cord syndrome, which usually occurs with a hyperextension injury or bleeding into the central canal, causes upper extremity loss of sensation and/or paralysis.** The lower extremities are either not involved or are minimally involved. Priapism (sustained erection) and poikilothermia (inability to regulate temperature control) occur with complete spinal cord injuries, not an incomplete one such as central cord syndrome.

 CENsational Pearl of Wisdom!

Brown-Sequard spinal cord injury is another incomplete spinal cord injury that involves hemisection of the cord in the anterior–posterior plane and occurs most often secondary to knife or gunshot wounds. This leaves the patient with paralysis on one side and paresthesia on the opposite side.

70. Answer: A

Nursing Process: Intervention

Rationale: **Oral steroids are an effective treatment for temporal arteritis because it is a vasculitis. If any**

visual deficits are noted, steroids should be administered intravenously. Anticonvulsants, muscle relaxants, and antihistamines will not be effective or necessary.

CENsational Pearl of Wisdom!

Patients with temporal arteritis will have pain and tenderness to the temporal area. An erythrocyte sedimentation rate (ESR) may be done and would reveal an ESR value greater than 80. The definitive diagnosis is made by temporal artery biopsy.

71. Answer: A

Nursing Process: Assessment

Rationale: **A cluster headache is characterized by pain episodes that are grouped or clustered together for a few days or a few weeks with long periods of remission. The headache is described as causing unilateral pain behind the eyes or near the temples. Associated symptoms include tearing, rhinorrhea, nasal congestion, and Horner's syndrome.** Fever, aphasia, and epistaxis are not associated with cluster headaches.

CENsational Pearl of Wisdom!

Horner's syndrome is a rare process that includes a combination of miosis, ptosis, and anhidrosis (lack of sweating) to one side of the face involving one eye.

72. Answer: C

Nursing Process: Evaluation

Rationale: **This patient is most likely experiencing a subarachnoid hemorrhage. The history of migraine headaches is not a risk factor for this catastrophic diagnosis. Patients with subarachnoid hemorrhage often state that the headache is the most severe they have ever had.** This is also a process that is a sudden onset. Often patients with cerebral aneurysms are asymptomatic until the time of bleeding. At the time of rupture, blood is forced into the subarachnoid space, causing symptoms of meningeal irritation, which would cause pain in the back of the neck when the head is moved in a forward (chin to chest) direction (nuchal rigidity). Other manifestations include nausea, vomiting, aphasia or other speech difficulties, photosensitivity, hypertension, and bradycardia. Other risk factors for this diagnosis are cocaine and amphetamine use and disease processes such as Marfan's syndrome and sickle cell disease.

CENsational Pearl of Wisdom!

Remember that all patients, even those who frequent our doors, are at risk for devastating events. No matter how many times patients have been treated, each one deserves to be heard and should be assessed based on their present complaint! Also, patients with a pending subarachnoid hemorrhage may have atypical headaches for the 2 weeks before rupture. Often, the first symptom is syncope and coma!

73. Answer: A

Nursing Process: Evaluation

Rationale: **One episode of hypotension, which drops the mean arterial pressure (MAP) below 70 mm Hg, can have devastating effects. The MAP should be maintained between 70 and 90 mm Hg. A blood pressure of 90/42 mm Hg creates an MAP of 58 mm Hg.** In a head injured patient, the cerebral perfusion pressure (CPP) should remain above 70 mm Hg. This is the end result of the formula, CPP = MAP − ICP. The patient in this question is within normal limits for a patient with head injury. To obtain this number, an intracranial catheter must be in place. Maintaining the serum osmolality below 320 mOsm is recommended, which is noted in this question. Urine output of 48 mL/hour is adequate output.

CENsational Pearl of Wisdom!

Although it is accepted to allow "permissive hypotension" in patient's suffering from hypovolemic shock, it is not permitted in the head injured patient. This will increase the patient's mortality and morbidity significantly!

74. Answer: C

Nursing Process: Evaluation

Rationale: **C-Collars can actually increase intracranial pressure (ICP). It is important to remove them as soon as possible once the C-spine has been appropriately cleared. This will help reduce the increasing intracranial pressure.** Maintaining the head in midline position, elevating the head of the bed to 30 degrees, and keeping the room quiet and dark are all ways to help keep intracranial pressure down. Other interventions that can assist in reducing ICP are to provide pain and sedating medications and administer osmotic diuretics. Hyperventilation should only be used as a short, temporary measure when the ICP is known to be elevated. Prophylactic hyperventilation is no longer performed.

75. Answer: D

Nursing Process: Assessment

Rationale: **The earliest indicator of neurologic status is the level of consciousness (LOC). A patient who exhibits altered mental status or decreased consciousness should be reevaluated.** Changes in the reaction and shape of pupils are late indicators of neurologic problems. Motor response appears as a delayed sign of neurologic status change. Capillary refill is an indicator of circulatory status.

References

Alzheimer's Association. (2018). *Frontotemporal dementia*. Retrieved from https://www.alz.org/alzheimers-dementia/what-is-dementia/types-of-dementia/frontotemporal-dementia (63)

AMBOSS. (2018). *Subarachnoid hemorrhage.* Retrieved from https://www.amboss.com/us/knowledge/Subarachnoid_hemorrhage (72)

American Heart Association. *Together to end stroke, 2015 guidelines*. Retrieved from https://www.strokeassociation.org/idc/groups/stroke-public/@wcm/@hcm/@sta/documents/downloadable/ucm_485538.pdf (41)

CRAM. (2010). *12 Cranial nerves*. Retrieved from https://www.cram.com/flashcards/12-cranial-nerves-1464273 (4)

Deranged Physiology. *Oculocephalic and cold caloric reflexes (CN III, VI, VIII)*. (2016). Retrieved from https://derangedphysiology.com/main/required-reading/neurology-and-neurosurgery/Chapter%20 4.6.7/oculocephalic-and-cold-caloric-reflexes-cn-iii-iv-vi-and-viii (26)

Drugs.com. (2018). *Phenytoin sodium*. Retrieved from https://www.drugs.com/monograph/phenytoin-sodium.html (2)

El Hussein, M. T., et al. (2017). The ABC's of managing increased intracranial pressure. *Journal of Nursing Education and Practice, 7*(4). Retrieved from http://www.sciedu.ca/journal/index.php/jnep/article/view/9788 (14)

Emergency Nurses Association. (2003). Pediatric emergency core curriculum (2nd ed.). Sudbury, Ontario, Canada: Jones & Bartlett Publishers (9, 21, 57, 58)

Emergency Nurses Association. (2014). Trauma nurse core course (7th ed.). Des Plaines, IL: Emergency Nurses Association. (1, 7, 8, 10, 13–16, 27, 30, 32, 36, 37, 39, 40, 41, 44, 55, 67, 75)

Emergency Nurses Association. (2017). Emergency nursing core curriculum (7th ed.). St. Louis, MO: Elsevier. (7, 24, 45, 47, 50, 53, 54, 56–66, 67, 70, 71, 75)

Emergency Nurses Association. (2018). Emergency nurse pediatric course (5th ed.). Des Plaines, IL: Emergency Nurses Association. (18, 19, 22, 32, 42, 43, 65, 66)

George, J. (2017). *An easier way to remember if succinylcholine is safe for your patient.* Retrieved from https://medium.com/@jstgeorge/can-you-remember-if-succinylcholine-is-safe-for-your-patient-58ef526dd349 (38)

Gondfim, F. A. A. (2015). *Spinal cord trauma and related diseases clinical presentation.* Medscape. Retrieved from https://emedicine.medscape.com/article/1149070-clinical (69)

Hammond, B., et al. (2013). Sheehy's manual of emergency care (7th ed.). St. Louis, MO: Elsevier. (3–6, 9, 13, 24, 28, 29, 31, 33, 35, 36, 45, 47, 50–52, 54–62, 64–68, 70–75)

Hauser, R. A. (2018). *Parkinson disease.* Medscape. Retrieved from https://emedicine.medscape.com/article/1831191-overview (48)

Howard, P. K., et al. (2010). Sheehy's emergency nursing principles and practice (6th ed.). St. Louis, MO: Elsevier. (11, 12, 16–20, 23, 44)

Jauch, E. C., (2017). *Acute Management of Stroke*, Medscape. Retrieved from: https://emedicine.medscape.com/article/1159752-overview#a7 (45)

Katz, K. D. (2018). *Organophosphate toxicity clinical presentation.* Medscape. Retrieved from https://emedicine.medscape.com/article/167726-clinical (12)

Kendra, C. (2018). *A guide to the anatomy of the brain.* Verywellmind. Retrieved from https://www.verywellmind.com/the-anatomy-of-the-brain-2794895 (25)

Kristina, D. (2018). *Can I use rubbing alcohol to bring down a fever?* Verywellhealth. Retrieved from https://www.verywellhealth.com/can-i-use-rubbing-alcohol-to-bring-down-a-fever-770595 (19)

Lafferty, K. A. (2018). *Rapid sequence intubation periprocedural care.* Medscape. Retrieved from https://emedicine.medscape.com/article/80222-periprocedure#b5 (32)

Lawrence, S. C. (2018). *Spinal cord injuries clinical presentation.* Retrieved from https://emedicine.medscape.com/article/793582-clinical (68)

Luzzio, C. (2018). *Multiple sclerosis.* Medscape. Retrieved from https://emedicine.medscape.com/article/1146199-overview (35)

Massage Therapy Reference. (2018). *Cranial nerves (names, mnemonics, testing)*. Retrieved from https://www.massagetherapyreference.com/cranial-nerves/ (3)

McDermott, M. L. (2018). 2018 AHA/ASA stroke early management guidelines. *American College of Cardiology*. Retrieved from https://www.acc.org/latest-in-cardiology/ten-points-to-remember/2018/01/29/12/45/2018-guidelines-for-the-early-management-of-stroke (61)

National Institute of Neurological Disorders and Stroke. (2019). Study of Tenecteplase (TNK) in acute ischemic stroke (TNK-S2B). Retrieved from https://www.ninds.nih.gov/Disorders/Clinical-Trials/Study-Tenecteplase-TNK-Acute-Ischemic-Stroke-TNK-S2B (61)

RXList. (2017). *Cerebyx*. Retrieved from https://www.rxlist.com/cerebyx-drug.htm#description (2)

Skidmore-Roth, L. (2018). 2019 Nursing drug reference (32nd ed.). St. Louis, MO: Elsevier. (46, 49)

SpinalCord.com. (2018). *T9–T12 spinal cord injuries*. Retrieved from https://www.spinalcord.com/t9-t12-vertebrae-thoracic-spinal-cord-injury (68)

Vandenakker-Albanese, C. (2018). *Brown-sequard syndrome*. Medscape. Retrieved from https://emedicine.medscape.com/article/321652-overview#a6 (73)

Weiner, D. L. (2018). *Reye syndrome clinical presentation*. Medscape. Retrieved from https://emedicine.medscape.com/article/803683-clinical (21)

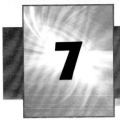

7 Medical and Communicable Diseases

Nancy Mannion Bonalumi, DNP, RN, CEN, FAEN

This chapter focuses specifically on medical emergencies and communicable diseases. On the test, these areas are included in the blueprint under "Psychosocial and Medical Emergencies" and "Environmental/Toxicology Emergencies/Communicable Diseases," and this portion of the actual test will comprise 25 total questions in the category of Psychosocial and Medical Emergencies and 15 questions in the category of Environmental/Toxicology Emergencies/Communicable Diseases spread across the spectrum of medical diseases and illnesses. Each of the following questions will be utilized both as a testing tool *and* as a teaching tool in the answer pages. Rationales for each correct answer and untrue answers are part of the teaching process. Additional information has been supplied in various areas.

1. Which of the following is the treatment of choice for anaphylaxis?
[ ] **A.** Pseudoephedrine
[ ] **B.** Epinephrine
[ ] **C.** Antihistamine
[ ] **D.** Corticosteroid

2. Which of the following body systems is most involved in anaphylaxis?
[ ] **A.** Gastrointestinal system
[ ] **B.** Respiratory system
[ ] **C.** Integumentary system
[ ] **D.** Neurologic system

3. Which of the following is a clinical indication of systemic inflammatory response syndrome (SIRS)?
[ ] **A.** Bradycardia
[ ] **B.** Slow, shallow respirations
[ ] **C.** Elevated white blood cell count
[ ] **D.** Hypertension

4. Goal-directed initial resuscitation measures for septic shock include which of the following?
[ ] **A.** Treating a state of hypoperfusion
[ ] **B.** Decreasing systemic vascular resistance (SVR)
[ ] **C.** Administrating epinephrine subcutaneously
[ ] **D.** Utilizing intravenous diuretic therapy

5. Sickle cell crisis is associated with a number of precipitants. Which of the following is **NOT** one of these precipitants?
[ ] **A.** Cold ambient temperature
[ ] **B.** Infection
[ ] **C.** Metabolic or respiratory alkalosis
[ ] **D.** High altitude

6. A nonresponsive, 64-year-old patient has the following findings in the emergency department: blood glucose 340 mg/dL, serum osmolality 320 mOsm/kg, and pH 7.2. The patient is taking deep, gasping respirations. The emergency nurse should suspect which of the following disease processes?
[ ] **A.** Hyperthyroid crisis (Storm)
[ ] **B.** Hyperosmolar hyperglycemic syndrome (HHS)
[ ] **C.** Syndrome of inappropriate antidiuretic hormone (SIADH)
[ ] **D.** Diabetic ketoacidosis (DKA)

7. An 11-month-old child is brought to the emergency department by his parents. His parents tell the emergency nurse he has been coughing and has had a runny nose for 1 day. He has a red rash on his face, a rectal temperature of 102.5° F (39.2° C), and bluish-white spots on his buccal mucosa. Which of the following conditions are these symptoms associated with?
[ ] **A.** Mumps
[ ] **B.** Measles (Rubeola)
[ ] **C.** Allergic reaction
[ ] **D.** Varicella (chicken pox)

8. When discharging a patient with sickle cell disease which of the following statements indicates the patient understands how to avoid precipitating a sickle cell crisis?
[ ] **A.** "I will self-manage flu-like symptoms for 48 hours before calling my physician."
[ ] **B.** "I can continue to participate in cold weather sporting events."
[ ] **C.** "When I am angry, I will keep my feelings to myself."
[ ] **D.** "I will drink at least 64 ounces of water every day."

9. A patient comes to the emergency department complaining of a nosebleed that began 2 hours before her arrival, and has not subsided, despite direct pressure. She has generalized ecchymosis, and states she has a history of idiopathic thrombocytopenia (ITP). Replacement therapy is indicated based on the diagnostic workup. Which of the following is the appropriate treatment?
[ ] **A.** Desmopressin (DDAVP)
[ ] **B.** IVIg (intravenous immunoglobulin)
[ ] **C.** Thrombin injection
[ ] **D.** Factor VIII

10. Which of the following is an electrocardiogram change consistent with hypercalcemia?
[ ] **A.** Prolonged QT interval
[ ] **B.** Inverted T waves
[ ] **C.** Ventricular tachycardia
[ ] **D.** Prolonged PR interval

11. Disseminated Intravascular Coagulation (DIC) is characterized by the following **EXCEPT**:
[ ] **A.** microvascular clots.
[ ] **B.** increased clotting factors.
[ ] **C.** decreased platelets.
[ ] **D.** impaired hemostasis.

12. An immunocompromised patient presents to the emergency department on the advice of a primary physician, based on which of the following physiologic criteria?
[ ] **A.** Elevated neutrophil count
[ ] **B.** Wound with purulent drainage
[ ] **C.** Warm, red, swollen insect bite
[ ] **D.** Temperature > 100.4° F/38° C

13. In sickle cell crisis, the red blood cells containing hemoglobin S change shape to become a/an:
[ ] **A.** crescent.
[ ] **B.** disc.
[ ] **C.** oblong.
[ ] **D.** figure 8.

14. Which of the following are clinical indicators of hypomagnesemia?
[ ] **A.** Muscle weakness
[ ] **B.** Prolonged QT interval
[ ] **C.** Loss of deep tendon reflexes
[ ] **D.** Muscle tetany

15. When administering intravenous magnesium, the emergency nurse should take which of the following actions?
[ ] **A.** Administer the infusion slowly.
[ ] **B.** Dilute the solution with normal saline only.
[ ] **C.** Administer narcotics at routine dose strength.
[ ] **D.** Monitor pulse and blood pressure every 4 hours.

16. A comatose patient arrives by ambulance to the emergency department. Assessment reveals a prolonged QT interval on electrocadiogram (ECG) and absent deep tendon reflexes.
Vital signs are as follows:

Blood pressure—86/52 mm Hg
Pulse—54 beats/minute
Respirations—8 breaths/minute
Temperature—98.2° F (36.7° C)
Pulse oximetry—94% on room air

The emergency nurse suspects which of the following electrolyte abnormalities?
[ ] **A.** Hypokalemia
[ ] **B.** Hyperkalemia
[ ] **C.** Hypermagnesemia
[ ] **D.** Hypomagnesemia

17. A patient without human immunodeficiency virus (HIV) infection has a tuberculin skin test (purified protein derivative [PPD]). Which of the following is considered a positive result?
[ ] **A.** Redness >10 mm
[ ] **B.** Induration >10 mm
[ ] **C.** Redness of 5 mm
[ ] **D.** Induration of 5 mm

18. Which of the following electrolyte abnormalities is commonly experienced by a patient in adrenal crisis?
[ ] **A.** Hypocalcemia
[ ] **B.** Hypernatremia
[ ] **C.** Hyperglycemia
[ ] **D.** Hyperkalemia

19. Which of the following statements would suggest that the patient diagnosed with mononucleosis understands their condition?

[ ] A. "I can share eating utensils with others as long as I don't have a fever."

[ ] B. "I need to avoid strenuous activity and contact sports for a month."

[ ] C. "A vaccination would have prevented me from contracting this."

[ ] D. "This is an inherited disease and there is nothing I can do about it."

20. Which of the following is the priority nursing intervention for a patient with bone pain related to leukemia?

[ ] A. Send blood for a complete blood count (CBC).

[ ] B. Place the patient in a private room.

[ ] C. Administer narcotics for pain control.

[ ] D. Send the patient for a computed tomography (CT) scan.

21. A 45-year-old patient arrives in the emergency department complaining of fever for the past 2 days. He is awake, alert, and oriented with the following vital signs:

Blood pressure—124/74 mm Hg
Heart rate—120 beats/minute
Respirations—22 breaths/minute
Pulse oximetry—94% on room air
Temperature—101.6° F (38.7° C)

He reports that he is HIV positive and taking antiviral medications. The emergency nurse should triage him at which acuity level using a 5-level system?

[ ] A. Level 1 (resuscitation or life-threatening)

[ ] B. Level 2 (high risk and/or emergent)

[ ] C. Level 3 (urgent)

[ ] D. Level 4/5 (nonurgent/nonemergent)

22. Which of the following is an age-specific consideration for children with sickle cell disease (SCD)?

[ ] A. Routine childhood vaccinations are not recommended.

[ ] B. Ischemic stroke is a high-frequency complication.

[ ] C. Symptoms of SCD are present at birth in affected children.

[ ] D. Attacks will decrease as the child enters adulthood.

23. An elderly patient arrives in the emergency department with a 3-cm laceration on the lower leg. The patient's history reveals daily intake of warfarin (Coumadin). Which of the following complications should the nurse educate the patient about?

[ ] A. Prolonged muscle weakness

[ ] B. Decreased prothrombin time

[ ] C. Prolonged wound healing

[ ] D. Decreased renal clearance

24. A petechial rash and fever are common symptoms of which of the following infectious diseases?

[ ] A. Lyme disease

[ ] B. Meningococcemia

[ ] C. Varicella zoster

[ ] D. Measles

25. Which of the following is the most serious complication associated with adrenal insufficiency (Addison's disease)?

[ ] A. Hypertensive crisis

[ ] B. Myocardial infarction

[ ] C. Intracranial bleed

[ ] D. Hypovolemic shock

26. Priority interventions for a patient with acute adrenal insufficiency (Addison's disease) include all of the following **EXCEPT**:

[ ] A. administration of intravenous (IV) antibiotics.

[ ] B. rapid infusion of a crystalloid solution.

[ ] C. continuous vital sign monitoring.

[ ] D. administration of intravenous (IV) hydrocortisone (Solu-Cortef).

27. A patient arrives in the emergency department with a potential anaphylactic reaction after eating peanuts. The patient has edematous lips, urticaria, and inspiratory stridor. Vital signs are as follows:

Blood pressure—86/60 mm Hg
Heart rate—116 beats/minute
Respirations—24 breaths/minute
Pulse oximetry—94% on room air
Temperature—98.4° F (36.8° C)

After administering epinephrine (Adrenaline), the emergency nurse can anticipate an order for which of the following types of medication?

[ ] A. Corticosteroid

[ ] B. Beta-blocker

[ ] C. Histamine-2 blocker

[ ] D. Antibiotic

28. Which of the following medications can interfere with the compensatory physiologic response to anaphylaxis?

[ ] A. Ceftriaxone (Rocephin)

[ ] B. Metoprolol (Lopressor)

[ ] C. Omeprazole (Prilosec)

[ ] D. Diphenhydramine (Benadryl)

29. Which of the following electrocardiogram (ECG) changes would the emergency nurse expect to see in a patient with a potassium level of 8.5 mEq/mL?
[ ] **A.** Tall P waves
[ ] **B.** Narrow QRS complex
[ ] **C.** Shortened PR interval
[ ] **D.** Peaked T waves

30. When discharging a patient from the emergency department with a diagnosis of hepatitis A, the emergency nurse knows the patient understands his condition based on which of the following statements?
[ ] **A.** "I got this disease from a dirty needle stick."
[ ] **B.** "I will be out of work for 14 days."
[ ] **C.** "I can donate blood in 4 weeks."
[ ] **D.** "My family can get vaccinated for hepatitis A."

31. Hemophilia A is characterized by a genetic deficiency of which clotting factor?
[ ] **A.** Factor IX
[ ] **B.** Factor VIII
[ ] **C.** Factor XI
[ ] **D.** Factor IV

32. Emergency nursing interventions for a hematoma or hemarthrosis due to hemophilia include all of the following **EXCEPT**:
[ ] **A.** application of warm packs.
[ ] **B.** immobilization of the area.
[ ] **C.** elevation of the extremity.
[ ] **D.** application of a compressive dressing.

33. A patient being discharged from the emergency department after treatment for hemophilia demonstrates understanding of his condition with which of the following statements?
[ ] **A.** "I can tell the gang that I can play touch football next weekend."
[ ] **B.** "If I need to I can take aspirin for my pain."
[ ] **C.** "I will arrange for prophylactic care prior to having dental treatments."
[ ] **D.** "I will avoid extremes of hot and cold weather."

34. Interventions for a post-organ transplant patient coming to the emergency department complaining of a fever include all of the following **EXCEPT**:
[ ] **A.** identification of the source of infection.
[ ] **B.** placing the patient in a private room.
[ ] **C.** restricting fluids and food.
[ ] **D.** initiating antibiotic therapy quickly.

35. Which of the following pharmacologic therapies should the emergency nurse anticipate administering to a patient with thyroid storm?
[ ] **A.** Aspirin
[ ] **B.** Propylthiouracil (PTU)
[ ] **C.** Levothyroxine (Synthroid)
[ ] **D.** Morphine sulfate

36. The classic presentation of thyroid storm includes all of the following **EXCEPT**:
[ ] **A.** fever.
[ ] **B.** tachycardia.
[ ] **C.** hot, dry skin.
[ ] **D.** mentation changes.

37. A patient is being seen in the emergency department with herpes zoster. The appropriate staff member to care for this patient would be a nurse who has never had:
[ ] **A.** pertussis.
[ ] **B.** chicken pox.
[ ] **C.** mumps.
[ ] **D.** measles.

38. Which of the following is a common finding in a patient experiencing hyperosmolar hyperglycemic syndrome (HHS)?
[ ] **A.** Glucosuria
[ ] **B.** Anuria
[ ] **C.** Hypertension
[ ] **D.** Bradycardia

39. Which of the following parenteral solutions should be used in the initial treatment of intracellular fluid deficit of a patient with hyperosmolar hyperglycemic syndrome?
[ ] **A.** D_5W with 0.9% normal saline (NS)
[ ] **B.** D_5W with 0.45% normal saline (NS)
[ ] **C.** 0.9% NS with 20 mEq potassium chloride
[ ] **D.** 0.9% normal saline (NS)

40. Which of the following is the most critical complication resulting from hypoglycemia?
[ ] **A.** Thiamine deficiency
[ ] **B.** Brain dysfunction
[ ] **C.** Acidosis
[ ] **D.** Hypothermia

41. Which of the following is an intrarenal cause of acute kidney injury (AKI)?
[ ] **A.** Episode of hypovolemia
[ ] **B.** Development of neurogenic bladder
[ ] **C.** Onset of renal calculi
[ ] **D.** Nonsteroidal anti-inflammatory drugs (NSAIDs)

42. Which of the following is the most significant early diagnostic test for acute kidney injury (AKI)?
[ ] **A.** Urinalysis
[ ] **B.** Creatinine
[ ] **C.** Hemoglobin
[ ] **D.** Potassium

43. Which of the following is a clinical feature of hypercalcemia?
[ ] **A.** Hyperreflexia
[ ] **B.** Weight loss
[ ] **C.** QT prolongation
[ ] **D.** Anuria

44. A patient in the emergency department is being evaluated for acute kidney injury (AKI) and appears very ill. A urinalysis and complete blood count (CBC) have been ordered. Which of the following additional tests would be most beneficial to determine the severity and acuity of renal failure and would require immediate life-saving interventions?
[ ] **A.** Intravenous pyelogram (IVP)
[ ] **B.** Blood urea nitrogen (BUN)
[ ] **C.** Renal arteriogram
[ ] **D.** Serum potassium

45. A patient's laboratory results indicate a sodium value of 106 mEq/mL. Which of the following would be the primary complication for the emergency nurse to anticipate?
[ ] **A.** Tetany
[ ] **B.** Seizure activity
[ ] **C.** Decreased urinary output
[ ] **D.** Profound bradycardia

46. A patient with chronic renal failure requires multiple units of packed red blood cells. The emergency nurse should monitor the patient for:
[ ] **A.** hypocalcemia.
[ ] **B.** hypokalemia.
[ ] **C.** increased white blood cell count.
[ ] **D.** decreased clotting time.

47. Which of the following should be performed by the emergency nurse caring for a patient with suspected Herpes Zoster (shingles)?
[ ] **A.** Place the patient in a negative-pressure room.
[ ] **B.** Administer postexposure prophylaxis.
[ ] **C.** Place the patient on contact precautions.
[ ] **D.** Wear an N-95 respiratory mask.

48. Which of the following two extracellular substances work together to regulate pH?
[ ] **A.** Sodium bicarbonate and acetic acid
[ ] **B.** Sodium bicarbonate and carbonic acid
[ ] **C.** Sodium bicarbonate and sodium hydroxide
[ ] **D.** Sodium bicarbonate and carbon dioxide

49. Which of the following is a true statement regarding the characterization of an acid and a base?
[ ] **A.** Acids release hydrogen (H^+) ions and bases accept H^+ ions.
[ ] **B.** Acids accept H^+ ions and bases release H^+ ions.
[ ] **C.** Both acids and bases can release and accept H^+ ions.
[ ] **D.** Acids can accept and release H^+ ions, and bases accept H^+ ions.

50. A patient demonstrates understanding of discharge instructions after being diagnosed with a latex allergy when stating "I know that I need to avoid many foods but its ok for me to eat:
[ ] **A.** kiwi."
[ ] **B.** bananas."
[ ] **C.** olives."
[ ] **D.** tomatoes."

51. Prerenal causes of acute kidney injury (AKI) include all of the following **EXCEPT**:
[ ] **A.** anaphylaxis.
[ ] **B.** sepsis.
[ ] **C.** heart failure.
[ ] **D.** renal artery stenosis.

52. Which of the following is the expected primary treatment outcome of postrenal acute kidney injury (AKI)?
[ ] **A.** Increase outflow of urine from the kidney
[ ] **B.** Increase renal artery perfusion
[ ] **C.** Increase systemic blood pressure
[ ] **D.** Decrease systemic blood pressure

53. Which of the following is the normal range for arterial blood pH?
[ ] **A.** 7.38 to 7.46
[ ] **B.** 7.40 to 7.52
[ ] **C.** 7.35 to 7.45
[ ] **D.** 7.28 to 7.38

54. An elderly patient has an elevated temperature, restlessness, confusion, and weakness after a radioactive iodine treatment. The physician suspects thyroid storm. Which treatment option should the emergency nurse anticipate?
[ ] **A.** Acetylsalicylate acid (Aspirin)
[ ] **B.** Propranolol (Inderal)
[ ] **C.** Atropine sulfate
[ ] **D.** Sodium bicarbonate

55. A patient with diabetes insipidus should be monitored for which of the following serum electrolyte imbalances?
[ ] **A.** Hypoglycemia
[ ] **B.** Hyponatremia
[ ] **C.** Hypernatremia
[ ] **D.** Hyperglycemia

56. Which of the following systems in the body works fastest to regulate pH in acid–base balance?
[ ] **A.** Renal
[ ] **B.** Respiratory
[ ] **C.** GI system
[ ] **D.** Endocrine

57. A mother brings her child in with a rash and fever and is diagnosed with measles. The mother is concerned about the children that she babysits for each day. Which of the following responses from the mother would indicate that proper education has been provided when the emergency nurse asks her to relay the proper incubation period for this disease process?
[ ] **A.** 1 to 2 days
[ ] **B.** 3 to 5 days
[ ] **C.** 4 to 7 days
[ ] **D.** 10 to 14 days

58. Which of the following is a complication of diphtheria?
[ ] **A.** Inability to open the jaw
[ ] **B.** Maculo-papular rash
[ ] **C.** Difficulty swallowing
[ ] **D.** Muscle spasms

59. While assessing a febrile patient, the nurse notes pain in the hamstring muscle when the patient flexes and contracts the leg. This is symptomatic of which of the following disease processes?
[ ] **A.** Guillain-Barré syndrome
[ ] **B.** Meningitis
[ ] **C.** Lumbar disc compression
[ ] **D.** Multiple sclerosis

60. A patient has been treated for diabetic ketoacidosis for the past 3 hours on an insulin drip. At present, the respiratory rate is 28 breaths/minute, as opposed to 44 breaths/minute on arrival, and the heart rate is 102 beats/minute instead of the initial 140 beats/minute. On asking the patient how she feels, the patient responds that she is better but is complaining of a headache with a pain rating of 7 on a scale of 1 to 10. Which of the following is the most important response by the emergency nurse regarding the new complaint at this time?
[ ] **A.** Obtain an order for acetaminophen (Tylenol).
[ ] **B.** Understand this is a normal reaction.
[ ] **C.** Check the blood sugar.
[ ] **D.** Take the patient's temperature.

61. Which of the following is the major cause of anaphylaxis?
[ ] **A.** Food products
[ ] **B.** Latex
[ ] **C.** Insect stings
[ ] **D.** Exercise

62. Which of the following would indicate treatment for pertussis (whooping cough) has been effective?
[ ] **A.** Resolution of characteristic "whooping" cough and fever
[ ] **B.** Completion of the prescribed antibiotic treatment
[ ] **C.** Negative nasopharyngeal swap for *Bordetella pertussis*
[ ] **D.** Negative reading of chest radiograph

63. Which of the following would indicate effective treatment for disseminated intravascular coagulopathy (DIC)?
[ ] **A.** Hematuria is noted after initiating treatment.
[ ] **B.** A venipuncture site does not bleed after 5 minutes.
[ ] **C.** The platelet count is decreased.
[ ] **D.** Coagulation times are increased.

64. Nursing care of a patient with disseminated intravascular coagulopathy (DIC) includes all of the following **EXCEPT**:

[ ] **A.** administration of medication via intramuscular route.

[ ] **B.** pressure dressings to active bleeding sites.

[ ] **C.** administration of intravenous heparin.

[ ] **D.** limiting the number of venipunctures.

65. All of the following are symptoms of *Clostridium difficile* infection **EXCEPT**:

[ ] **A.** bloody diarrhea.

[ ] **B.** fever.

[ ] **C.** crampy abdominal pain.

[ ] **D.** anorexia.

66. Patients suspected of *Clostridium difficile* infection should be placed in which of the following types of isolation?

[ ] **A.** Contact

[ ] **B.** Droplet

[ ] **C.** Airborne

[ ] **D.** No isolation is needed.

67. A vesicular rash and fever are indicative of which of the following infectious diseases?

[ ] **A.** Kawasaki disease

[ ] **B.** Varicella zoster

[ ] **C.** Lyme disease

[ ] **D.** Meningococcemia

68. Which of the following symptoms are indicative of measles?

[ ] **A.** Pruritic rash to the chest

[ ] **B.** Bluish-gray spots on the buccal mucosa

[ ] **C.** Parotid gland enlargement

[ ] **D.** Petechiae in the folds of the axilla

69. Allergic stings are most commonly caused by which of the following?

[ ] **A.** Hornets

[ ] **B.** Scabies

[ ] **C.** Bumble bees

[ ] **D.** Bed bugs

70. Causes of disseminated intravascular coagulation (DIC) include all of the following **EXCEPT**:

[ ] **A.** sepsis.

[ ] **B.** hemolytic transfusion reaction.

[ ] **C.** idiopathic thrombocytopenia.

[ ] **D.** transplant rejection.

71. Immunotherapy for anaphylaxis can be given to people with allergies to which of the following agents?

[ ] **A.** Peanuts

[ ] **B.** Insect stings

[ ] **C.** Milk

[ ] **D.** Latex

72. Which of the following is the hepatitis virus transmitted via the fecal-oral route?

[ ] **A.** Hepatitis A

[ ] **B.** Hepatitis B

[ ] **C.** Hepatitis C

[ ] **D.** Hepatitis D

73. Which of the following statements made by a patient being discharged with a diagnosis of hepatitis would indicate that the patient understood their instructions?

[ ] **A.** "I can eat anything I want even foods with high fat content."

[ ] **B.** "Other family members will not be able to use the same bathroom."

[ ] **C.** "It will be all right for me to drink alcohol every once in a while."

[ ] **D.** "I will need to reduce my calorie intake from now on."

74. A patient arrives in the emergency department with a slightly decreased level of consciousness and tachycardia. The glucometer reading is 42 mg/dL. He tells the emergency nurse that he has a past history of alcoholism, cirrhosis, coronary artery disease, and pneumonia. All of the following would be appropriate measures for this patient **EXCEPT**:

[ ] **A.** dextrose 50% intravenously.

[ ] **B.** glucagon intramuscularly.

[ ] **C.** place on cardiac monitor.

[ ] **D.** perform frequent vital signs.

75. Which of the following is the main route of transmission for infectious mononucleosis?

[ ] **A.** Blood

[ ] **B.** Skin lesions

[ ] **C.** Stool

[ ] **D.** Saliva

Answers/Rationales

1. Answer: B

Nursing Process: Intervention

Rationale: **Epinephrine is the treatment of choice in all cases of anaphylaxis. By stimulating vascular alpha-adrenergic receptors, epinephrine causes vasoconstriction, thereby increasing vascular resistance and blood pressure. Through its beta$_1$-receptor–stimulating actions, epinephrine increases the force and rate of myocardial contraction and relaxes bronchial smooth muscle, resulting in bronchodilation.** Pseudoephedrine is an alpha- and beta-adrenergic agonist that may also enhance release of norepinephrine. It has been used in the treatment of several disorders, including asthma, heart failure, rhinitis, and urinary incontinence, and for its central nervous system stimulatory effects in the treatment of narcolepsy and depression. Antihistamines work by physically blocking the H$_1$-receptors, stopping histamine from reaching its target. This decreases the body's reaction to allergens and therefore helps to reduce the troublesome symptoms associated with allergies. Corticosteroids are used mostly for their strong anti-inflammatory effects and in conditions that are related to the immune system function.

 CENsational Pearl of Wisdom!

Remember that diphenhydramine (Benadryl) and corticosteroids are used in the treatment of anaphylaxis, but epinephrine (Adrenaline) is the first-line drug because of its immediate action.

2. Answer: C

Nursing Process: Analysis

Rationale: **Anaphylactic reactions almost always involve skin manifestations. Pruritus (itching) and small or localized urticaria (hives) are often present with a minor allergic reaction. In anaphylaxis, widespread urticaria and itching may occur, along with angioedema.** Crampy abdominal pain, nausea, vomiting, or diarrhea rarely occurs, unless the reaction is triggered by a food allergy. Rhinorrhea, nasal congestion, hoarseness, throat tightness, cough, wheezing, and shortness of breath are respiratory symptoms found in about 60% of allergic/anaphylactic reactions. Neurologic symptoms (dizziness, blurred vision, headache, and seizure) are very rare and are secondary to the hypotension that occurs with anaphylaxis.

3. Answer: C

Nursing Process: Analysis

Rationale: **The signs of SIRS include tachycardia (elevated heart rate), tachypnea (elevated respiratory rate), an elevated temperature (or hypothermia), and an elevated white blood cell count and/or greater than 10% bands or immature neutrophils, also termed bandemia.** Hypertension is not considered a sign of SIRS. Hypotension commonly occurs in sepsis, but is not a SIRS criterion.

 CENsational Pearl of Wisdom!

The SIRS response is not only involved in sepsis, but also occurs with both infectious and noninfectious processes. SIRS with infection is sepsis.

4. Answer: A

Nursing Process: Intervention

Rationale: **Because septic shock is associated with a high mortality rate due to a state of severe hypoperfusion, early goal-directed resuscitation measures include treating the state of hypoperfusion. This includes fluid boluses, increasing the systemic vascular resistance (SVR) with vasopressor agents, and/or administering packed red blood cells (PRBCs) if needed.** These measures will decrease the risk of end organ damage often seen in cases of septic shock. Systemic vascular resistance is lowered in septic shock and treatment is aimed at increasing resistance. International guidelines recommend dopamine or norepinephrine as first-line vasopressor agents in septic shock, whereas epinephrine and vasopressin are considered as second-line agents. The effect of vasopressors will improve renal output; thus, there is no indication for diuretic therapy.

5. Answer: C

Nursing Process: Assessment

Rationale: **A state of acidosis, not alkalosis, can precipitate a sickle cell crisis. Acidosis results in a shift to the right on the oxyhemoglobin dissociation curve (Bohr effect), causing hemoglobin to desaturate (release oxygen) more readily.** Cold ambient temperature, infection, and high altitude are well-documented triggers of sickle cell crisis, and patients with this disease are instructed to take appropriate actions to avoid exposure to these triggers.

6. Answer: D

Nursing Process: Assessment

Rationale: **Most hyperglycemic emergencies are due to diabetic ketoacidosis (DKA). A decrease in available insulin increases the blood glucose level because it cannot be transported into cells. To meet the body's energy needs, the liver metabolizes fatty acids, which break down into ketone bodies. Dehydration, electrolyte losses, acidosis, and ketonuria ensue. Kussmaul respirations (deep, rapid breathing) are a compensatory mechanism to buffer the acidosis by reducing serum carbon dioxide levels.** Patients with thyroid storm will appear in a hyperdynamic state, with elevated heart rate, blood pressure, and temperature. Metabolic changes are not common. Hyperosmolar hyperglycemic syndrome (HHS) is characterized by blood glucose levels greater than 600 mg/dL and an absence of acidosis. Syndrome of inappropriate antidiuretic syndrome, due to oversecretion of the antidiuretic hormone, is characterized by decreased urinary output and sodium levels, lethargy, and confusion.

 CENsational Pearl of Wisdom!

Remember that the respiratory system is in control of the acid parameter of acid–base balance. When a situation of metabolic acidosis occurs, the body responds by blowing off the carbon dioxide, thus attempting to reduce the acid in the body.

7. Answer: B

Nursing Process: Assessment

Rationale: **The CDC immunization schedule for children is a first dose at age 12 to 15 months, followed by a second dose between ages 4 and 6 years, before the child enters school. An 11-month-old would not have had the vaccine yet. Koplik spots, small, red specks with a bluish-white center on the buccal mucosa, are a diagnostic lesion of measles. They appear approximately 2 days before the rash and disappear within 48 hours after the rash.** There is a difference between rubella (also known as 3-day measles) and rubeola (commonly known as measles). Mumps cause glandular enlargement of the parotid and salivary glands. There is no rash associated with mumps. In postpuberty males, the testes may be involved, producing orchitis and a risk of infertility. An allergic reaction may produce urticaria, hives, and a disseminated rash. The characteristic symptom of varicella is a vesicular rash that begins on the trunk and becomes generalized.

8. Answer: D

Nursing Process: Evaluation

Rationale: **Dehydration can precipitate a vaso-occlusive crisis in the capillary circulation. Microvascular occlusion leads to tissue ischemia and severe pain. Patients should ensure they have an adequate intake of fluids every day.** Infection is a precipitant of sickle cell crisis and patients should seek immediate medical attention at the first signs of malaise. Exposure to cold temperatures results in vasoconstriction of blood vessels in the skin, hands, feet, nose, and ears. This response is greatly exaggerated in the presence of sickle cell disease. Stressful events trigger the release of vasoactive hormones, which narrow blood vessels. This can lead to a vaso-occlusive crisis. Patients with sickle cell disease need strong coping mechanisms and communication skills to address stress.

9. Answer: B

Nursing Process: Intervention

Rationale: **In the patient with known idiopathic thrombocytopenia (ITP), an intravenous infusion of immunoglobulin (IVIg) is a first-line intervention, because it causes a rapid rise in the platelet levels. Platelet transfusion can also be considered if the count is less than 50,000 and in the presence of severe hemorrhage.** Desmopressin is a synthetic version of vasopressin, which increases the levels of factor VIIIc in the treatment of mild-to-moderate hemophilia. Factor VIII would be utilized in patients with hemophilia A. Thrombin causes blood coagulation by converting fibrinogen to fibrin. Thrombin is indicated for epistaxis, but is not a treatment for ITP.

 CENsational Pearl of Wisdom!

Another important thought—intramuscular injections should be avoided in patients with ITP.

10. Answer: A

Nursing Process: Analysis

Rationale: **Ions such as calcium are essential for conducting electrical current through the cardiac muscle. When ionized serum calcium levels increase, prolonged QT intervals occur.** T-wave inversion is a change seen in hypocalcemia. Patients with low magnesium levels will have ventricular dysrhythmias. A prolonged PR interval is a characteristic finding of hypokalemia.

 CENsational Pearl of Wisdom!

Hypercalcemia is usually seen in adult T-cell lymphoma and multiple myeloma. Additional causes include hyperparathyroidism, use of thiazide diuretics, hyperthyroidism, Addison's disease, renal failure, and excessive consumption of calcium. Treatment is aimed at identifying the underlying cause while preventing cardiac rhythm disturbances.

11. Answer: B

Nursing Process: Assessment

Rationale: **In Disseminated Intravascular Coagulopathy (DIC), both thrombosis and fibrin degradation occur simultaneously, leading to widespread bleeding along with abnormal clotting in the microcirculation.** DIC involves inappropriate and accelerated activation of the co-agulation cascade manifested by impaired hemostasis and a depletion of platelets and clotting factors.

12. Answer: D

Nursing Process: Assessment

Rationale: **The most significant indicator of infection in an immunocompromised person is fever. Thus, this population is instructed to seek medical care whenever the body temperature reaches 100.4° F/38° C.** Immunocompromised patients become neutropenic (decreased neutrophils) and leukemic (decreased total white blood cell count). The body's phagocytic response is suppressed, because the body does not recognize the presence of an infection by typical symptoms such as heat, redness, swelling, and pus at the site of infection.

 CENsational Pearl of Wisdom!

Patients who are immunocompromised are at greater risk of infection, even from normal body flora, as well as from an opportunistic source. These patients should be isolated from the main population of the ED, provided with a face mask to reduce inhaling potentially communicable diseases or, ideally, placed in reverse isolation. Neutropenic patients with fever are considered to be having a medical emergency, and the patient should be isolated from other patients and prioritized for medical evaluation in the ED setting. These patients should not be sent to the waiting room in a triage situation! The waiting room is full of infectious agents!

13. Answer: A

Nursing Process: Analysis

Rationale: **When cells containing hemoglobin S are deoxygenated, the cell changes its shape from a disc to a crescent. These cells become rigid, cannot travel through the microvasculature, and obstruct capillary blood flow, resulting in extensive tissue hypoxia which further exacerbates deoxygenation and increases sickling of the red blood cells.** Red blood cells with normal hemoglobin are disc-shaped. Red blood cells do not take an oblong or figure-8 shape.

 CENsational Pearl of Wisdom!

Oxygen can quickly reverse the sickling process in a large percentage of hemoglobin S–affected cells. Patients should be placed on supplemental oxygen as an immediate priority intervention. Hydroxyurea, a cytotoxic drug, can be used to treat sickle cell anemia. It creates hemoglobin F (HgbF), which is fetal hemoglobin and does not carry the mutation that causes the cells to sickle. Crises are less frequent and less severe with this medication.

14. Answer: D

Nursing Process: Assessment

Rationale: **When serum magnesium is low, the threshold for stimulation is decreased and nerve conduction velocity is increased, leading to an increase in the excitability of muscles and nerves. This can produce muscle cramps, fasciculations, and tetany.** Muscle weakness and loss of deep tendon reflexes, as well as prolonged QT interval in ECG, are indicative of hypermagnesemia.

15. Answer: A

Nursing Process: Intervention

Rationale: **Magnesium sulfate must be infused slowly at a rate not to exceed 125 mg/kg/hour to avoid potential cardiac or respiratory arrest.** Normal saline or 5% dextrose should be used to dilute the infusion. Caution should be used when administering CNS depressants such as narcotics and barbiturates because they potentiate the central nervous system depressant effect of magnesium. Patients being treated with intravenous magnesium sulfate should be placed on continuous cardiac/respiratory monitoring.

16. Answer: C

Nursing Process: Assessment

Rationale: **Elevated magnesium levels depress central and peripheral neuromuscular transmission affecting smooth, cardiac, and skeletal muscles, therefore displaying prolonged QT intervals and absent deep tendon reflexes. Depressed respirations, hypotension, and bradycardia are also part of this picture.** If magnesium levels are below normal, muscle spasms, including tetany, may be evident, along with hyperreflexia, ST depression/T-wave elevation, and hypertension. ECG changes associated with hypokalemia include ST segment and T-wave depression, premature atrial and ventricular contractions, and second- or third-degree heart block. In hyperkalemia, patients can be hyperexcitable, and ECG changes demonstrate peaked, elevated T waves, prolonged PR intervals, and a wide QRS complex.

17. Answer: B

Nursing Process: Evaluation

Rationale: **If a patient has HIV infection, induration of 5 mm or more is considered a positive result. Induration 10 mm or more is considered a positive PPD result in the absence of HIV infection.** Redness may be related to an allergic process but is not considered a positive PPD finding. If a patient has HIV infection, induration of 5 mm or more is considered a positive result.

18. Answer: D

Nursing Process: Assessment

Rationale: **Potassium elevation occurs in adrenal crisis because of an inability to regulate aldosterone, resulting in sodium and water depletion and retention of potassium. These patients frequently have hyponatremia in conjunction with hyperkalemia.** Patients with Addison's disease also have low cortisol production, inhibiting the breakdown of sugar into glucose, resulting in hypoglycemia. Hypocalcemia is related to low levels of mineralocorticoids, unrelated to aldosterone production.

 CENsational Pearl of Wisdom!

Addison's disease can be a very difficult to diagnosis because of the vagueness of the symptoms. The triad of laboratory results that can help to pinpoint this diagnosis is Hypoglycemia, Hyponatremia, and Hyperkalemia.

19. Answer: B

Nursing Process: Evaluation

Rationale: **Splenomegaly occurs frequently in mononucleosis. Because of the risk of injury to an enlarged spleen, strenuous activity and contact sports should be avoided for at least 4 weeks.** The virus is shared primarily via saliva and oropharyngeal route. Sharing eating utensils or food, kissing, and similar actions should be avoided during the incubation period of up to 60 days. There is no vaccine to prevent mononucleosis. It is a communicable virus, not a hereditary disorder.

 CENsational Pearl of Wisdom!

Aspirin is also contraindicated for those children diagnosed with mononucleosis. Remember that mononucleosis is a viral disease caused by the Epstein-Barr virus. The use of aspirin in children with a viral illness can cause Reye's syndrome.

20. Answer: B

Nursing Process: Intervention

Rationale: **Patients with leukemia are at high risk of contracting an infection, which can be lethal. Patients with such conditions should be immediately placed in reverse isolation to reduce the risk of infection.** Obtaining laboratory studies, administering pain medication, and obtaining radiology studies may be indicated, but are not an immediate priority of care.

21. Answer: B

Nursing Process: Assessment

Rationale: **Human immunodeficiency virus (HIV) positive patients with fever are at high risk for deterioration and should be prioritized to an immediate open bed. The patient requires a workup to determine the source of fever and should be protected from other patients who may have a communicable infectious condition.** This patient is not unresponsive, apneic, or in need of any life-saving interventions upon arrival, thus does not meet criteria for a level 1 acuity. Level 3 patients require two or more resources according to the Emergency Severity Index (ESI) algorithm, but his immunocompromised condition escalates his acuity to level 2. Level 4 patients require only one resource and this patient will clearly need multiple resources to identify the source of, and treat, the fever. In a 5-level system, level 5 requires no resources.

 CENsational Pearl of Wisdom!

On the actual test, questions may not be asked that are specific to the ESI; however, triage questions will be present. It is important to acknowledge proper understanding of triage priorities. Always remember to think "Is this patient high risk?" and move them up the scale. Also remember that any patient that requires "resuscitation," whether that is in the form of cardio-pulmonary resuscitation (CPR) or the need for immediate fluid resuscitation, airway management, and so on, is in the resuscitation category now.

22. Answer: B

Nursing Process: Analysis

Rationale: **In sickle cell disease (SCD), the crescent-shaped (sickled) cells become rigid when deoxygenated and cannot pass through the microcirculation, obstructing capillary blood flow. In the cerebral blood vessels, occlusion can lead to ischemic stroke.** Children with SCD are at high risk for infection and should receive all routine childhood immunizations. Fetal hemoglobin is protective during the first 6 months of life, after which SCD becomes evident. There is no evidence that SCD diminishes over time. A person may experience cluster attacks or go month or even years without an attack.

 CENsational Pearl of Wisdom!

Screening for HbS at birth is currently mandatory in the United States. This method of case finding allows institution of early treatment and control. Obtaining a series of baseline values on each patient to compare with those at times of acute illness is useful.

23. Answer: C

Nursing Process: Analysis

Rationale: **The aging process results in dermatologic changes, including a loss of subcutaneous fat, skin elasticity and strength, compounded by the increased bleeding time because of the warfarin. All of these factors contribute to extended wound healing time.** Muscle weakness develops in the elderly, but there is no indication it is a factor in this situation. The effect of warfarin is to prolong the prothrombin time (PT) by interfering with the synthesis of clotting factors. Renal clearance is not a direct complication of a laceration.

24. Answer: B

Nursing Process: Assessment

Rationale: **Meningococcemia is characterized by a rapid onset of fever, petechial rash, and purpura. Death can occur within hours of onset because of coagulopathies and sepsis.** Lyme disease symptoms become evident approximately 1 week after being bitten by an infected deer tick, typically a "bull's-eye" rash around the site of the bite and flu-like symptoms. A purulent vesicular rash that originates on the trunk before becoming generalized characterizes a varicella zoster infection. The onset of measles symptoms is between 7 and 14 days after exposure and is characterized by a high fever and the three "Cs" (cough, coryza, and conjunctivitis). The red, macular rash begins on the face and spreads to the trunk and extremities.

25. Answer: D

Nursing Process: Assessment

Rationale: **Patients with mineralocorticoid insufficiency may exhibit signs of sodium and volume depletion (for example, orthostatic hypotension and tachycardia). Additional symptoms include abdominal pain, fever,**

and confusion. Adrenal insufficiency is characterized by hypotension, not hypertension. Although conduction abnormalities such as prolonged PR or QT intervals may occur and alterations in serum potassium may produce a lethal dysrhythmia, myocardial infarction is not a primary complication. Intercranial bleeding is not associated with adrenal insufficiency.

26. Answer: A

Nursing Process: Intervention

Rationale: **Adrenal insufficiency is an endocrine disorder and does not require antibiotic therapy unless there is evidence of an underlying infection. It is not a priority intervention.** Hypovolemic shock is a life-threatening complication of acute adrenal insufficiency and requires aggressive fluid resuscitation. Additional priority interventions include administration of exogenous corticoids such as hydrocortisone (Solu-Cortef) or dexamethasone (Decadron). Vital signs should be continually monitored during the initial treatment phase.

 CENsational Pearl of Wisdom!

The administration of hydrocortisone (Solu-Cortef) could cause inaccuracies with a cortisol level if it is desired. This would be a diagnostic test to confirm the diagnosis. The administration of dexamethasone (Decadron) would not interfere with the test.

27. Answer: C

Nursing Process: Intervention

Rationale: **Studies have shown the combination of an H_1-blocker such as diphenhydramine (Benadryl) and an H_2-blocker such as famotidine (Pepcid) to be superior to an H_1-blocker alone in relieving the histamine-mediated symptoms of anaphylaxis.** Corticosteroids have no immediate effect on mitigating anaphylaxis. Beta-blockers may increase the risk of anaphylaxis and inhibit the therapeutic effect of epinephrine in treating anaphylaxis. There is no value to administration of antibiotics in treating anaphylaxis because it is not an infectious process.

28. Answer: B

Nursing Process: Analysis

Rationale: **Beta-blockers such as metoprolol (Lopressor) may increase the risk of anaphylaxis. They inhibit the therapeutic effect of epinephrine in treating anaphylaxis by not allowing the beta-receptors to accept the $beta_1$- and $beta_2$-adrenergic effects of epinephrine.** Ceftriaxone (Rocephin) is an antibiotic and has no effect on anaphylaxis.

Omeprazole (Prilosec) is a proton-pump inhibitor (PPI) that does not impact beta-receptors. Diphenhydramine (Benadryl) is an histamine-1 (H₁)-antihistamine and is used in the treatment of itching and hives associated with an allergic reaction.

 CENsational Pearl of Wisdom!

Patients taking beta-blockers who develop anaphylaxis may not respond to epinephrine administration, and refractory hypotension commonly occurs. Glucagon has inotropic and chronotropic effects that do not rely on beta-receptors and can be used. Use caution when administering glucagon, because it can induce vomiting. The emergency nurse should protect the patient's airway by placing them in the lateral recumbent position and have airway, suction and intubation equipment on hand.

29. Answer: D

Nursing Process: Assessment

Rationale: **Elevated serum potassium levels cause tall, peaked T waves on the electrocardiogram.** Elevated potassium can cause the P wave to disappear, not become tall. It also causes the QRS complex to widen, not narrow. PR intervals are lengthened when serum potassium is elevated.

30. Answer: D

Nursing Process: Evaluation

Rationale: **Hepatitis A vaccine is an inactivated (killed) vaccine that can be administered up to 21 days postexposure.** Hepatitis A is transmitted via the fecal-oral route. Hepatitis B and C can be transmitted through a dirty needle stick. Hepatitis A symptoms may last from 2 weeks to 6 months, and the infected person may be too ill to work. Blood banks will not accept blood during the acute phase of the illness, and up to 1 year in some cases.

 CENsational Pearl of Wisdom!

Hepatitis A vaccination requires 2 doses for long-lasting protection. These doses should be given at least 6 months apart. Children are routinely vaccinated between their first and second birthdays (12 through 23 months of age). Older children and adolescents can get the vaccine after 23 months. Adults who have not been vaccinated previously and want to be protected against hepatitis A can also receive the vaccine.

31. Answer: B

Nursing Process: Analysis

Rationale: **Hemophilia A is caused by a deficiency of functional plasma clotting factor VIII.** An absence of factor IX results in hemophilia B, also called Christmas disease. Hemophilia C, or Rosenthal syndrome, is caused by a deficiency of factor XI. Factor IV is ionized calcium and is required in many stages of the coagulation cascade.

 CENsational Pearl of Wisdom!

Von Willebrand's disease is a form of hemophilia that occurs due to a lack of von Willebrand's factor as well as deficiency of factor VIII in the clotting cascade. This form is unique in that females can have this genetic defect. They may have increased mucocutaneous bleeding as well as heavy menstrual periods.

32. Answer: A

Nursing Process: Intervention

Rationale: **Cold, not warm, packs, should be applied to hematomas or a joint with hemarthrosis to increase vasoconstriction and slow bleeding.** Immobilization of the affected area, elevation of an extremity, and the use of a mild compressive dressing are appropriate interventions.

33. Answer: C

Nursing Process: Evaluation

Rationale: **Hemophiliac patients should prepare for dental procedures such as extractions by consulting both the dentist and their hematologist for clotting factor replacement therapy, antifibrinolytic agents, and local hemostatic measures.** Patients with hemophilia should avoid contact sports. Over-the-counter medications containing aspirin or NSAIDs, which can precipitate or prolong bleeding, should be avoided. Temperature extremes do not influence hemophilia.

34. Answer: C

Nursing Process: Intervention

Rationale: **Fever can result in dehydration. Oral fluids as tolerated should be encouraged, and intravenous access should be initiated for administration of crystalloid solutions and medications.** Post-transplant patients face a lifetime of taking immunosuppressant medications to prevent organ rejection. It is important to isolate the patient from others in the emergency department environment.

Cultures of urine and blood and other likely sources of infection should be obtained. Antibiotics should be initiated within 1 hour of arrival in the emergency department.

35. Answer: B

Nursing Process: Intervention

Rationale: **Thyroid storm is characterized by extremes of hyperthyroidism. Propylthiouracil (PTU) blocks thyroid hormone synthesis.** Fever is a common symptom in thyroid storm and should be treated with cooling measures and antipyretics. However, aspirin should be avoided because it can increase thyroid hormone levels. Levothyroxine (Synthroid) is a synthetic replacement for thyroid hormone to treat hypothyroidism, not thyroid storm. Morphine sulfate is an opioid analgesic and is not indicated in the treatment of thyroid storm.

 CENsational Pearl of Wisdom!

PTU inhibits the synthesis of new thyroid hormone but is ineffective in blocking the release of thyroid hormone. Iodide will bind with existing thyroid hormone. Always wait 1 hour after the loading dose of PTU has been given to administer iodine to prevent the utilization of iodine in the synthesis of new thyroid hormone.

36. Answer: C

Nursing Process: Assessment

Rationale: **Patients in thyroid storm are heat-intolerant and sweat excessively, which, along with vomiting and fever, can exacerbate volume loss leading to hypovolemic shock.** Patients in thyroid storm typically have a core body temperature of 101.3° F (38.5° C) due to the body's increased metabolic rate. Hyperpyrexia (core temperature greater than 104° F [40° C]) can occur. Mental status changes, seizures, and coma are commonly seen in this condition. Tachycardia is a classic sign of thyroid storm.

37. Answer: B

Nursing Process: Analysis

Rationale: **Herpes zoster is caused by the reactivation of a dormant varicella (chickenpox) virus. Vesicular lesions develop along a nerve dermatome and contain the live virus. It is contagious to unvaccinated or susceptible hosts. A person who has not had chickenpox may be susceptible to the virus and become ill.** Pertussis is caused by the *Bordetella pertussis* organism. The measles and mumps viruses are not harbored in the body after the infection clears.

38. Answer: A

Nursing Process: Assessment

Rationale: **Excess glucose is excreted via the urine.** The patient will exhibit polyuria, not anuria, as the body draws out water to dilute the elevated blood glucose. The resulting dehydration will cause tachycardia and hypotension, leading to hypovolemic shock if untreated.

 CENsational Pearl of Wisdom!

Hyperosmolar hyperglycemic syndrome (HHS) is a complication of type 2 diabetes mellitus. Patients produce enough insulin to prevent ketosis but not enough to control blood glucose when HHS is triggered. This used to be called HHNC—Hyperosmolar Hyperglycemic Non-Ketotic Coma—but not everyone goes into a coma so they changed the terminology!

39. Answer: D

Nursing Process: Intervention

Rationale: **Fluid deficit can exceed 10 L in Hyperosmolar Hyperglycemic Syndrome (HHS). Rapid rehydration with 0.9 normal saline (NS) is required to prevent circulatory collapse.** Solutions containing dextrose are not indicated in the initial treatment of HHS but may be considered once serum glucose reaches 250 to 300 mg/dL. Serum potassium levels are generally within normal limits initially but should be monitored as the serum glucose levels decrease. Supplemental potassium can be added as needed.

40. Answer: B

Nursing Process: Analysis

Rationale: **Hypoglycemia is characterized by a reduction in plasma glucose concentrations. At low serum glucose levels, the brain is unable to extract oxygen, resulting in hypoxia, altered mental status, and potential brain damage.** Thiamine deficiency may result if the patient is malnourished, but it is not a primary complication. Acidosis is not a complication of hypoglycemia. Patients may develop hyperthermia or hypothermia because of a decreased serum glucose level, but it is not a critical complication.

41. Answer: D

Nursing Process: Analysis

Rationale: **Intrarenal acute kidney injury (AKI) is the result of damage to the body of the kidney because of prolonged hypoperfusion and immunologic or inflammatory** processes. **Chronic use of NSAIDs can be directly nephrotoxic to kidney tissue.** Decreased blood flow from hypovolemia is a prerenal cause of AKI, and neurogenic bladder and renal calculi, which obstruct the flow of urine out of the bladder or kidney, are postrenal causes of AKI.

42. Answer: A

Nursing Process: Analysis

Rationale: **An abnormal urinalysis, with a reddish-brown color, suggesting the presence of myoglobin or hemoglobin, red blood cells, uric acid, and calcium oxalate crystals, is an early finding of acute kidney injury (AKI).** An elevated serum creatinine, changes in hemoglobin levels, and alterations in serum potassium are later indications of AKI.

CENsational Pearl of Wisdom!

Watch your questions closely for words like "early"! These will make a difference in how the question will be answered. As in the above question all potential answers are correct but only one was the "early" sign.

43. Answer: B

Nursing Process: Assessment

Rationale: **Patients with hypercalcemia often complain of weight loss because of anorexia, nausea, vomiting, and constipation.** Hyperreflexia is a symptom of hypomagnesemia. QT prolongation is frequently observed in hypocalcemia. Anuria is defined in the adult population as a passage of less than 50 mL of urine/day and is a complication of acute kidney injury.

CENsational Pearl of Wisdom!

Hypercalcemic patients are often lethargic, confused, and hypertensive, and may have psychiatric manifestations such as psychotic episodes. They may also have impaired memory, feel fatigued, and have decreased muscle strength and reflexes.

44. Answer: D

Nursing Process: Assessment

Rationale: **The most common electrolyte imbalances seen in acute renal failure are hyperkalemia, hyponatremia, hypocalcemia, and hyperphosphatemia. Hyperkalemia is a life-threatening electrolyte disturbance requiring immediate treatment.** An intravenous

pyelogram visualizes abnormalities of the urinary system, including the kidneys, ureters, and bladder, and evaluates the flow of urine through the renal system. Renal angiography can be helpful in establishing the etiology of renal vascular diseases, including renal artery stenosis, but does not assist in determining the severity or acuity. An elevated blood urea nitrogen (BUN) is a hallmark of acute kidney injury but is not considered a life-threatening condition.

45. Answer: B

Nursing Process: Analysis

Rationale: **Normal sodium levels range between 135 and 145 mEq/mL. When serum sodium levels fall below 120 mEq/L, symptoms of hyponatremia appear. An altered level of consciousness ranging from confusion to coma and seizures are commonly seen.** Tetany is a serious complication of hypocalcemia. Decreased urinary output (less than 500 mL of urine/24 hours in an adult) is seen in both acute kidney injury and chronic renal failure. Tachycardia, not bradycardia, is seen in hyponatremia.

CENsational Pearl of Wisdom!

Hyponatremia can result from either a depletion of serum sodium or a dilution of sodium in the vascular system. Treatment of hyponatremia is to gradually replace sodium. The intravenous treatment is an IV infusion of 0.9% normal saline or hypertonic (3%) saline solution. Hypertonic saline can be dangerous! This is only given when sodium levels are extremely low (less than 110 mEq/mL) and needs to be stopped when symptoms are seen to be improving—not waiting for the numbers to return to normal!

46. Answer: A

Nursing Process: Analysis

Rationale: **Each unit of packed red blood cells (PRBCs) for transfusion contains approximately 3 mg of citrate as a preservative, which accumulates in the blood where it binds to circulating calcium, thereby reducing plasma calcium concentration. Patients receiving more than 5 units of PRBCs should have serum calcium levels checked. These patients may require intravenous calcium chloride of calcium gluconate.** A patient receiving multiple transfusions of PRBCs would be at risk of hyperkalemia due to the breakdown of blood cells that release potassium while it is being stored. White blood cell counts are not impacted with administration of packed red cells. Clotting times may be increased because packed red cells do not contain any clotting factors. Replacement of platelets and fresh frozen plasma (FFP) should be considered when multiple units of PRBCs are infused.

47. Answer: C

Nursing Process: Intervention

Rationale: **Herpes zoster is spread via direct contact with the herpetic lesions.** Negative-pressure isolation is indicated for airborne, not contact, isolation. A patient who is already symptomatic will not benefit from post-exposure prophylaxis. The N-95 respiratory mask is required for droplet infections such as tuberculosis.

CENsational Pearl of Wisdom!

Patients requiring contact isolation should be isolated in a single-patient area as soon as possible, caregivers should wear gloves and gown during direct care, and disposable or dedicated patient-care equipment should be used. Patient movement outside of the treatment room should be limited. If transport is necessary, the infected areas of the patient's body should be covered.

48. Answer: B

Nursing Process: Analysis

Rationale: **Sodium bicarbonate and carbonic acid are the two primary extracellular regulators of pH. pH is also further regulated by electrolyte composition within the intracellular and extracellular compartments.** Acetic acid is commonly known as vinegar and is not an extracellular substance in the human body. Carbon dioxide combines with water to form carbonic acid. Sodium hydroxide is lye or caustic acid and is not found in the body.

CENsational Pearl of Wisdom!

pH remains normal if a ratio of 20 base to 1 acid is maintained. Bicarbonate is the base parameter and carbonic acid (which creates carbon dioxide) is the acid component.

49. Answer: A

Nursing Process: Analysis

Rationale: **Acids are molecules that have the ability to release H^+ ions and bases are molecules that have the ability to accept or bind with H^+ ions.** Acids do not accept H^+ ions, and bases do not release H^+ ions.

50. Answer: C

Nursing Process: Evaluation

Rationale: **Approximately 50% of people with latex allergy have a history of another type of allergy. Food restriction for patients with latex allergies does not include olives.** Certain fruits and vegetables, such as bananas, chestnuts, kiwi, avocado, and tomato, can cause allergic symptoms in some latex-sensitive individuals because of a possible cross-sensitization of the latex product in these plants.

51. Answer: D

Nursing Process: Assessment

Rationale: **Renal artery stenosis produces localized ischemia because of narrowed renal artery perfusion within the kidney. It is considered an intrarenal or intrinsic cause of acute kidney injury (AKI).** Prerenal acute kidney injury results from decreased blood flow to the kidney, resulting in ischemia of the nephrons. Prolonged ischemia can lead to acute tubular necrosis and permanent renal damage. Profound, persistent systemic hypotension from anaphylaxis, sepsis, or heart failure are common causes of prerenal acute kidney injury.

52. Answer: A

Nursing Process: Evaluation

Rationale: **Postrenal acute kidney injury is the result of an obstruction of the urinary collection system from the calices of the kidney to the urethral meatus. Relief of the obstruction and allowing urine to flow out of the kidney is the intention of treatment interventions.** Increasing renal artery perfusion and increasing or decreasing systemic blood pressure are interventions which influence prerenal acute kidney injury.

53. Answer: C

Nursing Process: Assessment

Rationale: **Tight regulation of $[H^+]$ is crucial for normal cellular activities. The body requires a pH of 7.35 to 7.45 to maintain homeostasis.** pH values below 7.35 are reflective of acidosis and values in excess of 7.45 indicate alkalosis.

54. Answer: B

Nursing Process: Intervention

Rationale: **Propranolol is the mainstay of treatment for this problem. This will decrease the heart rate and also prevents conversion of T_4 to T_3. The T_3 state is the state in which thyroid hormone is utilized in the cells.**

Propranolol can be administered orally, via nasogastric tube, or intravenously. Intravenous dosing is 0.5 to 1.0 mg over a 10-minute period of time and then 1.0 to 2.0 mg every few hours depending on heart rate and blood pressure readings. Aspirin has antipyretic properties, which is usually indicated for controlling fever, but in thyroid storm, aspirin is contraindicated as it can free up more thyroid hormone in the T₃ state. Atropine would increase the heart rate. Anticholinergics such as atropine are ineffective in controlling the rapid heart rate of thyroid storm, as it is a hypermetabolic state because of excessive thyroid hormone release. Sodium bicarbonate is a buffer for the acid–base system. Acidosis may develop in patients with thyroid storm due to their hypermetabolic condition, but sodium bicarbonate is not a primary treatment of thyroid storm.

 CENsational Pearl of Wisdom!

Remember to avoid beta-blockers if the patient has asthma, chronic obstructive pulmonary disease, peripheral vascular disease, or decompensated heart failure. Also glucocorticoids are used in many of these crisis situations due to the increased use of cortisol, the stress hormone, during these episodes.

55. Answer: C

Nursing Process: Evaluation

Rationale: **Diabetes insipidus is caused by a defect in the secretion of antidiuretic hormone (ADH) or the kidney's ability to concentrate urine. The patient exhibits polyuria and polydipsia. This water disturbance results in dehydration and hypernatremia.** There is little to no effect on blood glucose values in diabetes insipidus. Patients with diabetes insipidus can pass large volumes (greater than 3 L/24 hour) of dilute urine, which concentrates serum sodium levels. Hyponatremia is not seen in this condition.

56. Answer: B

Nursing Process: Assessment

Rationale: **Both the respiratory and renal systems work to regulate pH in acid–base imbalance; however, the respiratory system works in a matter of minutes and reaches its peak within 12 to 24 hours of the onset of an acid–base imbalance.** The renal system also regulates acid–base balance; however, the onset of its effect is slower and the renal system will function for days to restore the pH to normal limits. The GI and endocrine systems have little or no effect on regulating acid–base balance.

 CENsational Pearl of Wisdom!

The kidneys are able to affect blood pH by excreting excess acids or bases. The kidneys have some ability to alter the amount of acid or base that is excreted, but because the kidneys make these adjustments more slowly than the lungs, this compensation generally takes several days. The nice thing is that this system can eventually correct an abnormal pH, but the respiratory system, which deals with the carbon dioxide (acid) component, will not be able to totally compensate.

57. Answer: D

Nursing Process: Evaluation

Rationale: **Measles is a highly contagious illness caused by the *Morbillivirus* and is spread by coughing and sneezing via close personal contact or direct contact with secretions. The average incubation period from exposure to onset of the measles is 10 to 14 day.** Patients are contagious from 1 to 2 days before the onset of symptoms. The patient can be infectious from 3 to 5 days before the appearance of the rash to 4 days after the onset of rash. The rash has an average duration of 4 to 7 days.

58. Answer: C

Nursing Process: Assessment

Rationale: **The toxins released by diphtheria set up the development of a localized or coalescing pseudomembrane, which can occur in any portion of the respiratory tract, leading to difficulty breathing. The pseudomembrane is characterized by the formation of a dense, gray debris layer comprising a mixture of dead cells, fibrin, red blood cells (RBCs), white blood cells (WBCs) and organisms.** The inability to open the jaw and muscle spasms are symptoms of tetanus, not diphtheria. Diphtheria does not produce a rash.

59. Answer: B

Nursing Process: Assessment

Rationale: **Meningeal irritation causes pain with flexion/extension of the leg (Kernig's sign).** Guillain-Barré is an acute peripheral neuropathy characterized by ascending muscle weakness and paralysis. There is no pain with flexion/extension of the hamstring muscle in Guillain-Barré. Lumbar disc compression is not accompanied by fever. Multiple sclerosis is characterized by intermittent episodes of neurologic symptoms such as paresthesia, weakness, and visual disturbances, but not fever. Flexion/extension of the hamstring muscles does not induce pain with this patient population.

CENsational Pearl of Wisdom!

Another sign of meningitis (besides Kernig's sign) is Brudzinski's sign. This is elicited by flexing the neck and the hips and knees flex automatically at the same time. Nuchal rigidity can also be seen. This causes the neck to not be able to bend to touch the chin to the chest. All three of these signs are great, but they are not always demonstrable in all patients with meningitis.

60. Answer: C

Nursing Process: Assessment

Rationale: **Blood glucose should be decreased at a rate of 75 to 100 mg/dL/hour. If the level is reduced too quickly, cerebral edema can occur. Blood glucose levels should be monitored hourly to make sure that the rate of decrease is not too great.** This is not normal for treatment for diabetic ketoacidosis (DKA). Tylenol (Acetaminophen) can help but is not the priority. Considering the temperature will not impact this problem.

61. Answer: A

Nursing Process: Analysis

Rationale: **Food is implicated in the largest percentage of anaphylactic episodes, causing approximately 13% to 65% of all episodes.** Latex is the cause of between 7% and 9% of anaphylactic reactions and has been steadily decreasing with the use of latex-free products, especially in the hospital setting. Insect stings account for 1% to 7% of episodes. Exercise-induced anaphylaxis is rare, occurring in less than 1% of the population.

CENsational Pearl of Wisdom!

In the Unites States, eight foods account for the majority of food allergy reactions: milk, egg, peanut, tree nuts, soy, wheat, fish, and shellfish.

62. Answer: C

Nursing Process: Evaluation

Rationale: **A negative swab is the only definitive evidence that treatment has been effective.** Despite resolution of fever and cough, pertussis infection may still

be present in the body. Pertussis requires an extensive course of antibiotics, often up to 3 weeks. Pertussis is not detected on a chest radiograph.

63. Answer: B

Nursing Process: Evaluation

Rationale: **Return of a normal clotting time is an indication that appropriate and effective treatment has occurred, which would be indicated by a venipuncture site that is not bleeding within this period of time.** Hematuria is a common physical finding in disseminated intravascular coagulation (DIC), along with hematemesis, occult blood in the stool, and prolonged bleeding from puncture sites. Platelets are decreased in DIC, and increasing the count is a goal of therapy. Coagulation times are prolonged in DIC. Goals of treatment are normal prothrombin time (PT) and partial thromboplastin time (PTT) values.

64. Answer: A

Nursing Process: Intervention

Rationale: **Intramuscular injections should be avoided to prevent bleeding and hematoma development at the injection site in a patient with disseminated intravascular coagulation (DIC).** Pressure dressings will slow bleeding until the coagulopathy is corrected. Heparin is the drug of choice for treatment of DIC. It acts to inhibit thrombin development, preventing clot formation in the microvasculature. Venipunctures, injections, and other interventions that may disrupt the integrity of the skin should be avoided to prevent additional bleeding.

CENsational Pearl of Wisdom!

The most important treatment for DIC is correcting the underlying cause. DIC is a secondary response to a primary problem and there is always a disease process that needs to be corrected. Other treatment options include the replacement of clotting factors through the use of platelets, cryoprecipitate, and fibrinogen.

65. Answer: A

Nursing Process: Assessment

Rationale: ***Clostridium difficile* infection is characterized by mild-to-moderate watery diarrhea that is rarely bloody.** It has a characteristic odor and may contain mucous. Common symptoms seen in patients with *C. difficile* infection include fever, especially in severe cases, crampy abdominal pain and a loss of appetite.

66. Answer: A

Nursing Process: Intervention

Rationale: **Clostridium difficile is categorized as a health care–acquired infection. The spores can live on inanimate objects for up to 5 months. Caregivers should use contact precautions to prevent exposure to themselves and inadvertent transmission to other patients.** Droplet precautions are indicated for patients known or suspected to be infected with pathogens transmitted by respiratory droplets that are generated by a patient who is coughing, sneezing, or talking. Use airborne precautions when caring for patients infected with known or suspected pathogens transmitted by the airborne route (tuberculosis, measles, chickenpox, herpes zoster, etc.).

 CENsational Pearl of Wisdom!

It is important to get patients placed into appropriate isolations as soon as possible! It takes more time and can be frustrating, but it most certainly needs to be done!

67. Answer: B

Nursing Process: Assessment

Rationale: **Varicella zoster lesions are fluid-filled vesicles, most commonly affecting the thoracic dermatome. The patient may have flu-like symptoms with or without fever.** A petechial rash of small, pinpoint lesions progressing rapidly to purpura is the characteristic manifestation of meningococcemia. Petechial and purpuric lesions develop from bleeding under the skin and do not blanch on applying pressure. Fever has a sudden onset and rises quickly. Kawasaki disease is a rare childhood illness, which presents with a fever and rash of poorly defined spots of various sizes, often bright red that blanch when pressure is applied. The rash of Lyme disease begins at the site of a tick bite after a delay of 3 to 30 days (average is about 7 days). It expands gradually over a period of days reaching up to 12″ or more (30 cm) across. As it enlarges, the center clears, resulting in a target or "bull's-eye" appearance.

68. Answer: B

Nursing Process: Assessment

Rationale: **Bluish-gray spots (Koplik spots) appear on the inside of the cheeks after 2 to 4 days of prodromal symptoms and are visible for up to 5 days. The rash of measles is maculopapular and first appears on the face.** A pruritic rash to the chest is indicative of varicella (chickenpox). Parotid gland enlargement is characteristic of mumps. Petechiae in the skin folds of the axilla and groin are found in scarlet fever.

69. Answer: A

Nursing Process: Analysis

Rationale: **Hornets, yellow jackets, and wasps are the leading cause of allergic stings. They are aggressive and can sting repeatedly with minimal provocation.** Scabies is an intensely itchy skin infestation caused by a mite. It does not produce an allergic reaction. Bumble bees can produce an allergic reaction but are much less aggressive and sting with much lower frequency. Bed bugs are parasitic insects that feed on blood. The bite produces a painless, pruritic lesion. Urticaria may develop from repeated exposure.

70. Answer: C

Nursing Process: Analysis

Rationale: **Idiopathic thrombocytopenia is a disease of increased peripheral platelet destruction, commonly seen in children several weeks after a viral infection such as chickenpox or rubella.** DIC is a thrombohemorrhagic disorder involving inappropriate and accelerated stimulation of the clotting cascade. Common causes include sepsis, a hemolytic transfusion reaction, transplant rejection as well as massive blood transfusions, major trauma, and obstetrical complications such as abruptio placentae and retained placenta.

71. Answer: B

Nursing Process: Intervention

Rationale: **Immunotherapy can provide significant improvements in allergic symptoms and reduce the need for additional pharmacotherapy of insect stings and environmental allergens such as pollen. Immunotherapy has proven to have long-term benefits and is effective for desensitizing a person as a means of preventing reactions to subsequent stings.** There are clinical trials using immunotherapy in peanut allergies, but it is not a proven therapy at this time. No specific immunologic therapy has been found to desensitize milk or latex allergies.

72. Answer: A

Nursing Process: Assessment

Rationale: **Hepatitis A is transmitted primarily through the fecal-oral route, usually by person-to-person contact or by ingesting contaminated water or food. It is infectious 2 weeks before and 2 weeks after symptom onset.**

Intravenous drug use and sexual contact are the primary transmission routes for hepatitis B. Blood transfusions are less frequently a source of transmission because of the careful screening of donated blood. Hepatitis C is also transmitted via IV drug use and from blood transfusions administered before testing of the blood supply. Hepatitis D is only found in patients with acute or chronic hepatitis B, because it is an incomplete virus and requires the hepatitis B virus to replicate. It is also transmitted via IV drug use or sexual contact.

 CENsational Pearl of Wisdom!

Remember that there are vaccines available for hepatitis A and B but not for hepatitis C!

73. Answer: B

Nursing Process: Evaluation

Rationale: **Family members and close personal contacts should avoid using the same bathroom as a patient with a diagnosis of hepatitis to avoid exposure to body substances and fluids. This exposure can potentially transmit the hepatitis virus.** Dietary instructions for a patient with hepatitis include a high-caloric, high-carbohydrate, low-fat diet. The patient should be instructed to eat small, frequent meals. Alcohol use is prohibited during the acute illness because it is metabolized in the liver.

74. Answer: B

Nursing Process: Intervention

Rationale: **With a past history of alcoholism and cirrhosis, glucagon will most likely not work for this patient. Glucagon stimulates the liver to produce glucose, and with the liver involvement in this patient, it will probably not work.** Providing intravenous glucose is appropriate. Patients with hypoglycemia should be placed on the cardiac monitor and have vital signs measured frequently in order to adequately watch the patient for signs of deterioration or improvement.

 CENsational Pearl of Wisdom!

Once hypoglycemia is treated and the patient responds, it is important to provide a meal so that the blood glucose level remains within a normal range. They need complex carbohydrates to maintain the sugar level.

75. Answer: D

Nursing Process: Analysis

Rationale: **The main causal agent of infectious mononucleosis is the Epstein-Barr virus. The usual route of transmission is oropharyngeal through saliva. Hence, its moniker as the "kissing disease."** The virus is not found in blood or stool. It is not passed by contact with skin lesions. Classic symptoms of mononucleosis include a flu-like prodromal period lasting 3 to 5 days followed by fever, pharyngitis, and lymphadenopathy. No rash is associated with mononucleosis.

References

Aberra, F. (2017, December 6). *Clostridium difficile colitis: Practice essentials, background, pathophysiology.* Retrieved from https://emedicine.medscape.com/article/186458-overview (66)

Acharya, S. S. (2018). *Pediatric Von Willebrand's disease, treatment and management.* Retrieved from https://emedicine.medscape.com/article/959825-treatment (31)

American Academy of Allergy, Asthma & Immunology. (n.d.). *Latex allergy.* Retrieved from https://www.aaaai.org/conditions-and-treatments/allergies/latex-allergy (50)

American College of Allergy, Asthma & Immunology. *Insect sting allergy.* (n.d.). Retrieved from https://acaai.org/allergies/types/insect-sting-allergies (69)

Avni, T., et al. (2015). Vasopressors for the treatment of septic shock: Systematic review and meta-analysis. *PLos One, 10*(8). doi:10.1371/journal.pone.0129305. (3, 4)

Benenson, I., et al. (2018). Sickle cell disease: Bone, joint, muscle, and motor complications. *Orthopaedic Nursing, 37*(4). doi:10.1097/NOR.0000000000000464. (22)

Bronfenbrener, R. (2017, January 7). *Acid-base interpretation: Reference range, interpretation, collection and panels.* Retrieved from https://emedicine.medscape.com/article/2058760-overview#a4 (48, 53, 56)

Brutsaert, E. F. (2017, February). *Hyperosmolar Hyperglycemic State (HHS)—Endocrine and metabolic disorders.* Retrieved from https://www.merckmanuals.com/professional/endocrine-and-metabolic-disorders/diabetes-mellitus-and-disorders-of-carbohydrate-metabolism/hyperosmolar-hyperglycemic-state-hhs (38, 39)

Campbell, R. L. (2018, July 24). *Anaphylaxis: Emergency treatment.* Retrieved from https://www.uptodate.com/contents/anaphylaxis-emergency-treatment (28)

Centers for Disease Control and Prevention. (2016, July 20). *Vaccine information statements (VISs).* Retrieved from https://www.cdc.gov/vaccines/hcp/vis/vis-statements/hep-a.html (30)

Centers for Disease Control and Prevention. (2017, August 7). *Pertussis (Whooping cough)*. Retrieved from https://www.cdc.gov/pertussis/php.html (62)

Centers for Disease Control and Prevention. (2017, February 28). *Transmission-based precautions*. Retrieved from https://www.cdc.gov/infectioncontrol/basics/transmission-based-precautions.html (65, 66)

Chen, S. S. (2018, June 27). *Measles: Practice essentials, background, pathophysiology*. Retrieved from https://emedicine.medscape.com/article/966220-overview (57, 68)

Cunha, B. A. (2018, April 23). *Epstein-Barr Virus (EBV) infectious mononucleosis (Mono): Background, pathophysiology, epidemiology*. Retrieved from https://emedicine.medscape.com/article/222040-overview (9)

Devarajan, P. (2018, April 23). *Oliguria: Background, etiology, epidemiology*. Retrieved from https://emedicine.medscape.com/article/983156-overview (43, 45)

Farrkh, A., et al. (2016). Dental surgical management of the patient with hemophilia. *General Dentistry, 64*(4), 14–17. Retrieved from https://www.agd.org/publications-and-news/general-dentistry/general-dentistry-details/july-august-2016 (33)

Hamdy, O. (2018). Diabetic ketoacidosis treatment. *Emedicine*. Retrieved from https://emedicine.medscape.com/article/118361-treatment#d9 (60)

Hamdy, O. (2018, July 2). *Hypoglycemia: Practice essentials, background, pathophysiology*. Retrieved from https://emedicine.medscape.com/article/122122-overview#a7 (40)

Javid, M. H. (2017, October 11). *Meningococcemia: Practice essentials, background, pathophysiology*. Retrieved from https://emedicine.medscape.com/article/221473-overview (24)

Javit, M. (2018, July 20). *Meningococcemia clinical presentation: History, physical examination*. Retrieved from https://emedicine.medscape.com/article/221473-clinical (67)

Khardori, R. (2018, April 27). *Diabetes insipidus: Practice essentials, background, etiology*. Retrieved from https://emedicine.medscape.com/article/117648-overview#a1 (55)

Klauer, K. M. (2017, October 10). *Adrenal crisis in emergency medicine: Background, pathophysiology, epidemiology*. Retrieved from https://emedicine.medscape.com/article/765753-overview (25, 26)

Levi, M. M., et al. (2018, April 22). *Disseminated intravascular coagulation*. Retrieved from https://emedicine.medscape.com/article/199627-overview (11)

Li, K., et al. (2015). Citrate metabolism in blood transfusions and its relationship due to metabolic alkalosis and respiratory acidosis. *International Journal of Clinical and Experimental Medicine, 8*(4), 6578–6584. (46)

Liess, B. (2018, April 5). *Immunotherapy for allergies: Background, indications, contraindications*. Retrieved from https://emedicine.medscape.com/article/1588289-overview#a1 (71)

Lo, B. (2018, August 1). *Diphtheria: Background, pathophysiology, epidemiology*. Retrieved from https://emedicine.medscape.com/article/782051-overview (58)

LoVerde D, et al. (2017, August). Anaphylaxis. *Contemporary Reviews in Critical Care Medicine*. doi:10.1016/j.chest.2017.07.033. (1, 2, 61)

Luciano, R., et al. (2017, March 1). *NSAIDS: Acute kidney injury (acute renal failure)*. Retrieved from https://www.uptodate.com/contents/nsaids-acute-kidney-injury-acute-renal-failure (41)

Maakaron, J. E. (2017, December 27). *Sickle cell anemia: Practice essentials, background, genetics*. Retrieved from https://emedicine.medscape.com/article/205926-overview (22)

Misra, M. (2018, June 6). *Thyroid storm treatment & management: Approach considerations, medical care, surgical care*. Retrieved from https://emedicine.medscape.com/article/925147-treatment#d7 (54)

Mustafa, S. S. (2018, July 20). *Anaphylaxis treatment & management: Approach considerations, initial emergency department interventions, administration of epinephrine*. Retrieved from https://emedicine.medscape.com/article/135065-treatment#d10 (28)

Samji, N. (2018, July 25). *Viral hepatitis*. Retrieved from https://emedicine.medscape.com/article/775507-overview (72, 73)

Schrag, E. D. (2018, July 18). *Hyperthyroidism, thyroid storm, and Grave's disease: Background, pathophysiology, epidemiology*. Retrieved from https://emedicine.medscape.com/article/767130-overview (35, 36)

Sheehy, S. B., et al. (2013). Sheehy's manual of emergency care. St. Louis, MO: Elsevier/Mosby. (5–8, 10, 12–20, 29, 31–40, 42–45, 51–58, 60, 63–64, 67, 70, 73–75)

Silverman, M. A. (2018, March 30). *Idiopathic Thrombocytopenic Purpura (ITP) in emergency medicine treatment & management: Prehospital care, emergency department care, consultations*. Retrieved May 17, 2018, from https://emedicine.medscape.com/article/779545-treatment#d2 (9)

Singer, M., et al. The third international consensus definitions for sepsis and septic shock (sepsis-3). *JAMA, 315*(8), 801–810. doi:10.1001/jama.2016.0287. (3, 4)

Staff, S. X. (2017, November 7). *Stress, fear of pain may be cause of painful sickle cell episodes*. Retrieved May

17, 2018, from https://medicalxpress.com/news/2017-11-stress-pain-painful-sickle-cell.html (3, 8)

Sweet, V. (2018). Emergency nursing: Core curriculum (7th ed.). St. Louis, MO: Elsevier. (1, 2, 5–8, 10, 12–21, 23–27, 32–53, 57–58, 60, 63–64, 67, 70, 73–75)

Tewari, S., et al. (2015). Environmental determinants of severity in sickle cell disease. *Haematologica, 100*(9), 1108–1116. doi:10.3324/haematol.2014.120030. (8)

The Free Dictionary. (n.d.). *Coagulation cascade & roles—of its various components.* Retrieved from https://medicaldictionary.thefreedictionary.com/coagulation factors (31)

Workeneh, B. (2018, July 9). *Acute kidney injury: Practice essentials, background, pathophysiology.* Retrieved from https://emedicine.medscape.com/article/243492-overview (42, 51, 52)

8 Respiratory Emergencies

Jaime Dahm, MSN, RN, CEN

Respiratory emergencies involve a wide variety of problems both medical- and trauma-related. On the test, there are 16 questions devoted to this body system. The following questions, answers, rationales, and CENsational Pearls of Wisdom should help to provide you with the tools that you will need to be successful on this part of the test. These questions can range from simple to complex and will include the scope of the nursing process—Assessment/Analysis/Intervention/Evaluation. This content is meant as a review of these concepts. Best of luck on this chapter!

1. An unrestrained passenger is thrown 20 feet (6 m) from a car that hit an embankment. On arrival to the emergency department, the patient is conscious and complains of shortness of breath. His vital signs are blood pressure 108/66 mm Hg, pulse 116 beats/minute with weak radial pulses, and respirations 26 breaths/minute and shallow. Capillary refill is delayed. The lungs are clear bilaterally with diminished breath sounds on the right. Paradoxical chest movement is noted on the right side. A chest radiograph shows a right pneumothorax and multiple rib fractures on the right (fourth to seventh). Which of the following potential injuries would be the trauma nurse's primary concern for this patient?
[ ] **A.** Flail chest
[ ] **B.** Tension pneumothorax
[ ] **C.** Ruptured diaphragm
[ ] **D.** Massive hemothorax

2. Which of the following assessment findings would **NOT** indicate a flail chest?
[ ] **A.** Paradoxical movement
[ ] **B.** Sucking chest wound
[ ] **C.** Respiratory distress
[ ] **D.** Pulmonary contusion

3. Which of the following drugs is safe for administration to the patient with asthma?
[ ] **A.** Beta-adrenergic blockers
[ ] **B.** Beta$_2$-agonists
[ ] **C.** Salicylates (Aspirin)
[ ] **D.** Nonsteroidal anti-inflammatory drugs (NSAIDs)

4. Which of the following findings is **NOT** consistent with blood loss greater than 1,500 mL in a patient with a hemothorax?
[ ] **A.** Mediastinal shift
[ ] **B.** Systolic blood pressure less than 80 mm Hg
[ ] **C.** Capillary refill greater than 4 seconds
[ ] **D.** Increased urinary output

5. After teaching the patient with asthma about inhalers, which of the following statements indicates the need for further instruction?
[ ] **A.** "I should hold the inhaler upright and shake it well."
[ ] **B.** "I should hold my breath for 5 to 10 seconds after each puff."
[ ] **C.** "I should hold the inhaler in my mouth with a good seal."
[ ] **D.** "I should hold my head back and forcefully exhale."

6. The first priority for a patient with a pulmonary embolus (PE) is:
[ ] **A.** correcting the hypoxia with oxygen.
[ ] **B.** administering heparin.
[ ] **C.** considering thrombolytic therapy.
[ ] **D.** administering morphine to treat pain.

7. Which of the following is **NOT** an appropriate intervention for the child with suspected epiglottitis?
[ ] **A.** Obtaining a throat culture
[ ] **B.** Providing supplemental oxygen
[ ] **C.** No invasive procedures
[ ] **D.** Lateral neck radiograph

8. Which of the following statements is **NOT** true regarding respiratory anatomical and physiologic differences in the pediatric patient?
[ ] **A.** The diaphragm is flatter and is the primary muscle for ventilation.
[ ] **B.** Pediatric alveoli are larger and result in increased surface area for gas exchange.
[ ] **C.** Abdominal muscles play a larger role in respiration.
[ ] **D.** Children have faster and deeper respiratory rates.

9. Which of the following is the priority intervention for a child with epiglottitis?
[ ] **A.** Providing oxygen by nasal cannula
[ ] **B.** Administering antibiotics
[ ] **C.** Assisting with intubation
[ ] **D.** Monitoring for dysrhythmias

10. Which of the following is the most serious injury associated with a fracture of the first or second rib?
[ ] **A.** Cervical spine injury
[ ] **B.** Aortic rupture
[ ] **C.** Tracheal tear
[ ] **D.** Clavicular fracture

11. A 24-year-old patient is in the early stage of an acute asthma attack. Knowing the pathology of asthma and the progression of an asthma attack and its correlation with arterial blood gases (ABGs), the nurse anticipates which of the following ABG results on this patient?
[ ] **A.** Normal pH, normal $PaCO_2$, and normal PaO_2
[ ] **B.** Elevated pH, decreased $PaCO_2$, and decreased PaO_2
[ ] **C.** Decreased pH, increased $PaCO_2$, and decreased PaO_2
[ ] **D.** Normal pH, normal $PaCO_2$, and decreased PaO_2

12. Which common laboratory test is used to assess for congestive heart failure?
[ ] **A.** Brain natriuretic peptide (BNP)
[ ] **B.** D-Dimer
[ ] **C.** Basic metabolic panel (BMP)
[ ] **D.** Troponin

13. An unrestrained patient who was involved in a high-speed motor vehicle collision is brought to the emergency department complaining of chest pain. The paramedic states that there was extensive damage to the steering column. Assessment of the patient's chest reveals a possible flail chest on the right side. The emergency nurse's knowledge of flail chest helps her/him understand that the patient is at risk for which of the following?
[ ] **A.** Myocardial contusion
[ ] **B.** Pneumonia
[ ] **C.** Rupture of the great vessels
[ ] **D.** Pulmonary contusions

14. A patient is brought to the emergency department with mild respiratory distress. His oxygen saturation is 95% on 3 liters of oxygen via nasal cannula, his respiratory rate is 28 breaths/minute, and his temperature is 101° F (38.3° C). He has decreased breath sounds over the base of the right lung and complains of a nonproductive cough. He has a history of tuberculosis. Based on these assessment findings, which of the following should the emergency nurse suspect?
[ ] **A.** Empyema
[ ] **B.** Transudative effusion
[ ] **C.** Exudative effusion
[ ] **D.** Pulmonary embolus

15. A patient with a previous medical history of stroke is brought to the emergency department with altered mental status. The patient's baseline mental status is alert and oriented to person, place, time, and event; however, at this time, the patient is responsive to painful stimuli only. Examination reveals hot, moist skin with a tympanic temperature of 102.2° F (39° C), adventitious lung sounds, and tachycardia. The emergency nurse suspects which of the following as a possible reason for these signs?
[ ] **A.** Congestive heart failure
[ ] **B.** Meningitis
[ ] **C.** Aspiration pneumonia
[ ] **D.** Stroke

16. Which of the following signs and symptoms may indicate that a patient has aspirated fluid?
[ ] **A.** Crackles and decreased mentation
[ ] **B.** Wheezing and poor skin turgor
[ ] **C.** Decreased urinary output and wheezing
[ ] **D.** Poor skin turgor and crackles

17. Which of the following is the best treatment for high-altitude pulmonary edema (HAPE)?
[ ] **A.** Acclimatization
[ ] **B.** Antibiotics
[ ] **C.** Decrease in altitude
[ ] **D.** No specific treatment exists

18. Which of the following is **NOT** a cause of noncardiac pulmonary edema?
[ ] **A.** Trauma
[ ] **B.** Aspiration
[ ] **C.** High altitude
[ ] **D.** Pneumothorax

19. When deciding interventions for patients exposed to carbon dioxide (CO_2), ethane, methane, propane, or other fuel gases, the emergency nurse bases her/his interventions on the knowledge that:

[ ] **A.** these gases bind to hemoglobin and require high-flow oxygen and occasionally hyperbaric treatment.

[ ] **B.** these gases do not bind to hemoglobin and often only require "fresh air" and supplemental oxygen.

[ ] **C.** each of these gases binds to hemoglobin differently and has an individual treatment and antidote.

[ ] **D.** exposure to each of these gases has no negative effects on the body and, therefore, requires no treatment.

20. A patient has extensive burns to his head, face, neck, and chest with much of his hair, including his eyebrows, burned off from an ignited flammable liquid. He is conscious, breathing, and in significant pain. He is noted to have a mildly hoarse voice. A baseline physical assessment has been completed. The most reliable additional assessment of the patient's breathing status would include:

[ ] **A.** arterial blood gases (ABGs).

[ ] **B.** complete blood count (CBC).

[ ] **C.** mixed venous blood gases.

[ ] **D.** oxygen saturation monitoring.

21. A patient was involved in a fire inside a backyard shed and sustained deep partial-thickness burns to his face, head, and neck with singed nasal hair. He arrives with a hoarse voice. Which of the following is the priority nursing management for this patient's airway?

[ ] **A.** Deliver high-flow oxygen by rebreather mask.

[ ] **B.** Monitor for increasing hoarseness of voice.

[ ] **C.** Prepare for emergent intubation.

[ ] **D.** Obtain equipment for emergency cricothyrotomy.

22. Which of the following is another sign of burn inhalation injury besides hoarseness?

[ ] **A.** Rapid easing of the work of respiration

[ ] **B.** Carbonaceous or black-tinged sputum

[ ] **C.** Persistent wet and productive cough

[ ] **D.** Moist mucous membranes

23. A patient has a history of heart failure and has been diagnosed with pneumonia. Audible, adventitious lung sounds are present. Which of the following sounds would the nurse **NOT** expect to hear?

[ ] **A.** Stridor

[ ] **B.** Crackles

[ ] **C.** Wheezing

[ ] **D.** Rhonchi

24. Which of the following is **NOT** a common sign or symptom of a pulmonary embolus (PE)?

[ ] **A.** Acute respiratory distress

[ ] **B.** Nonproductive cough

[ ] **C.** Bradycardia

[ ] **D.** Sudden chest pain

25. Which of the following laboratory tests would be the most important for a patient suspected of pneumonia?

[ ] **A.** D-Dimer

[ ] **B.** Sputum culture

[ ] **C.** Blood cultures

[ ] **D.** Prothrombin time (PT)

26. Which of the following findings indicates effective treatment of a tracheobronchial injury?

[ ] **A.** Respiratory rate of 36 breaths/minute

[ ] **B.** Jugular venous distension (JVD)

[ ] **C.** Repeat reading on pH of 7.42

[ ] **D.** Increased pulse pressure

27. Emergency medical service transports a 52-year-old patient in respiratory distress. Respiratory rate is 40 breaths/minute, and oxygen saturation is 86% on 10 L of oxygen/minute on a partial-rebreather mask. He cannot speak full sentences and the nurse determines that he has had previous visits to the emergency department because of hypoxemia and hypercarbia. Auscultation reveals wheezing and his secretions are thin and scant. Based on these assessment findings, which of the following is the most likely cause of this patient's symptoms?

[ ] **A.** Recurrence of chronic bronchitis

[ ] **B.** Acute exacerbation of emphysema

[ ] **C.** Acute exacerbation of asthma

[ ] **D.** Congestive heart failure

28. Which of the following is the initial treatment for a patient with a tracheobronchial injury?

[ ] **A.** Suctioning to maintain airway patency

[ ] **B.** Preparing for chest tube insertion

[ ] **C.** Intubating and providing mechanical ventilation

[ ] **D.** Preparing for surgical intervention

29. Which of the following arterial blood gas (ABG) readings is correct for the following results?

pH: 7.52
pCO_2: 22 mm Hg
HCO_3: 26 mEq/L
PaO_2: 92 mm Hg

[ ] **A.** Respiratory acidosis

[ ] **B.** Respiratory alkalosis

[ ] **C.** Metabolic acidosis

[ ] **D.** Metabolic alkalosis

30. Which of the following is the most likely intervention for a patient with a suspected diaphragmatic rupture?
[ ] A. Needle thoracostomy
[ ] B. Chest tube insertion
[ ] C. Preparation for surgery
[ ] D. Transfer to unit for observation

31. Which of the following is the treatment of choice for a patient with a pneumothorax?
[ ] A. Chest tube insertion
[ ] B. Emergency thoracotomy
[ ] C. Needle thoracostomy
[ ] D. Emergent intubation

32. Which of the following is the definitive diagnostic study for a patient with suspected esophageal disruption?
[ ] A. Chest radiograph
[ ] B. Transesophageal echocardiogram
[ ] C. Esophagography
[ ] D. Esophagoscopy

33. A patient with an open pneumothorax is admitted to the emergency department. A nonporous dressing was placed in the field. Which of the following findings suggests worsening of this patient's condition?
[ ] A. Respiratory rate of 24 breaths/minute
[ ] B. Decreased breath sounds on the affected side
[ ] C. Tracheal shift with jugular venous distension (JVD)
[ ] D. Blood pressure 120/80 mm Hg

34. Which of the following is the most appropriate treatment for a stable patient with an open pneumothorax?
[ ] A. Immediate chest tube insertion
[ ] B. Emergency thoracotomy
[ ] C. Autotransfusion
[ ] D. Intravenous dextrose 5% in water

35. The emergency nurse is caring for a patient who has an endotracheal (ET) tube and is on mechanical ventilation for respiratory failure. The nurse knows that the high-pressure alarm will sound for which of the following reasons?
[ ] A. Obstruction of the circuit tubing
[ ] B. ET tube disconnects from the ventilator
[ ] C. The ET tube becomes displaced
[ ] D. Decreased intrathoracic pressure

36. Which of the following is a life-threatening condition that occurs with penetrating chest wounds and results in impaired gas exchange and risk for deficient fluid volume?
[ ] A. Pulmonary contusion
[ ] B. Cardiac contusion
[ ] C. Open pneumothorax
[ ] D. Ruptured esophagus

37. Which of the following findings is consistent with a diagnosis of hyperventilation?
[ ] A. Increased mental acuity
[ ] B. Respiratory acidosis
[ ] C. Left arm pain
[ ] D. Carpopedal spasms

38. The presence of a barrel chest and cyanosis are indicative of which of the following respiratory pathologies?
[ ] A. Emphysema
[ ] B. Chronic bronchitis
[ ] C. Asthma
[ ] D. Pulmonary fibrosis

39. Administration of high levels of oxygen to a patient with chronic bronchitis as a subcategory of chronic obstructive pulmonary disease (COPD) can result in which of the following conditions?
[ ] A. Increased ventilatory drive
[ ] B. Diminished ventilatory drive
[ ] C. Ventilation/perfusion mismatch
[ ] D. Profound decrease in $PaCO_2$

40. Which of the following is most commonly associated with laryngotracheobronchitis (croup)?
[ ] A. Crackles
[ ] B. Barking cough
[ ] C. Wheezing
[ ] D. Friction rub

41. Which of the following is the most common cause of chest trauma–related deaths?
[ ] A. Falls
[ ] B. Assaults
[ ] C. Firearms
[ ] D. Motor vehicle crash

42. The patient with chronic bronchitis requires careful monitoring when receiving which of the following treatments?
[ ] **A.** Oxygen therapy
[ ] **B.** Increased fluids
[ ] **C.** Humidified air
[ ] **D.** Postural drainage

43. Which of the following return statements indicates successful education of a patient with acute bronchitis?
[ ] **A.** "As long as I limit my fluid intake, I shouldn't have further symptoms."
[ ] **B.** "I can continue smoking as long as I don't smoke in a closed area."
[ ] **C.** "I should take my antibiotic and that will cure my problem."
[ ] **D.** "I should use my bronchodilator to reduce symptoms."

44. Which of the following symptoms would a patient with a diagnosis of chronic bronchitis exacerbation most likely manifest?
[ ] **A.** Slight dry cough
[ ] **B.** Wet, productive cough
[ ] **C.** Inspiratory wheezing
[ ] **D.** Pursed lip breathing

45. A patient presents with a history of mild respiratory infection and a dry cough for the past week. The patient has recently developed a loose, productive cough. He is afebrile, appears nontoxic, and has had no difficulty eating or drinking. What is the most likely diagnosis for this patient?
[ ] **A.** Asthma attack
[ ] **B.** Acute bronchitis
[ ] **C.** Pneumonia
[ ] **D.** Chronic bronchitis

46. Treatment for a patient with a rib fracture includes which of the following?
[ ] **A.** Placing the patient in the supine position.
[ ] **B.** Taping the chest circumferentially to relieve pain.
[ ] **C.** Controlling pain to assist with breathing.
[ ] **D.** Forcing fluids to prevent dehydration.

47. Effective treatment of a patient with pulmonary contusion is best identified by which of the following?
[ ] **A.** Diminished breath sounds
[ ] **B.** Increased respiratory rate and effort
[ ] **C.** Decreased complaints of pain
[ ] **D.** Respiratory acidosis

48. Which of the following interventions is most appropriate for a patient with a pulmonary contusion?
[ ] **A.** Restrict intravenous fluid administration.
[ ] **B.** Provide supplemental humidified oxygen.
[ ] **C.** Position the patient to facilitate breathing.
[ ] **D.** Assist with removal of secretions.

49. Which of the following findings is commonly associated with a poor outcome in a patient with a pulmonary contusion?
[ ] **A.** Temperature of 100.4° F (38° C)
[ ] **B.** Crackles in lower lung fields
[ ] **C.** White blood cell count of 15,000 µL
[ ] **D.** Onset of hemoptysis

50. Which of the following is the most appropriate position to facilitate oxygen exchange in the patient with acute respiratory distress syndrome (ARDS)?
[ ] **A.** Side-lying position with the right lung down
[ ] **B.** Side-lying position with the left lung down
[ ] **C.** Prone position slightly on the right side
[ ] **D.** Semi-Fowler's position lying on the left side

51. Which of the following is the most important treatment for the patient with tension pneumothorax?
[ ] **A.** Elevate the head of the patient's bed.
[ ] **B.** Administer 100% oxygen.
[ ] **C.** Infuse intravenous normal saline slowly.
[ ] **D.** Assist with needle decompression.

52. Which of the following is the definitive therapy for a patient with a massive hemothorax?
[ ] **A.** Emergency thoracotomy
[ ] **B.** Chest tube insertion
[ ] **C.** Fluid resuscitation
[ ] **D.** Supplemental oxygenation

53. Which of the following is a true statement regarding emphysema?
[ ] **A.** Emphysema creates increased dead space in the lung fields.
[ ] **B.** An emphysemic patient is the one who develops cor pulmonale.
[ ] **C.** A stocky build is a normal body shape for emphysemic patients.
[ ] **D.** Respiratory infections are dominant in the patient with emphysema.

54. A patient is transported via EMS to the emergency department after having fallen from a roof. Upon assessment, the nurse notes lack of breath sounds on the left side. A chest tube is inserted in the left chest, but instead of releasing air, the catheter expels blood. What might be the reason for this?
[ ] **A.** Tension pneumothorax
[ ] **B.** Open pneumothorax
[ ] **C.** Hemothorax
[ ] **D.** Simple pneumothorax

55. Which of the following is the primary goal in the treatment of a patient with acute respiratory distress syndrome (ARDS)?
[ ] **A.** Treating the underlying condition
[ ] **B.** Maintaining nutritional requirements
[ ] **C.** Maintaining adequate tissue oxygenation
[ ] **D.** Preventing secondary infection

56. Which of the following findings indicates that a chest tube is **NOT** effective in the management of a pneumothorax?
[ ] **A.** Patient resting, pulse oximetry 96% on 2 L/nasal cannula
[ ] **B.** Breath sounds equal bilaterally, equal chest excursion
[ ] **C.** Patient anxious, respirations 36 breaths/minute
[ ] **D.** Trachea midline, jugular veins not distended

57. A patient is admitted to the emergency department after being involved in a single-car collision. On inspection, the emergency nurse finds tachypnea, bulging of the intercostal spaces on the left side, labored breathing with accessory muscle use, and jugular venous distension. There is left-sided hyperresonance on percussion and absent breath sounds on auscultation on the left. What is the most likely diagnosis based on these findings?
[ ] **A.** Tension pneumothorax
[ ] **B.** Flail chest
[ ] **C.** Ruptured diaphragm
[ ] **D.** Massive hemothorax

58. Which of the following interventions would be **LEAST** effective for a patient with rib fractures who is breathing deeply and coughing productively?
[ ] **A.** Incentive spirometry every 2 hours
[ ] **B.** Sitting in a chair at the bedside three times per day
[ ] **C.** Splinting the chest when coughing
[ ] **D.** Suctioning the patient every 2 hours

59. Which of the following is the most likely finding on a lateral neck radiograph in a child with epiglottitis?
[ ] **A.** Supraglottic narrowing
[ ] **B.** Steeple sign
[ ] **C.** Thickened mass
[ ] **D.** Subglottic narrowing

60. Measuring lung function by determining the patient's peak expiratory flow rate (PEFR) is an important step in determining the success of asthma management. Which of the following is the optimal PEFR?
[ ] **A.** PEFR greater than 80% of predicted or personal best
[ ] **B.** PEFR variability of 20% to 30%
[ ] **C.** PEFR less than 50% of predicted or personal best
[ ] **D.** PEFR variability of less than 30%

61. Air trapping, inflammation of smooth muscles, and mucus secretion are classic signs of which of the following respiratory illnesses?
[ ] **A.** Pulmonary effusion
[ ] **B.** Asthma attack
[ ] **C.** Chronic bronchitis
[ ] **D.** Acute respiratory distress syndrome

62. Right-sided heart failure can occur secondary to a pulmonary embolus (PE). Which of the following findings is consistent with this development?
[ ] **A.** Physiologic S_2 split heart sound
[ ] **B.** Peaked P wave on electrocardiogram (ECG)
[ ] **C.** Presence of expiratory wheeze
[ ] **D.** Pericardial friction rub

63. Which of the following diagnostic studies most accurately identifies the presence of a pulmonary embolus (PE)?
[ ] **A.** Bronchoscopy
[ ] **B.** Chest radiograph
[ ] **C.** Ventilation/perfusion (V/Q) scan
[ ] **D.** Pulmonary angiography

64. Diagnostic tests that might be helpful in supporting a diagnosis of pneumonia would include which of the following?
[ ] **A.** Complete blood count (CBC) and chest radiograph
[ ] **B.** Complete blood count (CBC) and lumbar puncture
[ ] **C.** Chest radiograph and serum sedimentation rate
[ ] **D.** Serum creatinine and electrolytes

65. Which of the following is the most common cause of traumatic pneumothorax?
[ ] **A.** Fractured ribs
[ ] **B.** Gunshot wound
[ ] **C.** Barotrauma
[ ] **D.** Central line insertion

66. A patient with chronic obstructive pulmonary disease (COPD) is given discharge instructions regarding nutritional support. Which of the following statements indicates the need for further teaching?
[ ] **A.** "I should eat five or six small meals each day."
[ ] **B.** "I will limit my fluid intake at mealtime."
[ ] **C.** "I should eat mostly carbohydrate foods."
[ ] **D.** "I should rest for 30 minutes before each meal."

67. Impaired pulmonary capillary permeability, high positive end-expiratory pressure (PEEP) on a ventilator, and an inability to maintain adequate oxygen saturation are signs of which of the following?
[ ] **A.** Emphysema
[ ] **B.** Pulmonary effusion
[ ] **C.** Chronic bronchitis
[ ] **D.** Acute respiratory distress syndrome

68. Which of the following is the most appropriate intervention for a patient with chronic obstructive pulmonary disease (COPD)?
[ ] **A.** Administer 100% oxygen via non-rebreather mask.
[ ] **B.** Obtain and monitor arterial blood gas (ABG) levels.
[ ] **C.** Restrict fluids to only at meal times.
[ ] **D.** Place the patient in a supine position.

69. Which of the following is the most likely laboratory finding in a patient with early acute respiratory distress syndrome (ARDS)?
[ ] **A.** Elevated CO level
[ ] **B.** Decreased PaO_2
[ ] **C.** Elevated $PaCO_2$
[ ] **D.** Decreased HCO_3^-

70. Which of the following is the definition of flail chest?
[ ] **A.** An unstable segment of the intercostal muscles.
[ ] **B.** A compressed rib cage with open chest wound
[ ] **C.** A fracture of two adjacent ribs, bilaterally
[ ] **D.** A fracture of two or more ribs in two or more places

71. A 10-year-old with a history of asthma is diagnosed with status asthmaticus. The emergency nurse knows this patient:
[ ] **A.** has severe expiratory wheezing.
[ ] **B.** has not responded to treatment.
[ ] **C.** has been taking antibiotics.
[ ] **D.** has underlying pneumonia.

72. A 15-month-old has been diagnosed with croup. Which of the following is most concerning?
[ ] **A.** Inspiratory stridor is heard
[ ] **B.** Mother cannot calm the child
[ ] **C.** Child has a barking cough
[ ] **D.** Child is restless when sleeping

73. A 4-year-old is brought to the emergency department by his mother who reports he swallowed a small toy. Which finding by the emergency nurse indicates complete airway obstruction?
[ ] **A.** Gagging
[ ] **B.** Coughing
[ ] **C.** Aphasia
[ ] **D.** Tachypnea

74. A child with cystic fibrosis (CF) has a cough and runny nose and has been diagnosed with an upper respiratory infection. Which action by the mother indicates appropriate learning?
[ ] **A.** Ensuring the patient eats a complete diet every day
[ ] **B.** Checking the child's temperature twice daily
[ ] **C.** Offering the child orange juice throughout the day
[ ] **D.** Increasing chest physiotherapy to four times per day

75. An infant with a history of a respiratory tract infection is brought to the emergency department and is diagnosed with bronchiolitis and respiratory syncytial virus (RSV). The emergency nurse institutes which of the following types of precautions?
[ ] **A.** Droplet
[ ] **B.** Standard
[ ] **C.** Contact
[ ] **D.** Airborne

Answers/Rationales

1. Answer: A

Nursing Process: Assessment

Rationale: **Fail chest is caused by two or more fractures of two to three or more adjacent ribs. These fractures do not move with the chest wall during respiration. Signs include paradoxical movement of the chest wall during inspiration and expiration, ineffective ventilation, and dyspnea.** Although flail chest can also cause a tension pneumothorax, this is not the primary concern for the trauma nurse. Classic signs of a tension pneumothorax include tracheal deviation, cyanosis, severe dyspnea, absent breath sounds on the affected side, distended jugular veins, and shock. The patient with a ruptured diaphragm will present with hypotension, dyspnea, dysphagia, shifted heart sounds, and bowel sounds in the lower to middle chest. A patient with a massive hemothorax will show signs of shock (tachycardia and hypotension), dullness on percussion on the injured side, decreased breath sounds on the injured side, respiratory distress and, possibly, a mediastinal shift.

 CENsational Pearl of Wisdom!

Flail chest leads to an inability to ventilate. In order to correct this, apply positive pressure ventilation—that is, intubation!

2. Answer: B

Nursing Process: Assessment

Rationale: **A sucking chest wound is indicative of an open pneumothorax.** All other findings are associated with flail chest.

 CENsational Pearl of Wisdom!

Although paradoxical movement of the chest wall is always the clue for flail chest, patients in the early phases of their trauma situation may not always demonstrate this phenomenon due to muscle spasms and splinting due to pain. Once pain control is administered, the flail segment will be more readily seen to move in a paradoxical fashion.

3. Answer: B

Nursing Process: Analysis

Rationale: **Beta$_2$-agonists are the first-line drugs of choice for the patient with asthma.** They relax bronchial smooth muscle and enhance mucociliary clearance. Beta-adrenergic blockers, salicylates (Aspirin), and NSAIDs can all worsen asthma.

4. Answer: D

Nursing Process: Analysis

Rationale: **The patient with a massive hemothorax will exhibit decreased urinary output due to decreased perfusion.** A mediastinal shift, systolic blood pressure less than 80 mm Hg, and a capillary refill greater than 4 seconds can all be associated with a hemothorax greater than 1,500 mL.

5. Answer: D

Nursing Process: Evaluation

Rationale: **A forced exhalation is not recommended during inhaler use because coughing, small-airway closure, and air trapping may result.** The correct technique for using an inhaler is as follows: The inhaler must be held upright and shook to ensure it is mixed thoroughly before administration. After inhalation of the medication, the patient should then hold his/her breath for 5 to 10 seconds to allow the medication to reach as far as possible into the lungs. If the patient has difficulty with this technique, a spacer device may be added to the inhaler. A good seal should also be part of the process.

 CENsational Pearl of Wisdom!

A spacer can be used to assist patients with using inhalers. A spacer provides a "space" for the medication to rest before being inhaled, leading to easier inhaler use. Spacers also mean less of the medication gets deposited into the mouth and throat, where it can lead to irritation.

6. Answer: A

Nursing Process: Intervention

Rationale: **Although all answers are appropriate interventions for the patient with a pulmonary embolus (PE), the priority is always airway, breathing, and** circulation. Providing high-flow oxygen by simple mask or non-rebreather will increase oxygenation.

> ### CENsational Pearl of Wisdom!
>
> *When treating a PE, a loading dose of heparin should be administered, followed by a continuous drip. The heparin should be titrated to an activated partial thromboplastin time (PTT) 1½ to 2 times the control. Heparin therapy is sufficient treatment for most patients with pulmonary emboli. For patients who present with significant hemodynamic compromise, streptokinase (Streptase) and tissue plasminogen activator (alteplase [Activase]) have been approved for use in pulmonary emboli. Pain increases oxygen demand and anxiety and should be treated with an appropriate dose of pain medication such as morphine.*

7. Answer: A

Nursing Process: Intervention

Rationale: **Obtaining a throat culture can lead to increased airway obstruction due to initiation of epiglottic spasm when irritated with the swab and, as such, would not be an appropriate intervention.** Epiglottitis is a true medical emergency due to the abrupt inflammation of the epiglottis causing airway obstruction. A lateral neck radiograph may indicate epiglottic and aryepiglottic swelling, referred to as the "thumbprint sign" and the "posterior triangle." The treatment goal is to maintain the airway until surgical capability in the operating room (OR) is possible. This is accomplished by providing supplemental oxygen as tolerated and performing no invasive procedures until the airway is secure.

8. Answer: B

Nursing Process: Analysis

Rationale: **Pediatric patients' alveoli are smaller than those of an adult and result in decreased surface area for gas exchange.** Pediatric patients also have increased respiratory rates which deplete limited reserves resulting in sudden decompensation. A pediatric patient's flatter diaphragm is the primary muscle for ventilation and their abdominal muscles play a larger role in respiration, meaning that abdominal trauma can impact a child's respiratory status.

9. Answer: C

Nursing Process: Intervention

Rationale: **Because children are at high risk for developing abrupt airway obstruction, the most important** intervention for a child with epiglottitis is airway management. Intubation should be performed as soon as possible in a controlled environment. Children need supplemental oxygen, but most are so anxious that they will not allow nasal cannula to stay in place. Provide humidified "blow-by" oxygen administered by the parent, if possible. The child needs antibiotics; however, the priority is airway management. The most common rhythm in this patient is sinus tachycardia related to compensation and, although important, cardiac monitoring is not a priority.

> ### CENsational Pearl of Wisdom!
>
> *Patients—whether pediatric or adult—are never discharged with a diagnosis of epiglottitis! And yes, more adults are now being diagnosed with this disease due to childhood vaccinations.*

10. Answer: B

Nursing Process: Analysis

Rationale: **Although a cervical spine injury, tracheal tear, or clavicular fracture can be associated with a fracture of the first or second rib, the most serious injury is aortic rupture, which often results in immediate death from severe hemodynamic compromise.** Suspect an aortic rupture in a trauma patient with motor, sensory, or pulse deficits in the lower extremities. Such deficits usually result from disruption of blood flow to the spinal cord. Other symptoms include unexplained hypotension and chest or back pain. A cervical spine injury can also be serious, especially if it involves a C_3, C_4, or higher lesion, which can result in respiratory depression. Tracheal tears lead to pneumomediastinum and have the potential for tension pneumothorax if undetected. Clavicular fractures cause great pain; however, they seldom cause more severe consequences.

11. Answer: B

Nursing Process: Analysis

Rationale: **Early in an acute asthma attack, respiratory alkalosis should be present, which should be evident with a pH greater than 7.45 and a decreased $PaCO_2$ (hypocarbia) because the carbon dioxide is being blown off at an increased rate. A low PaO_2 (hypoxemia) should be present if a true asthmatic event is occurring.** Acidosis indicated by a decreased pH (lower than 7.35) would be present in a patient with hypoventilation, which would be demonstrated by an increased $PaCO_2$. Normal readings on the arterial blood gas report would not indicate an asthma attack.

12. Answer: A

Nursing Process: Assessment

Rationale: **Brain naturetic peptide (BNP) is secreted in the ventricles in response to changes in pressure that occur when heart failure occurs and worsens.** A D-dimer is a nonspecific laboratory test to assess for the possibility of an embolus. A basic metabolic panel (BMP) will not assess for heart failure. The troponin T is a cardiac enzyme that assesses heart damage during a myocardial infarction.

13. Answer: D

Nursing Process: Analysis

Rationale: **A pulmonary contusion is a common result of nonpenetrating chest trauma, especially flail chest.** A myocardial contusion as well as rupture of the great vessels would be considered had the injury been on the left side. Also, rupture of the great vessels would lead to rapid cardiovascular instability and decline. Pneumonia would not be a direct result of chest trauma.

14. Answer: A

Nursing Process: Analysis

Rationale: **An empyema contains pus and can be caused by tuberculosis.** Transudative effusion is common with heart failure, renal, and liver disease, and exudative effusions are secondary to pulmonary malignancies, pulmonary embolus, and GI disease. Patients with pulmonary embolus often present with hypoxia and tachycardia and are afebrile.

CENsational Pearl of Wisdom!

If empyemas are not drained, they can solidify causing misdiagnoses via chest radiographs in the future.

15. Answer: C

Nursing Process: Assessment

Rationale: **Because a patient who has had a stroke may be at high risk for aspiration, the combination of warm, moist skin and adventitious lung sounds most likely results from aspiration pneumonia.** An acute onset of altered mental status may indicate a new stroke; however, the presence of a fever suggests an infectious process, ruling out congestive heart failure and a stroke. The adventitious lung sounds do not correlate with meningitis.

16. Answer: A

Nursing Process: Assessment

Rationale: **Aspirated fluid will enter the alveoli, causing crackles and decreased oxygenation, which in turn may cause altered mentation.** Wheezing is an adventitious lung sound caused by airway constriction, not aspiration. Aspiration does not affect urinary output. Skin turgor is a sign of dehydration and is not caused by aspiration.

17. Answer: C

Nursing Process: Intervention

Rationale: **A decrease in altitude is the best therapy for high-altitude pulmonary edema (HAPE) as it allows the body to initiate "self-correction" of many altitude-related physiologic processes, but acclimatization will rarely be sufficient without adjunctive therapy.** Getting "down off the mountain" is the most beneficial treatment option along with providing oxygen to the patient. The mechanisms of HAPE are not borne by bacteria and thus are not treated as pneumonia. There are several treatments that can be used for high-altitude sickness.

CENsational Pearl of Wisdom!

High-altitude sickness can occur in a variety of ways. Headache, nausea, and vomiting are common and can be treated with rest and fluids. In the South American country of Bolivia, coca tea, made from the leaves of the coca plant, is very useful for this. (No! It is not cocaine!) HAPE can occur as a pulmonary aspect of high-altitude illness manifesting as a noncardiac pulmonary edema and can also be treated with Lasix (Furosemide). HACE is the high-altitude form of cerebral edema. Dexamethasone (Decadron) is another useful medication for this. Diamox (Acetazolamide) can be used as both preventive therapy and treatment for these issues. Oxygen is one of the best treatments for high-altitude issues and in areas where this is common can often be purchased at airports and hotels. Some individuals experience the effects of high altitude as soon as the doors to the airplane open!

18. Answer: D

Nursing Process: Analysis

Rationale: **A pneumothorax would not cause fluid accumulation in the pleural space.** Trauma may cause rib fractures or thoracic compression, which can rupture alveoli. Aspiration may contribute to a collection of nonendogenous fluids in the alveoli. Sudden movement to a higher altitude may lead to high-altitude pulmonary edema (HAPE).

19. Answer: B

Nursing Process: Analysis

Rationale: **Getting the patient to fresh air, out of the source area of the gas, and supplemental oxygen is the treatment needed if the patient is conscious and breathing.** Methane, ethane, propane, CO_2, and other fuel gases do not react or bind to hemoglobin. These gases have the common effect of crowding out oxygen by reducing the oxygen percentage of the air that is taken in at high concentrations, essentially suffocating the victim.

20. Answer: A

Nursing Process: Assessment

Rationale: **Arterial blood gases (ABGs) provide a specific value for the PaO_2, a much more reliable number to ascertain oxygenation status.** An oxygen saturation monitor does not differentiate among oxygen, carbon monoxide, or any other toxic substance bound to the hemoglobin. Mixed venous blood gases do not yield as useful information as an ABG. A complete blood count (CBC) will provide the hemoglobin value important in oxygen transport; however, the hemoglobin is usually reported in the ABG results.

CENsational Pearl of Wisdom!

It is important to remember that any patient involved in a fire within an enclosed space may have inhaled several of the many products of incomplete combustion including carbon monoxide, cyanide-containing compounds, and other toxic compounds. Many of these substances, carbon monoxide being especially important, bind to hemoglobin and will give a false oxygen saturation reading.

21. Answer: C

Nursing Process: Intervention

Rationale: **The priority for inhalation burn injury is to secure the airway with intubation.** Burns of the face may indicate burns to the large and small airways. Although they initially appear stable, a burn will quickly swell and loss of the airway can occur rapidly. Waiting for the situation to worsen may delay intubation to the point at which intubation or even emergency cricothyrotomy is very difficult or impossible. Delivery of high-flow oxygen is appropriate but a rebreather mask does not secure an airway.

22. Answer: B

Nursing Process: Assessment

Rationale: **Black-tinged (carbonaceous) sputum from smoke generated in the fire is a hallmark sign of inhalation injury.** Respirations may become increasingly difficult as the injury matures. The mucous membranes of the burn-injured patient are commonly dry. The patient may have rales and rhonchi on auscultation, but the cough is dry and generally nonproductive.

23. Answer: A

Nursing Process: Assessment

Rationale: **Stridor is located in the upper airway and is a result of partial obstruction of the larynx or trachea.** Crackles, wheezing, and rhonchi are all possible with a patient experiencing an exacerbation of heart failure or pneumonia.

24. Answer: C

Nursing Process: Assessment

Rationale: **Tachycardia, not bradycardia, is seen with a pulmonary embolus (PE).** Acute respiratory distress, nonproductive cough, and chest pain are all signs and symptoms of a PE.

CENsational Pearl of Wisdom!

Always think of high-risk patients for pulmonary embolus! Sedentary lifestyles, long flights, extended car rides, and pregnant patients are all at high risk! Pregnant patients have high levels of fibrinogen and platelets, which create an elevated threat.

25. Answer: C

Nursing Process: Assessment

Rationale: **Blood cultures are considered the gold standard laboratory test to assess for specificity of organism-causing pneumonia.** A sputum culture may be ordered but is not always obtainable. A D-dimer assesses for protein fragments in the blood after blood clots are dissolved by fibrinolysis, and the prothrombin time (PT) assesses for clotting times.

26. Answer: C

Nursing Process: Evaluation

Rationale: **Findings consistent with improved status after tracheobronchial injury include vital signs within normal limits including a normal pulse pressure,**

decreased air leak, improved arterial blood gas (ABG) levels, improved tissue perfusion, and no increase in subcutaneous emphysema. The presence of jugular venous distension (JVD) could suggest a diagnosis consistent with a tension pneumothorax, a common complication of tracheobronchial injury.

CENsational Pearl of Wisdom!

Pulse pressure is the difference between systolic and diastolic readings. So, a blood pressure of 118/82 mm Hg would provide a pulse pressure of 36 mm Hg with the normal being under 40 mm Hg. A widening pulse pressure can be indicative of several diagnoses, including hypovolemia, bradycardias, increased intracranial pressure, thyrotoxicosis, valvular diseases, and aortic dissection. A narrowing of the pulse pressure can be caused by a decreased cardiac output as in cardiogenic shock and tachycardias.

27. Answer: B

Nursing Process: Assessment

Rationale: **This patient is having an exacerbation of emphysema.** The hallmark pathophysiology of emphysema and chronic bronchitis is hypoxemia and hypercarbia. Secretions, particularly thick secretions, are noted in a patient with chronic bronchitis, not emphysema. Emphysemic patients tend to have wheezing, whereas the chronic bronchitis patient usually exhibits rhonchi. White or pink, blood-tinged phlegm or frothy secretions are more indicative of heart failure. An acute episode of asthma is usually associated with hypocarbia as they are breathing rapidly and blowing off the carbon dioxide.

28. Answer: A

Nursing Process: Intervention

Rationale: **The priority intervention is to maintain airway patency, which is accomplished by immediate suctioning.** Chest tube insertion and surgical intervention will be necessary after the patient is stabilized. If the patient is intubated, the end of the endotracheal tube must be positioned distal to the injury. It is also advisable to monitor for possible pneumothorax.

29. Answer: B

Nursing Process: Analysis

Rationale: **Correct interpretation of these blood gas values is respiratory alkalosis.** The pH determines whether the reading is acidotic or alkalotic and because this is greater than 7.45, the patient is alkalotic. Normal pH is 7.35 to 7.45. The next determination is whether the problem is related to carbon dioxide or bicarbonate. The parameter that is not normal is the pCO_2 level with the bicarbonate level being within normal limits. Also, the pH and the respiratory components are opposite each other, that is, the pH is "up" and the CO_2 is "down." This meets criteria for a diagnosis of respiratory alkalosis. A common problem that creates this blood gas reading is hyperventilation. Metabolic problems are directly related to each other; thus, a metabolic alkalosis would show an increase in both the pH and the HCO_3. The PaO_2 is normal.

CENsational Pearl of Wisdom!

*There **will** be questions on simple blood gas analysis! Plan on it! A good mnemonic is "ROME"—Respiratory Opposite Metabolic Equal.*

30. Answer: C

Nursing Process: Intervention

Rationale: **Preparing a patient for surgical repair is the most important intervention for a ruptured diaphragm.** Needle thoracostomy and chest tube insertion are contraindicated in this patient because of the risk of puncturing the bowel and releasing its contents into the chest cavity. The potential for serious complications contraindicates transfer for observation. Intravenous (IV) fluids may become necessary if the bowel compresses large vessels causing a decrease in preload.

CENsational Pearl of Wisdom!

A gastric tube should be inserted in case of a ruptured diaphragm, but remember that the usual avenue of checking for placement of the gastric tube may not work in this situation! Listening for air over the epigastrium may provide a false-negative response because the tube may indeed be in the stomach—but the stomach is in the chest!!

31. Answer: A

Nursing Process: Intervention

Rationale: **A pneumothorax is treated with the insertion of a chest tube connected to an underwater seal;**

the tube remains in place until reexpansion of the lung is achieved. An emergency thoracotomy is reserved for a hemodynamically unstable patient. Needle thoracostomy is used in the treatment of tension pneumothorax. Most patients with a pneumothorax do not require emergent intubation.

32. Answer: D

Nursing Process: Assessment

Rationale: **The most definitive study is an esophagoscopy, used in a patient who has a negative esophagogram but is suspected of having esophageal disruption.** Chest radiographs often show mediastinal widening, which also occurs in aortic and tracheobronchial ruptures. Esophageal rupture is one of the possible complications of a transesophageal echocardiogram.

33. Answer: C

Nursing Process: Evaluation

Rationale: **The finding that suggests a worsening of the patient's condition is a tracheal shift with jugular venous distension (JVD) which indicates a tension pneumothorax.** The respiratory rate within normal limits and blood pressure 120/80 mm Hg are acceptable outcomes. The patient will have decreased breath sounds until reexpansion of the lung has been achieved.

34. Answer: A

Nursing Process: Intervention

Rationale: **If the patient's vital signs are stable with no signs of shock, the most appropriate intervention is chest tube insertion for reexpansion of the lung.** If the patient is unstable, an emergency thoracotomy is the definitive therapy. Autotransfusion may be used to stabilize the unstable patient until transportation to surgery. Lactated ringer's solution and normal saline are the only crystalloids acceptable for administration in traumatic emergencies.

35. Answer: A

Nursing Process: Assessment

Rationale: **Obstruction of the ventilator circuit tubing will increase expiratory pressure, which will sound the alarm.** Other causes of increased expiratory pressure include obstruction of the endotracheal tube (ET) (from biting the endotracheal tube when not properly sedated) or higher intrathoracic pressures. The ET tube becoming disconnected or displaced will result in a lowering pressure and would not sound the alarm.

 CENsational Pearl of Wisdom!

An interruption of the circuit from the ET tube will prevent the patient from being ventilated and the patient's oxygenation and SpO$_2$ will drop.

36. Answer: C

Nursing Process: Assessment

Rationale: **An open pneumothorax, which causes equalization of atmospheric and intrathoracic pressures, leads to lung collapse and impaired gas exchange.** A hemothorax is commonly associated with an open pneumothorax and results in a risk of fluid volume deficit. Cardiac and pulmonary contusions usually result from blunt trauma. A ruptured esophagus does have the risk of fluid volume deficit; however, the most serious complications result from infection.

37. Answer: D

Nursing Process: Assessment

Rationale: **Patients with hyperventilation exhibit carpopedal spasms, anxiety, jaw pain, tachypnea, diffuse chest pain, confusion, diaphoresis, and headache.** Patients with this process exhibit respiratory alkalosis because they are rapidly blowing off their carbon dioxide content (the acid component of arterial blood gases), not acidosis. Solitary left arm pain does not occur with hyperventilation.

 CENsational Pearl of Wisdom!

When blood gas readings return on hyperventilating patients, the expected outcome is respiratory alkalosis. If a low PaO$_2$ is also present, the etiology is not anxiety!! There are other causes of hyperventilation, including salicylate poisoning, diabetic ketoacidosis, and pulmonary embolus. Do not treat one of these patients with the same treatment for anxiety-driven hyperventilation!!

38. Answer: A

Nursing Process: Assessment

Rationale: **Barrel chest is a hallmark sign of emphysema because of the abnormal permanent enlargement of the air spaces distal to the terminal bronchioles. Emphysemic patients end up creating increased dead space (any place where air is transported but does not participate in diffusion of gases) and decreased functional lung tissue.** Barrel chest is not indicative of chronic bronchitis, asthma, or pulmonary fibrosis. Cyanosis can occur in many patients in which oxygen delivery is impaired.

39. Answer: B

Nursing Process: Evaluation

Rationale: **If high levels of oxygen are administered, the patient with chronic bronchitis can lose the hypoxic respiratory drive and respirations will decrease or even stop.** As respirations decrease, $PaCO_2$ levels rise, not fall. A patient with chronic bronchitis has had an elevated carbon dioxide level for a prolonged time and no longer depends on carbon dioxide level changes to regulate ventilations. Instead, the patient depends on hypoxia or lower PaO_2 level changes to regulate ventilations. This leads to a ventilation/perfusion mismatch. Increasing the oxygen level does not increase the ventilation/perfusion mismatch. Patients with chronic obstructive pulmonary disease (COPD) are further subdivided into the two categories of chronic bronchitis and emphysema, each with their own specific pathophysiologic changes and manifestations.

40. Answer: B

Nursing Process: Assessment

Rationale: **A barking cough occurs most commonly with croup; coughing frequency increases at night.** Crackles, or rales, are popping noises heard most often during inspiration. They indicate that fluid, pus, or mucus is in the smaller airways. A friction rub, caused by the two pleural surfaces rubbing together, is not heard with croup. Wheezing is a high-pitched musical sound. It can be heard during inspiration and expiration and usually accompanies an asthma attack or bronchospasm.

 CENsational Pearl of Wisdom!

When crackles or rales are heard, instruct the patient to cough and breathe deeply and then auscultate again. The sounds may have cleared!

41. Answer: D

Nursing Process: Analysis

Rationale: **Motor vehicle accidents account for two-thirds of all chest trauma–related deaths.** Other causes of thoracic injuries include falls, assaults, firearms, stabbings, crush injuries, and motor vehicle–pedestrian accidents.

42. Answer: A

Nursing Process: Evaluation

Rationale: **The patient with chronic bronchitis should be monitored closely when given low-flow oxygen to decrease the chances of depressing the respiratory drive because hypoxia becomes the stimulus to breathe for these patients.** Increasing fluids to liquefy secretions, humidifying the air, and performing postural drainage are also important therapies for a patient with chronic bronchitis.

43. Answer: D

Nursing Process: Evaluation

Rationale: **Medications prescribed for acute bronchitis may include bronchodilators, corticosteroids, expectorants, and antianxiety drugs.** The patient must increase fluid intake to liquefy secretions. Bronchitis is an inflammation resulting from irritation of the bronchial mucosa by pollen, smoking, or inhalation of irritating substances. Environmental irritants must be removed. Acute bronchitis is caused by a virus and therefore, antibiotics are not appropriate for this disease process.

 CENsational Pearl of Wisdom!

Overprescribing antibiotics for viral illnesses has been a major cause of the proliferation of superbugs. It is difficult sometimes for patients to understand this, but it is up to the health care providers to help educate the public about this. Be strong!!!

44. Answer: B

Nursing Process: Assessment

Rationale: **Patients with chronic bronchitis have an overproduction of sputum, which provides the basis for a wet and productive cough.** This is also a strong setup for infectious processes as bacteria have an inviting place to grow. Wheezing and pursed lip breathing are associated with emphysema. Emphysemic patients will have no cough. If they do cough, it is a minor dry, hacking-type cough.

 CENsational Pearl of Wisdom!

Patients with chronic obstructive pulmonary disease (COPD) can have aspects of both airway inflammation and airway collapse. Airway inflammation is manifested as chronic bronchitis, whereas airway collapse is manifested as emphysema. For each patient, one or the other will predominate. So, when a patient tells the nurse "I have COPD," it is important to determine which subclassification they have.

45. Answer: B

Nursing Process: Assessment

Rationale: **Patients with acute bronchitis initially have a dry cough that becomes more productive and they usually appear nontoxic.** Most patients with an acute asthma attack have exposure to allergens as an important history finding and are usually in acute respiratory distress with wheezing. A patient with pneumonia generally has an elevated temperature, productive cough, and coarse crackles. A patient with chronic bronchitis has a chronic productive cough.

 CENsational Pearl of Wisdom!

Infection is the most common cause of acute respiratory arrest in patients with asthma who appear toxic on admission.

46. Answer: C

Nursing Process: Intervention

Rationale: **Pain control for a patient with rib fractures is a priority to ensure adequate expansion of lung tissue and to facilitate turning, coughing, and deep breathing.** The patient should be placed in high Fowler's position to facilitate gas exchange and breathing. Avoid circumferential taping of the chest or rib belts because this predisposes the patient to atelectasis and pneumonia. The lung directly below the fractured rib is often bruised (pulmonary contusion). Fluids should be monitored closely to decrease the risk of acute respiratory distress syndrome (ARDS) which causes a noncardiac pulmonary edema.

 CENsational Pearl of Wisdom!

Patients with fractures of the first or second ribs should be thoroughly assessed for damage to underlying structures such as subclavian vein and artery lacerations and pulmonary tissue damage. There is a high mortality with these fractures due to these types of secondary damage.

47. Answer: C

Nursing Process: Evaluation

Rationale: **Effective treatment of a patient with pulmonary contusion is evidenced by decreased complaints of pain, equal bilateral breath sounds, and an improved respiratory rate, rhythm, depth, and effort.** Other indicators of effective treatment include vital signs within normal limits, arterial blood gases within acceptable limits, and improved skin and mucous membrane color.

48. Answer: A

Nursing Process: Intervention

Rationale: **If the patient is not exhibiting symptoms of hypovolemic shock, intravenous fluids should be restricted during initial care.** While providing supplemental oxygen, positioning the patient to facilitate breathing and assisting with removal of secretions are all treatments for pulmonary contusion; limiting IV fluid administration is associated with the best outcome for the patient.

49. Answer: B

Nursing Process: Assessment

Rationale: **Fluid overload, as evidenced by crackles in the lower lung fields, is consistently associated with a poor outcome in patients with pulmonary contusions.** A pulmonary contusion normally causes an inflammatory response that results in an increase in temperature and white blood cells. The patient with a pulmonary contusion is expected to have hemoptysis. The blood may be expectorated or suctioned from the endotracheal tube if the patient is intubated.

 CENsational Pearl of Wisdom!

Restriction of fluids, meticulous monitoring of intake and output, and monitoring of central venous pressure are appropriate interventions for a pulmonary contusion.

50. Answer: C

Nursing Process: Intervention

Rationale: **Research has shown that improved oxygenation parameters are seen when a patient with acute respiratory distress syndrome (ARDS) is placed in the prone position on the right side.** In ARDS, neither lung is functioning properly; therefore, the good lung down does not help determine positioning. Changing the patient's position at least every 2 hours is important. The nurse should allow 15 minutes after each turn for stabilization of parameters. If improvement is not seen, the patient should be turned to a more functional position.

 CENsational Pearl of Wisdom!

When positioning the ARDS patients for maximum oxygenation, the right lung down usually produces the best oxygenation parameters. This lung has three lobes and is not compressed by the heart.

51. Answer: D

Nursing Process: Intervention

Rationale: **All of the options listed are important in the treatment of tension pneumothorax, but the *most* important is needle decompression.** A 14-G needle inserted into the second intercostal space at the midclavicular line on the affected side is appropriate. A chest tube insertion should follow needle decompression.

 CENsational Pearl of Wisdom!

Research has found that in patients with large chest walls—muscular athletes, military individuals, or obese patients—the usual 14-G needle may not be long enough or stout enough to actually enter the pleural space. If this is used and the "whoosh" of air and improvement of the patient is not noted, an attempt may be made at the fifth intercostal space anterior line. Newer products have been developed that are longer and have greater strength. Also, important! *Insert the needle superior to the rib, not inferior where the nerves and blood vessels lie.*

52. Answer: A

Nursing Process: Intervention

Rationale: **The definitive treatment for a patient with a massive hemothorax is emergency thoracotomy.** It is imperative to identify and repair the source of bleeding. Temporary measures to stabilize the patient include chest tube insertion and, possibly, autotransfusion, fluid resuscitation (crystalloids and colloids), and supplemental oxygenation.

53. Answer: A

Nursing Process: Analysis

Rationale: **An increase in dead space occurs with emphysema due to destruction of alveolar walls and overdistension of the alveoli.** When this happens, these alveoli are no longer functional because they cannot participate in diffusion of gases. This increases dead space— a space where air is transported but does not assist with the work of the pulmonary system such as with the trachea. Cor pulmonale, right-sided heart failure caused by a pulmonary issue, is associated with chronic bronchitis. Chronic bronchitis patients usually have a stocky build as opposed to the thin extremities and barrel chest of the emphysema patient, and respiratory infections are more prone in the chronic bronchitis patient due to the increase in secretions.

54. Answer: C

Nursing Process: Analysis

Rationale: **A hemothorax is caused by free blood in the pleural space, usually caused by trauma, which will result in diminished or absent breath sounds on the affected side.** A tension pneumothorax or simple pneumothorax will not expel blood through the chest tube. An open pneumothorax will present with a bubbling, sucking noise at the site of injury but will not usually be associated with loss of blood.

 CENsational Pearl of Wisdom!

Remember that an open pneumothorax has a great potential to develop a tension pneumothorax! Removing a corner of the dressing may be necessary to save the patient's life if increasing respiratory distress along with hemodynamic instability is noted.

55. Answer: A

Nursing Process: Analysis

Rationale: **Identifying and treating the underlying condition is the *primary* goal.** If the condition causing acute respiratory distress syndrome (ARDS) is not treated, injury to the lung will continue, preventing adequate tissue oxygenation and predisposing the patient to a secondary infection. Later, the nurse should also provide adequate nutritional support in the form of increased protein and calories and limited carbohydrate intake.

56. Answer: C

Nursing Process: Evaluation

Rationale: **After chest tube insertion, the patient should be calm. A patient who is anxious with rapid respirations is showing signs of respiratory distress.** If the chest tube is effective, respirations and pulse oximetry reading should be within normal limits. Breath sounds should be heard in all lobes bilaterally with equal excursion of chest. The trachea should be midline without jugular venous distension.

57. Answer: A

Nursing Process: Assessment

Rationale: **Tension pneumothorax presents with severe respiratory distress, hypotension, diminished breath sounds over the affected area, hyperresonance, jugular venous distension and, eventually, tracheal shift to the unaffected side.** A finding of multiple rib fractures in a patient with respiratory distress verifies a diagnosis of flail chest. A patient with a ruptured diaphragm presents with hyperresonance on percussion, hypotension, dyspnea, dysphagia, shifted heart sounds, and bowel sounds in the lower to middle chest. A patient with massive hemothorax shows signs of shock (tachycardia and hypotension), dullness on percussion on the injured side, decreased breath sounds on the injured side, respiratory distress, and possibly, mediastinal shift.

58. Answer: D

Nursing Process: Evaluation

Rationale: **If the patient is effectively coughing productively and removing secretions, suctioning can be harmful.** Suctioning can cause mucosal trauma, hypoxemia, and even pulmonary infection. Incentive spirometry every 2 hours, sitting in a chair at the bedside three times per day, and splinting the chest wall to facilitate coughing are all measures to prevent pneumonia.

59. Answer: C

Nursing Process: Assessment

Rationale: **The lateral neck radiograph of a child with epiglottitis shows a thickened mass called the Thumbprint Sign.** The steeple sign is found in the patient with viral croup syndrome and is demonstrated with superior tapering in the trachea, often seen on the chest radiograph. Subglottic narrowing with membranous tracheal exudate is found in bacterial tracheitis. Supraglottic narrowing is not a diagnostic indicator.

 CENsational Pearl of Wisdom!

Epiglottitis is a supraglottic bacterial infection. Croup is a bacterial subglottic disease process. Remember that epiglottitis is an emergency diagnosis! Nothing should be done to the child until intubation equipment is at the bedside and there is access to an individual who is expert in intubating children. If the epiglottis is stimulated and it begins to spasm, there is very little chance of obtaining an airway on the child.

60. Answer: A

Nursing Process: Evaluation

Rationale: **The optimal peak expiratory flow rate (PEFR) is greater than 80% of predicted or personal best with a variability of less than 20%.** This is a simple bedside test. Monitoring PEFR helps assess the severity of obstruction. The nurse should evaluate the patient's response to treatment and detect changes in airflow. If PEFR is increasing

and subjective symptoms are decreasing, medication or dosage does not need to be changed. If PEFR is decreasing and symptoms are increasing, the patient can better judge his status and adjust medications appropriately.

61. Answer: B

Nursing Process: Assessment

Rationale: **Inflammation of smooth muscle leading to constriction of bronchioles and mucus production results in air trapping, respiratory acidosis, and hypoxemia, and are the classic symptoms of asthma.** Pulmonary effusion is caused by excessive fluid accumulation in the pleural space. Chronic bronchitis is a narrowing of the airway passages and an increase in mucus production, but it does not produce air trapping. Acute respiratory distress syndrome (ARDS) is an acute physiologic syndrome characterized by noncardiac pulmonary edema caused by increased pulmonary capillary permeability, high PEEP, and low oxygen saturation despite the use of supplemental oxygen.

62. Answer: B

Nursing Process: Assessment

Rationale: **Elevated pulmonary pressures resulting from pulmonary emboli can lead to dysfunction of the right heart, which, in turn, can lead to an increase in right atrial volume, showing an altered P wave on the ECG.** In lead II, the P wave is taller and more peaked than a normal P wave. A physiologic S_2 split is normal. When pulmonary pressures become severely elevated, the split becomes pathologic. Breath sounds are generally clear in a patient with pulmonary emboli. A pleural friction rub may be heard but is not due to the right-sided heart failure.

63. Answer: D

Nursing Process: Assessment

Rationale: **Although riskier than a V/Q scan, pulmonary angiography confirms the presence of a pulmonary embolus.** Bronchoscopy is typically used in differential diagnosis of pneumonia. A chest radiograph is usually done to rule out other pulmonary problems, such as pneumonia and atelectasis. A V/Q scan is used to locate the inadequately perfused area; however, results are not definitive. The most frequent diagnostic test used now is a computed tomography (CT) for pulmonary embolus.

 CENsational Pearl of Wisdom!

Be aware that patients can become a code blue candidate when undergoing a "CT for PE." Be watchful!!!

64. Answer: A

Nursing Process: Assessment

Rationale: **A complete blood count (CBC) is helpful in determining the presence of infection and identifying the microbial (viral, bacterial, or fungal) agent. A chest radiograph can identify the location of the pneumonia.** Sedimentation rate, electrolytes, serum creatinine and lumbar puncture do not assist in the differential diagnosis of pneumonia.

65. Answer: A

Nursing Process: Assessment

Rationale: **The most common cause of traumatic pneumothorax is fractured ribs.** Other common causes include penetrating trauma (gunshot or knife wound), insertion of a central venous pressure catheter or central line, barotrauma in mechanically ventilated patients, and closed pleural biopsy.

66. Answer: C

Nursing Process: Evaluation

Rationale: **The patient with chronic obstructive pulmonary disease (COPD) has a markedly increased need for protein, not carbohydrates, and calories to maintain an adequate nutritional status.** The patient's diet should be high in both protein and calories and should be divided into five or six small meals per day. Fluid intake should be maintained at 3 L/day unless contraindicated. Fluids should be taken between meals to reduce gastric distension and pressure on the diaphragm. The patient with COPD should rest for 30 minutes before each meal to conserve energy and decrease dyspnea.

 CENsational Pearl of Wisdom!

Encourage your patient with COPD to avoid exercise and breathing treatments for at least 1 hour before and after eating in order to conserve energy and decrease dyspnea.

67. Answer: D

Nursing Process: Assessment

Rationale: **Acute respiratory distress syndrome (ARDS) is an acute physiologic syndrome characterized by noncardiac pulmonary edema caused by increased pulmonary capillary permeability, high PEEP, and low oxygen saturation despite the use of supplemental oxygen.** Emphysema is a permanent condition that is caused by alveolar destruction. Pulmonary effusion is caused by excessive fluid accumulation in the pleura, and chronic bronchitis is a narrowing of the airway passages and an increase in mucus production.

 CENsational Pearl of Wisdom!

The addition of PEEP for a ventilated patient can be a good thing, but, it can also cause some problems for your patient! Barotrauma and a decreased cardiac output can occur with the addition of PEEP. The nurse may see a drop in blood pressure, indicating that PEEP should be subtracted, not added.

68. Answer: B

Nursing Process: Intervention

Rationale: **Monitoring arterial blood gas (ABG) levels is the appropriate intervention for the chronic obstructive pulmonary disease (COPD) patient.** The patient with COPD has abnormal ABG levels, which may predispose him to respiratory distress. The patient is hypoxemic with hypercapnia. Oxygen should be administered at low concentrations to maintain hypoxic drive. If the PaO_2 remains inadequate at low doses, the nurse should increase the oxygen while continuously monitoring the patient's respiratory status. A patient with COPD usually benefits from adequate hydration to liquefy secretions. Allow the patient to assume a position that facilitates ventilation, usually a forward-leaning high Fowler's position.

 CENsational Pearl of Wisdom!

Remember that your COPD patient may have a baseline oxygen saturation level below what is considered normal. Be sure to ask your patients what is their "normal."

69. Answer: B

Nursing Process: Assessment

Rationale: **Hypoxemia is a universal finding in acute respiratory distress syndrome (ARDS).** The $PaCO_2$ is low early in the disease because of hyperventilation, and rises later in the disease because of fatigue and worsening clinical status. The bicarbonate level may be low in ARDS and is related to reduced tissue oxygenation. Reduced oxygenation leads to anaerobic metabolism and accumulating lactate. HCO_3^- in the serum combines with the lactate, reducing circulating HCO_3^- levels. The carboxyhemoglobin level is increased in a patient with an inhalation injury, which commonly progresses to ARDS.

70. Answer: D

Nursing Process: Assessment

Rationale: **Flail chest is a fracture of two to three or more ribs (dependent on the reference used) in two or more places, resulting in a free-floating segment of the chest wall.** This instability causes paradoxical chest movement, which is commonly a sign of flail chest; however, until the chest muscles relax or pain relief is achieved, paradoxical movements are unlikely to be seen. The instability is in the rib cage itself not the intercostals. Flail chest is usually a closed injury. Bilateral injury is not required in flail chest. If bilateral injury is present, the risk of mortality increases drastically.

71. Answer: B

Nursing Process: Assessment

Rationale: **Status asthmaticus is asthma with moderate to severe airway obstruction that does not respond to initial treatment.** The child's wheezing stops when status asthmaticus develops because the airways are obstructed. Antibiotics are not treatment for asthma and the child has no signs of pneumonia.

 CENsational Pearl of Wisdom!

Treatment for status asthmaticus includes the use of low-dose magnesium acting as a smooth muscle relaxant. Also! Just because a patient is not wheezing, it does not mean they are not having an asthma attack! Wheezing after treatment is then a good thing!!

---

72. Answer: B

Nursing Process: Assessment

Rationale: **Inconsolability is cause for alarm in an infant.** In a child with respiratory problems, the inability of caregivers to soothe may be an indication of increasing hypoxia. Typical symptoms of croup include inspiratory stridor and a barking cough. Children are often restless when sleeping when they are ill.

73. Answer: C

Nursing Process: Assessment

Rationale: **With complete airway obstruction, the child cannot cough, speak, or breathe.** Tachypnea, gagging,

and coughing are signs of an incomplete obstruction. Other signs include vomiting, wheezing, cyanosis, and increased work of breathing.

74. Answer: D

Nursing Process: Evaluation

Rationale: **Increasing chest physiotherapy to four times a day is the appropriate intervention.** For a child with cystic fibrosis (CF), a simple upper respiratory infection may develop into pneumonia if the thick secretions are not loosened and removed by percussion and postural drainage. Making sure the child has an adequate diet, taking the child's temperature, and giving the child orange juice are important but not as vital as increasing the physiotherapy.

75. Answer: C

Nursing Process: Assessment

Rationale: **The child with respiratory syncitial virus (RSV) should be placed on contact precautions.** RSV is highly communicable and can live on surfaces for up to 6 hours. Standard precautions will not be enough to prevent spreading this organism. Gown and gloves should be worn when entering the room. Droplet and airborne precautions are not necessary.

References

Emergency Nurses Association. (2010). Sheehy's emergency nursing: principles and practice (6th ed.). St. Louis, MO: Elsevier. (1,3, 5, 6, 11, 12, 14–19, 23–25, 27, 37–40, 42–45, 50, 53, 61–64, 66–70, 74)

Emergency Nurses Association. (2012). Emergency nursing pediatric course: provider course (4th ed.). Des Plaines, IL: Emergency Nurses Association. (7, 8, 9, 59, 60, 71–73, 75)

Emergency Nurses Association. (2014). Trauma nursing core course: provider manual (7th ed.). Des Plaines, IL: Emergency Nurses Association. (1, 2, 4, 10, 13, 20–22, 26, 28–36, 41, 46–49, 51, 52, 54–58, 65, 70)

Marchione, V. (2017, December). *Widened pulse pressure may increase the risk of heart attacks and cardiovascular disease.* Retrieved from https://www.belmarrahealth .com/widened-pulse-pressure-increase-risk-heart-attacks-cardiovascular-disease/ (26)

Ren, X. (Mike). (2017, January). *Cardiogenic shock.* Medscape. Retrieved from https://emedicine.medscape.com/ article/152191-overview (26)

9 Orthopedic Emergencies

Tiffany Strever, BSN, RN, CEN, TCRN, FAEN

Orthopedic emergencies involve many types of injuries and complicating disease processes caused by the primary musculoskeletal damage. One of the major concerns when dealing with these emergencies is to make sure that tunnel vision does not take precedence! Do not become so intrigued with the bizarre presentation of these injuries that the basic ABC's take a back seat. When caring for these patients, take a step back and assess the primary and secondary survey to make sure nothing is missed. On the test, orthopedic questions are included in the categorical grouping of Maxillo-Facial, Ocular, Orthopedic, and Wound Care. There are 25 questions in this group.

1. A patient is brought to the emergency department by emergency medical services after being crushed while standing between a loading dock and a truck. The emergency nurse can anticipate which of the following injuries?

[ ] **A.** Humeral head fracture
[ ] **B.** Closed pelvic fracture
[ ] **C.** Humeral shaft fracture
[ ] **D.** Open-book pelvic fracture

2. Application of a pelvic binder in the patient with an open-book pelvic fracture may:

[ ] **A.** increase pain.
[ ] **B.** control hemorrhage.
[ ] **C.** displace the fracture.
[ ] **D.** decrease blood pressure.

3. Which of the following statements made by a patient would indicate to the emergency nurse that the patient does **NOT** understand discharge instructions for a sprained ankle?

[ ] **A.** "I should take the wrap off at night."
[ ] **B.** "I should keep my extremity down at all times."
[ ] **C.** "I should avoid use of my extremity."
[ ] **D.** "I should use ice for the first 48 hours, then heat."

4. A 16-year-old patient arrives at triage and states, "I was playing basketball, went to jump for a ball and felt a "sharp pain" in my heel." The patient is walking flat-footed. The emergency nurse should suspect which of the following?

[ ] **A.** Achilles tendon rupture
[ ] **B.** Grade II ankle strain
[ ] **C.** Grade III ankle sprain
[ ] **D.** Calcaneus fracture

5. A patient is brought to the emergency department following a motorcycle crash. Assessment reveals an open tibial fracture. Which of the following options would be the priority intervention for this patient?

[ ] **A.** Contact orthopedic surgeon
[ ] **B.** Obtain an appropriate radiograph
[ ] **C.** Administer prescribed intravenous antibiotics
[ ] **D.** Administer a tetanus injection

6. A patient presents to triage after a fall. The diagnosis is contusion of the lower leg. Which of the following is a true statement regarding a contusion?

[ ] **A.** Removal of the epithelium with dermis exposed
[ ] **B.** Collection of blood under the skin
[ ] **C.** Peeling of skin from underlying tissue
[ ] **D.** Complete separation of skin from underlying tissue

7. Which of the following is an appropriate intervention for a patient with a leg contusion?

[ ] **A.** Dependent positioning of the extremity
[ ] **B.** Application of pressure dressing
[ ] **C.** Application of ice pack
[ ] **D.** Intravenous pain medication

8. Which of the following would be an expected observation when assessing a patient with a suspected pelvic fracture?

[ ] **A.** Internal rotation of the leg
[ ] **B.** Blood at the urinary meatus
[ ] **C.** Evidence of neurogenic shock
[ ] **D.** Fecal incontinence

9. A patient is brought to the emergency department after jumping off of a 25-foot bridge. Which of the following types of vertebral injuries should the emergency nurse expect according to mechanism of injury?
[ ] **A.** Compression fracture
[ ] **B.** Chance fracture
[ ] **C.** Comminuted fracture
[ ] **D.** Fracture dislocation

10. Which of the following is **NOT** part of the vertebrae?
[ ] **A.** Spinous process
[ ] **B.** Transverse process
[ ] **C.** Facet
[ ] **D.** Spinal cord

11. The emergency nurse is discharging a patient with a diagnosis of gout. Which of the following statements made by the patient would indicate an understanding of the discharge instructions?
[ ] **A.** "I will start taking an aspirin daily."
[ ] **B.** "I should stop exercising."
[ ] **C.** "I will drink a glass of wine daily."
[ ] **D.** "I will take Allopurinol as directed."

12. A patient presents to triage after recent knee surgery with a painful swollen joint. Vital signs for this patient are as follows:

Blood pressure—112/82 mm Hg
Pulse—108 beats/minute
Respirations—16 breaths/minute
Temperature—98.4° F (36.8° C)
Pulse oximetry—96% on room air

The emergency nurse suspects which of the following types of joint effusion?
[ ] **A.** Blood
[ ] **B.** Bursitis
[ ] **C.** Gout
[ ] **D.** Septic arthritis

13. Excessive stretching or tearing of a ligament results in which of the following processes?
[ ] **A.** Dislocation
[ ] **B.** Avulsion
[ ] **C.** Strain
[ ] **D.** Sprain

14. Femoral head necrosis is a complication of hip dislocation. To prevent this complication, reduction of the dislocation should occur within which of the following hours?
[ ] **A.** 6
[ ] **B.** 8
[ ] **C.** 10
[ ] **D.** 12

15. A trauma patient arrives in the emergency department with an open ankle fracture. The emergency nurse should anticipate which of the following interventions?
[ ] **A.** Irrigation of the wound
[ ] **B.** Application of a traction splint
[ ] **C.** Application of a dry, nonsterile dressing
[ ] **D.** Administration of the appropriate tetanus dose

16. Which of the following is the leading cause of injury-related mortality in the elderly?
[ ] **A.** Motor vehicle crashes
[ ] **B.** Pedestrian hit by vehicle
[ ] **C.** Sports-related events
[ ] **D.** Accidental falls

17. A patient presents to the emergency department with a laceration of the lower arm and states that his little finger is numb. Grip strength to his hand is decreased. This indicates damage to which of the following nerves?
[ ] **A.** Median
[ ] **B.** Peroneal
[ ] **C.** Ulnar
[ ] **D.** Radial

18. A patient presents at triage and states, "I was playing racquet ball and twisted my ankle." There is mild tenderness and swelling of the ankle and the joint is stable. How would this sprain be classified?
[ ] **A.** Mild (grade I)
[ ] **B.** Moderate (grade II)
[ ] **C.** Severe (grade III)
[ ] **D.** Extreme (grade IV)

19. Treatment for lower grade sprains and strains is described by the mnemonic "RICE." The letters in this mnemonic does **NOT** include which of the following treatment options?
[ ] **A.** Ice
[ ] **B.** Rest
[ ] **C.** Exercise
[ ] **D.** Compression

20. A patient is diagnosed with a knee dislocation after a sporting event. The emergency nurse should consider which of the following additional injuries that is common with this primary injury?
[ ] **A.** Fibula fracture
[ ] **B.** Saphenous vein injury
[ ] **C.** Popliteal artery injury
[ ] **D.** Tibial nerve injury

21. A cast is being applied to a patient who has been diagnosed with a radial fracture. When applying the cast, the emergency nurse knows the elbow should be at what angle for proper cast application?
[ ] **A.** Flexed 30 degrees
[ ] **B.** Flexed 45 degrees
[ ] **C.** Flexed 90 degrees
[ ] **D.** No flexion

22. Which of the following is considered to be a "long" bone?
[ ] **A.** Carpal bone
[ ] **B.** Tarsal bone
[ ] **C.** Hip bone
[ ] **D.** Humerus bone

23. Which of the following is the name for the dense tissue that attaches muscles to bone and controls movement through extension and flexion?
[ ] **A.** Cartilage
[ ] **B.** Tendon
[ ] **C.** Ligament
[ ] **D.** Skeletal

24. A tennis player presents at triage with a swollen and painful elbow joint. The emergency nurse suspects which of the following types of joint effusion?
[ ] **A.** Septic arthritis
[ ] **B.** Gout
[ ] **C.** Blood
[ ] **D.** Bursitis

25. Which of the following would **NOT** be an appropriate treatment regimen for a patient with a shoulder dislocation?
[ ] **A.** Application of ice
[ ] **B.** Immobilization
[ ] **C.** Neurovascular assessment
[ ] **D.** Application of traction splint

26. Emergency medical services brings an 8-year-old who was struck by a car impacting the bumper. The emergency nurse should anticipate which of the following injuries?
[ ] **A.** Clavicle fracture
[ ] **B.** Ankle fracture
[ ] **C.** Femur fracture
[ ] **D.** Spinal cord injury

27. A radiograph demonstrates a "buckle" fracture of the arm. The emergency nurse knows this fracture is also known as which of the following types of fracture?
[ ] **A.** Torus
[ ] **B.** Greenstick
[ ] **C.** Compression
[ ] **D.** Comminuted

28. A trauma patient arrives in the emergency department with an open femur fracture. There is evidence of uncontrolled bleeding. Vital signs are as follows:

Blood pressure—96/64 mm Hg
Pulse—120 beats/minute
Respirations—28 breaths/minute
Temperature—99.2° F (37.3° C)
Pulse oximetry—94% on room air

Which of the following is the priority intervention for this patient?
[ ] **A.** Intravenous access
[ ] **B.** Obtain a radiograph
[ ] **C.** Direct pressure
[ ] **D.** Traction splint

29. A patient is transferred to a Level I trauma center with a crush injury to the forearm. Upon examination, the forearm is tense, has decreased sensation, and pain out of proportion to injury. Which of the following should the emergency nurse be suspicious for in this patient?
[ ] **A.** Radial nerve injury
[ ] **B.** Humeral fracture
[ ] **C.** Brachial artery injury
[ ] **D.** Compartment syndrome

30. A patient is diagnosed with a scaphoid fracture. The emergency nurse knows which of the following would be appropriate treatment?
[ ] **A.** Cast with the thumb in opposition
[ ] **B.** Sling with arm against body
[ ] **C.** Application of traction splint
[ ] **D.** Cast with elbow flexed 90 degrees

31. Which of the following statements indicates an understanding of discharge instructions after a posterior splint is placed?
[ ] **A.** The patient verbalized that he can walk short distances on the splint.
[ ] **B.** The patient states the need to follow up with the orthopedic surgeon.
[ ] **C.** The patient states that after 1 week he should return for splint removal.
[ ] **D.** The patient states they he can keep the leg dependent at all times.

32. A trauma patient sustained a severe crush injury to the lower extremity. When the urinary catheter is placed, the emergency nurse notes that the urine is dark brown in color. Which of the following should the nurse be most concerned about regarding this finding?
[ ] **A.** Compartment syndrome
[ ] **B.** Dehydration
[ ] **C.** Urinary tract infection
[ ] **D.** Rhabdomyolysis

33. An 86-year-old patient fell and sustained a pelvic fracture. This patient is given low-molecular-weight heparin to aid in prevention of which of the following complications?
[ ] **A.** Fat embolism
[ ] **B.** Pulmonary edema
[ ] **C.** Deep vein thrombosis
[ ] **D.** Congestive heart failure

34. Which of the following amputations is associated with the highest rate of successful reattachment rate?
[ ] **A.** Crush-like amputation
[ ] **B.** Amputation from a ripping force
[ ] **C.** Amputation from a blast force
[ ] **D.** Guillotine-type amputation

35. A 3-year-old is presented to the triage area with complaints of not using his left arm. The father states he jerked the child's arm to get him out of the street. The emergency nurse would suspect which of the following injuries?
[ ] **A.** Shoulder dislocation
[ ] **B.** Radial dislocation
[ ] **C.** Elbow fracture
[ ] **D.** Humeral fracture

36. A patient arrives in the emergency department with a swollen, tense forearm complaining of pain at a level of "10" on a scale of 1 to 10. This patient was discharged 4 hours before with a diagnosis of a sprained wrist. Which of the following would be the appropriate intervention at this time?
[ ] **A.** Apply an ice pack to the extremity.
[ ] **B.** Place the extremity at the level of the heart.
[ ] **C.** Place the patient in the waiting room to wait for a "fast-track" bed.
[ ] **D.** Have the patient go the urgent care center as the ED is very busy.

37. A trauma patient arrives in the emergency department via emergency medical services with bilateral femoral fractures. This patient has received 2 liters of lactated ringer intravenous fluids for resuscitation. Vital signs on arrival are as follows:

Blood pressure—76/40 mm Hg
Pulse—145 beats/minute
Respirations—32 breaths/minute
Temperature—99.6° F (37.5° C)
Pulse oximetry—90% on room air

These vital signs are indicative of a shock index of 1.9. Which of the following interventions is the priority for the emergency nurse caring for this patient?
[ ] **A.** Initiation of massive transfusion policy
[ ] **B.** Fluid bolus of lactated ringers
[ ] **C.** Place patient in Trendelenburg
[ ] **D.** Place bilateral traction splints

38. Which of the following intracompartmental pressures would be considered critical impairment?
[ ] **A.** Less than 10 mm Hg
[ ] **B.** 12 to 20 mm Hg
[ ] **C.** 21 to 30 mm Hg
[ ] **D.** Greater than 31 mm Hg

39. A traction splint would be used for which of the following fractures?
[ ] **A.** Humeral fracture
[ ] **B.** Ankle fracture
[ ] **C.** Forearm fracture
[ ] **D.** Femur fracture

40. Which of the following is a common complication of a pelvic fracture?
[ ] **A.** Muscle spasm
[ ] **B.** Hematochezia
[ ] **C.** Rhabdomyolysis
[ ] **D.** Urethral injury

41. A patient is being sent home on muscle relaxants. Which of the following statements made by the patient is indicative of a positive understanding of the discharge instructions?
[ ] **A.** "I will be able to drive while I am taking this medication."
[ ] **B.** "This will make me much more alert so that will be good."
[ ] **C.** "I understand this will make me restless and anxious."
[ ] **D.** "These pills can make me drowsy so I need to be cautious with them."

42. Which of the following would indicate to the emergency nurse that treatment for rhabdomyolysis has been effective?

[ ] **A.** Urine output is at least 100 mL/hour.

[ ] **B.** The urine is getting darker in color.

[ ] **C.** The creatine kinase levels are increasing.

[ ] **D.** There is increased muscle pain.

43. The emergency department has been holding a trauma patient for several hours when the patient suddenly develops pleuritic chest pain, hypoxemia, hemoptysis, and wheezes. The emergency nurse would suspect which of the following processes?

[ ] **A.** Fat embolism

[ ] **B.** Deep vein thrombosis

[ ] **C.** Pulmonary embolism

[ ] **D.** Pneumonia

44. Which of the following symptoms constitutes a medical emergency in a patient with acute lower back pain with suspected herniated lumbar disc?

[ ] **A.** Intermittent paresthesia

[ ] **B.** Sudden incontinence

[ ] **C.** Sciatic pain in legs

[ ] **D.** Back pain with sneezing

45. Which of the following is **NOT** a risk factor for a deep vein thrombosis?

[ ] **A.** Increasing age

[ ] **B.** Obesity

[ ] **C.** Increased mobility

[ ] **D.** Pregnancy

46. A patient comes to the emergency department with complaints of a burning and itching pain and intermittent numbness to the palm of the hand. The patient reports it is usually worse upon awakening in the morning. The emergency nurse notes decreased grip strength to the affected hand. Which of the following is the nerve most often responsible for this problem?

[ ] **A.** Ulnar

[ ] **B.** Median

[ ] **C.** Peroneal

[ ] **D.** Radial

47. Which of the following is a potential complication after manipulation of a long-bone fracture?

[ ] **A.** Deep vein thrombosis

[ ] **B.** Pulmonary embolism

[ ] **C.** Acute respiratory distress syndrome

[ ] **D.** Fat embolism

48. Which of the following is appropriate care of an amputated part?

[ ] **A.** Wrap part in dry dressing and place in a bag on ice.

[ ] **B.** Wrap part with moist dressing and place the part directly on ice.

[ ] **C.** Wrap part with moist dressing, place in a bag, and place the bag on ice.

[ ] **D.** Wrap part with dry dressing, place in a bag, and place the bag on ice.

49. A 3-year-old patient is brought to the emergency department by his parents. He fell down several steps and has a fracture of the forearm. Which of the following types of fractures would be the most concerning?

[ ] **A.** Epiphyseal

[ ] **B.** Transverse

[ ] **C.** Greenstick

[ ] **D.** Displaced

50. Parents are told that their child has sustained a fracture with a Salter–Harris classification of type II. The emergency nurse would understand that this is a grading for which of the following types of fractures?

[ ] **A.** Displaced

[ ] **B.** Spiral

[ ] **C.** Comminuted

[ ] **D.** Epiphyseal

51. An 82-year-old patient is brought to the emergency department by family with a concern regarding a possible fracture to his thoracic spine area after slipping in the living room and catching himself with the couch edge. He has no prior history and is on no medications. The emergency nurse knows that this patient may have fragile bones due to which of the following disease processes?

[ ] **A.** Paget's disease

[ ] **B.** Osteogenesis imperfecta

[ ] **C.** Legg–Perthes disease

[ ] **D.** Menkes kinky hair syndrome

52. Which of the following is the proper listing of the four types of blast injuries?

[ ] **A.** Primary, secondary, typical, quaternary

[ ] **B.** Principle, secondary, tertiary, quaternary

[ ] **C.** Principle, simple, tertiary, quaternary

[ ] **D.** Primary, secondary, tertiary, quaternary

53. Which of the following is the triad of symptoms that occur with fat embolism?
[ ] A. Muffled heart tones, distended neck veins, and hypotension
[ ] B. Decreased mental status, respiratory distress, and petechial rash
[ ] C. Absent breath sounds, distended neck veins, and tracheal deviation
[ ] D. Hypotension, tracheal deviation, and widened mediastinum

54. A caregiver brings a 6-month-old to triage and states "he fell out of the crib." The emergency nurse suspects maltreatment when radiographs reveal which of the following types of fracture?
[ ] A. Spiral
[ ] B. Comminuted
[ ] C. Avulsion
[ ] D. Greenstick

55. Which one of the following is **NOT** part of the six Ps of neurovascular checks?
[ ] A. Pain
[ ] B. Priapism
[ ] C. Pallor
[ ] D. Paresthesia

56. A patient presents to triage several hours after having a cast placed complaining of severe pain uncontrolled by pain medication. Which of the following would be the priority intervention for this patient?
[ ] A. Provide pain medication
[ ] B. Ultrasound for deep vein thrombosis
[ ] C. Bivalve the cast immediately
[ ] D. Check compartmental pressure

57. Which of the following injuries is caused by a primary blast force and is commonly overlooked?
[ ] A. Mild traumatic brain injury
[ ] B. Ruptured tympanic membrane
[ ] C. Intestinal rupture
[ ] D. Pulmonary barotrauma

58. Which of the following surgical interventions is the treatment for compartment syndrome?
[ ] A. Fasciotomy
[ ] B. Muscle flap
[ ] C. Debridement
[ ] D. Amputation

59. A patient arrives in the emergency department via emergency medical services (EMS) with a traction splint in place. Which of the following would be the priority intervention on patient arrival?
[ ] A. Remove the splint
[ ] B. Assess neurovascular status
[ ] C. Prepare patient for surgery
[ ] D. Administer antibiotics

60. A 4-year-old is seen with a diagnosis of a distal clavicular fracture. Which of the following is a true statement regarding this patient and fracture?
[ ] A. This is a normal fracture for this population of patients.
[ ] B. This usually occurs in the older pediatric patient.
[ ] C. There are usually no associated injuries with this fracture.
[ ] D. This can be a sign of child abuse in this age group.

61. A patient arrives in the emergency department with an open fracture of the tibia and fibula with a 6″ laceration and a closed femur fracture to the left leg. Which of the following would be the most important laboratory test to be ordered?
[ ] A. Potassium
[ ] B. Calcium
[ ] C. Type and crossmatch
[ ] D. Arterial blood gases

62. Which of the following injuries is most at risk for osteomyelitis?
[ ] A. Closed fracture of the tibia and fibula
[ ] B. Open fracture of the femur
[ ] C. Comminuted fracture of the humerus
[ ] D. Dislocation of the hip joint

63. Open fractures are graded using which of the following classifications?
[ ] A. Danis–Weber
[ ] B. Lauge–Hansen
[ ] C. Gustilo
[ ] D. Salter–Harris

64. A patient with an amputation of the hand from being caught in a machine at work presents with ongoing bleeding despite direct pressure and elevation of the extremity. Which of the following is the next appropriate interventional step?
[ ] A. Apply pressure dressing.
[ ] B. Insert an intravenous catheter.
[ ] C. Notify the physician.
[ ] D. Apply a tourniquet.

65. A patient with an open fracture of the elbow is now experiencing a fever of 101.6° F (38.7° C) and has yellowish drainage from the site. Which of the following organisms would be expected for this type of infectious process?

[ ] **A.** *Staphylococcus aureus*
[ ] **B.** *Escherichia coli*
[ ] **C.** *Streptococcus agalactiae*
[ ] **D.** *Serratia marcescens*

66. A patient is recovering from relocation of the patella. Which of the following interventions should the emergency nurse perform before discharge?

[ ] **A.** Apply local heat.
[ ] **B.** Apply a knee immobilizer.
[ ] **C.** Administer a tetanus shot.
[ ] **D.** Call the orthopedist.

67. A patient arrives to the emergency department after a motorcycle crash and is diagnosed with a forearm and femur fracture. Which of the following would be the potential least amount of blood loss that could occur for this patient?

[ ] **A.** 1.0 liter
[ ] **B.** 1.5 liters
[ ] **C.** 3.5 liters
[ ] **D.** 4.5 liters

68. Which of the following may be involved in a ligamentous injury of the knee?

[ ] **A.** Anterior cruciate ligament
[ ] **B.** Medial meniscus
[ ] **C.** Deltoid ligament
[ ] **D.** Anterior talofibular ligament

69. A patient is undergoing procedural sedation to relocate a shoulder dislocation. Which of the following is a priority assessment to be monitored during this procedure?

[ ] **A.** Intravenous site
[ ] **B.** Pain control
[ ] **C.** Respiratory status
[ ] **D.** Neurovascular status

70. The emergency nurse is aware that straw-colored effusion fluid withdrawn from a joint would most likely be which of the following types?

[ ] **A.** Blood effusion
[ ] **B.** Septic arthritis effusion
[ ] **C.** Bursitis effusion
[ ] **D.** Gout

71. When applying a splint on a patient with an Achilles tendon rupture, in which of the following positions should the foot be placed?

[ ] **A.** Plantar flexion
[ ] **B.** Dorsiflexion
[ ] **C.** Plantar extension
[ ] **D.** Medial rotation

72. Which of the following is the most common amputation seen in the pediatric population?

[ ] **A.** Small toe
[ ] **B.** Foot
[ ] **C.** Hand
[ ] **D.** Fingertip

73. A 16-year-old patient is seen in the emergency department with chest pain that is worse with deep inspiration. There is tenderness to the touch to the anterior right upper rib area. Which of the following would the emergency nurse expect to use for discharge information for this patient?

[ ] **A.** Exercise to strengthen muscles
[ ] **B.** Medication and exercise
[ ] **C.** Deep breathing and medications
[ ] **D.** Rest, medication, and deep breathing

74. A patient presents with a dislocated knee and decreased pedal and posterior tibialis pulses. The physician suspects vascular injury. The emergency nurse would anticipate which of the following diagnostic procedures?

[ ] **A.** Vascular angiography
[ ] **B.** Computed tomography (CT)
[ ] **C.** Lateral knee radiograph
[ ] **D.** Magnetic resonance imaging (MRI)

75. All of the following are examples of definitive stabilization **EXCEPT** a/an:

[ ] **A.** open reduction.
[ ] **B.** traction.
[ ] **C.** casting.
[ ] **D.** sling.

Answers/Rationales

1. Answer: D

Nursing Process: Assessment

Rationale: **In this scenario, the anticipated mechanism of injury would be an open-book pelvic fracture because the patient was crushed between two objects in a standing position.** Because the patient was standing, it is unlikely his humerus or humeral head would be impacted by the crush. Closed pelvic fractures are generally caused by lateral compression from motor vehicle crashes.

 CENsational Pearl of Wisdom!

An open-book fracture occurs when the pelvic ring is disrupted. With this injury, there is an anterior injury that creates a widened pubic symphysis and a posterior injury involving a fracture or ligamental disruption.

2. Answer: B

Nursing Process: Intervention

Rationale: **Open-book pelvic fractures have the potential to bleed significantly. Application of pelvic binders (or a folded sheet) may improve alignment, control hemorrhage, and provide comfort.** With placement of the binder, there may actually be an improvement in the blood pressure secondary to the hemorrhage control.

3. Answer: B

Nursing Process: Evaluation

Rationale: **Keeping the extremity dependent can lead to additional swelling. The extremity should be elevated.** Removing the wrap, resting the extremity, and using ice for swelling in the first 48 hours are all correct.

 CENsational Pearl of Wisdom!

The RICE mnemonic is useful for sprains and strains.
R = Rest—Don't use it!
I = Ice—For 48 hours then heat!
C = Compression—Take the bandage off twice daily and at night!
E = Elevate—Keep it up!

4. Answer: A

Nursing Process: Assessment

Rationale: **Classic symptoms of an Achilles tendon rupture include sharp pain or "pop" in the heel, and walking flat-footed. The rupture can be precipitated by jumping or pushing off.** Strains and sprains share similar signs and symptoms. Sprains, however, involve the ligament around the joint, whereas strains involve muscle or tendon. With sprain and strain there is swelling, pain, and possible joint instability depending on the grade of injury. With a calcaneal fracture, the patient would not be able to walk on the foot.

 CENsational Pearl of Wisdom!

With an Achilles tendon rupture, the patient would not be able to plantar flex the foot when the posterior aspect of the lower leg is squeezed. The patient can be in a prone position or lying on their abdomen with the feet hanging off of the bed.

5. Answer: C

Nursing Process: Intervention

Rationale: **The standard of care for open fractures is quick administration of antibiotics. This should occur within the first hour and preferably within the first 30 minutes. The American College of Surgeons has set the standard of 30 minutes for initiation of the first antibiotic.** Obtaining an radiograph, administering tetanus vaccine, and contacting an orthopedic specialist are appropriate, but they are not as time-sensitive.

 CENsational Pearl of Wisdom!

In cases of open fractures, advocate for early antibiotic administration!

6. Answer: B

Nursing Process: Assessment

Rationale: **A contusion is a collection of blood under the skin.** An avulsion consists of a peeling of the skin away from the associated tissue. A degloving injury is removal of or complete separation of skin from underlying tissue. An abrasion involves removal of the epithelium.

7. Answer: C

Nursing Process: Intervention

Rationale: **Application of ice would follow the "RICE" mnemonic along with elevation, not dependent positioning for this type of injury.** Intravenous pain medications would not be the preferred choice of pain control. Pressure dressings would not be utilized on this injury as it could encourage the development of compartment syndrome.

8. Answer: B

Nursing Process: Assessment

Rationale: **Blood at the urinary meatus is an indication of a pelvic fracture due to laceration or disruption of the urethra. Urinary catheter placement should be delayed pending further evaluation.** Legs are usually externally rotated. Patients with pelvic fractures can bleed significantly, so they would demonstrate signs and symptoms of hypovolemic shock not neurogenic shock. Fecal incontinence would occur with a spinal cord injury, not a pelvic fracture.

 CENsational Pearl of Wisdom!

If there is a disruption of the urethra, the prostate gland would either be "high-riding," inability to palpate, or feel "boggy." In this circumstance, the ED nurse should not insert a urinary catheter. Hand the catheter to the trauma surgeon or primary physician caring for the patient and have them insert it. A retrograde urethrogram should be done first before the insertion takes place in these instances.

9. Answer: A

Nursing Process: Analysis

Rationale: **Compression fractures occur with axial loading. The loading of the vertebral column can occur with diving or in this case jumping.** A Chance fracture (involves fracture through the spinous process, the pedicles, and the vertebral body) is seen with hyperflexion and usually occurs in the thoracolumbar region. Comminuted (or burst) fractures are associated with vertical axial compression and fracture dislocations require extreme flexion.

10. Answer: D

Nursing Process: Analysis

Rationale: **The spinal cord is not part of the vertebrae but it runs through the vertebra and is protected in this way.** The facet, spinous, and transverse processes are all parts of the vertebrae.

11. Answer: D

Nursing Process: Evaluation

Rationale: **Allopurinol is one of the main medications utilized to treat gout. Allopurinol works to reduce the production of uric acid. This along with nonsteroidal anti-inflammatory drugs, Colchicine, Probenecid, and Anturane, are medications used to treat acute gout.** Both aspirin and alcohol should be avoided because they can stop the excretion of uric acid. Increasing activity may actually help decrease symptoms.

12. Answer: A

Nursing Process: Assessment

Rationale: **A blood effusion is seen after surgery or trauma to the joint.** Bursitis is from overuse and inflammation of the bursa sac. Gout is an alteration in the uric acid production, and septic arthritis is caused by bacteria entering the joint from the bloodstream, tissue, or a wound. Both gout and septic arthritis are usually associated with a fever, which this patient does not have.

13. Answer: D

Nursing Process: Analysis

Rationale: **A sprain occurs due to stretching or tearing of a ligament.** A strain is stretching or tearing of the muscle or tendon. A dislocation follows an injury that creates a disruption in the joint and pulls the bones out of their normal positioning. An avulsion is a pulling or tearing away of skin, tissue, or bone.

 CENsational Pearl of Wisdom!

Sprains are considered to be first, second, or third degree. This is determined based on the severity and the amount of disruption to the joint. For instance, a third-degree ankle sprain would create an unstable joint and, although not fractured, would still require a posterior splint and crutches. Follow-up with orthopedic specialty would also be necessary.

14. Answer: A

Nursing Process: Intervention

Rationale: **Reduction of dislocations should be done as soon as possible, and within a 6-hour timeframe.** Any time over 6 hours is incorrect because the longer the dislocation remains, the greater the risk of necrosis.

15. Answer: D

Nursing Process: Intervention

Rationale: **Next to early antibiotic administration, assessment and administration of tetanus immunization is a priority.** Irrigation of the ankle should be done in the operating room due to potential joint involvement. Traction splints are for femur fractures and should never be placed with an open ankle fracture. The dressing should be moist and sterile.

 CENsational Pearl of Wisdom!

This is a good example of reading the question carefully! A dressing would be a good option but the type of dressing is wrong. When reading the question, be careful to read every word and make sure that you take each of those words into account.

16. Answer: D

Nursing Process: Analysis

Rationale: **Falls are a leading cause of death in all ages but is the number one cause in the elderly. Due to changes in perception, balance, eye sight, and hearing, they are more likely to fall. Additionally, comorbidities can complicate recovery.** Motor vehicle crashes, pedestrians hit by a vehicle, and playing sports are all mechanisms of injury but not the leading cause for this population.

17. Answer: C

Nursing Process: Assessment

Rationale: **When the ulnar nerve is affected, grip strength can be affected as well as causing numbness to the little and ring fingers. Other manifestations include inability to have coordinated hand movement and weakness to the hand.** Median nerve injury results in inability to touch the thumb to the base of the small finger. Peroneal nerve injuries cause decreased sensation to the leg and can cause foot drop as well as a "slapping" type of gait. If the radial nerve is affected, the patient will not be able to give the "thumbs-up" sign or the "hitchhiker's" sign.

18. Answer: A

Nursing Process: Analysis

Rationale: **The symptoms presented are those of a minor sprain; there is no tearing and the joint is stable.** A grade II sprain would involve tearing without joint instability. Grade III sprains result in an unstable joint. There is no grade IV in the grading of sprains.

19. Answer: C

Nursing Process: Intervention

Rationale: **Exercise is a contraindication for a sprain. The "E" in this mnemonic stands for elevate.** The "R" is for rest, "I" is for ice, and the "C" stands for compression, which would be like an Ace wrap.

 CENsational Pearl of Wisdom!

Mnemonics are wonderful tools! Use them to help remember facts that help us care for our patients. The hard part is remembering which mnemonic goes with which part of the body!!

20. Answer: C

Nursing Process: Assessment

Rationale: **Popliteal artery injury is a frequent and significant high risk complication with a dislocated knee. All patients including those who relocate spontaneously before arrival to the emergency department should be assessed for this event. Some can maintain pulses for a time due to collateral flow.** Fibula fracture and tibial nerve injuries are not usually associated with knee dislocation. The saphenous vein is in the lower leg away from the knee.

21. Answer: C

Nursing Process: Intervention

Rationale: **The elbow should be flexed 90 degrees for position of healing. Additionally, the wrist should remain in a neutral position and not be dependent so a sling would also be necessary.** Positioning the elbow straight or less than 90 degrees would not be correct position.

22. Answer: D

Nursing Process: Analysis

Rationale: **Long bones include the femur, tibia, and fibula and, in this case, the humerus, as well as the radius and ulna.** Carpal (wrist bones) and tarsal bones (hindfoot and midfoot) are classified as short bones and are cube-shaped. The hip bone is classified as an irregular bone and is complex-shaped.

23. Answer: B

Nursing Process: Analysis

Rationale: **Tendons are dense, fibrous tissues made up of collagen that attach bones to muscle.** Cartilage provides a cushioning for bones. Cartilage also takes many forms and is commonly replaced by bone as infants and children grow. However, adults have cartilage in many places as well. Ligaments are connective tissues holding bones together at joints. Skeletal muscles are attached to the bone by tendons. Skeletal muscle allows movement through contraction.

24. Answer: D

Nursing Process: Assessment

Rationale: **Bursitis is an inflammation of the bursa sac of a joint from overuse.** Blood in the joint occurs with trauma or surgery. Gout arises from an alteration in the production of uric acid. Septic arthritis is sudden in onset and occurs from bacteria entering the joint through the blood stream, tissue, or a puncture wound.

 CENsational Pearl of Wisdom!

Septic arthritis can be caused by sexually transmitted illnesses such as Neisseria gonorrhoeae, and can also occur due to other infectious agents and etiologies. Some of these etiologies are as follows: intravenous illicit drug use, prosthetic joints, immunosuppression, Lyme disease, and traumatic injuries. Other organisms such as fungi and viruses can also create a septic joint.

25. Answer: D

Nursing Process: Intervention

Rationale: **Traction splints are utilized for stabilizing long-bone fractures, most commonly the femur.** Shoulder dislocations should be immobilized with the arm close to the body with a sling. Neurovascular assessment is important for all orthopedic injuries. Ice should be applied to reduce swelling.

 CENsational Pearl of Wisdom!

Here is another example of reading your questions very carefully! A traction splint would be used for a femur/hip fracture, but if there is a tibial or fibular fracture on the same leg, then it would be contraindicated! If the patient were lying in front of you, you would know not to put a traction splint on that leg! But, in reading questions you might miss that information. Word of caution—read your questions methodically and study every word!

26. Answer: C

Nursing Process: Assessment

Rationale: **A femur fracture is a common injury with a school-aged child being hit by a vehicle due to bumper height. Whereas an adult may attempt to turn from an impact, children do not, thus resulting in being struck straight on.** Because of the height of children, the ankle and clavicle are not points of impact with the bumper of the car. The spinal cord may be injured but not from the initial impact.

27. Answer: A

Nursing Process: Analysis

Rationale: **A "buckle" fracture is also known as a torus fracture.** This is demonstrated by no disruption of the cortex. In a "greenstick" fracture, the cortex does show disruption on the involved side. Both torus and greenstick fractures are breaks that involve one side of the bone, but there is a difference. In compression fractures, the bone collapses onto itself, and in comminuted fractures, the bone is splintered or fragmented with two or more fragments of bone involved. This can commonly occur with gunshot wounds, but can also be direct blunt trauma.

28. Answer: C

Nursing Process: Intervention

Rationale: **The priority for this patient is to control the hemorrhage with direct pressure. If direct pressure does not work, consider the use of a tourniquet.** Establishing intravenous access should be accomplished, but active bleeding must be stopped first. A traction splint may be appropriate, but should be done after hemorrhage control. Obtaining radiographs is not a priority.

 CENsational Pearl of Wisdom!

Uncontrolled hemorrhage is a leading cause of death in trauma patients. A major movement to educate the public about this potentially fatal complication is called "Stop the Bleed." This national campaign created for interested lay individuals teaches the basic concepts of hemorrhage control, including the use of tourniquets in appropriate circumstances.

29. Answer: D

Nursing Process: Assessment

Rationale: **Crush injuries have the potential to develop compartment syndrome resulting from cellular** destruction. **Symptoms include tense swelling, altera-tion in neurovascular assessment, and pain dispro-portionate to the injury.** Radial nerve injury would be identified by inability to demonstrate the "thumbs-up" sign. The humerus is an upper arm bone and is not noted to be involved. Brachial artery injury may cause alteration in neurovascular status, but not the disproportionate pain.

CENsational Pearl of Wisdom!

The arm and the leg both have multiple compart-ments. It depends on which compartment is in-volved regarding the potential loss of pulses and capillary refill time.

30. Answer: A

Nursing Process: Intervention

Rationale: **The scaphoid bone, also known as the navic-ular bone, lies between the hand and the forearm on the radial side of wrist. It is located in the anatomical snuff box. To ensure correct healing, the thumb must be placed in the correct position, or that of opposition.** Application of a sling would be important for shoulder dislocations or humeral fractures. Traction splints are used to stabilize long-bone fractures. A cast with the elbow flexed 90 degrees is proper treatment for forearm fractures.

31. Answer: B

Nursing Process: Evaluation

Rationale: **Verbalizing the need for follow-up with the orthopedist indicates understanding of the discharge instructions.** The patient should not walk on the splint, return for its removal, or keep the extremity dependent. Those responses would indicate a lack of understanding of the provided instructions.

CENsational Pearl of Wisdom!

Remember that casts are not applied in the ED. Splints are placed so that there is room for swell-ing to occur. Casts are applied later in the pro-cess. Splints should never completely encircle the extremity!

32. Answer: D

Nursing Process: Assessment

Rationale: **Rhabdomyolysis is a potential complication of a crush injury. As myoglobin is released, the urine**

will become dark brown or reddish in color. Compart-ment syndrome is a swelling of the compartment of an injured extremity. Dehydration will decrease urine out-put and the color will be dark, but will be a dark amber color. A urinary tract infection causes urine color to be cloudy.

CENsational Pearl of Wisdom!

One of the major sequelae of rhabdomyolysis is renal failure! The myoglobin can actually cause an obstruction in the renal tubules and there are toxins that are released.

33. Answer: C

Nursing Process: Intervention

Rationale: **Immobility that would be involved with an elderly patient who has sustained a pelvic fracture can cause stasis and development of a thrombus.** This venous thrombosis can then progress to a pulmonary em-bolus. Low-molecular-weight heparin would be an appro-priate preventive intervention. Pulmonary edema results from fluid overload. Congestive heart failure may develop in patients with cardiac history when over-resuscitated. Fat embolisms occur in patients who have manipulation of long-bone fractures. This can also happen with pelvic fractures, but preventive measures with low-molecular-weight heparin have not been shown to prevent this com-plication from fat emboli.

34. Answer: D

Nursing Process: Assessment

Rationale: **Guillotine-type amputations have the high-est success rate as the tissue is preserved and cleanly severed.** The other injuries listed have tissue, nerve, and vessel destruction and/or loss that make reimplantation less successful.

35. Answer: B

Nursing Process: Analysis

Rationale: **Dislocation of the radial head, also known as Nurse Maid's elbow, is a common injury in young children. It occurs as a result of an arm that is jerked or pulled, and the hallmark symptom is nonuse of the extremity by the child.** Shoulder dislocations, elbow, or humeral fractures usually occur from a fall or other trau-matic event. A fracture would require greater force than a simple jerking on an arm, especially in a child as the bones are more pliable.

36. Answer: B

Nursing Process: Intervention

Rationale: **Placing the affected extremity at the level of the heart would be the most appropriate action for this patient as the manifestations are consistent with compartment syndrome. Elevating the extremity would be counterproductive for the desired outcome.** Ice should not be used as it will further constrict the neurovascular integrity. This patient should not wait as time is an important factor in saving this extremity. Necrosis of tissue can occur within 4 to 6 hours and the clock is already ticking by the time the patient arrives in the ED. Patients should not be sent to urgent care centers without a medical screening examination, which cannot be done by the triage nurse.

CENsational Pearl of Wisdom!

Do not get into the habit of underestimating potential injuries or processes because of "frequent flyers" or concern about drug seeking behavior! Assess every patient each time they come to the ED according to their chief complaint and important background information. Be cautious about being too judgmental as it may get in the way of your objectivity!

37. Answer: A

Nursing Process: Intervention

Rationale: **This patient is clearly in hypovolemic shock. A femoral fracture can bleed significantly and, in this case, is multiplied due to the bilateral situation. Each fractured femur can lose 1 to 2 liters of blood. This patient has already received crystalloid resuscitation and has not responded. Therefore, activation of massive transfusion protocol is appropriate.** Giving additional crystalloids will dilute the already-depleted blood volume and can pop off developed clots, dilute the red blood cells which provide the oxygen-carrying capacity and dilute clotting factors as well as contribute to hypothermia. Trendelenburg is not a definitive intervention. Shock position or modified Trendelenburg would be more appropriate in the hypovolemic patient; however, it would be difficult to perform this with the sustained injuries. Splints are appropriate but correcting shock status is the highest priority.

CENsational Pearl of Wisdom!

Shock index is a great indicator for the need to initiate massive transfusion protocol. The formula for this is heart rate divided by systolic blood pressure. A reading of 0.5 to 0.7 is considered normal. Value greater than 1.5 indicates that massive transfusion policy should be started.

38. Answer: D

Nursing Process: Analysis

Rationale: **Normal compartment pressure can range from less than 10 mm Hg to less than 15 or 20.** These numbers are dependent on the author. Most authors will agree that measurements greater than 30 to 31 mm Hg indicates a critical level and that measures must be instituted immediately to save the limb. Another way to determine the number of criticality is to use the delta number. This number is derived by subtracting the intracompartmental pressure from the diastolic pressure. Readings of less than 30 on this reading are indicative of compartment syndrome. Therefore, if a reading of 25 was present for the intracompartmental pressure and the blood pressure was 102/82 mm Hg, the delta number would be 57 and would rule out compartment pressure.

39. Answer: D

Nursing Process: Intervention

Rationale: **Traction splints are used to stabilize the femur.** The other fractures benefit from splinting but not traction splints.

40. Answer: D

Nursing Process: Assessment

Rationale: **Urethral injury is a common complication of a pelvic fracture.** Muscle spasms are seen with femur fractures. Hematochezia is blood in the stool and should not be associated with a pelvic fracture. Rhabdomyolysis is acute destruction of muscle tissue and not a complication of a pelvic fracture.

41. Answer: D

Nursing Process: Evaluation

Rationale: **Muscle relaxants have the potential to make the patient drowsy, so this statement verbalized by the patient indicates good understanding and effective education of medication side effects.** If the patient understood that muscle relaxants can result in drowsiness, then driving would be contraindicated, as would stating they will be more alert. Muscle relaxants do not generally cause anxiety or restlessness.

42. Answer: A

Nursing Process: Evaluation

Rationale: **To clear myoglobin and preserve kidney function, urine output needs to be at least 100 mL/hour.** If urine is getting darker, fluid resuscitation is inadequate. Increasing muscle pain and creatine kinase levels also indicate the condition is not improving. Creatinine kinase levels should be decreasing. An elevated creatinine kinase level is one of the hallmark findings of rhabdomyolysis. Muscle pain, especially in the lower back, is one of the common signs.

43. Answer: C

Nursing Process: Assessment

Rationale: **The signs in this scenario are those of pulmonary embolism. Sudden onset of shortness of breath, pleuritic chest pain, hemoptysis, and wheezing as well as signs of hypoxemia all point to the development of a pulmonary embolus.** Deep vein thrombosis would manifest with symptoms of swelling, warmth, and pain in the extremity harboring the clot. A fat embolism will have symptoms of decreased mental status, respiratory distress, and a petechial rash. Pneumonia would take longer to appear and would carry a fever and cough with it.

44. Answer: B

Nursing Process: Assessment

Rationale: **Incontinence is a medical emergency, possibly indicating cauda equina syndrome. Immediate evaluation is indicated.** Surgical intervention must occur in a short period of time in order to not have a negative outcome. Leg pain, intermittent paresthesias, and pain with sneezing are nonemergent symptoms of a herniated disc.

45. Answer: C

Nursing Process: Assessment

Rationale: **A patient who is fully mobile or has increased mobility is at low risk for deep vein thrombosis because immobility is one cause of this complication.** Older patients, bariatric, and pregnant patients are all at greater risk for development of deep vein thrombosis.

46. Answer: B

Nursing Process: Analysis

Rationale: **The median nerve is responsible for movement of the small muscles of the hand and sensation in the palm. This is the nerve involved in carpal tunnel syndrome. This nerve runs through the middle of the wrist into the hand. The space available for it in the carpal tunnel becomes minimized and symptoms then appear.** The ulnar nerve allows for abduction of the fingers and supplies sensation to the little finger. The radial nerve provides the ability to extend the thumb and delivers sensation to the dorsum of the thumb. Both of these nerves can be involved in carpal tunnel syndrome, but are not the cause. The peroneal nerve is located in the foot and causes extension of the foot and great toe and sensation to the first web space.

47. Answer: D

Nursing Process: Analysis

Rationale: **Fat embolism is a potential complication when long-bone fractures are manipulated. This complication may occur within 12 hours.** This is why immediate immobilization is so important. Deep vein thrombosis develops from immobility, which may then lead to pulmonary embolism. This can then progress to adult respiratory distress syndrome.

48. Answer: C

Nursing Process: Intervention

Rationale: **Amputated parts should be wrapped in a moist saline-soaked dressing, placed in a sealed plastic bag and placed on ice.** Placing the part directly on ice could cause the part to freeze, making it unable to be reimplanted. A moist dressing prevents the tissues from drying out.

 CENsational Pearl of Wisdom!

It is highly important that the amputated part be placed on ice so that reimplantation can occur after a longer period of time. If not placed on ice, this "warm ischemia" time only allows for 4 to 6 hours for reimplantation. Cool ischemia time provides a wider window of opportunity for reimplantation— up to 18 hours depending on the damage to the tissues. So, ice is good—just not directly on the ice!!!

49. Answer: A

Nursing Process: Analysis

Rationale: **Fractures of the epiphyseal plate can affect healing and growth.** This area is where the bones grow; thus, major problems can be expected as the child matures. Whereas the others would need proper care and healing, they are not as concerning as the sequelae that can occur with an epiphyseal plate injury.

50. Answer: D

Nursing Process: Assessment

Rationale: **An epiphyseal plate fracture has a Salter–Harris classification. These range from 1 to 5, and those that are 3 and above will usually require surgical intervention in order to maintain blood supply to the area to avert future growth problems.** A "displaced" fracture is a type of classification because fractures can be nondisplaced or displaced. All fractures can then be classified depending on whether they are open (compound) or closed and stable or unstable as well as the displacement criteria. Comminuted and spiral fractures do not have specific classifications.

 CENsational Pearl of Wisdom!

When children have epiphyseal plate injuries, radiographs will often be taken of the opposite side so that providers and radiologists will understand what the area should look like at that point in the child's growth.

51. Answer: A

Nursing Process: Analysis

Rationale: **Paget's disease causes weak and brittle bones due to an interruption in the bone recycling process in older males. This can create a situation in which pathologic fractures, fractures that occur due to weakness in the structural composition of bones, take place.** Osteogenesis imperfecta is an inherited, genetic defect that causes brittle bones along with other symptoms. This condition is diagnosed at or shortly after birth and causes fractures throughout the child's life. Legg–Perthes disease is a disease of childhood that causes a disruption of blood supply to the hip joint. This progresses to avascular necrosis. Menkes kinky hair syndrome is genetic defect in the utilization of copper. With this disease process the child has very sparse, brittle hair and an array of other symptoms including neuromuscular defects and weakened bones.

52. Answer: D

Nursing Process: Analysis

Rationale: **The correct classifications of blast injuries are primary, secondary, tertiary, and quaternary.** Understanding these phases help the nurse determine potential injuries patients may sustain in the event of a blast event.

 CENsational Pearl of Wisdom!

Blast injuries can occur with any type of explosion. The following are the four types of injuries associated with blasts or explosions.
Primary: *Initial impact—examples are blast lung, middle ear damage, tympanic membrane rupture, globe rupture, concussion.*

Secondary: *Objects flying through the air—examples are penetrating injuries from pieces that were involved in the bomb or missile.*
Tertiary: *Body being thrown—examples are fractures, amputations, and brain injuries.*
Quaternary: *Injuries/illnesses not due to the first three types—examples are burns, asthma, chronic obstructive pulmonary disease, angina, hyperglycemia, and crush-type injuries.*

53. Answer: B

Nursing Process: Assessment

Rationale: **Decreased mental status, respiratory distress, and petechial rash are the triad of symptoms associated with fat embolism.** Muffled heart tones, distended neck veins, and hypotension are known as Beck's triad, indicating pericardial tamponade. Absent breath sounds, distended neck veins, and tracheal deviation indicate tension pneumothorax. An aortic disruption will have symptoms of hypotension, tracheal deviation to the right side, and a widened mediastinum on radiograph.

54. Answer: A

Nursing Process: Analysis

Rationale: **A spiral fracture results from a twisting action and should elevate the nurse's suspicion for maltreatment.** Greenstick fractures are a buckling type of fracture and are common in the pediatric population. Comminuted fractures occur when bone splinters and there are two or more fragments, and an avulsion fraction is when a small part of the bone is torn away at the point where the muscle attaches to the bone after a muscular contraction.

55. Answer: B

Nursing Process: Assessment

Rationale: **Priapism is a sustained erection and is an indication of spinal cord injury, and not part of the "six Ps."** The Ps are: **P**ain/**P**allor/**P**ulselessness/**P**aresthesias/**P**aralysis/**P**ressure. Two more that can be added are: Tem**P**erature and Ca**P**illary Refill.

56. Answer: C

Nursing Process: Intervention

Rationale: **The most important priority intervention for this patient is to bivalve the cast. Nothing can be done until the area can be visualized.** Sometimes just removing the cast can take care of the pain. Compartment syndrome is a major concern, but the pressure cannot be checked until the cast is removed. This can be caused by an external force such as a cast and pain disproportionate to injury is an indication of this complication. Deep vein thrombosis is painful but not disproportionate. Pain control may be an issue, but again the hallmark symptom in this scenario is the report of disproportionate pain to injury.

57. Answer: A

Nursing Process: Assessment

Rationale: **Mild traumatic brain injury is often missed as symptoms are subtle.** Injuries such as ruptured tympanic membrane, pulmonary barotrauma, and intestinal rupture are usually diagnosed easily. These are all primary blast forces that affect gas-filled organs.

58. Answer: A

Nursing Process: Intervention

Rationale: **Fasciotomy is the emergency surgical intervention for compartment syndrome to relieve the pressure and salvage the tissue and/or limb.** A muscle flap may be used to reconstruct the extremity after fasciotomy. Debridement is performed as treatment for dirty wounds or necrotic tissue. Amputation may result if fasciotomy is not performed promptly.

59. Answer: B

Nursing Process: Intervention

Rationale: **Assessing neurovascular status with a splint in place is important to evaluate the current status of the limb and to compare with the prior reported condition.** The splint should remain in place unless directed otherwise. The patient may go to surgery but assessment of current status is priority. Administration of antibiotics would be important but the assessment of neurovascular integrity is the first priority.

   CENsational Pearl of Wisdom!

One type of traction splint that is used is a HARE traction splint. Nurses who are not comfortable with application of this type of splint should practice before they need this in a trauma situation. Find someone in the department who has experience and ask for their help! The patient will be in a great deal of pain during the application, but relief is realized once traction is applied resulting in the reduction of muscle spasms and realignment of the extremity. Provide comfort to the patient during this procedure!

60. Answer: D

Nursing Process: Analysis

Rationale: **A distal clavicular fracture can be a sign of child abuse as the perpetrator may be grabbing the child from behind.** The normal fracture site associated with clavicle breaks is mid-shaft for all age groups. There can be associated subclavian vein or artery lacerations and hemo/pneumothoraces.

61. Answer: C

Nursing Process: Analysis

Rationale: **Musculoskeletal injuries can cause major blood loss. In this scenario, a femoral fracture can cause the loss of at least 1 to 2 liters of blood. An associated open fracture of the tibia and fibula can increase that amount of blood loss. Type and crossmatch would be important because this patient may require blood products due to the potential hemorrhage from fractures and large lacerations.** Potassium leaks may occur with significant tissue destruction, but not hemorrhage. It would be important to know the baseline of the potassium and calcium if the patient were to receive large amounts of packed red cells; however, the most important out of these options would be the type and crossmatch. Arterial blood gases may be done, but these assess respiratory/hypoxia status.

   CENsational Pearl of Wisdom!

Remember that when blood products are given, elevated potassium levels can occur due to the breakdown of cells as blood products sit on the storage shelves. Knowledge of the baseline potassium level would be important. Hypocalcemia can also occur with large amounts of blood products due to the preservative citrate combining with available calcium. Watch for these electrolyte abnormalities when giving blood!

62. Answer: B

Nursing Process: Assessment

Rationale: **Osteomyelitis is a potential complication of an open fracture due to the potential of contamination.** Closed fractures have no communication with the environment and carries little risk for contamination. Comminuted fractures have splintered fragments and do not have a higher risk of contamination. The major complication of hip dislocation is femoral head necrosis.

63. Answer: C

Nursing Process: Assessment

Rationale: **Gustilo is the classification for open fractures. These classifications are grade I, II, and III. Grade III fractures are further subclassified as IIIA, IIIB, and IIIC.** Danis–Weber is the classification for fibula fractures. Lauge-Hanse is the classification system for ligament injury and Salter–Harris classification is for growth plate fractures.

 CENsational Pearl of Wisdom!

Remember, we already talked about Salter–Harris classification! You should have been able to at least rule that one out as a potential correct answer. When you know for sure something does not match with the question, rule it out and ignore it. That should cut down the potential for answering the question incorrectly!

64. Answer: D

Nursing Process: Intervention

Rationale: **Controlling the hemorrhage is the highest priority. Application of a tourniquet would be the next step because direct pressure and elevation of the extremity has not stopped the bleeding.** Application of a pressure dressing would most likely not help because direct pressure has not worked. Starting an intravenous catheter and notifying the physician are important, but hemorrhage control is the priority.

 CENsational Pearl of Wisdom!

Remember that direct pressure is always the first option. Tourniquets should be used when direct pressure has not contained the bleeding, massive bleeding is occurring, the patient is exsanguinating, and there is enough of a stump left to apply the tourniquet.

65. Answer: A

Nursing Process: Analysis

Rationale: **Osteomyelitis is an infection of the bone, most often as a result of an open fracture with direct contamination. *Staphylococcus aureus* is found on human skin and is the main causative bacteria.** *Escherichia coli* and *Streptococcus agalactiae* are common in the gastrointestinal tract and *Serratia marcescens* is found in water.

66. Answer: B

Nursing Process: Intervention

Rationale: **The appropriate intervention after knee relocation is application of an immobilizer.** Ice should be used for the first 48 hours to reduce swelling, not heat. Tetanus immunization is not indicated unless there is an open wound, and calling for orthopedic follow-up is not a priority intervention postreduction. The patient or family members should actually make this type of call because they know their own schedule. The ED nurse does not know the best time for an office visit for this patient.

67. Answer: B

Nursing Process: Analysis

Rationale: **Blood loss with orthopedic injuries is a huge potential. The forearm can lose from 0.5 to 1.5 liters and the femur can lose from 1.0 to 2.0 liters. Therefore, the least amount potential blood loss would be 1.5 liters.** The highest amount that could potentially lost would be 3.5 liters. A pelvic fracture could bleed out 1.5 to 4.5 liters.

68. Answer: A

Nursing Process: Assessment

Rationale: **The anterior cruciate ligament is one of the commonly injured ligaments of the knee.** The medial meniscus is cartilage, not a ligament. The deltoid ligament is in the shoulder and the anterior talofibular ligament is located in the ankle.

69. Answer: C

Nursing Process: Assessment

Rationale: **Priority assessment during procedural sedation is an ongoing evaluation of the patient's respiratory status.** Monitoring the intravenous site and pain control are important aspects, but respiratory status is, of course, the priority. Neurovascular status is a pre- and postprocedure assessment.

 CENsational Pearl of Wisdom!

Remember!!! Airway is always the first priority! You cannot go wrong with airway!

70. Answer: C

Nursing Process: Analysis

Rationale: **Straw-colored effusion fluid is most likely from a bursitis.** A blood effusion would have bloody return of the aspirate. White blood cells would be present with septic arthritis and gout would produce urate crystals.

71. Answer: A

Nursing Process: Intervention

Rationale: **The correct position for the foot when applying a splint for an Achilles tendon rupture is plantar flexion to allow the tendon to rest and prevent further overstretching and injury.** Dorsiflexion and planter extension will result in excessive tension. The foot/ankle should not be rotated in either direction.

72. Answer: D

Nursing Process: Assessment

Rationale: **The fingertip is the most common amputation for children due to the finger being shut in car doors.** There may be amputations of toes, hands, or feet, but these areas are not common.

73. Answer: D

Nursing Process: Intervention

Rationale: **This patient is demonstrating symptoms of costochondritis. Treatment for this diagnosis includes rest, medication, and deep breathing.** Exercise may exacerbate symptoms. Medications and deep breathing alone are not appropriate.

74. Answer: A

Nursing Process: Analysis

Rationale: **Peripheral vascular angiography is the best diagnostic test to evaluate vascular injury. Computed tomography (CT)** assesses musculoskeletal trauma and surrounding organ injury. A lateral radiograph does not demonstrate vascular injury. Magnetic resonance imaging (MRI) would provide excellent information about organs and other structures but would not assist with vascular data.

75. Answer: D

Nursing Process: Intervention

Rationale: **A sling would allow for movement and not provide stabilization.** Open reduction, traction, and casting are all forms of definitive stabilization of a fracture.

 CENsational Pearl of Wisdom!

An easy one to end on! Remember to pick out the word "definitive" in this last question!

References

American Academy of Orthopaedic Surgeons. (2018). *Sprains, strains and other soft-tissue injuries.* OrthoInfor. Retrieved from https://orthoinfo.aaos.org/en/diseases--conditions/sprains-strains-and-other-soft-tissue-injuries/ (3, 4, 13, 18, 19)

American Association of Neurological Surgeons. (2018). *Cauda equina syndrome.* Retrieved from http://www.aans.org/Patients/Neurosurgical-Conditions-and-Treatments/Cauda-Equina-Syndrome (44)

American College of Surgeons. (2012). Advanced trauma life support: the ninth ed. *The Journal of Trauma and Acute Care Surgery, 74,* 1363–1366. (5, 28, 32, 48)

American College of Surgeons. *Best practices in the management of orthopaedic trauma.* Trauma Quality Improvement Program. Retrieved from https://www.facs.org/~/media/files/quality%20programs/trauma/tqip/tqip%20bpgs%20in%20the%20management%20of%20orthopaedic%20traumafinal.ashx (5, 33)

Athwal, G. S., et al. (2018). *Dislocated shoulder.* OrthoInfo. Retrieved from https://orthoinfo.aaos.org/en/diseases--conditions/dislocated-shoulder/ (25)

Brusch, J. L. (2017). *Septic arthritis.* Emedicine. Retrieved from https://emedicine.medscape.com/article/236299-overview (24)

Brusch, J. L. (2018). *Septic arthritis clinical presentation.* Emedicine. Retrieved from https://emedicine.medscape.com/article/236299-clinical (12)

Centers for Disease Control and Prevention. (2018). *Explosions and blast injuries a primer for clinicians.* Retrieved from https://www.cdc.gov/masstrauma/preparedness/primer.pdf (52)

De Falla, K. (2018). *Common risks and side effects of muscle relaxants.* Retrieved from https://www.spine-health.com/treatment/pain-medication/common-risks-and-side-effects-muscle-relaxants (41)

Egol, K. A., et al. (2010). Handbook of fractures (4th ed.). Philadelphia, PA: Wolters Kluwer. (40, 71)

Emergency Nurses Association. (2012). Emergency nursing pediatric course (4th ed.). Des Plaines, IL: Emergency Nurses Association. (26, 31, 34, 49, 54, 72)

Emergency Nurses Association. (2014). Trauma nurse core course (7th ed.). Des Plaines, IL: Emergency Nurses Association. (1, 2, 8, 9, 15, 16, 22, 23, 27, 36, 37, 39, 42, 43, 45, 47, 50, 51, 53, 57–64, 69, 74, 75)

Emergency Nurses Association. (2017). Emergency nursing core curriculum (6th ed.). St. Louis, MI: W.B. Saunders Company. (36, 73)

Haddad, S. L., et al. (2018). *Sprained ankle.* OrthoInfo. Retrieved from https://orthoinfo.aaos.org/en/diseases--conditions/sprained-ankle/ (18)

Jennings, C. D., et al. (2018). *Carpal tunnel syndrome*. Retrieved from https://orthoinfo.aaos.org/en/diseases--conditions/carpal-tunnel-syndrome/ (46)

Kishner, S., et al. (2018). *Osteomyelitis*. Retrieved from https://emedicine.medscape.com/article/1348767-overview (65)

Life in the Fast Lane. (2018). *Compartment syndrome*. Retrieved from https://lifeinthefastlane.com/compartment-syndrome/ (38)

Mayo Clinic. (2018). *Legg-Calve-Perthes disease*. Retrieved from https://www.mayoclinic.org/diseases-conditions/legg-calve-perthes-disease/symptoms-causes/syc-20374343 (51)

Mayo Clinic. (2018). *Paget's disease of bone*. Retrieved from https://www.mayoclinic.org/diseases-conditions/pagets-disease-of-bone/symptoms-causes/syc-20350811 (51)

Patel, A. (2018). *Knee dislocations*. Ortho Bullets. Retrieved from https://www.orthobullets.com/trauma/1043/knee-dislocation (20)

Saglimbeni, A. J. (2018). *Achilles tendon injury: Clinical presentation*. Emedicine. Retrieved from https://emedicine.medscape.com/article/309393-clinical#b3 (4)

Sharma, R., et al. (2018). *Greenstick fracture*. Radiopaedia. Retrieved from https://radiopaedia.org/articles/greenstick-fracture (27)

Sheil, W. C., Jr. (2018). *Costochondritis*. Retrieved from https://www.emedicinehealth.com/costochondritis/article_em.htm (73)

Shlamovitz, G. Z. (2018). *Urethral catheterization in men*. Emedicine. Retrieved from https://emedicine.medscape.com/article/80716-overview (8)

Solheim, J. (2014). Certified emergency (CEN) review course. Retrieved from https://solheim-enterprises.teachable.com/p/onlinecen (3, 4, 6, 7, 11, 12, 14, 19, 21, 24, 30, 35, 38, 52, 55, 56, 66, 67, 70)

Spoonamore, M. J. (2018). *Spine anatomy*. Retrieved from http://www.uscspine.com/spine-health-education/spinal-anatomy.cfm (10)

U.S. National Library of Medicine. (2017). *Menkes disease*. Retrieved from https://medlineplus.gov/ency/article/001160.htm (51)

U.S. National Library of Medicine. (2018). *Osteogenesis imperfect*. Retrieved from https://ghr.nlm.nih.gov/condition/osteogenesis-imperfecta (51)

Werdo, B., et al. (2018). *Knee injury*. Retrieved from https://www.emedicinehealth.com/knee_injury/article_em.htm (68)

Williams, B. R. (2018). Peripheral nerves of the upper extremity. Orthopaedics One Clerkship. In: *Orthopaedics One—The Orthopaedic Knowledge Network*. Retrieved from https://www.orthopaedicsone.com/x/Q4DEAg (17)

Young, C. C. (2017). *Ankle sprain clinical presentation*. Emedicine. Retrieved from https://emedicine.medscape.com/article/1907229-clinical#b4 (13)

10 Maxillofacial and Ocular Emergencies

Melissa L. Weir, MS, BSN, RN, CEN, CPEN

Maxillofacial and ocular emergencies can be life- and vision-threatening to the patient and therefore, are a high priority. On the Certified Emergency Nurse (CEN) test, remember that airway is always the answer and maxillo-facial injuries can impact this a great deal! This chapter is dedicated to these emergencies and involves both medical and traumatic injuries. CENsational Pearls of Wisdom have been added to enhance the learning process as well as rationales that deal with both the correct and incorrect answers. The CEN test will have 21 questions on this aspect and is included with orthopedic and wound management questions.

1. While examining a patient who sustained a direct blow to the eye, the emergency nurse notes a tear-drop-shaped pupil. The nurse prepares interventions for which of the following?
[ ] **A.** Ruptured globe
[ ] **B.** Glaucoma
[ ] **C.** Hyphema
[ ] **D.** Orbital fracture

2. A patient presents to triage after splashing drain cleaner in the eyes. The priority intervention for the emergency nurse is to:
[ ] **A.** assess visual acuity.
[ ] **B.** patch the affected eye(s).
[ ] **C.** initiate eye flushing.
[ ] **D.** initiate ophthalmology consult.

3. A patient reports spontaneous painless loss of vision in one portion of the left eye and occasionally seeing flashing lights bilaterally. What additional assessment should be completed by the emergency nurse?
[ ] **A.** Determine the sensation of floaters in the left eye.
[ ] **B.** Inquire about unprotected eye exposure to ultraviolet light.
[ ] **C.** Prepare for fluorescein examination.
[ ] **D.** Assess for pupil dilation in the affected eye.

4. A patient presents with unilateral painless loss of vision and is being evaluated for central retinal artery occlusion. Priority intervention by the emergency nurse includes which of the following?
[ ] **A.** Digital ocular massage
[ ] **B.** Patch the affected eye
[ ] **C.** Facilitate mild hyperventilation
[ ] **D.** Assist the patient to supine position

5. Upon examination of a patient exhibiting eye pain with extraocular movement (EOM), the emergency nurse finds pain on palpation of the sinuses and nasal quality to the voice. For which of the following conditions will the nurse continue to assess?
[ ] **A.** Conjunctivitis
[ ] **B.** Orbital cellulitis
[ ] **C.** Iritis
[ ] **D.** Uveitis

6. Which of the following statements made by a patient indicates the need for further instruction about the treatment of bacterial conjunctivitis?
[ ] **A.** "I can use disposable daily contact lenses since starting antibiotic ointment."
[ ] **B.** "I will discard all of my old eye makeup and clean my makeup brushes."
[ ] **C.** "I will avoid use of eye makeup until the infection is gone."
[ ] **D.** "Warm compresses will help to remove discharge from my eyelids."

7. Which of the following actions by the emergency nurse should be questioned regarding treatment for acute angle-closure glaucoma?
[ ] **A.** The nurse requests an order for an antiemetic.
[ ] **B.** A stat dose of a topical beta-blocker is administered.
[ ] **C.** Miotic eye drops such as pilocarpine are administered immediately upon arrival, before other medication.
[ ] **D.** Stat intravenous access is obtained in preparation for administration of acetazolamide (Diamox).

8. A patient has purulent, yellow discharge from the eyes. The emergency nurse recognizes this presentation as being consistent with which of the following?
[ ] **A.** Conjunctivitis
[ ] **B.** Blepharitis
[ ] **C.** Hordeolum
[ ] **D.** Chalazion

9. Which of the following is the priority intervention for a patient presenting with a penetrating foreign body eye injury?
[ ] **A.** Application of an eye patch
[ ] **B.** Administration of antibiotics
[ ] **C.** Administration of analgesics
[ ] **D.** Application of a rigid shield

10. A patient has the appearance of bright red blood to the lateral portion of the sclera. The patient states he noticed the redness after continuous harsh coughing yet denies recent trauma and pain. The emergency nurse suspects this patient will be diagnosed with which of the following?
[ ] **A.** Retinal hemorrhage
[ ] **B.** Ultraviolet keratitis
[ ] **C.** Subconjunctival hemorrhage
[ ] **D.** Eight-ball hyphema

11. The emergency nurse knows that the patient understood discharge instructions for an uncomplicated orbital fracture when they state:
[ ] **A.** "The bruising around my eye should go away in a day or so."
[ ] **B.** "Antibiotics will be prescribed so I don't get an infection."
[ ] **C.** "I will use warm packs for the pain."
[ ] **D.** "I will try to avoid blowing my nose."

12. Which of the following eye complaints stated by a patient does the triage nurse recognize as emergent?
[ ] **A.** Facial numbness and inability to look upward
[ ] **B.** Bloody appearance to the sclera
[ ] **C.** Perception of five to six floaters in the eye
[ ] **D.** Pain on the surface of the eye and excessive tearing

13. When assessing a patient with an eyelid laceration, the emergency nurse concludes that the patient has a deep laceration with injury to the levator muscle due to which of the following alterations?
[ ] **A.** Inability to close the eyelid
[ ] **B.** Inability to open the eyelid
[ ] **C.** Bleeding to the eyelid
[ ] **D.** Visual disturbance

14. A patient presents after being hit in the face with a baseball. The patient states he has "bloody vision" and assessment reveals decreased visual acuity. What other assessment data confirms the presence of a hyphema?
[ ] **A.** Patient describes perception of a curtain coming down over his eye
[ ] **B.** Visualization of blood covering the lower half of the iris
[ ] **C.** Limitation in extraocular eye movements
[ ] **D.** Severe pain when blinking the eye

15. A patient reports acute onset of loss of partial vision described as a cloudy veil over the top portion of the eye. The patient denies pain. The emergency nurse prepares for which of the following diagnostic evaluations which will confirm the diagnosis?
[ ] **A.** Tonometry for intraocular pressure measurement
[ ] **B.** Fluorescein stain for examination of the cornea
[ ] **C.** Pupil dilation for fundal examination
[ ] **D.** Computed tomography (CT) of the orbits

16. The emergency nurse is providing discharge instructions to a patient treated for corneal abrasion from contact lenses. Which of the following instructions is **NOT** appropriate for this patient?
[ ] **A.** Instillation of topical ophthalmic antibiotic drops
[ ] **B.** Avoid wearing contact lenses until reevaluation by a provider.
[ ] **C.** Use of an eye patch until pain is resolved.
[ ] **D.** Rest the eyes by avoiding eye strain and direct sunlight.

17. Which of the following does the emergency nurse prepare the patient for in the treatment of iritis?
[ ] **A.** Instillation of antibiotic ophthalmic ointment
[ ] **B.** Eye flush with normal saline
[ ] **C.** Cold compress to the eye
[ ] **D.** Instillation of ophthalmic steroids

18. A patient presents with sudden onset of deep unilateral eye pain, blurry vision, halos around lights, and nausea. The emergency nurse recognizes this ocular emergency as:
[ ] **A.** ultraviolet keratitis.
[ ] **B.** closed-angle glaucoma.
[ ] **C.** central retinal artery occlusion.
[ ] **D.** retinal detachment.

19. A child has a bean in the ear. Which of the following is the most appropriate initial action for the emergency nurse to implement?
[ ] **A.** Attempt to suction the bean out of the ear canal.
[ ] **B.** Irrigate the ear canal with water.
[ ] **C.** Use forceps to attempt removal of the bean.
[ ] **D.** Apply lidocaine drops to the ear canal.

20. A patient experiences hearing loss, swelling, erythema, and severe itching to the ear. The emergency nurse prepares for which of the following interventions?
[ ] **A.** Insertion of an ear wick
[ ] **B.** Intravenous access
[ ] **C.** Otic administration of mineral oil
[ ] **D.** Irrigation of the ear canal

21. A patient has a live insect in the ear. Which action does the emergency nurse take first?
[ ] **A.** Perform ear irrigation with lukewarm water.
[ ] **B.** Gather equipment for manual extraction.
[ ] **C.** Prepare for moderate sedation for the extraction.
[ ] **D.** Administration of mineral oil in the ear canal.

22. Which of the following objects, if lodged in a child's nose, must be removed emergently?
[ ] **A.** Plastic toy part
[ ] **B.** Small disc battery
[ ] **C.** Rubber pencil eraser
[ ] **D.** Cashew nut

23. A patient has profuse bleeding from the nose that has persisted despite application of firm pressure to the nostrils. Which of the following diagnostic evaluations is the priority test?
[ ] **A.** Activated partial thromboplastin time (aPTT)
[ ] **B.** Complete blood count (CBC) and prothrombin time (PT)
[ ] **C.** International normalized ratio (INR)
[ ] **D.** Hematocrit count and type and crossmatch

24. A patient is being discharged after treatment for epistaxis. Which of following statements indicates the patient understood the instructions?
[ ] **A.** "I will take ibuprofen for pain from the nasal packing."
[ ] **B.** "I will avoid taking hot showers when possible."
[ ] **C.** "I will instill phenylephrine nose drops for 10 days."
[ ] **D.** "I will blow my nose to clear out scabs that form."

25. A patient presents with postauricular pain, drooling, inability to blink one eye, and unilateral facial paralysis. Which of the following will be used to confirm the diagnosis?
[ ] **A.** Facial radiograph
[ ] **B.** Electromyography (EMG)
[ ] **C.** Computed tomography (CT)
[ ] **D.** Clinical presentation

26. Appropriate discharge instructions for the patient diagnosed with Bell's palsy includes which of the following?
[ ] **A.** Lubricant eye drops at night
[ ] **B.** Use of ophthalmic antibiotics
[ ] **C.** Prescription for antiepileptic drugs
[ ] **D.** Bed rest until symptoms resolve

27. The emergency nurse is preparing a patient for discharge after incision and drainage of an auricular hematoma. Which of the following reflects accurate discharge teaching?
[ ] **A.** Maintain the compression dressing until follow-up.
[ ] **B.** Follow-up for reevaluation of the ear in 7 days.
[ ] **C.** Antibiotics will not be indicated as there is no infection.
[ ] **D.** Take nonsteroidal anti-inflammatory drugs to manage pain.

28. A patient presents with high fever and the following signs and symptoms affecting the right ear: swelling, erythema and pain to the pinna, otorrhea, and decreased hearing. The emergency nurse prepares interventions for which of the following?
[ ] **A.** Ruptured tympanic membrane
[ ] **B.** Parotitis
[ ] **C.** Otitis externa
[ ] **D.** Mastoiditis

29. Which of the following disorders does the emergency nurse **NOT** expect as a complication of mastoiditis?
[ ] **A.** Bell's palsy
[ ] **B.** Tooth abscess
[ ] **C.** Hearing loss
[ ] **D.** Labyrinthitis

30. A patient involved in a motor vehicle accident is being evaluated for a zygomatic fracture. Which of the following complaints indicates the presence of a zygomatic fracture?
[ ] **A.** Altered sensation to the mandible
[ ] **B.** Feeling of numbness to the ear
[ ] **C.** Lack of feeling to the cheek
[ ] **D.** Lack of movement to the chin

31. A patient has a suspected zygomatic fracture. The nurse prepares the patient for which of the following diagnostic tests that will confirm this diagnosis?
[ ] **A.** Facial ultrasound
[ ] **B.** Lateral facial radiograph
[ ] **C.** Waters view radiograph
[ ] **D.** Facial computed tomography (CT)

32. Which of the following is the highest priority for ongoing monitoring of the patient with a nasal fracture?
[ ] **A.** Bleeding is controlled
[ ] **B.** Pain score decreased to 0 (zero)
[ ] **C.** Extent of periorbital ecchymosis
[ ] **D.** Development of fever

33. A patient was punched in the jaw. Which of the following assessment findings is consistent with mandibular fracture?
[ ] **A.** Numbness to the cheek
[ ] **B.** Sublingual hematoma
[ ] **C.** Avulsed tooth
[ ] **D.** Blowout fracture

34. A patient describes a fall resulting in hitting the chin on a table. He now complains of inability to open the mouth, malocclusion, and bleeding at the gum line. The emergency nurse suspects the patient has sustained which of the following fractures?
[ ] **A.** Mandibular
[ ] **B.** Zygomatic
[ ] **C.** Basilar skull
[ ] **D.** LeFort II

35. Otorrhea and rhinorrhea are **NOT** typically associated with which of the following injuries?
[ ] **A.** Basilar skull fracture
[ ] **B.** LeFort III
[ ] **C.** LeFort II fracture
[ ] **D.** LeFort I fracture

36. The emergency nurse is caring for a patient who sustained significant blunt force trauma to the face. The nurse observes free-floating movement of the nose and infraorbital rim. Which of the following injuries is consistent with this presentation?
[ ] **A.** LeFort I
[ ] **B.** LeFort II
[ ] **C.** Craniofacial disjunction
[ ] **D.** Zygomatic fracture

37. A patient is being discharged after treatment for temporomandibular joint (TMJ) dislocation. The emergency nurse concludes that the patient needs additional instructions if he/she states which of the following?
[ ] **A.** "This can reoccur if I open my mouth too wide or grind my teeth."
[ ] **B.** "I should take muscle relaxants for continued pain."
[ ] **C.** "I will continue on a liquid diet until the follow-up visit."
[ ] **D.** "Soft foods for the next few days are the best option for eating."

38. A patient complains of unilateral ear pain, inability to close the mouth completely, neck pain, and a clicking sound every time he moves his jaw. The emergency nurse will prepare for interventions for which of the following?
[ ] **A.** LeFort II fracture
[ ] **B.** Nasal fracture
[ ] **C.** Temporal mandibular joint dislocation
[ ] **D.** Ruptured tympanic membrane

39. The emergency nurse is preparing a patient for diagnostic evaluation of a suspected fractured larynx. Which of the following is most appropriate related to patient preparation for definitive testing?
[ ] **A.** Place topical anesthetic spray at the bedside
[ ] **B.** Secure intravenous access
[ ] **C.** Check the patient's creatinine (Cr)
[ ] **D.** Prepare end-tidal CO_2 monitoring

40. A patient with a fractured larynx is hoarse, has neck pain, and the oxygen saturation is decreasing. Which of the following interventions should the emergency nurse implement at this time?
[ ] **A.** Insert a nasopharyngeal airway.
[ ] **B.** Prepare for immediate cricothyrotomy.
[ ] **C.** Have the patient suck on ice chips.
[ ] **D.** Place the patient in a supine position.

41. A college student presents with anxious appearance, drooling, muffled voice, high fever, and dyspnea. The emergency nurse prepares for which of the following?
[ ] **A.** Intravenous access
[ ] **B.** Immediate needle cricothyrotomy
[ ] **C.** Throat swab for group A Streptococci
[ ] **D.** Assess immunization status

42. A patient is being evaluated for epiglottitis. Which of the following diagnostic tests is **NOT** the priority?
[ ] **A.** Complete blood count (CBC)
[ ] **B.** Blood culture
[ ] **C.** Lateral soft-tissue neck radiograph
[ ] **D.** Complete metabolic panel (CMP)

43. The emergency nurse is completing an assessment for a patient with sinusitis. Which of the following is a predisposing factor for sinusitis?
[ ] **A.** Recurrent episodes of epistaxis
[ ] **B.** Recent viral upper respiratory infection
[ ] **C.** Recent fitting for dentures
[ ] **D.** Recurrent migraine headache

44. Treatment of the patient with sinusitis includes which of the following?
[ ] **A.** Follow-up with Ear–Nose–Throat (ENT) provider
[ ] **B.** Use of a cool compress over sinuses
[ ] **C.** Nasal decongestant sprays for 10 days
[ ] **D.** Humidifier in areas where patient spends most time

45. Diagnostic evaluation of the patient with acute uncomplicated sinusitis includes which of the following?
[ ] **A.** Nasal swab for cultures
[ ] **B.** Complete blood count (CBC)
[ ] **C.** Palpation of the sinuses
[ ] **D.** Magnetic resonance imaging (MRI)

46. Which of the following statements indicates that a patient understood discharge instructions for sinusitis?
[ ] **A.** "I will be sure to drink more water while I have this infection."
[ ] **B.** "I will be sure to use the antibiotics until the symptoms are gone."
[ ] **C.** "I can use the nose drops for 2 weeks, until my follow-up appointment."
[ ] **D.** "Cool compresses should help with the stuffiness and headache."

47. A patient with poor dentition presents with high fever, agitation, malodorous breath, edematous tongue, and inability to completely close the mouth. On assessment, the ED nurse notes firm swelling below the mandible extending to the lower neck. The emergency nurse prepares for diagnostic testing for which of the following?
[ ] **A.** Ludwig's angina
[ ] **B.** Vincent's angina
[ ] **C.** Epiglottitis
[ ] **D.** Dental abscess

48. The emergency nurse recognizes which of the following pathophysiologic alterations occurring with Ludwig's angina takes the highest priority?
[ ] **A.** Tripod position and limited range of motion to the jaw
[ ] **B.** Invasion of B-hemolytic streptococcus bacteria into the submandibular region of the neck
[ ] **C.** Elevation and posterior displacement of the tongue
[ ] **D.** Temperature: 102° F (38.9° C); pulse: 106 beats/minute; respirations: 24 breaths/minute

49. A patient has muffled voice, difficulty opening the mouth, and significant firm swelling with crepitus below the jaw extending to the neck. Vital signs are as follows:

> Blood pressure—118/64 mm Hg
> Pulse—102 beats/minute
> Respirations—24 breaths/minute
> Temperature—101.5° F (38.6° C)
> Pulse oximetry—94% on room air

The patient is placed on humidified oxygen via face mask. Which of the following is the next priority intervention?
[ ] **A.** Prepare for emergency cricothyrotomy
[ ] **B.** Radiology for computed tomography (CT)
[ ] **C.** Administer oral antipyretics
[ ] **D.** Administer intravenous antibiotics

50. A patient with a history of poor dental hygiene and recent completion of chemotherapy presents with fever, mouth pain, swelling and bleeding to the gums, and malodorous breath. Which of the following actions would **NOT** be appropriate?
[ ] **A.** Initiate dental consult
[ ] **B.** Suction the oropharynx
[ ] **C.** Intravenous access
[ ] **D.** Antibiotic administration

51. A patient has fever, gingival pain, bleeding gums, and foul breath. The patient is suspected of having trench mouth. Which of the following is another term for this disorder?
[ ] **A.** Ludwig's angina
[ ] **B.** Vincent's angina
[ ] **C.** Pericoronitis
[ ] **D.** Dental abscess

52. Which of the following statements made by a patient diagnosed with Vincent's angina indicates the need for further instruction?
[ ] **A.** "I will eat a well-balanced diet."
[ ] **B.** "I know to take all the antibiotics as directed."
[ ] **C.** "I should rinse my mouth with antiseptic mouthwash."
[ ] **D.** "I will brush my teeth with a hard-bristle toothbrush."

53. The emergency nurse understands that the condition in which bacteria or viruses cause inflammation of the cochlea and other structures of the inner ear is referred to as which of the following?
[ ] **A.** Vertigo
[ ] **B.** Sinusitis
[ ] **C.** Meniere's
[ ] **D.** Labyrinthitis

54. The emergency nurse prepares to administer all of the following to the patient diagnosed with labyrinthitis **EXCEPT**:
[ ] **A.** promethazine (Phenergan).
[ ] **B.** meclizine (Antivert).
[ ] **C.** pseudoephedrine (Sudafed).
[ ] **D.** lorazepam (Ativan).

55. Which of the following does the emergency nurse inquire about in the history of a patient with labyrinthitis?
[ ] **A.** Otitis media
[ ] **B.** Sinusitis
[ ] **C.** Epistaxis
[ ] **D.** Mastoiditis

56. The emergency nurse is preparing for diagnostic evaluation of the patient with labyrinthitis. Which of the following is expected to assist with confirmation of this disorder?
[ ] **A.** Caloric testing will reveal increased response on the affected side.
[ ] **B.** Audiogram will reveal hypersensitivity to low- and high-pitch sounds.
[ ] **C.** Caloric testing will reveal decreased or absent response on affected side.
[ ] **D.** Magnetic resonance imaging (MRI) will reveal a mass as the cause of symptoms.

57. A 55-year-old patient reports episodes of the sensation that the room is rotating, inability to walk without falling, nausea, and a roaring sensation in the ear. The emergency nurse prepares for treatment of which of the following?
[ ] **A.** Mastoiditis
[ ] **B.** Meniere's disease
[ ] **C.** Sinusitis
[ ] **D.** Otitis media

58. Which of the following does the emergency nurse expect to be in the treatment plan for a patient with Meniere's disease yet not for labyrinthitis?
[ ] **A.** Administration of antiemetic medication
[ ] **B.** Instructions to change positions slowly
[ ] **C.** Instructions to avoid operation of heavy machinery
[ ] **D.** Administration of diuretic medication

59. Which of the following pharmaceutical treatments does the emergency nurse prepare as a priority for the patient with Meniere's disease?
[ ] **A.** Erythromycin (E-Mycin)
[ ] **B.** Phenylephrine
[ ] **C.** Meclizine (Antivert)
[ ] **D.** Ibuprofen (Advil)

60. Which of the following patients is at highest risk for complete airway compromise?
[ ] **A.** Retropharyngeal abscess
[ ] **B.** Trigeminal neuralgia
[ ] **C.** Vincent's angina
[ ] **D.** Bell's palsy

61. The emergency nurse is assessing a child who has torticollis, high fever, and swollen lymph nodes to the neck. The emergency nurse suspects this child has which of the following diagnoses?
[ ] **A.** Epiglottitis
[ ] **B.** Laryngitis
[ ] **C.** Retropharyngeal abscess
[ ] **D.** Streptococcal pharyngitis

62. Which of the following diagnostic tests is the highest priority for the patient with retropharyngeal abscess?
[ ] **A.** Chest radiograph
[ ] **B.** Lateral neck radiograph
[ ] **C.** Blood specimen for white blood count
[ ] **D.** Computed tomography (CT) of the neck

63. The emergency nurse examines a patient with a complaint of sore throat and notes uvular deviation, muffled voice, and foul odor to breath. Which of the following diagnoses is the highest probability with these manifestations?
[ ] **A.** Peritonsillar abscess
[ ] **B.** Retropharyngeal abscess
[ ] **C.** Tonsillitis
[ ] **D.** Pharyngitis

64. A patient is being evaluated for a peritonsillar abscess. For which of the following should the emergency nurse prepare?
[ ] A. Computed tomography (CT)
[ ] B. Neck radiograph
[ ] C. Throat swab
[ ] D. Incision and drainage

65. A patient describes sudden onset of unilateral face pain after chewing a hard candy. The pain is described as an electric shock. The emergency nurse proceeds to evaluate the patient for:
[ ] A. fractured tooth.
[ ] B. Bell's palsy.
[ ] C. ruptured tympanic membrane.
[ ] D. trigeminal neuralgia.

66. The emergency nurse understands that trigeminal neuralgia is a disorder that affects which of the following cranial nerves?
[ ] A. Seventh (Facial)
[ ] B. Fifth (Trigeminal)
[ ] C. Second (Optic)
[ ] D. Third (Oculomotor)

67. Which of the following principles does the emergency nurse use to determine triage acuity for a patient with an avulsed tooth?
[ ] A. Tooth that is affected
[ ] B. Formation of clots
[ ] C. Time of injury
[ ] D. Solution tooth is in

68. A parent reports her 18-month-old child had sudden onset of a persistent cough. The child is afebrile and has mild stridor on assessment. The emergency nurse prepares for further evaluation of which of the following?
[ ] A. Upper airway obstruction
[ ] B. Peritonsillar abscess
[ ] C. Nasal foreign body
[ ] D. Ludwig's angina

69. The emergency nurse is providing instructions to a patient with parotitis. Which of the following is the rationale for instructing the patient to gently massage the parotid gland?
[ ] A. Help to dry up secretions from the gland.
[ ] B. Relieve pain associated with infection of the gland.
[ ] C. Facilitate drainage of secretions from the gland.
[ ] D. Minimize loss of muscle function around the gland.

70. Which of the following disease processes would possibly place the patient at risk for a thermal burn to the globe?
[ ] A. Bell's palsy
[ ] B. Hyphema
[ ] C. Conjunctivitis
[ ] D. Ludwig's angina

71. The emergency nurse observes purulent drainage from a patient's ear. The patient complains of decreased hearing and a sensation of the room spinning. The emergency nurse prepares interventions for which of the following?
[ ] A. Otitis externa
[ ] B. Suppurative otitis media
[ ] C. Labyrinthitis
[ ] D. Ruptured tympanic membrane

72. A patient is being evaluated for a ruptured tympanic membrane. Which of the following preexisting conditions is **NOT** related to the diagnosis?
[ ] A. Head trauma with blood behind the tympanic membrane
[ ] B. Concurrent sinusitis and frequent airline travel
[ ] C. Swimmer's ear
[ ] D. Otitis media

73. A patient has extreme itching to the ear and swollen pre- and postauricular lymph nodes. The emergency nurse suspects the patient has:
[ ] A. otitis externa.
[ ] B. otitis media.
[ ] C. mastoiditis.
[ ] D. Meniere's disease.

74. A parent describes the infant as grabbing at the ear, history of fever, irritability, and decreased appetite. The emergency nurse prepares interventions for which of the following?
[ ] A. Otitis externa
[ ] B. Otitis media
[ ] C. Foreign body in the ear
[ ] D. Ruptured tympanic membrane

75. The emergency nurse suspects a patient has otitis media. Which of the following would be an appropriate diagnostic evaluation tool?
[ ] A. Culture of the ear canal
[ ] B. Blood specimen
[ ] C. Whisper voice test
[ ] D. Otoscopic examination

Answers/Rationales

1. Answer: A

Nursing Process: Assessment

Rationale: **Globe rupture is an ophthalmic emergency caused by severe blunt or penetrating trauma to the eye and may result in permanent loss of vision. Classic presentation of ruptured globe includes a peaked or tear-drop-shaped pupil, vitreous humor leakage, enophthalmos (posterior displacement of eye due to loss of integrity), loss of vision, and pain.** Glaucoma is the result of increased intraocular pressure and distinct change in pupil shape is not a classic sign. Hyphema is blood in the anterior chamber of the eye and does not result in change in pupil shape or size. Orbital fracture is a fracture of the supporting structures of the globe and does not result in change in pupil shape or size, unless accompanied by a ruptured globe.

 CENsational Pearl of Wisdom!

If the tip of the tear drop can be seen, this is the point of perforation.

2. Answer: C

Nursing Process: Intervention

Rationale: **Immediate intervention is to irrigate the eye with normal saline or lactated ringer solution to stop the burning and minimize permanent damage to the eye.** The longer the substance remains in contact with the eye, the more the damage will occur. Alkali substances may require up to 1 hour of flushing to neutralize the substance. Assessments and interventions, which may delay eye flushing, should be deferred or done concurrently with eye flushing. A detailed assessment should occur after eye flushing. There is no therapeutic value to patching the eye in the case of ocular burns. Systemic analgesics and topical cycloplegic drops may be administered, and ophthalmology will be consulted yet neither intervention should delay eye flushing.

3. Answer: A

Nursing Process: Assessment

Rationale: **This presentation is most consistent with retinal detachment, which occurs when vitreous humor or blood seeps in-between retinal layers. The loss of sight occurs to a visual field and is painless because the retina lacks pain fibers. Photopsia (sensation of flashing light) may occur in the affected and the unaffected eye, whereas floaters (often described as black spots) occur in the affected eye.** Unprotected exposure to ultraviolet light results in delayed onset of severe pain to the eyes. Fluorescein examination is indicated with suspected foreign body in the eye or corneal inconsistency. Unilateral pupil dilation may occur with narrow-angle (closed-angle) glaucoma.

4. Answer: D

Nursing Process: Intervention

Rationale: **Central retinal artery occlusion results from an embolus lodged in the retinal artery. Vision loss is sudden and painless. Priority interventions are geared toward restoring circulation within 90 minutes of symptom onset to prevent permanent blindness. Supine position optimizes circulation.** A temporary measure of having the patient rebreathe carbon dioxide (brown bag or administration of carbogen gas) may facilitate mild vasodilation. Ocular massage should be reserved for a provider and may increase circulation or dislodge a clot. An eye patch is indicated in conditions in which eye movement is prohibited to promote healing and decrease pain. Hyperventilation will result in loss of carbon dioxide, which may result in vasoconstriction.

5. Answer: B

Nursing Process: Assessment

Rationale: **Orbital cellulitis is an infection of the soft tissues of the orbit posterior to the orbital septum. It is most commonly caused by ethmoid sinusitis. Presentation includes decreased visual acuity, proptosis (bulging eye), pain with eye movement, diffuse swelling and erythema of the lid and periorbital area, and serous discharge.** The other conditions may cause eye pain, yet they are not typically associated with sinus infection.

 CENsational Pearl of Wisdom!

Orbital cellulitis may result in blindness and is potentially life-threatening because the infection may extend into the brain. Rapid identification of the infection, including differentiation from periorbital cellulitis (preseptal superficial infection of the lid and periorbital area), is imperative. This is one of the patients that triage nurses must keep from leaving without being seen! It is vital that they be treated with intravenous antibiotics!

6. Answer: A

Nursing Process: Evaluation

Rationale: **Contact lenses should not be worn at all during a bout with conjunctivitis.** Bacterial conjunctivitis is highly contagious. Infection control measures include handwashing, instillation of antibiotic ophthalmic ointment, eye cleansing procedure, avoiding use of eye makeup, and discarding previously used eye makeup.

7. Answer: C

Nursing Process: Intervention

Rationale: **Pilocarpine is a cholinergic miotic which causes contraction of the ciliary muscle resulting in pupil constriction. The action facilitates the outflow of aqueous humor, which subsequently decreases intraocular pressure. Pressure-induced ischemic paralysis of the ciliary muscle will prevent the medication from working; therefore, pilocarpine should be administered 1 hour after administration of other agents to decrease intraocular pressure.** Nausea and vomiting will result in increased intraocular pressure; therefore, an antiemetic will be helpful. Topical beta-blockers, such as timolol and diuretics decrease aqueous humor production.

8. Answer: A

Nursing Process: Assessment

Rationale: **Conjunctivitis, also referred to as pink eye, is a bacterial or viral invasion of the conjunctiva. Classic presentation includes the sensation of something in the eye, discharge, reddened sclera, and itching.** Signs and symptoms of blepharitis are similar to conjunctivitis, yet the eyelid is involved resulting in lid inflammation and possible loss of eyelashes. Hordeolum, also referred to as a sty, results in isolated abscess of an eyelid follicle. Chalazion is inflammation of the meibomian gland on the inner surface of the eyelid and presents with a mass beneath the lid.

CENsational Pearl of Wisdom!

The type of conjunctivitis can often be determined by the type of discharge. Purulent discharge is associated with bacterial infection, serous discharge is associated with viral infection and allergic reaction, and pruritis is associated with allergic reaction.

9. Answer: D

Nursing Process: Intervention

Rationale: **Priorities of care for the person presenting with a penetrating eye injury include securing the impaled object and shielding the injured eye to minimize manipulation of the object in the eye, which will lead to further injury.** Placing additional pressure on the injured eye should be avoided; therefore, patching the eye is contraindicated. Antibiotics and analgesics will likely be indicated, yet securing the impaled object is the priority to minimize further damage to the eye.

CENsational Pearl of Wisdom!

With penetrating foreign body eye injury, the unaffected eye should also be patched to minimize consensual movement of the eyes.

10. Answer: C

Nursing Process: Assessment

Rationale: **Subconjunctival hemorrhage is a benign condition that occurs when blood vessels of the conjunctiva rupture and blood is trapped between the subconjunctiva and the sclera. Some cases are idiopathic, yet it frequently occurs due to increased pressure to the area secondary to coughing, straining, forceful vomiting, or vigorous rubbing of the eye. Subconjunctival hemorrhage occurs suddenly, and other than the appearance, the patient is usually asymptomatic.** Hyphema indicates blood in the anterior chamber of the eye resulting from trauma. An eight-ball hyphema occurs when the entire anterior chamber is covered in blood. Retinal hemorrhage occurs in association with other eye injuries and/or head trauma. Both hyphema and retinal hemorrhage results in visual disturbances. Ultraviolet keratitis is a type of corneal burn, which may have delayed symptom onset from the time of the exposure to ultraviolet light.

11. Answer: D

Nursing Process: Evaluation

Rationale: **An uncomplicated orbital fracture is an isolated disruption of the orbital rim followed by blunt trauma to the eye. The patient should minimize any actions that place pressure on the eye, such as blowing the nose, to minimize further eye injury and prevent reinjury.** Periorbital bruising may take days to weeks to resolve. Antibiotics may not be prescribed if there is no disruption to the skin around the eye or involvement of the globe. Ice packs should be used to decrease swelling.

12. Answer: A

Nursing Process: Analysis

Rationale: **Facial numbness and inability to look upward are consistent with fracture to the orbital floor, also referred to as a blowout fracture. The signs and symptoms are consistent with entrapment of extraocular muscles and the infraorbital nerve, indicating a blowout fracture.** Subconjunctival hemorrhage results in bloody appearance of the sclera and is typically a benign uncomplicated presentation. Floaters in the eye may be seen with retinal detachment; yet when the patient counts the number of floaters, it is usually benign and not associated with retinal hemorrhage. Corneal abrasion results in significant eye irritation and pain with excessive tearing, yet is not considered an emergent presentation.

13. Answer: B

Nursing Process: Assessment

Rationale: **Ptosis occurs with eyelid lacerations affecting the levator muscle, which is located under the upper lid, above the globe.** This muscle is responsible for raising the upper lid. Bleeding may occur with any laceration and should be controlled. Visual disturbances may occur with eyelid lacerations with concurrent injury such as hyphema or globe disruption.

 CENsational Pearl of Wisdom!

Protrusion of orbital fat with an associated eyelid laceration is consistent with septum involvement and injury to the levator muscle. Eyelid lacerations affecting the lacrimal structures should be repaired by an ophthalmologist.

14. Answer: B

Nursing Process: Assessment

Rationale: **Visualization of blood in the anterior chamber of the eye is the definition of a hyphema.** Hyphema may occur secondary to blunt or penetrating trauma and any portion of the anterior chamber of the eye may be affected, evidenced by a blood fluid line across the iris or blacked-out appearance in an eight-ball hyphema. The patient will experience blurry vision, blood-tinged vision, pain, and decreased visual acuity. Retinal detachment gives the perception of floaters, flashing lights, or a veil or curtain across a visual field. Orbital fractures, leading to entrapment of the extraocular muscles, results in the inability to move the eye. Corneal abrasions result in pain with lid or globe movement.

 CENsational Pearl of Wisdom!

A hyphema has a chance of rebleed within 2 to 5 days. This will put the patient at high risk for the development of secondary glaucoma.

15. Answer: C

Nursing Process: Analysis

Rationale: **Painless loss of vision accompanied by the perception of floaters, flashing lights, cloudy smoky vision, or a veil or curtain over the vision are classic presentations for retinal detachment. Retinal detachment is separation of the layers of the retina and subsequent fluid or blood pooling between the retinal layers. Retinal detachment can occur spontaneously or secondary to trauma. The condition is diagnosed by dilated posterior eye examination of the fundus.** Tonometry is indicated for glaucoma and iritis. Fluorescein stain is indicated for assessment of corneal irregularities such as abrasions or ulcerations. Computed tomography (CT) is indicated in orbital fracture, sinusitis, and associated facial trauma.

16. Answer: C

Nursing Process: Evaluation

Rationale: **There is no therapeutic indication for patching the eye. Corneal abrasion is a defect on the surface of the cornea.** Common causes are contact lenses, foreign body in the eye, exposure to chemical irritant in the eye, or direct scratch to the eye. Complications of corneal abrasions include infection, corneal ulceration, and delayed healing. Use of topical ophthalmic antibiotics, resting the eye, avoiding eye strain such as with computer use, and avoiding instillation of anything in the eye are important to avoid complications.

17. Answer: D

Nursing Process: Intervention

Rationale: **Iritis is an inflammatory process that may be idiopathic or secondary to systemic inflammatory disorders. Instillation of topical ophthalmic steroids and cycloplegic agents is indicated to treat the inflammation and reduce ciliary spasms.** Warm compresses and resting the eye by darkening the environment is indicated. There is no therapeutic benefit of instilling antibiotic ointment or flushing the eyes, because neither of these interventions will directly decrease the inflammation.

18. Answer: B

Nursing Process: Assessment

Rationale: **Closed-angle, also referred to as narrow-angle glaucoma, occurs when the angle between the iris and the cornea becomes blocked. The condition can lead to permanent loss of sight due to pressure on the optic nerve. Classic presentation includes painful loss of vision, blurred vision, halos around lights, photophobia, nausea, vomiting, and intense headache. The globe will feel rock hard, the cornea appears hazy, and the pupil is poorly reactive or fixed.** Ultraviolet keratitis presents with local symptoms, including the sensation of something in the eye, profuse tearing, photophobia, and blurred vision, yet systemic symptoms are not usually present. Central retinal artery occlusion and retinal detachment typically present with painless loss of vision.

 CENsational Pearl of Wisdom!

Closed-angle glaucoma is a true ophthalmic emergency. If treatment is not initiated within hours of symptom onset, permanent blindness can occur. Open-angle glaucoma is the more common form occurring idiopathically in the geriatric population.

19. Answer: A

Nursing Process: Intervention

Rationale: **Rubber-tipped suction is a safe effective method to attempt removal of organic foreign bodies from the ear canal.** Liquids should be avoided because organic material may swell, further obstructing the ear canal. Alligator forceps may be used by an experienced provider to attempt removal of a foreign body. In this situation with a child, suction is the safer option of those presented.

20. Answer: A

Nursing Process: Intervention

Rationale: **The symptoms suggest otitis externa, also referred to as swimmer's ear, which is an infection of the external ear canal. An ear wick facilitates topical antibiotic administration into the swollen canal.** Intravenous access may be needed for the administration of antibiotics if mastoiditis is suspected. Administration of mineral oil and ear irrigation are indicated for foreign body in the ear.

21. Answer: D

Nursing Process: Intervention

Rationale: **Removal of live insects should be attempted by drawing the insect toward the light using an otoscope or flashlight. If this fails, the insect should be killed using lidocaine or mineral oil before manual removal or flushing.** Ear irrigation and manual extraction take place once the insect is dead. The procedure does not require sedation.

 CENsational Pearl of Wisdom!

Live insects in the ear are definitely an "emergency" to the patient! It is very unsettling for the patient!

22. Answer: B

Nursing Process: Intervention

Rationale: **Any object in the nasal passage may become dislodged resulting in obstructed airway. A disc battery lodged in the ear or nose can cause tissue necrosis in as little as 4 hours.** Organic materials such as rubber, wood, or food tend to be very irritating to the mucosa causing symptoms earlier as compared with inorganic material such as metal or plastic items.

23. Answer: D

Nursing Process: Analysis

Rationale: **The priority is to maintain a patent airway and ensure hemodynamic stability. Monitoring the amount of blood loss and preparing for blood replacement are interventions that meet those priorities. Type and crossmatch are essential to prepare for blood volume replacement, if needed.** Complete blood count (CBC), international normalized ratio (INR), partial thromboplastin time (aPPT), and prothrombin time (PT). are all important to determine clotting status and blood loss; however, the hematocrit and type and crossmatch are the priority tests.

 CENsational Pearl of Wisdom!

Uncontrolled persistent epistaxis is indicative of a posterior bleed. Posterior bleeds originate in the posterior nasal or nasopharyngeal cavity and are typically arterial bleeds requiring nasal packing.

24. Answer: B

Nursing Process: Evaluation

Rationale: **Discharge instructions for patients with epistaxis include avoiding anything that may contribute to continued bleeding or rebleed.** Specific precautions include use of saline nasal spray, a humidifier, and taking warm showers to keep the nasal mucosa moist. They should also avoid hard blowing or sneezing, digital manipulation, and aspirin and nonsteroidal anti-inflammatory drugs. Phenylephrine nasal spray may be used as a vasoconstrictor, yet should not be used continuously for prolonged periods of time.

25. Answer: D

Nursing Process: Analysis

Rationale: **There is no definitive diagnostic test to confirm Bell's palsy, and diagnosis is confirmed based on clinical presentation of the hallmark signs and symptoms.** Facial radiology may confirm bone deformities and masses in the sinuses. Computed tomography (CT) is used to rule out intracranial bleed but does not confirm the diagnosis of Bell's palsy. Electromyography (EMG) is used as part of the comprehensive evaluation to assess nerve and motor function.

26. Answer: A

Nursing Process: Interventions

Rationale: **Bell's palsy is caused by damage to the facial nerve (cranial nerve VII), often from herpes virus. Treatment includes administration of antivirals, corticosteroids, analgesics, eye lubricants, and facial massage.** Bell's palsy is not caused by bacterial infection. Antiepileptic drugs are used for treatment of trigeminal neuralgia. There is no therapeutic indication for strict bed rest.

27. Answer: A

Nursing Process: Intervention

Rationale: **Auricular, also referred to as perichondrial hematoma, is a complication from shearing forces to the anterior auricle resulting in hematoma formation between the skin and cartilage of the ear. It occurs from direct blunt force trauma to the ear and is a common injury seen in wrestling. A compression dressing is indicated to minimize the reformation of hematoma after incision and drainage procedure.** The ear must be evaluated every 24 hours for several days. Antibiotics prophylaxis will be administered, and nonsteroidal anti-inflammatory drugs should be avoided to minimize bleeding risk. Inadequate treatment or healing may result in a permanent deformity referred to as cauliflower ear.

 CENsational Pearl of Wisdom!

Even though a pressure-type dressing is used, cover the ear with fluffed 4 × 4 gauzes to protect the cartilage in the ear. Pad the ear well.

28. Answer: D

Nursing Process: Assessment

Rationale: **Acute mastoiditis is an inflammatory process secondary to bacterial infection of the mastoid air cells of the temporal bone. It may occur with an associated otitis media. Presentation includes fever, inflammation and erythema to the mastoid and auricle, otorrhea, hearing loss, and deep, localized pain behind the ear.** Ruptured tympanic membrane may result in impaired hearing, vertigo, and drainage (blood) from the ear. Parotitis is inflammation of the parotid gland and presents with unilateral swelling below the ear and jaw. Otitis externa is an infection and inflammation of the auditory canal and may present with itching of the ear canal and external ear, pain with movement of the ear and swelling of the ear canal. Fever is not a classic symptom of otitis externa.

29. Answer: B

Nursing Process: Evaluation

Rationale: **Tooth abscess is not an expected complication of mastoiditis.** Complications include hearing loss, facial nerve palsy, osteomyelitis, labyrinthitis, meningitis, subdural empyema, and abscess formation to the bones and soft tissue near the mastoid.

30. Answer: C

Nursing Process: Assessment

Rationale: **The cheek, side of the nose, upper lip, teeth, and gums are all supplied by the infraorbital nerve as it exits through the zygoma, the main bone bridging the maxilla to the temporal bone. Paresthesia to those areas innervated by that nerve would be expected.** The mandible and chin are supplied by the inferior alveolar nerve, which is a branch of the mandibular nerve. Ear numbness can be caused by sensory nerve damage.

 CENsational Pearl of Wisdom!

High-velocity motor vehicle accidents are a common mechanism of injury for comminuted fractures of the zygomatic process and often involve orbital rim fractures. A step-off deformity or flattened cheek is one of the manifestations that accompanies zygomatic fractures. Diplopia can also occur due to entrapment of one of the muscles that move the eyeball.

31. Answer: D

Nursing Process: Analysis

Rationale: **Computed tomography (CT) is the preferred diagnostic imaging for zygomatic fracture.** Waters view (occipitomental) radiographs, Caldwell view (occipitofrontal) radiographs, and ultrasound can be used to screen for (not diagnose) zygomatic fractures. Lateral facial radiograph is not indicated for zygomatic fracture.

32. Answer: A

Nursing Process: Evaluation

Rationale: **The highest priorities for ongoing evaluation of the patient with nasal fracture are patency of airway and maintenance of hemodynamic status. Monitoring for control of bleeding achieves the priority goal of hemodynamic stability.** Control of pain is a priority and assessment should determine a pain score that is realistically tolerable for the patient. Yet a pain score of 0 (zero) may not be realistic. Periorbital ecchymosis is expected and may get worse immediately after the trauma, with bruising dissipating days after the trauma. Septal hematoma leading to infection and necrosis is a complication of nasal fracture. The hematoma may need to be drained. The patient should also be placed on antibiotics and monitored for fever.

33. Answer: B

Nursing Process: Assessment

Rationale: **Mandibular fractures may manifest with sublingual bleeding or hematoma, trismus, malocclusion, bleeding gums, loose teeth, paresthesia of the lower lip, and ruptured tympanic membrane.** Numbness to the cheek is consistent with maxillary or zygomatic fractures. Avulsed teeth occur with direct trauma to the teeth. Blowout fracture is a fracture to the orbital floor from direct trauma to the orbit or is seen in association with LeFort, maxillary, or zygomatic fractures.

 CENsational Pearl of Wisdom!

Mandibular fractures can be an avenue for possible airway obstruction. The tongue can be displaced posteriorly due to the loss of bony support, and the growing sublingual hematoma can also cause a greater amount of posterior displacement.

34. Answer: A

Nursing Process: Analysis

Rationale: **Inability to open the mouth due to spasms, also referred to as trismus, malocclusion, bleeding at the gum line, and sublingual hematoma are classic**

signs of mandibular fracture. **Mandibular fractures occur with direct trauma to the jaw or chin.** Zygomatic fractures occur following a blow to the zygoma and presents with altered sensation to the face. Basilar skull fractures and LeFort fractures occur with direct trauma to the front of the face.

35. Answer: D

Nursing Process: Analysis

Rationale: **LeFort I, a transverse fracture across the maxilla, is not typically associated with cerebrospinal fluid (CSF) leaks.** CSF leaks, as evidenced by otorrhea (drainage from the ear) and rhinorrhea (drainage from the nose), are seen in basilar skull fractures and LeFort II and LeFort III fractures.

 CENsational Pearl of Wisdom!

The highest concern for LeFort fractures is airway obstruction. Especially with LeFort II and III, massive damage is done to the face and obstruction of the airway with broken teeth, blood, and clots, and emesis is an important aspect of care. Suctioning and airway control are of utmost importance! Also, patients with these types of fractures should be evaluated for head, neck, and multisystem trauma due to the significant force required.

36. Answer: B

Nursing Process: Analysis

Rationale: **LeFort II fracture is a pyramidal fracture across the bridge of the nose and involves the maxillary segment of the zygomatic, nasal and orbital bones. This can lead to the free-floating appearance of the nose and infraorbital rim.** LeFort I fracture is a transverse fracture across the maxilla and the patient will present with malocclusion. LeFort III fracture is complete craniofacial disjunction and the patient will present with significant facial asymmetry and subcutaneous emphysema. Zygomatic fractures may have an associated orbital rim fracture, yet does not include a nasal fracture.

 CENsational Pearl of Wisdom!

LeFort II and III fractures require early ocular examination as these fractures will cause periorbital swelling and may delay the ability to examine the eyes.

37. Answer: C

Nursing Process: Evaluation

Rationale: **Discharge instructions for the patient treated for temporal mandibular joint (TMJ) dislocation include a soft diet for 3 to 4 days, avoiding anything that may cause stress on the joint (that is, excessive yawning and teeth grinding), and taking muscle relaxants as needed.** A liquid diet is not indicated.

 CENsational Pearl of Wisdom!

TMJ dislocation is anterior and superior displacement of the jaw resulting in spasms that prevent the condyles from returning to normal position. It can occur unilaterally or bilaterally from something as simple as opening the mouth too wide.

38. Answer: C

Nursing Process: Analysis

Rationale: **Presentation consistent with temporomandibular joint dislocation includes history of wide and prolonged mouth opening followed by malocclusion, trismus, headache, otalgia, neck pain, and a snap, click, or pop sensation with jaw movement.** A LeFort II fracture is a pyramidal fracture across the bridge of the nose. LeFort II and nasal fractures are accompanied by epistaxis, nasal swelling, and asymmetry. Ruptured tympanic membrane presents with localized signs and symptoms of the ear such as decreased hearing, ear drainage, and otalgia.

39. Answer: A

Nursing Process: Analysis

Rationale: **The most definitive diagnostic test for suspected laryngeal fracture is intranasal fiberoptic laryngoscopy. The procedure can be done at the bedside, and a topical anesthetic spray will be used to suppress the gag reflex during the procedure.** Intravenous access may be warranted, yet contrast dye computed tomography (CT) may not be indicated unless there is a need to evaluate for associated neck injuries. Assessment of blood urea nitrogen (BUN) and creatinine is indicated before any scanning that requires contrast dye. While pulse oximetry is important for monitoring the patient at this time, ETCO$_2$ monitoring, indicated for moderate sedation, may not be needed.

40. Answer: B

Nursing Process: Intervention

Rationale: **A surgical airway is required for patients with a fractured larynx who are losing their airway. This patient will require oxygen due to the decreasing oxygen saturation, and the hoarseness and neck pain are indicators that a patent airway is not present.** The patient should be NPO and the head of the bed should be elevated 30 to 45 degrees. Nothing should be placed in the nasal/oral-pharyngeal space due to potential stimulation of the gag reflex.

 CENsational Pearl of Wisdom!

If the patient with a fractured larynx requires supplemental oxygen, humidified oxygen is recommended because it is less irritating to the airway compared with oxygen that is not humidified.

41. Answer: A

Nursing Process: Intervention

Rationale: **Intravenous (IV) access is a priority intervention for blood specimen collection (complete blood count, blood culture), intravenous fluid, and antibiotic administration due to this patient exhibiting signs of acute epiglottitis.** Epiglottitis is an infection and inflammation of the epiglottitis most frequently caused by *Haemophilus influenzae* type B (HiB) and group A streptococci. Classic signs and symptoms of epiglottitis include extreme anxiety, drooling, dyspnea, sore throat, acute onset of high fever, tripod position, and stridor. The patient should be placed in a high-visibility bed near an emergency airway cart. Nothing should be placed in the mouth due to the potential laryngospasm. Obtaining a complete history is important to determine the immunization status, yet IV access is the priority. Needle cricothyrotomy is reserved for when the airway patency is severely compromised.

 CENsational Pearl of Wisdom!

The cardinal signs of epiglottitis include the three Ds—dyspnea, dysphagia, and drooling. Stridor is considered a late sign! No patient with drooling should ever be sent back to the waiting room!

42. Answer: D

Nursing Process: Analysis

Rationale: **Diagnostic evaluation for the patient with suspected epiglottitis includes complete blood count (CBC), blood culture, and portable lateral soft-tissue radiograph.** The CBC differential will show a shift to the left as an indication of bandemia consistent with a bacterial infection. The neck radiograph will reveal a positive thumb print sign consistent with a swollen epiglottis. Blood cultures are necessary as bacteremia is a potential with an epiglottitis diagnosis. Positive blood cultures are present in the adult patient approximately 25% of the time. A complete metabolic panel (CMP) is not immediately indicated.

CENsational Pearl of Wisdom!

Epiglottitis used to be a pediatric disease process. It is now seen more in adults than in the pediatric population due to vaccinations against Haemophilus influenzae type B. In the adult patient, other organisms are often seen.

43. Answer: B

Nursing Process: Assessment

Rationale: **The most common history associated with sinusitis is recent viral upper respiratory tract infections, with up to 90% of patients having had one.** A small percentage (5% to 10%) of patients have bacterial superinfection requiring antimicrobial treatment. Invasive dental procedures, such as treatment for dental abscess, can be a risk factor for sinusitis; however, denture fittings are not considered to be risk factors. The patient with a migraine headache may experience sinus pain but does not constitute sinusitis. Epistaxis should be evaluated to ensure the patient does not develop a septal hematoma, which can lead to infection but is not a risk factor for sinusitis.

44. Answer: D

Nursing Process: Intervention

Rationale: **Patient education for the patient with sinusitis includes nasal decongestants for 3 to 5 days, elevation of head of bed, application of heat to the face, and use of a humidifier.** Consultation to an ENT may occur if the patient has recurrent sinusitis or sinusitis that is not responding to treatment. Consultation from the emergency department is not indicated.

45. Answer: C

Nursing Process: Analysis

Rationale: **Acute uncomplicated sinusitis is a clinical diagnosis in which presenting signs and symptoms are coupled with inspection and palpation techniques of the sinuses.** Nasal swabs are rarely performed in the emergency setting, yet may be indicated when chronic recurrent sinusitis exists. A complete blood count (CBC) may be within normal range, unless the infection has become systemic. Magnetic resonance imaging (MRI) is valuable for evaluation of soft tissue of the sinuses, yet it is of little value in the diagnosis of sinusitis.

46. Answer: A

Nursing Process: Evaluation

Rationale: **The patient with sinusitis should increase their fluid intake to facilitate liquification of nasal secretions.** The full course of antibiotics, if prescribed, should be completed. Antibiotics should not be taken only until symptoms are gone. Typically, phenylephrine nasal spray may be used as a decongestant for short periods of time, maximum of 3 days due to the potential for rebound congestion. Warm compresses should be used to relieve nasal pressure and stuffiness by loosening secretions, which will then result in decreased sinus pain.

47. Answer: A

Nursing Process: Analysis

Rationale: **Ludwig's angina is a bacterial infection of the submandibular space. Classic presentation includes high fever, agitation, malodorous breath, edematous tongue, inability to completely close the mouth, dyspnea, drooling, upward and backward displacement of the tongue, trismus, and marked swelling below the mandible extending to the lower neck.** History often includes poor dental hygiene, including dental abscess and other comorbidities such as immunosuppressive disorders. Vincent's angina, also referred to as trench mouth or acute ulcerative gingivitis, results in mouth and gum bleeding and pain. Epiglottitis is an infection of the epiglottis, resulting in dyspnea, dysphagia, and drooling. Of the named disorders, only Ludwig's angina results in swelling to the mandible, neck, and mediastinum.

48. Answer: C

Nursing Process: Analysis

Rationale: **Progressive infection of the submandibular region, neck, and mediastinum results in upward and** posterior displacement of the tongue. **Severe upper airway obstruction can occur secondary to tongue displacement and should be considered the highest priority when planning care.** The care team should be prepared for advanced airway management with nasal or oral airway insertion, laryngeal mask airway, or surgical airway (tracheostomy). Abnormal vital signs are consistent with infection of B-hemolytic streptococci bacteria. Tripod positioning is a compensatory position assumed by the patient to facilitate breathing. Trismus (inability to open/close the mouth due to spasms) occurs causing limited range of motion of the jaw and the tripod positioning helps to overcome this as well.

49. Answer: D

Nursing Process: Intervention

Rationale: **Airway patency and adequate oxygenation are the highest priorities in a patient with Ludwig's angina. The patient is able to vocalize, and humidified oxygen is being administered. The next priority intervention is securing intravenous access for specimen collection and administration of fluids and antibiotics.** Diagnostic testing is indicated to confirm the infection and determine the degree of airway compromise; however, initiation of treatment should not be delayed and should be based on the clinical diagnosis. Nothing should be administered orally. Emergency tracheostomy would be a preferred advanced airway over cricothyrotomy due to severe airway swelling.

 CENsational Pearl of Wisdom!

Ludwig's angina is an airway emergency. The patient should be immediately placed in a high-visibility bed, near an airway cart. Airway compromise is the leading cause of death in those with Ludwig's angina.

50. Answer: B

Nursing Process: Intervention

Rationale: **Airway compromise is not an expected finding and there is no indication that the airway is not patent; therefore, suctioning is not indicated.** Vincent's angina, also referred to as acute necrotizing ulcerative gingivitis or trench mouth, is a bacterial infection of the gums. History typically includes immunosuppression, malnourishment, and poor dental hygiene. Classic presentation of Vincent's angina includes bleeding, painful and swollen gums, fever, halitosis, and gray pseudomembranous ulcers on the pharynx. Intravenous access

should be obtained for specimen collection, intravenous fluids, and antibiotic administration. The patient should be seen by a dentist for definitive management.

 CENsational Pearl of Wisdom!

Another piece of information about chemotherapy patients—remember that these patients should never go back to the waiting room! The waiting room is full of contagious organisms. Any patient who is considered to be neutropenic (low white blood cell count) should not be around others with possible contagious diseases. It does not matter what the patient is presenting with—they cannot go back to the waiting room!

51. Answer: B

Nursing Process: Assessment

Rationale: **Vincent's angina, also referred to as acute necrotizing ulcerative gingivitis or trench mouth, is a bacterial infection of the gums.** Classic presentation of Vincent's angina includes bleeding, painful and swollen gums, fever, halitosis, and gray pseudomembranous ulcers on the pharynx. Ludwig's angina is bacterial invasion of the submandibular structures. Pericoronitis is inflammation of the gingival tissue around the crown of an erupting or impacted tooth. Dental abscess is the localized accumulation of pus in various regions of the tooth and gum. Dental abscess can lead to complications of Vincent's or Ludwig's angina.

52. Answer: D

Nursing Process: Evaluation

Rationale: **Vincent's angina is a bacterial infection of the gums, resulting in bleeding and painful and swollen gums. Once brushing can be tolerated, a soft-bristle toothbrush should be used or the patient can gently wipe the gums.** The patient should be instructed to eat nutritious food, take antibiotics as prescribed, and rinse the mouth with an antiseptic mouthwash in the acute phase of the infection.

53. Answer: D

Nursing Process: Assessment

Rationale: **Labyrinthitis is an inflammatory process of the structure of the inner ear, the labyrinth.** Meniere's disease is a disorder affecting the inner ear and is thought to be due to increased fluid and pressure in the endolymphatic system. Sinusitis is an inflammatory process of the sinuses secondary to infection. Vertigo is the feeling of spinning and is associated as a manifestation with both labyrinthitis and Meniere's disease.

54. Answer: C

Nursing Process: Intervention

Rationale: **Pseudoephedrine (Sudafed) is a decongestant that is not typically indicated for the treatment of labyrinthitis as nasal stuffiness is not part of the typical presentation.** Meclizine (Antivert) is an antihistamine used to treat vertigo—one of the main symptoms of labyrinthitis. Promethazine (Phenergan) is an antiemetic that has sedative effects and may help with symptoms of nausea and vertigo. Lorazepam (Ativan) is a benzodiazepine, which may assist with resolving vertigo and diminish general anxiety experienced due to all symptoms.

55. Answer: A

Nursing Process: Assessment

Rationale: **Preexisting disorders for labyrinthitis include bacterial ear infections, recent viral infections, barotrauma, migraine headaches, Meniere's syndrome, meningitis, arteriosclerosis, and systemic autoimmune disorders such as systemic lupus erythematous.** Sinusitis and mastoiditis, although may be concurring with labyrinthitis, are not typically preexisting conditions. Epistaxis is not associated with labyrinthitis.

56. Answer: C

Nursing Process: Assessment

Rationale: **Caloric reflex testing, a test of the vestibulo–ocular reflex, is performed by instilling cool water onto the tympanic membrane and evaluating for nystagmus. A person with labyrinthitis would be expected to have a decreased or absent response on the affected side.** An audiogram will reveal some degree of conductive or sensorineural hearing loss. The patient may be sensitive to loud sounds, yet audiography is not needed to determine this finding. Magnetic resonance imaging (MRI) may be used to rule out the presence of a mass as seen in other conditions that may cause similar symptoms. MRI may also be used to confirm labyrinthitis as the cochlea, vestibule, and semicircular canals will show changes post contrast but would be done at a later time.

 CENsational Pearl of Wisdom!

Before caloric testing, one must visually inspect the tympanic membrane to ensure it is intact. A ruptured tympanic membrane is a contraindication of testing.

57. Answer: B

Nursing Process: Assessment

Rationale: **Meniere's disease, also referred to as endolymphatic hydrops, is thought to be caused by increased fluid and pressure in the inner ear resulting in destruction of the vestibular and cochlear apparatus. It occurs most frequently in those between 50 and 60 years of age. The classic presentation includes episodic rotational vertigo, ataxic gait, tinnitus (roaring or ringing in the ears), nausea, diaphoresis, and sensorineural hearing loss.** The exact cause is unknown, yet it may be associated with trauma, infection, or degeneration of the inner ear. Otitis media would present with ear pain and fever. Mastoiditis would have manifestations of pain in the mastoid area associated with swelling, fever, and headache. Sinusitis symptoms would include fever, pain and tenderness in the sinus areas, and drainage.

58. Answer: D

Nursing Process: Intervention

Rationale: **Diuretics and low sodium diet are part of the treatment plan for the patient with Meniere's disease to decrease the fluid and pressure build up in the endolymphatic system.** Labyrinthitis is due to viral or bacterial infections, leading to inflammation of the labyrinth. Nausea and vertigo are experienced in both disorders. Hence, the need for antiemetics and instructions to manage vertigo and maintain safety.

59. Answer: C

Nursing Process: Intervention

Rationale: **Meclizine (Antivert) is an antihistamine used to treat vertigo—a major symptom of Meniere's disease.** Meniere's disease is not caused by bacterial infection; therefore, erythromycin, a macrolide antibiotic, will not be indicated. Phenylephrine is used as a nasal decongestant for sinusitis and other disorders affecting the nasal passages, such as rhinitis and is not indicated in the treatment of Meniere's disease. Although an analgesic such as ibuprofen may be taken for discomfort (headache and feeling of fullness in the ear) experienced from Meniere's disease, treating the debilitating symptoms of vertigo and nausea are higher priorities.

60. Answer: A

Nursing Process: Evaluation

Rationale: **A retropharyngeal abscess is an infection in the deep space of the neck, posterior to the pharynx, nasopharynx, and oropharynx. An infection can result in an abscess large enough to cause obstruction to the airway.** Trigeminal neuralgia is a repetitive firing of the trigeminal nerve and results in painful spasms to the face. Vincent's angina is necrotizing gingivitis and results in bleeding, painful gums. Bell's palsy is paralysis of the facial nerve and results in unilateral palsy of the face.

61. Answer: C

Nursing Process: Assessment

Rationale: **Retropharyngeal abscess results in significant neck stiffness and pain, fever, sore throat, cough, drooling, and cervical lymphadenopathy. The severe neck stiffness and pain can result in the infant or child tilting the head to one side with the chin tilted in the opposite direction.** Epiglottitis more commonly affects adolescents and young adults and presents with high fever, dyspnea, dysphagia, and drooling. Tonsillitis presents with fever, sore throat, referred pain to the ear, and exudate on the tonsils. Laryngitis presents with hoarseness and difficulty swallowing. Torticollis and cervical lymphadenopathy are not classic signs of epiglottitis, tonsillitis, or laryngitis.

62. Answer: B

Nursing Process: Analysis

Rationale: **Widening of the retropharyngeal soft tissues, which can be easily seen on lateral neck radiograph and is consistent with retropharyngeal abscess in a large percentage of cases is the priority diagnostic test.** A small percentage of patients with retropharyngeal abscess will have a normal white blood cell count; therefore, this test cannot be used to rule out the diagnosis. A chest radiograph to assess for concurrent infection or complications such as mediastinitis and pneumonia should be done, yet are not exclusively diagnostic for retropharyngeal abscess. Computed tomography (CT) may be indicated after a lateral neck radiograph to determine the extent of the infection and assist with treatment options.

63. Answer: A

Nursing Process: Assessment

Rationale: **Peritonsillar abscess results from infection to the tonsillar capsule and results in uvular deviation, "hot potato" (muffled) voice, drooling, dysphagia, and halitosis.** Retropharyngeal abscess, tonsillitis, and pharyngitis are all infectious processes that cause sore throat, yet none cause uvular deviation and the classic "hot potato" quality to the voice.

64. Answer: D

Nursing Process: Intervention

Rationale: **Incision and drainage of the abscess is indicated so that cultures can be obtained and to provide immediate relief of symptoms by removing pus and decreasing** the size of the abscess. Computed tomography may be indicated if direct visualization of the area is not possible. Neck radiograph and throat swab do not provide information about the type of purulent drainage in the abscess.

65. Answer: D

Nursing Process: Assessment

Rationale: **Trigeminal neuralgia is repetitive firing of the trigeminal nerve resulting in painful spasms to the face. The pain is usually unilateral and is described as an excruciating, stabbing, electric shock. It is triggered by chewing, brushing teeth, or touching the face. A** fractured tooth may result from chewing on something hard and results in sensitivity to air or temperature variations. Patients with Bell's palsy may complain of pain near the ear, yet the quality is not described as electric shock. A ruptured tympanic membrane can result in significant ear pain, especially if it occurs secondary to trauma, yet the quality is not described as electric shock.

66. Answer: B

Nursing Process: Assessment

Rationale: **Trigeminal neuralgia is a disorder that affects the fifth (Trigeminal) cranial nerve, resulting in repetitive firing of the nerve that then cause painful spasms to the face.** The seventh (Facial) cranial nerve is affected in Bell's palsy. The second (Optic) cranial nerve is responsible for the sensory function of visual acuity. The third (Oculomotor) cranial nerve is responsible for the motor function of the eye, including pupil constriction and dilation.

 CENsational Pearl of Wisdom!

Just as a follow-up on the cranial nerves—remember that when assessing extraocular eye movements, EOMs, the nerves involved are three (Oculomotor), four (Trochlear), six (Abducens). This is often on the test! On the test, the cranial nerves are usually listed by number and by name. So for this question, it made it awfully easy, right?

67. Answer: C

Nursing Process: Evaluation

Rationale: **An avulsed tooth is an emergency because teeth reimplanted within 30 minutes have a better chance of survival.** The specific tooth that is avulsed does not determine triage acuity. Primary teeth are not reimplanted because it can result in injury to the permanent tooth. Bleeding that cannot be controlled with pressure, such as biting down on a gauze, should be considered for up-triage. Avulsed teeth should be placed in milk or saline solution. Caution should be taken to not handle the root of the tooth.

68. Answer: A

Nursing Process: Assessment

Rationale: **Most foreign body aspirations occur in children younger than 3 years of age. Any young pediatric patient with an acute onset of persistent cough, wheeze, or stridor should be evaluated for foreign body in the airway. Foreign body aspirations usually go into the right bronchus. It is straighter, wider, and has greater airflow.** Peritonsillar abscess will result in stridor, yet the patient will be febrile. A pediatric patient with a nasal foreign body will likely have pain, swelling, and a foul odor or drainage from the nose. Ludwig's angina is a deep infection to the soft tissue of the neck resulting in high fever and dyspnea, yet not a persistent cough.

69. Answer: C

Nursing Process: Intervention

Rationale: **Parotitis is inflammation of the parotid gland, the largest salivary gland. Inflammation can occur secondary to viral or bacterial invasion, or calculi formation. Massaging the gland helps to promote drainage.** The patient should also be instructed to increase fluid intake and use agents such as lemon drops to increase saliva production. Massaging would not dry secretions, relieve the pain, or affect muscle function.

70. Answer: A

Nursing Process: Analysis

Rationale: **Thermal burns rarely involve the actual eye globe because the eyelid protects the globe. In Bell's palsy, the patient is unable to close the eyelid and, therefore, would place the patient at risk for injury to the globe.** Exophthalmos, a bulging globe associated with Grave's disease, would also be a situation in which the globe would not be protected. A hyphema, conjunctivitis, and Ludwig's angina would not affect the ability of the eyelid to close and protect the eye.

71. Answer: D

Nursing Process: Assessment

Rationale: **Ruptured tympanic membrane is a complication of otitis media as fluid accumulates and pressure builds in the inner ear. Bloody or purulent discharge, decreased hearing, tinnitus, and vertigo are classic presentations of ruptured tympanic membrane.** It is not common for tinnitus and vertigo to occur with otitis media or otitis externa. Purulent drainage is not common in labyrinthitis.

72. Answer: C

Nursing Process: Assessment

Rationale: **Otitis externa, referred to as swimmer's ear, results in closure of the ear canal, yet does not typically result in ruptured tympanic membrane. The most common cause of ruptured tympanic membrane is infection.** Trauma to the head, face, or ear, resulting in hemotympanum and barotrauma secondary to change in altitude, can result in ruptured tympanic membrane.

73. Answer: A

Nursing Process: Assessment

Rationale: **Otitis externa, referred to as swimmer's ear, is an inflammatory process of the external ear canal and the auricle. Classic presentation includes pruritis, erythema, swelling, pain around the auricle, and swollen lymph nodes. The swelling can be severe and result in complete closure of the ear canal.** Otitis media results in ear pain, pulling or tugging on the ear, and a sensation of fullness to the ear. Mastoiditis results in pain, erythema, and swelling to the mastoid bone. Meniere's disease is characterized by vertigo, tinnitus, nausea, and vomiting.

74. Answer: B

Nursing Process: Assessment

Rationale: **Otitis media is a common childhood infection, and classic presentation in infants includes pulling, grabbing or placing their finger in the ear, fever, irritability, and decreased appetite. Older children or adults may complain of the sensation of fullness in the ear and decreased hearing.** Otitis externa is characterized by swelling and intense itching of the external auditory canal. Ruptured tympanic membrane is characterized by drainage from the ear, tinnitus, transient vertigo, and decreased hearing. Foreign body in the ear is characterized by sensation of something in the ear and possible drainage from the ear, yet fever is not to be expected.

75. Answer: D

Nursing Process: Evaluation

Rationale: **Otitis media is an infection of the middle ear and is diagnosed with otoscopic examination to provide direct visualization of the tympanic membrane (TM). The TM may appear yellow, white, or have erythemic discoloration, be bulging or retracted, or have purulent discharge, or a visible fluid line.** The infection is local; therefore, blood specimen collection to look for systemic infection is not indicated. Culture of the ear canal may be indicated in otitis externa. The whisper voice test may be done to test for gross hearing, yet is not diagnostic for otitis media.

References

Barak, M., et al. (2015, June 16). Airway management of the patient with maxillofacial trauma: Review of the literature and suggested clinical approach. *Biomed Research International, 2015*, 724032. Retrieved from https://www.ncbi.nlm.nih.gov/pmc/articles/PMC4486512/ (33)

Boston, M. E. (2017, January 23). *Labyrinthitis*. Medscape. Retrieved from https://emedicine.medscape.com/article/856215-overview (53–56)

Brook, I. (2018, March 1). *Acute sinusitis*. Medscape. Retrieved from https://emedicine.medscape.com/article/232670-overview#a1 (43–46)

Candamourty, R., et al. (2012, July–December). Ludwig's angina—An emergency: A case report with literature review. *Journal of Natural Science, Biology and Medicine, 3*(2). doi: 10.4103/0976-9668.101932 (46–48)

Dersu, I. I. (2018, July 27). *Hyphema glaucoma*. Medscape. Retrieved from https://emedicine.medscape.com/article/1206635-overview#a5 (14)

Devan, P. (2018, February 15). *Mastoiditis*. Medscape. Retrieved from https://emedicine.medscape.com/article/2056657-overview (28, 29)

Emergency Nurses Association. (2019). Emergency nurses pediatric course provider manual (5th ed.). Burlington, MA: Jones & Bartlett Learning. (19, 20)

Freedman, J. (2017, April 13). *Acute angle-closure glaucoma in emergency medicine treatment & management*. Medscape. Retrieved from https://emedicine.medscape.com/article/798811-treatment#d10 (7, 18)

Gompf, S. G. (2018, April 10). *Epiglottitis workup*. Emedicine. Retrieved from https://emedicine.medscape.com/article/763612-workup#c11 (42)

Gorovoy, I. R. (2015). Pearls in ophthalmology for the emergency nurse. *Journal of Emergency Nursing, 41*(1), 19–22. doi: 10.1016/j.jen.2014.06.006n. (3)

Hammond, B. B., et al. (Eds.). (2013). Sheehy's manual of emergency care (7th ed.). St. Louis, MO: Mosby Elsevier. (1, 2, 4, 6–9, 13–19, 30, 33, 34, 41, 42, 67, 68)

Harrington, J. M. (2017, September 13). *Orbital cellulitis*. Medscape. Retrieved from https://emedicine.medscape.com/article/1217858-overview (11, 12)

Kahn, J. H. (2018, October 5). *Retropharyngeal abscess*. Medscape. Retrieved from https://emedicine.medscape.com/article/764421-overview (60–62)

Lent, G. S. (2018). *Complex ear laceration*. Medscape. Retrieved from https://emedicine.medscape.com/article/83294-overview#a6 (27)

Leybell, I. (2018, May 10). *Auricular hematoma drainage*. Medscape. Retrieved from https://emedicine.medscape.com/article/82793-overview (27)

Mathur, N. N. (2018, April 25). *Orbital fracture treatment and management*. Medscape. Retrieved from https://emedicine.medscape.com/article/867985-treatment (5)

Murchison, A. P. (2017). *Ocular burns*. Merck Manual. Retrieved from https://www.merckmanuals.com/professional/injuries-poisoning/eye-trauma/ocular-burns#v1112322 (70)

Nguyen, Q. A. (2018, April 24). *Epistaxis*. Medscape. Retrieved from https://emedicine.medscape.com/article/863220-overview (22, 23)

Oman, K. S., et al. (Eds.). (2007). Emergency nursing secrets (2nd ed.). St. Louis, MO: Mosby Elsevier. (10–12, 35, 36)

Pancholi, S. S. (2018, August 10). *Laryngeal fractures*. Medscape. Retrieved from https://emedicine.medscape.com/article/865277-overview (39, 40)

Seiff, S. (2016, August 31). *Zygomatic complex fractures*. Medscape. Retrieved from https://emedicine.medscape.com/article/1218360-overview (30, 31)

Sorenson, M., et al. (2019). Pathophysiology: Concepts of human disease. Hoboken, NJ: Pearson Education. (1, 3, 8, 15, 16, 18, 42, 66)

Sweet, V. (Ed.). (2017). Emergency nursing core curriculum (7th ed.). St Louis, MO: Saunders. (1, 2, 4, 6, 7, 9, 11–19, 31, 33–38, 41, 42, 45–50, 57–59, 60, 62, 69, 71–75)

Tarlan, B., et al. (2013). Subconjunctival hemorrhage: Risk factors and potential indicators. *Clinical Ophthalmology (Auckland, N.Z.), 7*, 1163–1170. doi: 10.2147/OPTH.S35062. (10)

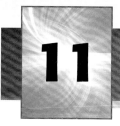

11 Psychosocial Emergencies

Aaron Wolff, RN, BSN, CEN

Psychosocial emergencies comprise a large range of subjects and are mixed together in the Certified Emergency Nurse (CEN) blueprint with medical questions. As a grouping, there will be a total of 25 questions on the test (psychosocial and medical). Questions involving psychosocial issues can be difficult because they are harder to write and answer. Read the questions carefully and take your time! Enjoy answering these questions and understanding the CENsational Pearls of Wisdom that others have learned over the years as well as having this additional information included in this and other chapters.

1. Which of the following is the most important action to ensure patient safety before rooming the patient who is suicidal?
[ ] A. Ensure there are no items present that could be used to harm themselves.
[ ] B. Talk with family members regarding patient statements and actions.
[ ] C. Ask the patient to commit to no self-harm while in the ED.
[ ] D. Thoroughly review the patient's history for past suicide attempts.

2. Anxiety is a manifestation of:
[ ] A. increased parasympathetic nervous system stimulation.
[ ] B. decreased parasympathetic nervous system stimulation.
[ ] C. increased sympathetic nervous system stimulation.
[ ] D. decreased sympathetic nervous system stimulation.

3. The level of anxiety at which a patient loses their ability to think logically is:
[ ] A. level I: mild.
[ ] B. level II: moderate.
[ ] C. level III: severe.
[ ] D. level IV: panic.

4. During a manic episode, a patient with bipolar disorder may:
[ ] A. present withdrawn and depressed.
[ ] B. present unkempt with poor hygiene.
[ ] C. display poor social judgment.
[ ] D. refuse to answer questions.

5. The postpartum patient with a history of bipolar disorder has an increased risk of:
[ ] A. eclampsia.
[ ] B. psychosis.
[ ] C. hemorrhage.
[ ] D. fatigue.

6. Human trafficking victims are unlikely to solicit assistance from the emergency nurse because:
[ ] A. they are psychologically abused and manipulated.
[ ] B. they are voluntary participants in their circumstances.
[ ] C. their psychological needs are being fulfilled.
[ ] D. they are safe in their home environment.

7. Lithium, a drug used to treat bipolar disorder, is known to have which of the following characteristics?
[ ] A. Wide therapeutic window
[ ] B. Little risk for overdose
[ ] C. Potentially dangerous in the dehydrated patient
[ ] D. Used to treat many nonpsychological diagnoses

8. Atypical antipsychotic drugs affect the dopamine and serotonin receptors and have lower _____ compared with typical antipsychotic medications.
[ ] A. daily compliance
[ ] B. extrapyramidal syndromes
[ ] C. financial burden
[ ] D. therapeutic benefits

9. A family member who has immediately and unexpectedly experienced the death of a loved one in the emergency department may manifest all of the following **EXCEPT**:

[ ] **A.** depression.

[ ] **B.** grief.

[ ] **C.** denial.

[ ] **D.** anger.

10. The majority of completed suicides are in which of the following populations?

[ ] **A.** Men

[ ] **B.** Women

[ ] **C.** Nonveterans

[ ] **D.** Children

11. Common physical manifestations of eating disorders include all of the following **EXCEPT**:

[ ] **A.** dehydration/nutritional imbalances.

[ ] **B.** cardiac arrhythmias/electrolyte imbalances.

[ ] **C.** acute renal or hepatic failure.

[ ] **D.** progressive vision loss/diplopia.

12. When assisting someone who has just experienced the death of their family member and is in a state of acute grief, which of the following is **NOT** an appropriate statement by the emergency nurse?

[ ] **A.** "I'm so sorry for your loss."

[ ] **B.** "We gave all the care one could hope for."

[ ] **C.** "You are a strong person and will get through this."

[ ] **D.** "I'm sorry your husband died."

13. When assessing for medical clearance (medical stability), which of the following should **NOT** prevent transfer to psychiatric services?

[ ] **A.** Hypoglycemia

[ ] **B.** Adverse drug event

[ ] **C.** Dehydration

[ ] **D.** Homelessness

14. When first-generation antipsychotic medications are used in the medication naive patient, which of the following may be used to prevent/reverse dystonic reactions?

[ ] **A.** Haloperidol (Haldol)

[ ] **B.** Diphenhydramine (Benadryl)

[ ] **C.** Droperidol (Inapsine)

[ ] **D.** Lorazepam (Ativan)

15. Which of the following does **NOT** call for a high index of suspicion for child maltreatment?

[ ] **A.** Bruising on a child who is less than 4 months of age

[ ] **B.** Bruises on the ears, neck, or thorax on a child of any age

[ ] **C.** Discolorations on the back/buttocks on a child less than 3 years old

[ ] **D.** Patterned bruises on the backs of the legs of a toddler

16. The psychiatric condition with the highest mortality rate is:

[ ] **A.** anorexia nervosa.

[ ] **B.** bipolar disorder.

[ ] **C.** dementia.

[ ] **D.** psychotic depression.

17. When discharging the depressed patient from the emergency department, the most important intervention is:

[ ] **A.** administering a first dose of a selective serotonin reuptake inhibitor (SSRI).

[ ] **B.** verifying social contacts are present outside of the emergency department.

[ ] **C.** encouraging that nutritional needs are met.

[ ] **D.** assessing the home environment for weapons.

18. The suicidal patient is at greater risk of attempting suicide in all of the following situations **EXCEPT**:

[ ] **A.** access to weapons.

[ ] **B.** intoxication.

[ ] **C.** recent social stressors.

[ ] **D.** friend/family presence.

19. Potential nonpsychiatric causes of acute agitation and behavior changes include all of the following **EXCEPT**:

[ ] **A.** hypoxia.

[ ] **B.** thyroid disorders.

[ ] **C.** stroke.

[ ] **D.** dementia.

20. After identifying an adult victim of human trafficking, the emergency nurse should do all of the following **EXCEPT**:

[ ] **A.** force the victim to remain in the ED against their will.

[ ] **B.** collaborate with police and other community aid resources.

[ ] **C.** discretely offer assistance resources to victim.

[ ] **D.** appropriately treat all medical needs of the patient.

21. Which of the following would **NOT** be an expected outcome following the administration of ketamine?

[ ] **A.** Decrease in chronic depressive behaviors and thoughts

[ ] **B.** Relief of suicidal ideation thoughts and actions

[ ] **C.** Reduction of symptoms in patients with excited delirium

[ ] **D.** Diminished aggressive behavior in the acute grieving process

22. When discussing the potential risks and benefits of caring for a victim of sexual assault, all of the following are true statements **EXCEPT**:

[ ] **A.** there are risks and benefits to all medications that may be appropriately offered.

[ ] **B.** there is potential need for follow-up care and treatment if prophylactic care is refused.

[ ] **C.** the patient has the right to accept or refuse all or parts of the offered care.

[ ] **D.** refusal of treatments will prevent prosecution of the crime.

23. The dementia patient is most likely at risk of receiving suboptimal emergency care for an acute hip fracture because:

[ ] **A.** their vascular sufficiency may be compromised and impede healing.

[ ] **B.** their ability to interpret and communicate pain may be compromised.

[ ] **C.** they are not competent to consent to a surgical treatment.

[ ] **D.** it is impossible to keep them in the bed for a thorough evaluation.

24. The peak frequency of onset and diagnosis of schizophrenia is in which of the following age groups?

[ ] **A.** 5 to 14 years

[ ] **B.** 15 to 24 years

[ ] **C.** 25 to 34 years

[ ] **D.** 35 to 44 years

25. When caring for a patient who is acutely agitated and presenting a risk to self and others, which of the following is an appropriate intervention?

[ ] **A.** Administer enough medication to get them to sleep.

[ ] **B.** Place them in a seclusion room with a sitter or status checks every 15 minutes.

[ ] **C.** Immediately implement four-point leather restraints.

[ ] **D.** Begin with the least restrictive means necessary to keep them and others safe.

26. Which of the following is a true statement regarding restraining a patient when necessary?

[ ] **A.** Utilize a trained and coordinated team approach.

[ ] **B.** Have the strongest members of the staff overpower the patient.

[ ] **C.** Direct the patient to cooperate or law enforcement will be called.

[ ] **D.** Engage family members to physically assist.

27. Acute Stress Disorder (ASD) differs from Post-Traumatic Stress Disorder (PTSD) because the:

[ ] **A.** triggering events are of a different magnitude.

[ ] **B.** length of time since the life-changing event is different.

[ ] **C.** emergent needs of patients during each crisis differ.

[ ] **D.** pathophysiologic stress response is different.

28. Schizoaffective disorder involves at least one schizophrenic-like episode lasting more than 2 weeks plus a diagnosis of _____ during a nonschizophrenic-like period.

[ ] **A.** post-traumatic stress disorder

[ ] **B.** an episode of dementia

[ ] **C.** a major mood disorder

[ ] **D.** suicidal ideation

29. Delusional Disorder involves the presence of delusions, often nonbizarre and potentially plausible while not actual, that persists for:

[ ] **A.** a few days.

[ ] **B.** at least 1 month.

[ ] **C.** more than 1 month.

[ ] **D.** at least 1 year.

30. During the initial treatment of a patient with a medication overdose, the priority assessment is identification of:

[ ] **A.** the ingested substance.

[ ] **B.** the motivating trigger.

[ ] **C.** the time of the ingestion.

[ ] **D.** life-threatening conditions.

31. A priority in caring for a family member grieving the acute loss of a loved one includes:

[ ] **A.** determining where to disposition the body.

[ ] **B.** assisting with making family notifications.

[ ] **C.** expressing acknowledgment of the reality of the death.

[ ] **D.** securing social support for the grieving person.

32. The emergency nurse's priority for a patient in police custody who are seeking medical clearance after alleged bizarre and criminal behavior is to:

[ ] A. facilitate rapid disposition so there is no emergency department disruption.

[ ] B. delay history gathering until the officer is present to take notes.

[ ] C. accept the patient's request to refuse care without any examination.

[ ] D. thoroughly assess the patient for signs of illness or injury.

33. Emergency department operational efficiency that minimizes waits for triage and bedding and shortens length of stay does all the following **EXCEPT**:

[ ] A. decreases workplace stress.

[ ] B. decreases patient anxiety.

[ ] C. makes patients feel care was less thorough.

[ ] D. helps staff establish trust with patients.

34. When assessing a victim of domestic violence, a priority for the emergency nurse should be:

[ ] A. gaining access to the patient without the presence of family.

[ ] B. asking the family if the patient is safe at home.

[ ] C. discussing with the family concerns for patient safety.

[ ] D. ensuring a safe discharge environment.

35. The parent most likely to experience a child death due to Sudden Infant Death Syndrome (SIDS) has a child of what age?

[ ] A. 1 to 7 days

[ ] B. 1 to 16 weeks

[ ] C. 4 to 12 months

[ ] D. 1 to 1½ years

36. Discharge teaching after a dystonic reaction includes ensuring the patient recognizes that:

[ ] A. symptoms may return for several days as medication wears off.

[ ] B. the emergency department medications are all that is needed to prevent reoccurrence.

[ ] C. the next time they receive the causative drug, they may not have a reaction.

[ ] D. they do not need to include the causing drug on their allergy list.

37. When treating an acutely psychotic patient, all of the following are appropriate **EXCEPT**:

[ ] A. reorienting them back to reality as frequently as necessary.

[ ] B. policy requirement of mandatory seclusion or four-point restraints.

[ ] C. comprehensive assessment for potential medical causes to their psychosis.

[ ] D. escalation of restrictive intervention to protect the patient and others from harm.

38. Which of the following is **NOT** a typical intervention for a patient demonstrating manifestations of mania?

[ ] A. Evaluate for a therapeutic lithium level

[ ] B. Assess for a panel of drugs of abuse

[ ] C. Reorient them to their physical limitations

[ ] D. Report their condition to family without their consent

39. Which of the following classes of medications would most likely **NOT** be prescribed in an emergency care environment due to their slow onset of effectiveness?

[ ] A. Typical antipsychotic

[ ] B. Atypical antipsychotic

[ ] C. Benzodiazepine

[ ] D. Selective serotonin reuptake inhibitor (SSRI)

40. In the event of an intentional overdose of lorazepam (Ativan), which concomitant condition would prompt you to question an order to administer a reversal agent?

[ ] A. Seizure history

[ ] B. Bipolar disorder

[ ] C. Opioid allergy

[ ] D. History of angioedema

41. A patient with a history of alcoholism presents to the emergency department with agitation and hallucinations after reportedly abstaining from alcohol for 48 hours. Appropriate interventions include all the following **EXCEPT**:

[ ] A. benzodiazepines.

[ ] B. continued abstinence from alcohol.

[ ] C. vitamin B_1.

[ ] D. watchful waiting.

42. Delirium unrelated to alcohol withdrawal is **NOT** typically treated with which of the following pharmacologic interventions?

[ ] A. Haloperidol (Haldol)

[ ] B. Atypical antipsychotic medications

[ ] C. Benzodiazepines

[ ] D. Ziprasidone (Geodon)

43. Which of the following would indicate an improvement in a patient with a diagnosis of Serotonin Syndrome?
[ ] **A.** Increased heart rate
[ ] **B.** Normothermia
[ ] **C.** Mydriasis
[ ] **D.** Dry mucous membranes

44. The most significant side effect of tricyclic antidepressants (TCAs) is:
[ ] **A.** cardiac toxicity in overdose.
[ ] **B.** high abuse potential when taken recreationally.
[ ] **C.** withdrawal syndromes when stopped abruptly.
[ ] **D.** sedation in overdose situations.

45. A dangerous side effect of Monoamine Oxidase Inhibitor (MAOI) antidepressant overdose is:
[ ] **A.** hypotension.
[ ] **B.** hypertension.
[ ] **C.** sedation.
[ ] **D.** severe agitation.

46. Treatment of Monoamine Oxidase Inhibitor (MAOI) accidental overdose includes all of the following **EXCEPT**:
[ ] **A.** administration of phentolamine.
[ ] **B.** cooling measures.
[ ] **C.** dietary cautions.
[ ] **D.** lying supine.

47. Neuroleptic Malignant Syndrome (NMS), a rare but potentially fatal side effect of antipsychotic drugs, is associated with all of the following **EXCEPT**:
[ ] **A.** fever.
[ ] **B.** muscle rigidity.
[ ] **C.** tremors.
[ ] **D.** urinary retention.

48. The most common time of onset of neuroleptic malignant syndrome (NMS) is associated with which of the following regarding the prescription use of Monoamine Oxidase Inhibitors (MAOIs)?
[ ] **A.** Within the first 2 weeks of starting an MAOI
[ ] **B.** After abrupt cessation of an MAOI
[ ] **C.** After decreasing a patient's MAOI dose
[ ] **D.** After taking an MAOI for many years

49. In which of the following circumstances does a psychiatric patient have the right to refuse treatment?
[ ] **A.** They are under conservatorship and the decision maker agrees to the treatment.
[ ] **B.** The patient is below 18 years of age and the parent consents to treatment.
[ ] **C.** They are voluntarily receiving care, but they are refusing a medication.
[ ] **D.** An injury is reasonably believed to have impaired their ability to consent.

50. Which of the following is **NOT** a predisposing factor influencing psychosocial health?
[ ] **A.** Sociocultural influences
[ ] **B.** Developmental factors
[ ] **C.** Biologic components
[ ] **D.** Social stressors

51. If a patient presents a significant threat to others, the nurse has a duty to do which of the following?
[ ] **A.** Warn the at-risk individual
[ ] **B.** Protect the at-risk individual
[ ] **C.** Protect patient confidentiality
[ ] **D.** Violate confidentiality law

52. Secondary traumatic stress is a form of Post-Traumatic Stress Disorder (PTSD) seen in what percentage of emergency nurses?
[ ] **A.** Less than 10%
[ ] **B.** Approximately 25%
[ ] **C.** Up to 50%
[ ] **D.** More than 50%

53. Notification to a child of the death of their sibling is most therapeutically delivered by:
[ ] **A.** the on-duty physician.
[ ] **B.** the patient's nurse.
[ ] **C.** a chaplain or social worker.
[ ] **D.** a trusted family member.

54. Which of the following statements made by the wife of a patient who was an unsuccessful resuscitation attempt would most indicate that her presence during the attempt was a positive experience?
[ ] **A.** "I wonder if more medicine would have helped?"
[ ] **B.** "I will never get over seeing the screen show that flat line."
[ ] **C.** "I feel like nothing more could have been done."
[ ] **D.** "I wish I had had someone to explain things to me."

55. A patient with acute onset of visual hallucinations is most likely experiencing which of the following situations?
[ ] **A.** Acute delirium
[ ] **B.** Chronic fatigue
[ ] **C.** Chronic psychosis
[ ] **D.** Psychotic break

56. Which of the following is **NOT** associated with opiate withdrawal?
[ ] **A.** Yawning
[ ] **B.** Bradycardia
[ ] **C.** Piloerection
[ ] **D.** Nausea

57. Acute toxicity of hallucinogenic substances is manifested with all of the following symptoms **EXCEPT**:
[ ] **A.** central nervous system (CNS) depression.
[ ] **B.** central nervous system (CNS) stimulation.
[ ] **C.** general excitation.
[ ] **D.** general agitation.

58. Upon initial interaction with the agitated patient, the most appropriate response would include which of the following?
[ ] **A.** Medication intervention
[ ] **B.** Isolation initiation
[ ] **C.** Restraint preparation
[ ] **D.** Verbal de-escalation

59. Compulsive bathing is associated with chronic use of which of the following drugs?
[ ] **A.** Marijuana
[ ] **B.** Opiates
[ ] **C.** Benzodiazepines
[ ] **D.** Methamphetamines

60. Pediatric psychiatric patients are at high risk for which of the following?
[ ] **A.** Completed suicide
[ ] **B.** Maltreatment/abuse
[ ] **C.** Acute drug intoxication
[ ] **D.** Therapeutic drug toxicity

61. Which of the following is **NOT** a detrimental social determinant of care?
[ ] **A.** Homelessness
[ ] **B.** Unemployment
[ ] **C.** Addiction
[ ] **D.** Obesity

62. After the death of a child, the probability of divorce:
[ ] **A.** increases slightly.
[ ] **B.** increases significantly.
[ ] **C.** decreases slightly.
[ ] **D.** decreases significantly.

63. Which of the following processes does **NOT** typically present during childhood?
[ ] **A.** Autism
[ ] **B.** Tourette's disorder
[ ] **C.** Schizophrenia
[ ] **D.** Pica

64. Which of the following is one of the strongest risk factors for the abuse of spouses in adulthood?
[ ] **A.** Parental violence during childhood
[ ] **B.** Low socioeconomic status
[ ] **C.** High socioeconomic status
[ ] **D.** Alcohol use in the home

65. The adolescent patient may manifest feelings of depression in which of the following manners?
[ ] **A.** Regressive behavior
[ ] **B.** Use of alcohol/drugs
[ ] **C.** Hyperactivity
[ ] **D.** "I don't know" answers

66. A patient appears younger than her stated age. She looks to the person with her before answering any assessment questions. Which of the following does **NOT** increase the emergency nurse's suspicion this patient is being trafficked?
[ ] **A.** She does not make eye contact with the nurse.
[ ] **B.** She has a small symbol tattooed on her wrist.
[ ] **C.** She has a large tattoo on her lower back.
[ ] **D.** She is not able to state her address.

67. Which of the following is most likely to be a complication of physical restraints in an agitated patient?
[ ] **A.** Pulmonary embolus
[ ] **B.** Heart failure
[ ] **C.** Bowel obstruction
[ ] **D.** Femoral dislocation

68. Approximately half of all people diagnosed with Post-Traumatic Stress Disorder (PTSD) also suffer from which of the following processes?
[ ] **A.** Major depression
[ ] **B.** Schizophrenia
[ ] **C.** Narcissism
[ ] **D.** Agoraphobia

69. Approximately one of four people in America will experience which of the following disorders?
[ ] **A.** Depression
[ ] **B.** Anxiety
[ ] **C.** Eating
[ ] **D.** Bipolar

70. During the acute phase of crisis, specifically, the first 72 hours, therapeutic actions should focus on all the following **EXCEPT**:
[ ] **A.** patient safety.
[ ] **B.** increased isolation.
[ ] **C.** situational support.
[ ] **D.** symptom management.

71. Which of the following is **NOT** a balancing factor for resolution of psychosocial crisis?
[ ] A. The precipitating event
[ ] B. Adequate coping mechanisms
[ ] C. Ample situational support
[ ] D. Realistic perception of the event

72. Which of the following is a true statement regarding the catharsis technique of crisis intervention?
[ ] A. It begins with medication.
[ ] B. It is initiated after a period of isolation.
[ ] C. It delivers positive responses to adaptive behaviors.
[ ] D. It emphasizes active listening.

73. Which of the following is the appropriate therapeutic response in a threatening situation?
[ ] A. Aggression
[ ] B. Passivity
[ ] C. Assertiveness
[ ] D. Indifference

74. Which of the following is **NOT** a predictor for aggressive behavior?
[ ] A. Active psychotic symptoms
[ ] B. Low socioeconomic status
[ ] C. Substance abuse disorders
[ ] D. History of violence

75. A patient with an anxiety disorder asks about complementary and alternative therapies during discharge. Evidence-based recommendations includes which of the following?
[ ] A. Eye movement desensitization and reprocessing
[ ] B. The practice of yoga
[ ] C. The utilization of acupuncture
[ ] D. The addition of therapeutic touch

Answers/Rationales

1. Answer: A

Nursing Process: Intervention

Rationale: **Ensuring patient safety is a primary responsibility of the nurse.** Although establishing rapport (committing to no self-harm) is typically the first step in nursing care, clearing the room of potential hazards after the patient is present could impede rapport while also allowing the patient a means and opportunity to harm self or others. Reviewing the history is an appropriate step of the patient assessment after patient privacy is secured. Talking to family members regarding their presenting actions and statements is also important; however, the priority is patient safety in the initial stages of care.

CENsational Pearl of Wisdom!

Verifying means to ensure personal safety is also a concern for emergency nurses when caring for patients experiencing psychosocial issues. This is usually done at the same time when the initial care is in progress. Always make sure that you—the nurse—are safe from harm! Have an escape out of the room available and never situate yourself in a position in which the patient is between you and the door!

2. Answer: C

Nursing Process: Analysis

Rationale: **Anxiety is the result of increased sympathetic nervous system stimulation (fight or flight).** Increased parasympathetic stimulation (rest and digest) would counter sympathetic stimulation. Both decreased sympathetic and decreased parasympathetic stimulation would allow a return to baseline.

3. Answer: D

Nursing Process: Assessment

Rationale: **Level IV anxiety is typified by an inability to solve problems or think logically and obligates the nurse to identify safety plans for the patient and others as the patient may experience changes in their personality.** Patients with level I anxiety are aware of their environmental stimuli and can rationally problem-solve. Level II anxiety is associated with a heightened focus on immediate concerns while the patient remains cooperative with care providers. Level III anxiety patients do not engage with the full spectrum of their situation and demonstrate regressive behaviors while often needing repetitive direction.

CENsational Pearl of Wisdom!

Level IV: While a level 5 triage acuity patient may express anxiety over a long lobby wait, this dysfunctional expectation is a situational anxiety response, not an anxiety disorder.

4. Answer: C

Nursing Process: Assessment

Rationale: **During a manic phase, the patient with bipolar disorder often has poor social judgment, which can manifest as sexual inappropriateness, becomes hypersocial, with rapid, verbose speech without allowing opportunity for reciprocal communication, and/or displays grandiosity of thought and ideas.** The manic phase is the opposite of the depressed phase, which may manifest with social withdrawal. The manic patient is more likely to display flamboyant personal style and dress rather than be unkempt. Patients in a manic episode will usually be more than willing to answer questions—often providing long and rambling explanations to questions. It will be difficult to keep them on task and to elicit appropriate answers from them.

 CENsational Pearl of Wisdom!

When patients are in the manic phase, be sure to provide a safe environment for them. They may need to pace or move about. They must be closely observed at all times.

5. Answer: B

Nursing Process: Assessment

Rationale: **Although postpartum psychosis occurs in only 1 to 2 per 1,000 births, the bipolar patient is at increased risk for this process.** The psychotic patient typically has difficulty sleeping rather than increased fatigue. Eclampsia has no known correlation with bipolar disorder. There is no known risk of hemorrhage due to bipolar disorder; however, there may be risk related to the medication profile of each patient.

 CENsational Pearl of Wisdom!

The desire for pickles and ice cream is not a symptom of abnormal behavior or suggestive of developing psychosis. This is normal in pregnancy! Health care professionals should watch closely, however, for manifestations of mental health issues that might exacerbate or escalate in the pregnant and postpartum patient.

6. Answer: A

Nursing Process: Analysis

Rationale: **Victims of human trafficking are held captive through psychological manipulation using treats and fear of reprisal against themselves and others by their captor.** Although they may feel they entered the circumstances voluntarily initially, their physical and psychological needs are not being appropriately met and their safety and possibly the safety of others is at risk if they pursue escape.

7. Answer: C

Nursing Process: Intervention

Rationale: **Lithium hemoconcentrates when patients become dehydrated, resulting in a relative elevation in the blood level.** Given the narrow therapeutic window, these relative elevations can result in symptoms of overdose spanning nausea, muscle twitching, convulsions, and coma. Although no longer a first-line treatment, lithium is used primarily in the treatment of bipolar disorders and less frequently for schizophrenia and major depressive disorders.

8. Answer: B

Nursing Process: Evaluation

Rationale: **Extrapyramidal side effects are diminished compared with typical antipsychotics and therefore have increased compliance.** The atypicals also demonstrate benefits in reducing symptoms associated with psychosis such as hostility, violence, and suicidal behavior. This class of drug is relatively more expensive when compared with typical antipsychotic medications.

 CENsational Pearl of Wisdom!

Atypical versus Typical Antipsychotics: Atypical antipsychotics are also known as second generation. This group of antipsychotics cause less extrapyramidal symptoms than the first-generation or typical antipsychotics. Examples of atypical (second generation) antipsychotic medications includes clozapine (Clozaril), lurasidone (Latuda), olanzapine (Zyprexa), quetiapine (Seroquel), risperidone (Risperdal), ziprasidone (Geodon), and aripiprazole (Abilify).

Typical antipsychotics include thioridazine (Mellaril), haloperidol (Haldol), thiothixene (Navane), and chlorpromazine (Thorazine).

9. Answer: A

Nursing Process: Analysis

Rationale: **A diagnosis of depression is not indicated until a compilation of at least five persistent symptoms such as loss of interest, depressed mood, appetite changes with weight change, sleep disturbances, decreased cognition, fatigue, psychomotor changes, and recurrent thoughts of death or feelings of worthlessness persist distinctly from an event such as a family death.** Denial as well as anger are normal phases of grief, as is depression, but defining a response as depression immediately is not appropriate.

10. Answer: A

Nursing Process: Analysis

Rationale: **Although women attempt suicide more frequently than men, 80% of all suicides are completed by men.** Older adult males who are widowed or divorced are at highest risk of successful suicide. Veterans are recognized as being high risk for suicide. Child suicide attempts, although significant, are uncommon.

11. Answer: D

Nursing Process: Assessment

Rationale: **Dehydration and nutritional abnormalities are present in 47% of admissions, followed by electrolyte imbalances for 34%, cardiac dysrhythmias in 24%, and 4% presenting with renal or hepatic failure.** Visual impairment is not a complication.

 CENsational Pearl of Wisdom!

The emergency nurse should be suspicious for eating disorders in order to help in the identification of this psychosocial disorder. The other major component for emergency nurses is to be aware of pathophysiologic complications that may cause life-threatening issues. Be suspicious!

12. Answer: C

Nursing Process: Intervention

Rationale: **Encouraging the grieving person does not acknowledge the significance of the loss and grief that is normal.** Although it is important to demonstrate support of the survivor, during the acute event, it is a time to focus on assimilating the event reality. Now is not the time to try to list their vision beyond the current situation. Acknowledging their loss is a genuine empathy, which acknowledges and reinforces the permanence of the event. Stating you did all you could assists with questions or doubts about what may have been done differently. Words such as "death" and "died" provide concrete meaning and are to be used in place of descriptions such as "passed" or "have gone to a better place."

13. Answer: D

Nursing Process: Assessment

Rationale: **Homelessness is a social determinant of health that may contribute to mental illness.** It is not a medical condition that can be definitively treated in the emergency department (ED). All other conditions provided are within the scope and duties of ED treatment and therefore must be resolved before transfer to definitive psychiatric care.

14. Answer: B

Nursing Process: Intervention

Rationale: **Diphenhydramine (Benadryl) is therapeutic in preventing and treating dystonic reactions.** Haloperidol (Haldol) and droperidol (Inapsine) can cause dystonic reactions. Lorazepam (Ativan) may be palliative for a patient experiencing the effect, but does not reverse it.

 CENsational Pearl of Wisdom!

Dystonic reactions are very scary for patients! Be calm! A little Benadryl will fix them right up! This reaction involves extremely strong muscular contractions to the neck or torso, which causes the patient's head and body to be held in contorted and abnormal positions. The eyes are also often affected (known as oculogyric crisis), causing the patient to not be able to look downward or they may maintain a deviated gaze. The mouth is unable to be closed and the tongue may protrude involuntarily. These reactions are a type of extrapyramidal symptoms.

15. Answer: C

Nursing Process: Assessment

Rationale: **Blue/green discolorations on the back/buttocks, called melanocytic nevus (Mongolian spots), can be present from birth up to 3 years old.** Bruising under the age of 4 months is rare because of lack of mobility and should be cause for concern. Bruises on the ears, neck, and thorax can be normal but are rare and deserve additional consideration. Patterned bruises in a child of any age, especially on the backs of the legs which are rarely bruised compared with the front of legs due to the hazards of collisions during typical forward movement, are also red flags.

 CENsational Pearl of Wisdom!

As an emergency nurse, be suspicious for Munchausen's syndrome by Proxy, also known as Factitious Disorder by Proxy. In this abusive situation, the perpetrator (usually the mother) creates illness and injury in the child for secondary gain. They receive a great deal of praise and recognition from others for being a "great parent." Watch for "frequent flyers" in the ED. They may be there because of abusive situations—no matter the age.

16. Answer: A

Nursing Process: Analysis

Rationale: **Anorexia Nervosa has the highest mortality rate due to metabolic complications and concomitant risk of suicidal ideation.** Although all other mentioned diagnoses have mortality risks, anorexia has the highest risk of all psychiatric diagnoses.

17. Answer: B

Nursing Process: Intervention

Rationale: **Social interaction in the most effective and urgent need for the depressed patient.** Selective serotonin reuptake inhibitor (SSRI) medications are not acutely effective and may take weeks to reach a therapeutic effect. Nutritional care is important in the long-term recovery plan and may require ongoing intervention, but that is not the most urgent need. A depressed patient is at risk for becoming suicidal, in which case access to weapons may be indicated, but the timeliest means of preventing such escalation is to connect the patient with social resources.

18. Answer: D

Nursing Process: Intervention

Rationale: **Engaging friends/family in care diminishes risk of suicide.** Ensuring the removal of access to weapons, resolving/preventing intoxication, and diminishing social stressors are all appropriate interventions to decrease suicidal risk.

19. Answer: D

Nursing Process: Analysis

Rationale: **Dementia can result in acute agitation related to confusion and amplified sensory stimulation**

in the emergency department but is not the cause of the initial presenting symptom. All the other conditions are considerations for medical causes of agitation, which may be part of the decision making before a patient is "medically cleared" for psychiatric treatment. Both hypothyroidism and hyperthyroidism are causes of behavioral issues that can appear to be psychiatric in nature.

 CENsational Pearl of Wisdom!

Always be concerned about medications that the patient is on or is supposed to be taking—and the dosing regimen—when determining potential medical reasons for psychosocial presentations. Sometimes interactions between medications or side effects can be a cause of the behavior!

20. Answer: A

Nursing Process: Intervention

Rationale: **The adult victim of human trafficking cannot be detained against their will and attempting to do so may be harmful to them or others.** It is appropriate to access adult protective services and other regional resources. Discretely offering resources can be helpful, but the key to success is in not putting the patient at risk by delivering the aid in a way that alerts the captor. Treating all medical needs is of primary importance.

21. Answer: D

Nursing Process: Evaluation

Rationale: **Ketamine is an old medication with new uses in the mental health field. It does not have properties that help when an individual is in a situational crisis causing them to utilize defensive and aggressive mechanisms instead of their usual coping mechanisms.** It is now being used and explored in this field to treat depression, suicidal ideation, and excited delirium.

22. Answer: D

Nursing Process: Intervention

Rationale: **Refusing treatment has no implication to the ability to prosecute the crime, but refusal of the collection of evidence can impede prosecution.** Example: Refusal of prophylactic antibiotics is inconsequential to prosecution, whereas refusal to collect a swabbed fluid specimen may complicate prosecutorial efforts. All other answer options are appropriate nursing care.

23. Answer: B

Nursing Process: Analysis

Rationale: **The dementia patient may have impaired ability to assess their own pain and communicate their symptoms.** It is incumbent upon the nurse to dedicate adequate attention to objective signs of discomfort such as body posture and vital sign changes. Chronic vascular pathology will not impact emergency care, but attentive monitoring of distal circulation may be a heightened concern due to communication challenges with the patient. If the patient is incompetent to consent to treatment themselves, a surrogate decision maker is indicated. Sedation and/or a bedside sitter may be necessary to ensure patient safety, and adequate pain control will facilitate safe care.

CENsational Pearl of Wisdom!

Elder patients and those with dementia may benefit from the use of the FLACC scoring system that was created for the pediatric patient.

24. Answer: B

Nursing Process: Analysis

Rationale: **The highest frequency of onset/diagnosis of schizophrenia is in the age group of 15 to 24 years.**

CENsational Pearl of Wisdom!

All patients presenting to the emergency department with psychiatric symptoms should have a Mental Status Examination (MSE) performed. The pieces and parts of this examination include the following: General Appearance/Rate and Tone of Speech/Subjective Mood/Objective Affect/Intellect/Short-Term or Long-Term Memory Loss/Abnormal Thought Processes (flight of ideas/thought blocking)/Hallucinations or Illusions/Insight and Judgment. (Do they know they are ill or need help?)

25. Answer: D

Nursing Process: Intervention

Rationale: **Keeping the patient and others safe during a period of crisis is the priority and should be achieved using the least restrictive yet effective means.** This may include a combination of medications and changes to the physical environment and their mobility, but it must be implemented in a measured fashion that may involve escalating restriction and medication modalities with the goal of being effective, not excessive and never punitive or because it is just too hard to care for them short of sedation until asleep.

26. Answer: A

Nursing Process: Intervention

Rationale: **This is a high-risk situation for both the patient and staff. A trained team approach, which has been practiced outside of emergent circumstances, is indicated.** Attempting to use the strongest staff approach is likely to harm both the patient and the provider. Threatening the patient with police intervention is abusive and not likely to result in a therapeutic result. Family should not be allowed to participate in such an intervention.

CENsational Pearl of Wisdom!

It is no longer appropriate to refer to a therapeutic intervention of restraint as a "takedown."

27. Answer: B

Nursing Process: Analysis

Rationale: **Acute stress disorder (ASD) is the condition that occurs within the first 30 days after the life-changing event. During this phase, the patient is still working through the actual event experience.** After 30 days, if the social and physiologic stress persists, the condition becomes post-traumatic stress disorder (PTSD) and symptoms result from triggering of the memory of the event. The needs of the patient for reassurance and safety remain unchanged in the emergency department.

28. Answer: C

Nursing Process: Analysis

Rationale: **Schizoaffective disorder involves the presence of two conditions: A major mood disorder (mania or major depression) occurring independent of a schizophrenic-like psychosis lasting more than 2 weeks.** Although serious, the other choices are unrelated to the diagnosis of schizoaffective disorder.

29. Answer: B

Nursing Process: Analysis

Rationale: **Delusions must be present for more than 1 month to qualify for diagnosis as Delusional Disorder.**

CENsational Pearl of Wisdom!

Although the emergency nurse may feel the patient's request for three hydrocodone (Norco) refills may be

delusional, it does not reflect the gravity of psychiatric delusion. Delusions can take many forms such as being persecutory, grandiose, romantic, catastrophic, or somatic. Examples of these false beliefs would be believing that some horrible event was imminent or that someone was being followed. These delusions are built around the concept that they could be a reality and are potentially believable.

30. Answer: D

Nursing Process: Assessment

Rationale: **The priority assessment should be the identification of the need for immediate lifesaving interventions (that is, airway, breathing, and circulation).** The timing and type of ingestion are important for anticipating potential changes in the patient's condition, but life-threatening symptomatology and concerns must be addressed first. Motivation behind the ingestion (attempted suicide or accidental overdose) will be a priority for care before discharge or inpatient care planning.

31. Answer: C

Nursing Process: Intervention

Rationale: **Ensuring the family member accepts the reality of the circumstances is the first step toward healing.** Disposition of the deceased is an administrative necessity, which can proceed after care of the family. Urgently making notifications is not time-sensitive and can distract the family from internalizing the reality. Securing social support is important before discharge but is not an immediate need.

32. Answer: D

Nursing Process: Analysis

Rationale: **Due to the reported bizarre behavior, it is incumbent upon the nurse to assess for medical and psychiatric illness.** History gathering is a critical part of the patient assessment and should be a priority regardless of officer attention. The potential of cognitive impairment may preclude the patient's right to refuse care. Seeking rapid disposition can be a therapeutic priority after medical needs are ruled out.

 CENsational Pearl of Wisdom!

Good relationships with law enforcement are common in emergency departments in general, and such relationships can be sustained through collegial communications without compromising our professional commitment to the patient.

33. Answer: C

Nursing Process: Analysis

Rationale: **Decreased operational efficiency, *not positive operational efficiency*, can make patients feel that they are not being cared for properly.** Effective operations are valuable contributors to nursing self-care. Long waits increase frustrations of patients, which can diminish trust and prolong the process of establishing rapport with the patient. Proper functioning of the emergency department will decrease patient anxiety and help to create a positive experience for the patient and significant others.

 CENsational Pearl of Wisdom!

Little else can be more straining on a career in the service of emergency department patients than poorly managed operations. Your local grocery store has figured out how to keep waiting tolerable. The professional nurse should recognize there is more to good operations than adding more staff. Challenge your department to figure out better ideas than adding people at what could be a process design problem.

34. Answer: A

Nursing Process: Analysis

Rationale: **It may not be possible to gather an accurate history and physical examination with a potential perpetrator present.** The patient, not the family, should be the subject of questions regarding their personal safety. Ensuring a safe discharge is of critical importance, but, is an aspect of care later in the visit.

35. Answer: B

Nursing Process: Intervention

Rationale: **Although sudden infant death syndrome (SIDS) may occur anytime between 1 week and 1 year of birth, the peak incidence is before 4 months.** These parents will need coping resources before release from the emergency department.

36. Answer: A

Nursing Process: Evaluation

Rationale: **Due to the long duration of action of most medications that can cause dystonia, symptoms may recur.** Redosing of treatment is likely needed as the emergency dosing may not be adequate to prevent these reoccurrences. Once the patient experiences the reaction, the recurrent use of the causative agent will result in the same reaction. Although not a true allergic reaction, placing this medication, which causes significant negative reactions on the "allergy" list, is appropriate.

37. Answer: B

Nursing Process: Intervention

Rationale: **Policy requirement of mandatory seclusion or restraints for a diagnosis is not appropriate.** The acutely psychotic patient may require frequent reorientation to reality. Ruling out medical causes of psychosis is a standard of care. The decision for the level of restraint necessary should be borne in assessment of the patient and should progress from the least restrictive to the level necessary to protect the patient and others.

 CENsational Pearl of Wisdom!

When you think seclusion is the answer, consider if the patient needs it or if you may just be well past a reasonable opportunity to reorient yourself to reality with a break.

38. Answer: D

Nursing Process: Intervention

Rationale: **In general, unless patients are being held and admitted under a "hold," they maintain all their civil rights, including their right to patient privacy.** A subtherapeutic lithium level may be the cause of their manic episode. Toxicity of drugs of abuse may masquerade as mania. The manic patient may perceive powers and abilities that exceed reality.

 CENsational Pearl of Wisdom!

When answering questions on the test, remember that situations and circumstances are discussed in general terms because nurses from all parts of the country are being tested. Different aspects of care can be termed differently in different regions; for instance, a psychiatric hold may be called a "96-hour hold" in one part of the nation but called a "5150 hold" in another, and there may be nuances particular to different areas and jurisdictions. Be careful to not get caught answering questions "just as we do it."

39. Answer: D

Nursing Process: Intervention

Rationale: **While frequently effective after days or weeks of use, the SSRI (selective serotonin reuptake inhibitor) medications are not an acutely beneficial emergency department intervention.** All the other drugs have an onset, which may be beneficial during a typical emergency department stay.

40. Answer: A

Nursing Process: Analysis

Rationale: **Seizures cannot be effectively treated with benzodiazepines after administration of a benzodiazepine reversal agent.** The patient may best be cared for using supportive respiratory care until the overdose wears off. Another appropriate intervention would be exploring for therapeutic levels of antiseizure medications. The other conditions are not associated with increased risk from a reversal agent.

41. Answer: D

Nursing Process: Intervention

Rationale: **Watchful waiting is not a typical treatment for acute alcohol withdrawal syndrome resulting in delirium tremens.** All the other interventions are within the standard of care. Benzodiazepines are helpful in decreasing the severity of the withdrawal and in preventing potential seizure activity. Thiamine (vitamin B_1) is useful in preventing Wernicke's encephalopathy/Wernicke–Korsakoff syndrome. Thiamine is necessary for the successful metabolism of glucose in the brain. Alcohol should not be taken during the course of treatment for alcohol withdrawal.

 CENsational Pearl of Wisdom!

Patients in alcohol withdrawal can progress to delirium tremens (DT). This can be a dangerous situation and should not be considered to be an uncomplicated process. Act early to begin true therapy so this patient does not become a boarder because the floor feels they cannot handle a disruptive sobering patient.

42. Answer: C

Nursing Process: Intervention

Rationale: **Benzodiazepine administration is not appropriate for nonalcohol-related delirium and may exacerbate the symptoms.** The most common cause of delirium is due to drug ingestion. Haloperidol (Haldol) and atypical antipsychotics such as Ziprasodone (Geodon) may prove effective.

43. Answer: B

Nursing Process: Evaluation

Rationale: **Hyperthermia is a trademark symptom of Serotonin Syndrome, therefore, normothermia would indicate an improvement in this patient.** Other manifestations include tachycardia, dilated pupils (mydriasis), and dry mucous membranes as well as agitation, hyperreflexia, diaphoresis, and flushed skin.

CENsational Pearl of Wisdom!

Always make sure providers are aware of all medications a patient is taking! Serotonin Syndrome occurs when too much serotonin is dumped out into the body. This can happen when patients are taking two medications that produce the same results—an increase in serotonin production. It can also happen with one of these medications in a patient who has hypersensitivity to serotonin. These medications include SSRIs Selective Serotonin Reuptake Inhibitors (SSRIs). Taking a monoamine oxidase inhibitor (MAOI) with an SSRI can have disastrous results. Another serotonin-releasing drug is St. John's Wort. Be careful with seemingly "simple" herbal remedies!

44. Answer: A

Nursing Process: Assessment

Rationale: **Life-threatening cardiac arrhythmias can occur in TCA overdose.** These are not commonly abused, except as a means in attempted suicide. Withdrawal syndromes can occur with abrupt cessation, but symptoms are not life-threatening and are prevented with tapering over a few days. Sedation in overdose is a known side effect, but it is not as significant a concern as the cardiotoxic effects.

CENsational Pearl of Wisdom!

Patients with tricyclic antidepressant overdoses as a suicidal gesture are candidates for a high success rate. Recognize the significant risk of success from these overdoses and ensure aggressive management.

45. Answer: B

Nursing Process: Assessment

Rationale: **Severe hypertension can result from monoamine oxidase inhibitors (MAOIs) overdoses, which blocks the metabolism of norepinephrine.** Hypotension, sedation, and severe agitation are not associated with MAOI overdose.

46. Answer: D

Nursing Process: Intervention

Rationale: **Overdoses of monoamine oxidase inhibitors (MAOIs) cause severe hypertension, and lying flat increases cerebral blood pressure.** Cooling measures may be required as the overdose can elevate temperature. Many foods, such as cured, pickled or fermented food and drink (especially red wine), can potentiate the effect of MAOIs. Phentolamine blocks the action of norepinephrine, the causative agent behind the overdose-associated hypertension.

CENsational Pearl of Wisdom!

An example of an monoamine oxidase inhibitor (MAOI) is phenelzine (Nardil). This class of medication are older drugs and are not the first-line medications for antidepressant use. These were some of the first antidepressants utilized.

47. Answer: D

Nursing Process: Assessment

Rationale: **Neuroleptic malignant syndrome (NMS) is the result of autonomic nervous system dysfunction, and bowel and bladder sphincters may relax causing incontinence rather than retention.** The body's ability to regulate primarily unconsciously controlled functions such as muscle and temperature control occur. Temperature elevation is due to an increase in muscle activity.

48. Answer: A

Nursing Process: Assessment

Rationale: **The most common onset of neuroleptic malignant syndrome is between 4 and 14 days after starting the medication.** Cessation and decreasing the dose is associated with decreased risk of NMS. The risks of NMS after a therapeutic dose has been achieved are low, but dehydration can result in increased risk due to relative concentration of the drug level.

CENsational Pearl of Wisdom!

Find out your facility policy for procurement of medications to treat this condition. Many facilities have a strong process backed by policy between the Operating Room and the Pharmacy because these treatments are very high-cost drugs. The policy should include the ED, and practicing the request/delivery process is well worth the effort.

49. Answer: C

Nursing Process: Analysis

Rationale: **A patient who is not under involuntary hold has the right to refuse aspects of or all of care.** Conservatorship appoints another to make decisions for the patient. The parent is the legal decision maker for a patient under the age of 18, but the nurse should be aware that a therapeutic rapport is critical in working with a patient who is resistant to care. Care may be administered in the event of an injury, which can be reasonably believed to impair the ability of the patient to decide for themselves; however, those administering the treatment must reasonably believe the treatment will benefit the patient. In other words, if the nurse does not feel it is appropriate, they should not administer the order.

50. Answer: D

Nursing Process: Assessment

Rationale: **Social stressors are precipitating factors that are related to psychosocial health, not predisposing factors.** Precipitating factors cause a person to experience disruption from their norms or trigger a maladaptive response. Predisposing factors occur early in life and contribute to the potential for development of a psychological disorder.

51. Answer: B

Nursing Process: Intervention

Rationale: **The nurse has the duty to protect those at risk, which may include assisting with transfer to inpatient care of the psychiatric patient.** This standard is frequently misunderstood as simply a duty to warn those at risk. The rights of the patient do not include confidentiality when they are posing a genuine risk to others. Such disclosures and actions to protect others are not a violation of confidentiality law. This is referred to as Tarasoff's law.

 CENsational Pearl of Wisdom!

Few Emergency Departments have timely access to inpatient psychiatric resources, so our profession needs to build skills in this expertise. At one point in time, we were not always as exceptional as we are now in the treatment of Acute Myocardial Infarction and Stroke, but once we accepted it as our interest, we became very good at delivering great outcomes. We must all step up to this new challenge.

52. Answer: D

Nursing Process: Analysis

Rationale: **Significant symptoms of stress have been found in 64% of studied Emergency Department nurses.** Symptoms are understood to be the result of repeated exposure to traumatic and stressful care events common to the emergency care environment. Attention to self-care as well as recognition of symptoms and prompt intervention is key to the long-term health of the emergency department nurse.

53. Answer: D

Nursing Process: Analysis

Rationale: **Such a traumatic message is best received from a trusted friend or family member who can sustain interaction with the sibling.** The other individuals are very important in the process, but the best person to deliver this information is the trusted friend or family member.

54. Answer: C

Nursing Process: Evaluation

Rationale: **The Emergency Nurses Association (ENA) as well as other international emergency nurse associations (and national emergency care organizations) support family presence during resuscitation. Family members who are in the room can see all of the things that are being done for their loved one. This is a positive outcome for those who are left behind.** It is difficult for them to see the reality of the death, but it can help the grieving process to begin. Staff members should always be present when this is done. That staff member's total responsibility is the family member. Family members should have this support or they should not be allowed into the resuscitation room.

55. Answer: A

Nursing Process: Analysis

Rationale: **Visual hallucinations are most commonly associated with acute delirium. Chronic fatigue is not associated with acute visual hallucinations.** Both acute and chronic psychosis are more commonly associated with auditory rather than visual hallucinations.

 CENsational Pearl of Wisdom!

This sort of detailed knowledge may be the first step in leading your psychiatric patients to the types of outcomes we strive to deliver.

56. Answer: B

Nursing Process: Assessment

Rationale: **Tachycardia, not bradycardia, is associated with opiate withdrawal.** All other options are associated with opiate withdrawal.

CENsational Pearl of Wisdom!

Piloerection is "goose bumps." This is caused by a sympathetic response that allows small muscles, arrector pili muscles, to contract, which then pulls the hair in an upright position. This goes along with the "Fight or Flight" reaction.

57. Answer: B

Nursing Process: Assessment

Rationale: **A common effect of hallucinogenic substances includes central nervous system (CNS) depression as well as general social excitability and agitation.** Symptoms of CNS stimulation are uncommon.

58. Answer: D

Nursing Process: Intervention

Rationale: **It is appropriate to initiate interventions with the agitated patient with the least invasive means.** It is appropriate to escalate the level of intervention in response to ineffective therapeutic effect through isolation, medication, or as a last resort restraint.

 CENsational Pearl of Wisdom!

Working with law enforcement is an important aspect of care of the psychosocial patient in the emergency department. Be sure to utilize this group of professionals in the best way possible for a positive outcome for your patients. Work together—not against—each other.

59. Answer: A

Nursing Process: Assessment

Rationale: **Cannabinoid Hyperemesis Syndrome is an increasingly common condition associated with chronic consumption of modern marijuana and products of marijuana origin.** Patients typically present with abdominal pain, nausea, and vomiting and have a compulsion to bathe multiple times a day with hot water because it helps to relieve the symptoms. The other choices are not associated with this combination of symptoms.

 CENsational Pearl of Wisdom!

We have all heard of the antiemetic effects of marijuana, but who would have anticipated this scientifically validated syndrome?

60. Answer: B

Nursing Process: Assessment

Rationale: **Pediatric psychiatric patients have high incidences of maltreatment.** Although suicide attempts can be common in this population, completion is uncommon. Drug intoxication and therapeutic toxicity can be acute; however, the larger, more often missed concern is the need to assess for signs of maltreatment.

 CENsational Pearl of Wisdom!

It cannot be stated enough times that the emergency department nurse must be suspicious for child abuse. There are many red flags including the caregiver paying more attention to the behavior of the child rather than the injury itself and the bypassing of closer emergency departments. This should raise suspicion.

61. Answer: D

Nursing Process: Analysis

Rationale: **Obesity is not identified as a social determinate of care, although it is associated as a risk factor for many medical conditions.** All of the other options are considered social determinants that should be evaluated.

62. Answer: B

Nursing Process: Analysis

Rationale: **The death of a child has profound implications for the dynamics of individuals and the family unit and is associated with significant increases in divorce rates.**

63. Answer: C

Nursing Process: Assessment

Rationale: **A diagnosis of schizophrenia most commonly occurs in early adulthood.** All the other choices typically present before adulthood.

 CENsational Pearl of Wisdom!

Pica is the act of eating or chewing on something that has no nutritional value such as ice, dirt, or clay. This is sometimes a culturally accepted norm in some groups of people.

64. Answer: A

Nursing Process: Assessment

Rationale: **Abuse is considered a cyclical problem because the dysfunctional coping activity is often a learned response gained through observation in childhood.** The dysfunction knows no socioeconomic boundaries. Although alcohol use is commonly involved, it is not a causative factor.

 CENsational Pearl of Wisdom!

It is always best practice to ask every person who comes to the ED for care if they are safe at home. One of the best clues that something may be amiss is a moment of hesitation before responding to the nurse.

65. Answer: B

Nursing Process: Assessment

Rationale: **The adolescent may manifest depression in a variety of ways, including the use of alcohol or drugs, delinquency, traumatic injuries (from risk-taking behaviors), sexual promiscuity, or other manners of acting out type of behavior.** Children may show regressive or hyperactive type of behavior as well as enuresis. The older adult may answer orientation questions without difficulty, but when asked how things are in general, for instance, may reply with "I don't know," which can translate to "I don't care."

66. Answer: C

Nursing Process: Analysis

Rationale: **Large tattooing of the lower back is most commonly associated with a patient's independent choice.** However, tattooing may be used to "brand" a trafficked individual to an abductor and is usually found on the wrist. Refusal to make eye contact could be a sociocultural norm, but it could also be suggestive that the patient is looking to their captor for acceptable answers. Not knowing or refusal to disclose their address may be a signal that they are held against their will and either do not know the answer or are forbidden to disclose the answer by their captor.

67. Answer: A

Nursing Process: Analysis

Rationale: **Individuals who are physically restrained for periods of time have the potential to develop deep vein thrombosis, which can then escalate to a pulmonary embolus.** Always be aware of this possibility. The other potential options are not usual complications from the restraining process.

68. Answer: A

Nursing Process: Analysis

Rationale: **Major Depression is a common concomitant diagnosis for patients with post-traumatic stress disorder (PTSD).** The other choices, while possible, are not noted in the literature as being strongly correlated.

 CENsational Pearl of Wisdom!

Agoraphobia is a condition of anxiety causing avoidance of certain places or situations that might create a feeling of helplessness or of feeling trapped. Many different fears can be involved, including increased anxiety in crowds or being around any type of large groups of people, but, it can also be associated with both open and enclosed areas.

69. Answer: B

Nursing Process: Analysis

Rationale: **Approximately 25% of Americans experience clinically diagnosable anxiety during their life span.** Depression, eating disorders, and bipolar disorder are far less common.

70. Answer: B

Nursing Process: Intervention

Rationale: **Isolation is not a strong therapy for the duration of an acute psychiatric manifestation.** The other options are all strong contributors to successful outcomes during the early phase of the psychosocial nursing intervention.

 CENsational Pearl of Wisdom!

Crisis Stabilization Facilities emphasize safety, support, and symptom management during the first 72 hours of a psychosocial patient's need. By front-loading these therapies, these care milieus are often able to prevent the need for inpatient psychiatric care.

71. Answer: A

Nursing Process: Analysis

Rationale: **The precipitating event is a causative factor associated with a mental health crisis.** All the other answers are considered balancing factors, which facilitate resolution or prevention of a crisis.

72. Answer: D

Nursing Process: Intervention

Rationale: **Catharsis involves active listening to the patient as they "tell their story" and is identified as a therapeutic intervention.** Medication as a therapeutic adjunct to care may be indicated, but it is not a precursor to catharsis. Isolation is the inverse of catharsis. Positive reinforcement of adaptive behaviors is appropriate but is independent of catharsis.

73. Answer: C

Nursing Process: Intervention

Rationale: **Professional assertiveness is an appropriate and often effective response.** Aggression is not a professional response and can escalate the circumstances. Passivity is not effective and can result in increased risk for the nurse. Indifference does not facilitate a therapeutic relationship.

 CENsational Pearl of Wisdom!

When dealing with aggressive individuals, for whatever reason, speak in a low tone of voice and do assume a power position over them too quickly. This can put them in a defense mode. The health care provider may indeed need to assume this at some point; however, do not rush to this play. Use slow movements, provide limits that are held to, and use simple, concrete expressions.

74. Answer: B

Nursing Process: Analysis

Rationale: **There is no socioeconomic status that is predictive of aggressive behavior.** The other choices are known to be predictive for increased aggressive potential.

75. Answer: C

Nursing Process: Intervention

Rationale: **Acupuncture is an evidence-based treatment for anxiety, depression, and substance use disorders.** Eye Movement Desensitization is an evidence-based treatment for post-traumatic stress disorder (PTSD). Yoga and therapeutic touch may hold therapeutic benefit but do not have adequate research to be identified as evidence-based options.

References

Barnhorst, A., et al. (2014, November). Pulmonary embolism in a psychiatric patient. *Clinical Case Conference, American Journal of Psychiatry, 171,* 11. Retrieved from https://ajp.psychiatryonline.org/doi/pdf/10.1176/appi.ajp.2013.13040494 (67)

Bourgeois, J. A. (2017, November). *Delusional disorder.* Retrieved from https://emedicine.medscape.com/article/292991-overview (29)

Burns, M. J. (2018). *What is the role of thiamine in the treatment of delirium tremens (DTs)?* Medscape. Retrieved from https://www.medscape.com/answers/166032-46134/what-is-the-role-of-thiamine-in-the-treatment-of-delirium-tremens-dts (41)

Chan, V. (2017, January 4). Schizophrenia and psychosis. *Child and Adolescent Psychiatric Clinics of North America,* 341–366. (24)

Chapa, D. A. (2017). Psychosocial aspects of high acuity and critical care. In *Core curriculum for high acuity, progressive, and critical care nursing* (pp. 700–724). St. Louis, MO: Elsevier Health Sciences. (27, 41, 42)

Coshal, S. E. (2017, January 9). Evaluations of depression and suicidal patients in the emergency room. *Psychiatric Clinics of North America,* 363–377. (17, 18)

Deal, N. E. (2015, January 11). Stabilization and management of the acutely agitated or psychotic patient. *Emergency Medicine Clinics of North America,* 739–752. (19, 32, 37)

Delgadillo, D. (2017, January 7). When there is no sexual assault nurse examiner: Emergency nursing care for female adult sexual assault patients. *Journal of Emergency Nursing,* 308–315. (21, 22)

Emergency Nurses Association. (2012). Sheehy's manual of emergency care. St. Louis, MO: Elsevier Health Science. (25, 30, 31, 41)

Emergency Nurses Association. (2018). Emergency nursing core curriculum. St. Louis, MO: Elsevier. (1–12)

Frankenberg, F. R. (2018). *Schizophrenia medication*. Retrieved from https://emedicine.medscape.com/article/288259-medication#2 (8)

Guthrie, K. (2016, May 24). *Stiff and twisted*. Retrieved from https://lifeinthefastlane.com/toxicology-conundrum-030/ (14)

Hammond, B., et al. (2013). Sheehy's manual of emergency care (7th ed.). St. Louis, MO: Mosby Elsevier. (43)

Killian, M. A. (2016). Medical evaluation of the behavioral health emergency patient. *Journal of Emergency Nursing*, 78–80. (13)

Leetch, A. E. (2015). Evaluation of child maltreatment in the emergency department. *Child and Adolescent Psychiatric Clinics of North America*, 41–64. (15, 16)

Manton, A. (2016, January 3). Human trafficking and the emergency nurse. *Journal of Emergency Nursing*, 99–100. (20)

Normandi, P. A., et al. (2016, January). Use of intranasal ketamine for the severely agitated or violent ED patient. *Journal of Emergency Nursing, 42*(1), 61–63. (21)

Killian M, Valdez A. Medical evaluation of the behavioral health emergency patient. *Journal of Emergency Nursing*. 2016;42(1):78–80.

Sikka, V. A. (2015, January 11). Psychiatric emergencies in the elderly. *Emergency Medicine Clinics of North America*, 825–839. (23)

The Light Program. (2016, February 10). *How to spot 5 signs of depression in teen-agers*. Retrieved from https://thelightprogram.pyramidhealthcarepa.com/how-to-spot-5-signs-of-depression-in-teenagers/ (65)

Wiscarz-Stuart, G. (2013). Principles and practice of psychiatric nursing. St. Louis, MO: Elsevier Mosby. (14, 26, 28, 29, 36, 38–41, 43–50, 61–75)

Cardiovascular Emergencies

Geraldine F. Muller, MSN, RN, CEN, TCRN

Cardiovascular issues are many and varied and range from the patient with angina to traumatic injuries. On the Certified Emergency Nurse (CEN) test, this system covers 20 questions. Understanding the basic anatomy and physiology of the heart can help you comprehend questions for which you may not have immediate recall. Study the flow of blood through the heart to help remember the basics of right- and left-sided heart failure. Recognize the essentials of electrocardiogram (ECG) lead placement and what each set of leads tells you. There will most likely be a few rhythm strips on the test to identify, and emergency medications are often present as well.

1. The decrease in cardiac output from right ventricular infarction can be explained by:
[ ] **A.** vasospasms of coronary arteries.
[ ] **B.** inflammation and destruction of cardiac muscle.
[ ] **C.** ventricular dilatation and decreased contractility.
[ ] **D.** interstitial volume overload.

2. Which of the following is the most critical intervention during the first minutes of ventricular fibrillation?
[ ] **A.** Advanced airway
[ ] **B.** Epinephrine 0.1 mg IV/IO
[ ] **C.** Immediate cardiac compressions
[ ] **D.** Electrical defibrillation

3. Which of the following is a reversible cause of pulseless electrical activity (PEA)?
[ ] **A.** Hypoglycemia
[ ] **B.** Hypotension
[ ] **C.** Hypernatremia
[ ] **D.** Hypoxia

4. Which of the following is an absolute contraindication for thrombolytic therapy in acute coronary syndrome?
[ ] **A.** Seizure at onset with residual neurological impairments
[ ] **B.** Gastrointestinal hemorrhage within previous 21 days
[ ] **C.** History of previous intracranial hemorrhage
[ ] **D.** Major serious trauma within previous 14 days

5. Which of the following would the emergency nurse anticipate for a patient with an aortic dissection?
[ ] **A.** Emergent surgery
[ ] **B.** Chest tube insertion
[ ] **C.** Immediate intubation
[ ] **D.** Pericardial decompression

6. Nitroglycerin is a vasodilator that reduces myocardial oxygen demand by decreasing preload and improving coronary blood flow. Contraindications to nitrate administration in acute coronary syndromes include which of the following?
[ ] **A.** ST-segment depression on electrocardiogram (ECG)
[ ] **B.** Dyspnea (respiratory rate greater than 20 breaths/minute)
[ ] **C.** Hypotension (systolic blood pressure less than 90 mm Hg)
[ ] **D.** Tachycardia (heart rate greater than 100 beats/minute)

7. A patient is complaining of chest pain, light-headedness, shortness of breath, and sweating. The emergency nurse should suspect which of the following conditions?
[ ] **A.** Pericarditis
[ ] **B.** Myocardial ischemia
[ ] **C.** Heart failure
[ ] **D.** Endocarditis

8. A patient arrives with a gunshot wound to the left chest. The patient is alert, complaining of pain, and has difficulty breathing. Objective data includes hypotension, muffled heart sounds, jugular vein distension (JVD), tachycardia, tachypnea, and an open wound to the left chest. Oxygen via non-rebreather and two large-bore intravenous catheters have been placed.

Vital signs on arrival were as follows:

  Blood pressure—80/50 mm Hg
  Pulse—125 beats/minute
  Respirations—32 breaths/minute
  Pulse oximetry—80% on room air
  Temperature—98.6° F (37.0° C)

Which of the following should the emergency nurse anticipate to prepare for next?

[ ] **A.** Assist with a resuscitative thoracotomy.
[ ] **B.** Prepare for massive blood transfusion.
[ ] **C.** Assist with a pericardiocentesis.
[ ] **D.** Prepare for aggressive ventilatory support.

9. Which of the following is an indication for an emergency resuscitative thoracotomy?

[ ] **A.** Patients sustaining penetrating abdominal injuries
[ ] **B.** Blunt trauma with no signs of life
[ ] **C.** Penetrating thoracic wound with recent loss of vital signs
[ ] **D.** Qualified trauma surgeon is not available.

10. Which of the following is **NOT** a classic manifestation of the triad of symptoms that accompanies a right ventricular infarction?

[ ] **A.** Hypotension
[ ] **B.** Jugular venous distension
[ ] **C.** Tachycardia
[ ] **D.** Clear lungs

11. A patient with a history of Marfan's syndrome presents with the following symptoms: tearing retrosternal back pain, hypertension, right- and left-arm blood pressure variation of 20 mm Hg, and decreased level of consciousness. The emergency nurse should consider which of the following conditions as the primary process?

[ ] **A.** Pericardial tamponade
[ ] **B.** Thoracic trauma
[ ] **C.** Aortic dissection
[ ] **D.** Ruptured diaphragm

12. Which of the following changes on the electrocardiogram would the emergency nurse recognize as being indicative of an acute myocardial infarction?

[ ] **A.** ST-segment depression
[ ] **B.** Dynamic T-wave inversion
[ ] **C.** Nondiagnostic changes in ST segment
[ ] **D.** ST-segment elevation

13.

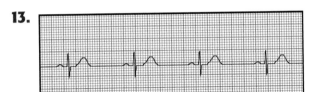

Treatment for the abovementioned rhythm in a symptomatic adult would include which of the following interventions?

[ ] **A.** Cardioversion at 50 to 100 joules
[ ] **B.** Beta-blocker or calcium channel blocker
[ ] **C.** Atropine 0.5 mg bolus given intravenously
[ ] **D.** Intravenous nitroglycerin, titrate to effect

14. A patient is complaining of chest pain unrelieved with rest. The electrocardiogram shows T-wave inversion and there is no elevation in troponin. The emergency nurse suspects which of the following disease entities?

[ ] **A.** Stable angina
[ ] **B.** Unstable angina
[ ] **C.** Non-ST elevation myocardial infarction (Non-STEMI)
[ ] **D.** ST elevation myocardial infarction (STEMI)

15. A patient arrives pulseless and apneic. The cardiac monitor shows asystole. Which of the following medications would the emergency nurse anticipate?

[ ] **A.** Amiodarone (Cordarone)
[ ] **B.** Epinephrine (Adrenaline)
[ ] **C.** Atropine sulfate
[ ] **D.** Dopamine (Intropin)

16. The emergency nurse realizes that the student nurse understands premature atrial contractions when the student makes which of the following statements?

[ ] **A.** "Premature atrial complexes may precede supraventricular tachycardia, atrial flutter, or atrial fibrillation."

[ ] **B.** "Premature atrial complexes may occur in a saw-toothed pattern and are called flutter waves."

[ ] **C.** "Premature atrial complexes are characterized by a chaotic atrial rhythm and an irregular ventricular response."

[ ] **D.** "Premature atrial complexes occur with accessory conduction system pathways that predispose to reentrant rhythms."

17. Atrial fibrillation is clinically significant for which of the following reasons?

[ ] **A.** Atrial fibrillation may initiate ventricular fibrillation when it is multifocal.

[ ] **B.** There is a complete absence of conduction between the atria and the ventricles.

[ ] **C.** This increases the risk of life-threatening ventricular dysrhythmias.

[ ] **D.** The loss of atrial contraction causes stroke volume to decrease by 20% to 30%.

18. Which of the following is the first intervention for new-onset third-degree atrioventricular block with serious signs and symptoms?

[ ] **A.** Initiate a dopamine (Intropin) infusion 2 to 20 μg/minute.

[ ] **B.** Application of a transcutaneous pacemaker

[ ] **C.** Administer adenosine (Adenocard) 6 mg intravenously.

[ ] **D.** Prepare for amiodarone (Cordarone) 300 mg intravenous.

19. A pediatric patient is unstable, with poor perfusion, hypotension, and supraventricular tachycardia with a rate of 300 beats/minute. Immediate treatment would include which of the following?

[ ] **A.** Administer adenosine intravenously using the port closest to the infusion site.

[ ] **B.** Apply ice to the child's face for 10 to 15 seconds.

[ ] **C.** If the child is older, consider vagal maneuvers, such as coughing.

[ ] **D.** Initiate synchronized cardioversion with 0.5 to 1 joules/kg.

20. Immediate post-cardiac arrest care in comatose patients after return of spontaneous circulation (ROSC) includes which of the following?

[ ] **A.** Maintaining a ventilatory PETCO$_2$ between 55 and 60 mm Hg

[ ] **B.** Maintaining a minimum systolic blood pressure of 80 mm Hg

[ ] **C.** Maintaining a target temperature of 32° C to 36° C (89.6° F to 96.8° F)

[ ] **D.** Maintaining arterial oxygen saturation of 90% or greater

21. Magnesium sulfate 1 to 2 g mixed in 50 mL of 0.9% sodium chloride and administered over 5 to 60 minutes intravenously is recommended in which of the following situations?

[ ] **A.** Alternative to amiodarone with pulseless ventricular tachycardia or ventricular fibrillation

[ ] **B.** Second-line drug of choice for treatment of symptomatic bradycardia

[ ] **C.** First-line drug of choice for most forms of narrow-complex supraventricular tachycardia

[ ] **D.** Only if torsade de pointes, digitalis toxicity, or suspected hypomagnesemia is present

22. Anginal equivalents, particularly in women, diabetics, and the elderly may include which of the following sets of symptoms?

[ ] **A.** Shortness of breath, fatigue, palpitations, near-syncope, nausea, vomiting

[ ] **B.** Chest burning, pressure, tightness, discomfort, distress

[ ] **C.** Prior myocardial infarction, stent placement, pacemaker presence

[ ] **D.** Altered level of consciousness, muffled heart sounds, jugular venous distension

23. A 65-year-old patient complains of nocturnal dyspnea, orthopnea, dyspnea on exertion, and ankle swelling. The emergency nurse knows these may be signs of a/an:

[ ] **A.** impending myocardial infarction.

[ ] **B.** episode of unstable angina.

[ ] **C.** mild to moderate heart failure.

[ ] **D.** spontaneous pneumothorax.

24. A patient is brought to the emergency department by emergency medical services in asystole. Cardiopulmonary resuscitation (CPR) was performed en route. Which of the following are the recommended interventions for asystole?

[ ] **A.** CPR and atropine

[ ] **B.** Defibrillation and atropine

[ ] **C.** CPR and epinephrine

[ ] **D.** Defibrillation and epinephrine

25. A patient complains of a headache, drowsiness, confusion, and chest pain. Vital signs are as follows:

Blood pressure—220/130 mm Hg
Pulse—120 beats/minute
Respirations—22 breaths/minute
Pulse oximetry—95% on room air
Temperature—98.6° F (37° C)

The nurse suspects which of the following conditions?
[ ] **A.** Pericarditis
[ ] **B.** Acute arterial occlusion
[ ] **C.** Hypertensive emergency
[ ] **D.** Decompensated heart failure

26. A 75-year-old patient arrives with symptoms of dizziness, near-syncope, shortness of breath, and chest pain. There is a history of an implantable electronic device. The nurse should prepare for immediate:
[ ] **A.** stat 12-lead electrocardiogram.
[ ] **B.** magnet application.
[ ] **C.** interrogation of the pacemaker.
[ ] **D.** cardiology consult.

27.

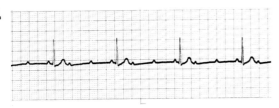

The emergency nurse recognizes the above rhythm as:
[ ] **A.** first-degree heart block.
[ ] **B.** second-degree heart block, Type I.
[ ] **C.** second-degree heart block, Type II.
[ ] **D.** third-degree heart block.

28. A patient complains of acute shortness of breath, frothy pink-tinged sputum, and chest pain. Crackles and wheezes are present. Past medical history includes diabetes, hypertension, and heart failure. The emergency nurse suspects which of the following disease processes?
[ ] **A.** Pericardial tamponade
[ ] **B.** Pneumothorax
[ ] **C.** Pulmonary embolus
[ ] **D.** Pulmonary edema

29. A patient arrives in the emergency department complaining of a low-grade fever, weight loss, night sweats, fatigue, and pleuritic-type chest pain. He has a past medical history of rheumatic heart disease, intravenous drug abuse, and has several body piercings and tattoos. The nurse notices Janeway lesions on the palms of both hands and clubbing. The emergency nurse suspects which of the following problems?
[ ] **A.** Cardiac vessel disease
[ ] **B.** Infective endocarditis
[ ] **C.** Pericarditis
[ ] **D.** Myocarditis

30. The emergency nurse anticipates which of the following interventions for a patient with cardiomegaly?
[ ] **A.** B-type natriuretic peptide (BNP), chest radiograph, ECG, furosemide
[ ] **B.** Metabolic panel, chest radiograph, ECG, nitroprusside
[ ] **C.** Troponin, chest radiograph, ECG, metoprolol
[ ] **D.** Coagulation profile, chest radiograph, ECG, anticoagulants

31. Which of the following would indicate successful use of thrombolytic therapy?
[ ] **A.** T-wave inversion
[ ] **B.** Decreased ST segment
[ ] **C.** Prolonged QT intervals
[ ] **D.** Pathologic Q waves

32. Objective assessment of an acute aortic dissection would include which of the following?
[ ] **A.** Manual blood pressure taken in both arms
[ ] **B.** Inspection for petechial rash to extremities
[ ] **C.** Inspection for extremity edema, anasarca, and ascites
[ ] **D.** Auscultation of heart sounds for prominent apical pulse / S3, S4

33. Complete the following statement with the appropriate phrase. Myocarditis is a/an:
[ ] **A.** narrowing or occlusion of arteries caused by arteriosclerosis.
[ ] **B.** inflammation and destruction of cardiac muscle.
[ ] **C.** disease of the endocardium and heart valves.
[ ] **D.** inflammation of the pericardium that is frequently idiopathic.

34. A patient arrives in the emergency department with the following signs and symptoms: worsening dyspnea, tachypnea, cough, edema, fatigue, and distended neck veins. The emergency nurse suspects which of the following as a primary diagnosis?
[ ] **A.** Pulmonary embolism
[ ] **B.** Heart failure
[ ] **C.** Cardiac tamponade
[ ] **D.** Tension pneumothorax

35. Which of the following explanations is true regarding Raynaud's disease?
[ ] **A.** A narrowing or occlusion of the arteries outside the heart as a result of thickening of the intimal wall
[ ] **B.** Severely reduced blood flow as a result of vasospasm of the digits in response to cold, stress, and/or smoking
[ ] **C.** An inflammatory disorder that decreases blood flow first in the hands and feet that results in ischemia and pain
[ ] **D.** A type of hardening caused by the accumulation of fats and cholesterol that creates plaque in the arteries

36. An unrestrained driver arrives in the emergency department after a rollover crash at 80 miles/hour. Which of the following are the most common causes of pulseless electrical activity (PEA) rhythm for this patient?
[ ] **A.** Hypovolemia and hypoxia
[ ] **B.** Thrombosis and toxins
[ ] **C.** Hydrogen ion acidosis and hypothermia
[ ] **D.** Hypoglycemia and syncope

37. Cardiogenic shock is the result of myocardial pump failure, decreased cardiac output (CO), and inadequate tissue perfusion, most commonly caused by myocardial infarction (MI) or ischemia. Signs and symptoms would include which of the following?
[ ] **A.** Tachypnea, crackles, hypotension, and pale, clammy skin
[ ] **B.** Dyspnea, stridor, wheezing, bronchospasm, erythema
[ ] **C.** Bradycardia, hypotension, and warm, dry skin
[ ] **D.** Tachycardia, altered level of consciousness, uncontrolled external bleeding

38. Pericardial tamponade and tension pneumothorax are examples of which type of shock?
[ ] **A.** Hypovolemic
[ ] **B.** Cardiogenic
[ ] **C.** Neurogenic
[ ] **D.** Obstructive

39. Which of the following is a true statement regarding the diagnosis of Spontaneous Coronary Artery Dissection (SCAD)?
[ ] **A.** SCAD usually occurs in young women.
[ ] **B.** SCAD is associated with atherosclerotic heart disease.
[ ] **C.** SCAD usually occurs at rest.
[ ] **D.** SCAD requires thrombolytic therapy.

40. A construction worker fell from the 10th floor at work. He arrives restless, with severe chest discomfort, hypotension, tachycardia, tachypnea, chest wall ecchymosis, and paraplegia. The emergency nurse anticipates which of the following plans for appropriate tests and subsequent intervention?
[ ] **A.** Transesophageal echo, computed tomography (CT) scan, surgery
[ ] **B.** Echocardiography, pericardiocentesis or pericardial window
[ ] **C.** Chest radiograph, chest tube insertion, and closed chest drainage
[ ] **D.** Chest radiograph, cover open wound, needle thoracentesis

41. Signs and symptoms of acute arterial occlusion include which of the following symptoms?
[ ] **A.** Pain, pallor, pulselessness, paresthesia, paralysis
[ ] **B.** Chest pain, tachycardia, tachypnea, elevated temperature
[ ] **C.** Severe pain, blood pressure variation in arms, peripheral cyanosis
[ ] **D.** Chest pain, dyspnea, nausea, diaphoresis, fatigue

42. Long QT syndrome may precipitate which of the following?
[ ] **A.** Torsade de pointes
[ ] **B.** Atrial fibrillation
[ ] **C.** Complete heart block
[ ] **D.** Supraventricular tachycardia

43. Cardiac output (CO) is a product of which of the following formulas?
[ ] **A.** Preload × Afterload
[ ] **B.** Zone 1 × Zone 2
[ ] **C.** Heart rate × Stroke volume
[ ] **D.** (Age in years)/ 4 + 4

44. The emergency nurse identifies a condition that precipitates sudden cardiac death from blunt trauma to the left anterior chest wall that occurs predominantly in young, healthy, male athletes as:

[ ] **A.** long QT syndrome.

[ ] **B.** commotio cordis.

[ ] **C.** point of maximal impulse.

[ ] **D.** Kawasaki disease.

45. The most common cause of trauma-related cardiogenic shock is:

[ ] **A.** uncontrolled external hemorrhage.

[ ] **B.** pneumothorax and cardiac tamponade.

[ ] **C.** injury or ischemia to cardiac tissue.

[ ] **D.** spinal cord injury and loss of vascular tone.

46. All of the following would indicate reperfusion after thrombolytic therapy **EXCEPT**:

[ ] **A.** relief of chest pain.

[ ] **B.** onset of dysrhythmia.

[ ] **C.** ST-segment normalization.

[ ] **D.** Osborn wave.

47. A patient arrives with a history of surgery 3 weeks ago and now has complaints of leg swelling, redness, warmth, and tenderness. The emergency nurse suspects which of the following?

[ ] **A.** Post-thrombotic syndrome (PTS)

[ ] **B.** Thromboangiitis obliterans (Buerger's disease)

[ ] **C.** Peripheral venous thrombosis

[ ] **D.** Raynaud's disease

48. Diaphragmatic injury most often results from penetrating injury to the thorax or from high-speed deceleration forces common in motor vehicle crashes. With which of these signs and symptoms for diaphragmatic injury would the nurse have a high index of suspicion with that history?

[ ] **A.** Initially asymptomatic, Kehr's sign, dyspnea

[ ] **B.** Impending doom, severe chest pain, severe dyspnea

[ ] **C.** Increasing restlessness, tachycardia, tachypnea, hypoxia

[ ] **D.** Anxiety, signs of shock, decreased breath sounds

49. Injury to the aorta would require which of the following types of medications as an emergent intervention?

[ ] **A.** Vasopressors to maintain systolic blood pressure greater than 100 mm Hg

[ ] **B.** Beta-blockers to decrease heart rate and mean arterial pressure

[ ] **C.** Antiarrythmics to prevent development of rhythm disturbances

[ ] **D.** Antibiotics as prophylaxis for infectious processes

50. Cardiac tamponade occurs when blood or fluid accumulates in the pericardial sac. The emergency nurse would anticipate assisting with which of the following interventions?

[ ] **A.** Needle thoracentesis

[ ] **B.** Chest tube insertion

[ ] **C.** Pericardiocentesis

[ ] **D.** Thoracotomy

51. Treatment for a patient with venous thrombosis would include:

[ ] **A.** calcium channel blockers or adrenergic blocking agents and nonnarcotic analgesia.

[ ] **B.** inotropic support with dobutamine if 1 to 2 L of fluid fails to improve cardiac output.

[ ] **C.** heparin, low-molecular-weight heparin, analgesia, compression stockings.

[ ] **D.** anti-inflammatory agents, antipyretics, antibiotics, and colchicine.

52. A patient arrives with a persistent narrow, regular tachyarrhythmia causing hypotension, altered mental status, signs of shock, and ischemic chest discomfort. Which of the following is the recommended intervention?

[ ] **A.** Synchronized cardioversion starting at 50 to 100 joules

[ ] **B.** Vagal maneuvers, adenosine, beta-blocker, or calcium channel blocker

[ ] **C.** Adenosine 6 mg rapid intravenous push, followed with a 20 mL normal saline flush

[ ] **D.** Amiodarone 150 mg over 10 minutes, repeat as needed

53. Which of the following is a true statement regarding synchronized shocks?

[ ] **A.** Electrical shock will be delivered as soon as the operator pushes the shock button.

[ ] **B.** Caution is needed because these shocks use higher energy levels.

[ ] **C.** Used for an unstable patient when polymorphic ventricular fibrillation is present

[ ] **D.** The actual shock avoids delivery during cardiac repolarization.

54. When a post-cardiac arrest, comatose patient achieves return of spontaneous circulation (ROSC), which of the following would the emergency nurse anticipate performing immediately?

[ ] **A.** Elevate the head of the bed.
[ ] **B.** Maintain administration of 100% oxygen.
[ ] **C.** Hyperventilate the patient via ET tube.
[ ] **D.** Administer warm fluid boluses.

55. The emergency nurse recognizes which of the following as common causes or precipitants of supraventricular tachycardia?

[ ] **A.** Digoxin, beta-blockers and calcium channel blockers
[ ] **B.** Hypoxia, ischemia, heart failure, myocardial infarction, caffeine, and alcohol
[ ] **C.** Hypertension, atherosclerosis, chronic cocaine use, and cardiac surgery
[ ] **D.** Thrombosis, vasospasm, cocaine use, and chemotherapeutic agents

56. Patients with cardiomyopathy may present with a past medical history of hypertension, angina, coronary artery disease, anemia, thyroid dysfunction, or breast cancer. The emergency nurse would expect to see which of the following symptoms?

[ ] **A.** Chest pain, changes on electrocardiogram (ECG), and aphasia
[ ] **B.** Fatigue, dyspnea on exertion, orthopnea, and edema
[ ] **C.** Fever, night sweats, arthralgia, dyspnea, cough, pain
[ ] **D.** Hypotension, clear lung sounds, increased jugular venous pressure

57. The patient with a past medical history of atrial fibrillation arrives with complaints of sudden-onset severe lower limb pain and paresthesia. The emergency nurse palpates the limb and finds it pale, pulseless, and cold. Which of the following plans of care would the nurse expect the provider to prescribe?

[ ] **A.** Smoking cessation, daily exercise, healthy diet, control blood pressure
[ ] **B.** Compression leg garments, exercise therapy, prevent tissue injury
[ ] **C.** Systemic anticoagulation, intravenous fluid therapy, intra-arterial thrombolysis
[ ] **D.** Anticoagulation, ambulation, rest, and D-dimer and other laboratory studies

58. A patient presents with a narrow-complex tachycardia. Vital signs are as follows:

Blood pressure—110/82 mm Hg
Pulse—180 beats/minute
Respirations—20 breaths/minute
Pulse oximetry—95% on room air
Temperature—98.6° F (37° C)

Which of the following initial outcomes will be expected with the successful use of the proper medication to treat this patient?

[ ] **A.** Third-degree AV block
[ ] **B.** Burst of atrial fibrillation
[ ] **C.** Ventricular tachycardia
[ ] **D.** Period of asystole

59. The emergency nurse recognizes that cardiac resynchronization therapy (CRT) is/uses:

[ ] **A.** an extracorporeal mechanical pump implanted to assist or replace the function of either the left or right ventricle.
[ ] **B.** an electronic device that delivers low-voltage pacing pulses to relieve or prevent symptomatic bradycardia.
[ ] **C.** a biventricular pacemaker to treat the conduction defects that cause uncoordinated contraction of the ventricles.
[ ] **D.** an electronic device that monitors heart rhythm and sends a shock to the heart if the rhythm detected is ventricular fibrillation.

60. Current recommendations for acute coronary syndrome reperfusion therapy include which of the following?

[ ] **A.** Door-to-needle time of 30 minutes for fibrinolytic therapy and door-to-balloon time of 90 minutes for percutaneous coronary perfusion.
[ ] **B.** Fibrinolytics should be administered within 24 hours of presentation with qualifying electrocardiogram (ECG), if PCI is not available within 90 minutes of first medical contact.
[ ] **C.** PCI can be offered to patients presenting to non–PCI-capable centers if PCI can be initiated within 3 hours of first medical contact.
[ ] **D.** Patients who present more than 3 hours after the onset of symptoms or patients with ST-segment depression are ineligible for fibrinolytics.

61.

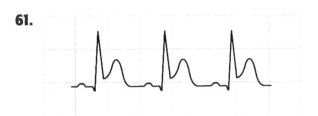

Which of the following identifies the significance of the above rhythm?

[ ] **A.** Hyperkalemia; tall, peaked T waves; early hyperacute sign

[ ] **B.** T-wave inversion, ischemia, T wave appears deep and symmetrical

[ ] **C.** Injury pattern, elevation above the isoelectric line indicates acuteness of injury

[ ] **D.** Pathologic Q wave, appears within 24 hours of infarct, may remain permanent

62. Which of the following would be a red flag regarding the potential for long QT syndrome in youth?

[ ] **A.** Dysrhythmias associated with rest

[ ] **B.** Difficulty with palpating radial pulses

[ ] **C.** Sudden syncope with exercise

[ ] **D.** Sudden death during sleep

63. A pulsus paradoxus greater than 12 mm Hg in a patient with a large pericardial effusion predicts cardiac tamponade with sensitivity of 98% and specificity of 83%. Which of the following is a definition of pulsus paradoxus?

[ ] **A.** Beat-to-beat variability of the pulse amplitude on waveform

[ ] **B.** Fall in systolic pressure of greater than 10 mm Hg with inspiration

[ ] **C.** A difference of less than 10 mm Hg between simultaneous blood pressure measurement in both arms

[ ] **D.** A fall in blood pressure of more than 20 mm Hg systolic when moving from supine to standing position

64. A patient arrives in the emergency department with complaints of a viral infection within the past 2 weeks, now complaining of fever, fatigue, dyspnea, chest pain, and malaise. Electrocardiogram (ECG) reveals sinus tachycardia with decreased QRS amplitude and transitory Q-wave development. Vital signs are as follows:

Blood pressure —90/60 mm Hg
Heart rate—135 beats/minute
Respiratory rate—28 breaths/minute
Pulse oximetry—95% on room air
Temperature—100.4° F (38.0° C)

Which of the following disease processes should the emergency nurse suspect?

[ ] **A.** ST-segment myocardial infarction

[ ] **B.** Myocarditis

[ ] **C.** Pericarditis

[ ] **D.** Endocarditis

65. Ninety percent of acute aortic dissections occur in the ascending aorta. The emergency nurse knows that the most important predisposing risk factor for this process is which of the following?

[ ] **A.** Trauma

[ ] **B.** Cardiac surgery

[ ] **C.** Hypertension

[ ] **D.** Cocaine use

66. Labetalol (Normodyne) would be contraindicated in all of the following patients **EXCEPT**:

[ ] **A.** a 68-year-old with congestive heart failure.

[ ] **B.** a 45-year-old with blood pressure of 210/118 mm Hg.

[ ] **C.** an 82-year-old with heart rate of 40 beats/minute.

[ ] **D.** a 28-year-old with recent asthmatic attack.

67. Which of the following is a potential complication of nitroprusside (Nipride) administration?

[ ] **A.** Hypertension

[ ] **B.** Asthma attack

[ ] **C.** Restless leg syndrome

[ ] **D.** Cyanide toxicity

68. Which of the following medications should be avoided in a patient with a right ventricular myocardial infarction?

[ ] **A.** Opioids, diuretics

[ ] **B.** Aspirin, clopidogrel (Plavix)

[ ] **C.** Atropine, statin therapy

[ ] **D.** Dopamine (Intropin), dobutamine

69. Which of the following statements made by a patient being discharged with a diagnosis of Raynaud's phenomenon would indicate that the discharge instructions were understood?

[ ] **A.** "I will wear gloves to keep warm and work hard on stopping smoking."

[ ] **B.** "I will keep my arm elevated on a pillow and apply ice to my hand."

[ ] **C.** "I have an elastic bandage at home that I can wear when I am on the computer."

[ ] **D.** "I will drink plenty of fluids and take aspirin for the pain."

70. A patient arrives in the emergency department with complaints of chest pain for the past 30 minutes after mowing the lawn. He also reports nausea, dyspnea, and dizziness. The 12-lead electrocardiogram shows greater than 2 mm ST elevation in leads V_1, V_2, and V_3. This indicates injury to which of the following areas of the heart?
[ ] **A.** Inferior
[ ] **B.** Lateral
[ ] **C.** Anterior
[ ] **D.** Posterior

71. Which of the following would be the proper lead placement to definitively diagnose a right ventricular infarct?
[ ] **A.** Fourth intercostal space left sternal border
[ ] **B.** Fifth intercostal space right midclavicular line
[ ] **C.** Fifth intercostal space posterior axillary line
[ ] **D.** Fourth intercostal space right sternal border

72. Which of the following is **NOT** a cardiovascular consequence of cocaine use?
[ ] **A.** Acute myocardial infarction
[ ] **B.** Aortic dissection
[ ] **C.** Hypertensive crisis
[ ] **D.** Pericarditis

73. Which of the following is the most common and concerning electrolyte imbalance associated with digoxin toxicity?
[ ] **A.** Hyponatremia
[ ] **B.** Hypercalcemia
[ ] **C.** Hypomagnesemia
[ ] **D.** Hyperkalemia

74. Which of the following should be potentially withheld in an infant with a patent ductus arteriosus?
[ ] **A.** Formula
[ ] **B.** Breast milk
[ ] **C.** Warmth
[ ] **D.** Oxygen

75. Which of the following is the most common area of rupture in traumatic cardiac injury?
[ ] **A.** Aortic arch
[ ] **B.** Pulmonary vein
[ ] **C.** Ligamentum arteriosum
[ ] **D.** Right coronary artery

Answers/Rationales

1. Answer: C

Nursing Process: Analysis
Rationale: **Injury to the right ventricle causes right ventricular dilatation and decreased contractility. The inability to pump venous blood forward into the pulmonary vasculature reduces blood flow to the left ventricle, which leads to a drop in cardiac output.** Inflammation and destruction of cardiac muscle is seen in myocarditis. Prinzmetal's angina (also known as variant angina) is the result of coronary artery vasospasms. Interstitial volume overload is characteristic of heart failure.

2. Answer: C

Nursing Process: Intervention
Rationale: **CPR performed early can double or triple survival from witnessed sudden cardiac arrest. For every minute that passes between collapse and defibrillation, the chance of survival from a witnessed ventricular fibrillation declines by 7% to 10% per minute if no bystander cardiopulmonary resuscitation is provided.** A major emphasis of the 2015 American Heart Association (AHA) Guidelines Update for Cardiopulmonary Resuscitation (CPR) and Emergency Cardiac Care (ECC) is high-quality chest compressions with minimal interruption and a decreased emphasis on early placement of an advanced airway; providers may defer insertion of an advanced airway until the patient fails to respond to initial CPR and defibrillation attempts or demonstrates return of spontaneous circulation (ROSC). The optimal number of cycles of CPR and shocks required before starting pharmacologic therapy remains unknown; however, epinephrine should be given when IV/IO access is accomplished. Defibrillation should be performed as soon as it can be accomplished and immediate CPR should be performed while waiting to shock.

3. Answer: D

Nursing Process: Analysis
Rationale: **As less oxygen reaches the heart, the heart rate slows and contractility becomes less effective;**

placement of an advanced airway is theoretically more important during pulseless electrical activity (PEA) and might be necessary to achieve adequate oxygenation or ventilation. According to the American Heart Association, hypoglycemia, hypotension, and hypernatremia are not reversible causes of pulseless electrical activity.

4. Answer: C

Nursing Process: Analysis

Rationale: **History of previous intracranial hemorrhage is an absolute exclusion criterion for thrombolytic therapy.** Seizure at onset with residual neurological impairments, gastrointestinal hemorrhage within previous 21 days, and major serious trauma within previous 14 days are relative exclusion criteria.

 CENsational Pearl of Wisdom!

A provider with expertise in acute stroke care may elect to treat with thrombolytic therapy after weighing the risks and benefits.

5. Answer: A

Nursing Process: Intervention

Rationale: **Definitive treatment of an acute aortic dissection consists of surgical repair of the rupture.** Chest tube placement is indicated for pneumothoraces or hemothorax. The priority is to move the patient to definitive care; intubation can be accomplished in the operating room. Pericardial decompression is indicated for pericardial tamponade.

 CENsational Pearl of Wisdom!

There are three major types of aneurysms. A fusiform aneurysm is caused by a weakening of the medial layer, the middle layer, of the artery. This type of aneurysm completely encircles the vessel. A saccular aneurysm, also caused by a weakening of the middle layer, is a dilatation of one area of the circumference of the involved artery. A dissecting aneurysm is caused by a tear in the intima or innermost layer of the vessel, which then creates a false lumen and starts ripping the layers apart as more and more blood fills this false lumen.

6. Answer: C

Nursing Process: Intervention

Rationale: **Nitroglycerin reduces myocardial oxygen demand by decreasing preload and improving coronary blood flow; therefore, it is contraindicated in patients with inadequate preload, represented by hypotension.** It effectively reduces ischemic chest discomfort in coronary syndromes which may include symptoms of ST depression, dyspnea, and tachycardia.

 CENsational Pearl of Wisdom!

One side effect of nitroglycerin that does not occur very often is reflex tachycardia. This happens because of the vasodilation, thus causing a sympathetic response of tachycardia. The "hose" is too large for the amount of blood that it is holding, so the body identifies it as a shock state and attempts to compensate for the event. Rates in this situation can be as high as 140 to 160 and is short-lived.

7. Answer: B

Nursing Process: Analysis

Rationale: **Symptoms suggestive of ischemia include chest pain, pressure, discomfort spreading to shoulders, neck, one or both arms, or into the jaw, between the shoulder blades, light-headedness, dizziness, fainting, sweating, nausea or vomiting, and shortness of breath.** Patients with pericarditis may present with fever, chest pain that is relieved by sitting forward, pleuritic chest pain, and can have a pericardial friction rub. Heart failure symptoms include crackles with auscultation, blood-tinged sputum, dyspnea, and extremity swelling. Signs and symptoms of endocarditis would include fever, pleuritic pain, hemoptysis, and arthralgia/myalgias.

8. Answer: C

Nursing Process: Intervention

Rationale: **Beck's triad, which consists of hypotension, muffled heart sounds, and jugular venous distension, along with tachycardia, dyspnea, cyanosis, and a history of penetrating trauma are signs of a pericardial tamponade, a collection of blood in the pericardial sac. As blood accumulates in the noncompliant pericardial sac, it exerts pressure on the heart, inhibiting ventricular filling and, therefore, cardiac output. A pericardiocentesis will aspirate the blood out of the sac** and relieve the pressure on the heart. A resuscitative thoracotomy is indicated with a traumatic cardiac arrest. Massive blood transfusion is not indicated at this point. Ventilatory support may be necessary when the patient goes in for surgical repair, but the first priority is relieving pressure on the heart to improve cardiac output.

 CENsational Pearl of Wisdom!

When assisting with a pericardiocentesis, the emergency nurse should watch the monitor/ECG for ST elevation and premature ventricular contractions (PVCs) caused by the needle being inserted beyond the pericardial sac into the ventricle. Once the needle is retracted into the sac, these manifestations will go away.

9. Answer: C

Nursing Process: Intervention

Rationale: **Penetrating thoracic wounds with recent loss of vital signs is an indication for an emergency thoracotomy in order to determine the site of injury and stop persistent hemorrhage.** Penetrating abdominal injuries and blunt trauma with no signs of life are not indications for an emergency thoracotomy. A qualified surgeon who *is* available as backup is an indication for emergency thoracotomy to take the patient to the operating room for definitive repair.

10. Answer: C

Nursing Process: Assessment

Rationale: **Patients with a right ventricular infarction usually have bradycardic rhythms. This malady is associated with inferior myocardial infarctions, which involve the right coronary artery. This artery supplies the inferior myocardial wall as well as the SA and AV nodes.** Classic manifestations of a right ventricular infarction, which accompanies an inferior MI at least 30% to 40% of the time, are hypotension, jugular venous distension (JVD), and clear lungs.

 CENsational Pearl of Wisdom!

Patients experiencing a right ventricular infarction have a decreased preload. Small boluses of fluid will help in this situation. Avoid the use of nitrates, morphine sulfate, or diuretics which would decrease preload even more.

11. Answer: C

Nursing Process: Analysis

Rationale: **Past medical history of Marfan's syndrome, tearing retrosternal back pain, hypertension, right- and left-arm blood pressure variation of 20 mm Hg, and decreased level of consciousness are classic symptoms of acute aortic dissection.** Marfan's syndrome is a genetic connective tissue disorder that predisposes the patient to aortic dissection due to weakening of the aorta. Pericardial tamponade would present with jugular venous distension, dyspnea, and tachycardia in addition to chest pain. Thoracic trauma is not specific. Ruptured diaphragm would present with chest pain radiating to the left shoulder, abdominal pain, and decreased breath sounds on the affected side.

12. Answer: D

Nursing Process: Assessment

Rationale: **ST-segment elevation is strongly suspicious for myocardial injury for ST elevation myocardial infarction (STEMI).** ST-segment depression and dynamic T-wave inversion are suspicious or ischemia. Nondiagnostic changes in ST segment or T wave are low/intermediate risk for acute coronary syndrome.

13. Answer: C

Nursing Process: Intervention

Rationale: **Atropine 0.5 mg bolus given intravenously is a first-line treatment for symptomatic bradycardia.** (The clue in this question is the fact that it is symptomatic!) Cardioversion at 50 to 100 joules is recommended for conversion of atrial flutter and supraventricular tachycardia. Beta-blockers and calcium channel blockers will slow the heart rate and are used for symptomatic narrow-complex tachyarrhythmias. Intravenous nitroglycerin is contraindicated in patients with marked bradycardia because nitroglycerin will lower the amount of venous return to the heart. This, in addition to the low heart rate, could compromise cardiac output.

14. Answer: B

Nursing Process: Assessment

Rationale: **Unstable angina is characterized by the classic signs of continued chest pain despite rest or nitroglycerin and no elevation of troponin.** Stable anginal pain goes away with rest. Non-STEMI is defined as ST depression or T-wave inversion with elevation of cardiac biomarkers. STEMI (ST elevation myocardial infarction) definition requires ST elevation in two or more contiguous leads or new left bundle branch block and troponin elevation beyond the 99th percentile of the upper reference limit.

CENsational Pearl of Wisdom!

When talking to patients regarding potential chief complaints of chest pain, always remember to make sure they understand that tightness and heaviness are "equal" to pain. Many will say "Not really" to the question "Are you having chest pain?" but are still rubbing or holding their chest. When the nurse says "But does it feel tight or heavy?" the answer is so often "Yes, that's how it feels." They need to know that this is considered "pain" to us!

15. Answer: B

Nursing Process: Intervention

Rationale: **Epinephrine 1 mg every 3 to 5 minutes is recommended for asystole in addition to beginning high-quality cardiopulmonary compressions and identifying a reversible cause.** Amiodarone is the first-line antiarrhythmic drug given in ventricular fibrillation or pulseless ventricular tachycardia. Atropine and then dopamine are indicated for symptomatic bradycardia.

16. Answer: A

Nursing Process: Evaluation

Rationale: **Premature atrial complexes may precede supraventricular tachycardia, atrial flutter, or atrial fibrillation. These complexes appear on the electrocardiogram as identical to the patient's PQRST complexes but are "premature" or early in the pattern.** Flutter waves occur in atrial flutter and appear as a sawtooth pattern which can be variable. Atrial fibrillation is characterized by a chaotic atrial rhythm associated with an irregular ventricular response. Supraventricular tachycardia is common in the pediatric population, some of whom are born with accessory conduction system pathways that predispose them to reentrant rhythms.

17. Answer: D

Nursing Process: Analysis

Rationale: **The loss of normal atrial contraction and atrial "kick" causes stroke volume to decrease by 20% to 30%. The atria are unable to expel the normal amount of blood during an episode of atrial fibrillation. Atrial "kick" provides for an increase in blood volume in the left ventricle at the end of diastole. Without this extra "kick" at the end of the filling time, there is loss of volume and, therefore, decreased cardiac output.** Premature ventricular contractions (PVCs) may initiate ventricular fibrillation when they are multifocal and also increase the risk for life-threatening ventricular dysrhythmias or sudden cardiac death. Absence of conduction between the atria and the ventricles is called third-degree heart block.

CENsational Pearl of Wisdom!

Another major problem with atrial fibrillation is the development of thrombi in the atria and the potential for a major cerebrovascular accident (CVA) event. This occurs because the atria never completely empty and blood pools causing clotting and embolic release. Anticoagulation is a must for these patients.

18. Answer: B

Nursing Process: Intervention

Rationale: **New-onset third-degree atrioventricular block with manifestations (especially with a wide-QRS complex) is an indication for insertion of a transvenous pacemaker; transcutaneous pacing is a temporizing measure until the transvenous pacemaker is placed.** Dopamine or epinephrine infusions are also temporizing measures before insertion of a transvenous pacemaker, but application of a transcutaneous pacemaker should be done first. Adenosine is indicated for stable narrow-complex supraventricular tachycardia. Amiodarone is indicated as second-line treatment for ventricular fibrillation or pulseless ventricular tachycardia after shock, CPR, and a vasopressor.

19. Answer: D

Nursing Process: Intervention

Rationale: **Initiating synchronized cardioversion with 0.5 to 1 joules/kg is initial treatment for unstable infants or children with supraventricular tachycardia. The patient in this scenario is hypotensive and has evidence of poor perfusion.** Adenosine, application of ice to the face, and other vagal maneuvers are attempted in children (and adults) who are hemodynamically stable.

20. Answer: C

Nursing Process: Intervention

Rationale: **Maintaining a constant target temperature between 32° C and 36° C (89.6° F to 96.8° F) for 24 hours has been demonstrated to improve neurologic recovery.** Ventilation should be titrated to a PETCO$_2$ of 35 to 45 mm Hg or a PaCO$_2$ of 40 to 45 mm Hg. Hypotension (blood pressure ≤ 90 mm Hg) should be treated with fluid bolus or vasopressor infusion. Oxygen delivery should be titrated to the lowest FiO$_2$ required to achieve an arterial oxygen saturation of 94% to 99% to avoid potential oxygen toxicity.

21. Answer: D

Nursing Process: Intervention

Rationale: **Administration of magnesium is recommended only if torsades de pointes, digitalis toxicity, or suspected hypomagnesemia is present. Hypomagnesemia can cause a prolonged Q-T interval and the magnesium will help shorten the Q-T interval to its normal. In digitalis toxicity, the administration of magnesium for replacement may be vital to decrease dysrhythmias and can act indirectly as an antagonist of digoxin.** Lidocaine 1 to 1.5 mg/kg is an alternative to amiodarone in cardiac arrest from pulseless ventricular tachycardia or ventricular fibrillation. Dopamine infusion is the second-line drug for symptomatic bradycardia after atropine. Adenosine 6 mg given rapidly over 1 to 3 seconds followed by a normal saline bolus of 20 mL is the first drug for narrow-complex supraventricular tachycardia.

22. Answer: A

Nursing Process: Assessment

Rationale: **In the three populations listed, chest pain can be absent or atypical. Shortness of breath, fatigue, palpitations, near-syncope, nausea, and vomiting are anginal equivalents and may be present in women, diabetics, and the elderly instead of the classic chest pain that is usually expected.** Burning, pressure, tightness, discomfort, and distress are words patients use to describe chest pain of cardiac origin, and so is not a "set of symptoms." Prior myocardial infarction, stent placement, and pacemaker presence are risk factors for cardiovascular disease, not symptoms. Altered level of consciousness, muffled heart sounds, and jugular venous distension are signs of an aortic arch dissection.

23. Answer: C

Nursing Process: Assessment

Rationale: **Nocturnal dyspnea, orthopnea, dyspnea on exertion, and ankle swelling are signs of mild-to-moderate heart failure. Severe heart failure occurs when patients are unable to perform their usual physical activity and have symptoms at rest. Increased physical activity causes increased symptomatology.** Although dyspnea on exertion may be present with myocardial infarction, unstable angina and pneumothorax, ankle swelling, nocturnal dyspnea, and orthopnea would not be expected in these disease processes.

24. Answer: C

Nursing Process: Intervention

Rationale: **CPR and epinephrine are recommended for asystole.** Available evidence suggests that the routine use of atropine during pulseless electrical activity (PEA) or asystole is unlikely to have a therapeutic benefit and has been removed from the Adult Cardiac Arrest Algorithm. Likewise, in all outcomes studied, including return of spontaneous circulation (ROSC) and survival, there was a worse outcome for shock delivery with asystole; therefore, electrical delivery is not recommended for asystole.

25. Answer: D

Nursing Process: Analysis

Rationale: **Hypertensive emergency is defined as a systolic blood pressure over 180 mm Hg or a diastolic blood pressure over 120 mm Hg with evidence of impending end-organ damage, in this case cerebrovascular impairment.** Signs of pericarditis are cardiac in nature, along with a possible elevated body temperature and a friction rub. Acute arterial occlusion would result in pain, pallor, pulselessness, paresthesia, or paralysis of the affected limb. Decompensated heart failure may have hypertension present, but symptoms would also include possible jugular venous distension, dyspnea, peripheral edema, nausea, and crackles.

 CENsational Pearl of Wisdom!

Remember that not all hypertension is dropped immediately! There are some disease processes in which the blood pressure must be decreased quickly, such as with an aneurysm or aortic dissection; however, in instances of cerebrovascular accident (CVA), the blood pressure is maintained at a higher level to perfuse the brain and not cause an increase in the size of the infarct. Cerebral perfusion pressure must be maintained at a level of at least 60 to 70 in the adult to perfuse the brain. The formula is: CPP = MAP − ICP. The mean arterial pressure (MAP) must keep up with the intracranial pressure (ICP) to maintain the cerebral perfusion pressure.

---

26. Answer: A

Nursing Process: Intervention

Rationale: **All of the interventions may be required; however, an emergent 12-lead electrocardiogram (ECG) and rhythm strip to determine whether the implantable cardioverter defibrillator (ICD) is functioning correctly should be done initially.** The magnet inactivates the sensing function so that during magnet mode, the pacemaker will pace asynchronously. Magnet application may be done later to identify battery depletion or malfunction of the ICD. Interrogation of the ICD should be done by the emergency department, cardiology department, or the device manufacturer. A consult to cardiology would be needed also.

27. Answer: C

Nursing Process: Assessment

Rationale: **Second-degree heart block, Type II is characterized by a constant PR interval that is followed by a nonconducted P wave.** First-degree heart block is the most common conduction disturbance and is characterized by a PR interval that is greater than 0.20 seconds and rarely requires treatment. Type I second-degree heart block (Mobitz I or Wenckebach) is slower and slower impulse conduction through the AV node and is seen as gradual prolongation of the PR interval until one depolarization from the atria is completely blocked. Third-degree heart block results from injury to the cardiac conduction system, so that no impulses are conducted from the atria to the ventricles; the atrial contractions are faster and independent of the slower beating ventricles.

CENsational Pearl of Wisdom!

Plan on identifying a few heart dysrhythmias on the test. They may be embedded within the question or simply asked such as in this question. Become proficient in identifying rhythms. It will be good for your test taking and important for your patients!

28. Answer: D

Nursing Process: Assessment

Rationale: **The symptoms presented are typical of acute pulmonary edema related to heart failure.** Pericardial tamponade has muffled heart sounds, distended neck veins, and hypotension (Beck's triad). Breath sounds would be decreased on the affected side in a pneumothorax. Pulmonary embolus causes nonspecific signs, but dyspnea, tachypnea, syncope, or cyanosis are most common.

CENsational Pearl of Wisdom!

Pulmonary edema is associated with left-sided heart failure. It causes a backup of fluid in the pulmonary system. Edema of the ankles and feet is associated with right-sided heart failure because it causes a backup of fluid in the venous system. Think about how the flow of blood goes through the heart. That will help you remember the manifestations of right- and left-sided heart failure. Blood returns to the heart through the superior and inferior vena cava and empties into the right atrium. After entering the right ventricle, the deoxygenated blood flows into the pulmonary system through the pulmonary artery. Once oxygen is picked up (and carbon dioxide is dropped off to be breathed off), blood reenters the heart via the

pulmonary veins into the left atrium. It then is passed into the left ventricle and pumped out to the body through the aorta. Therefore, right-sided heart failure is manifested by a back up of blood into the venous system and left-sided heart failure presents as pulmonary edema as it backs up fluid in the lungs. Usually, these symptoms occur simultaneously due to how interconnected the right and left sides of the heart function.

29. Answer: B

Nursing Process: Analysis

Rationale: **Low-grade fever, weight loss, night sweats, fatigue, arthralgia, and pleuritic chest pain are signs and symptoms of infective endocarditis. Risk factors include a history of rheumatic heart disease, intravenous drug use, body piercings, and tattoos. Janeway lesions (small reddened macular-like nodules found on the hands and feet) and clubbing are classic signs of infective endocarditis.** Cardiac vessel disease is not specific for these signs and symptoms. Pericarditis presents with pleuritic chest pain that radiates to the left shoulder, causes increased pain in the supine position, and may be relieved by sitting up and leaning forward. Viral infection is the most common cause of myocarditis, including parvovirus, herpesvirus 6, and coxsackievirus B. Clinical myocarditis often is self-limiting unless the host immune response is overwhelming or inappropriate.

CENsational Pearl of Wisdom!

The potential for endocarditis which causes infection and destruction of the heart valves is the reason that those patients who are IV drug abusers are not considered good candidates for cardiac organ donation.

30. Answer: A

Nursing Process: Intervention

Rationale: **B-type natriuretic peptide (BNP), chest radiograph, ECG, and furosemide is the plan of care for a patient with cardiomegaly. Patients with cardiomegaly present with symptoms of heart failure, manifested by a reduction in left ventricular contractility and cardiac output.** Metabolic panel, chest radiograph, ECG, and nitroprusside are recommended for hypertensive crisis. Troponin, chest radiograph, ECG, and metoprolol are indicated in myocardial infarction. Coagulation profile, chest radiograph, ECG, and anticoagulants are treatment for venous thromboembolisms.

31. Answer: B

Nursing Process: Evaluation

Rationale: **Thrombolytic therapy should open closed coronary arteries and reperfuse the heart. Reperfusion** would be indicated by ST segments falling back to normal levels. **Elevated ST segments indicate injury to the heart muscle.** T-wave inversion would demonstrate ischemia. Prolonged QT intervals are a negative finding and can be a forerunner of torsade de pointes. Pathologic Q waves are indicative of necrosis in the heart wall.

32. Answer: A

Nursing Process: Assessment

Rationale: **Manual blood pressures taken in both arms would be the correct objective assessment parameter. The primary event in an aortic dissection is a tear in the aortic intima which allows blood to pass into the aortic media, thereby creating a false lumen; pressure within this false channel can compress the true aortic lumen and reduce blood flow. A considerable variation greater than 20 mm Hg systolic may be seen when comparing the blood pressure in the arms with this diagnosis.** Inspection for petechiae related to microemboli is performed for a suspected acute arterial occlusion. Edema of the extremities, anasarca (generalized swelling), or ascites would be assessed for heart failure. Prominent apical pulse and the presence of S3 or S4, is found in hypertensive crises cases.

33. Answer: B

Nursing Process: Analysis

Rationale: **Myocarditis causes an inflammation and destruction of the actual cardiac muscle. Patients may present nearly asymptomatic, in severe heart failure, or with sudden death from dysrhythmias. Causes of myocarditis are numerous and include infectious, toxic, and immunologic.** Arteriosclerosis can cause both peripheral vascular disease which contains the arteries outside of the heart and cardiac disease within the coronary arteries. Endocarditis is an infection that generally affects normal heart valves and can be caused by many different bacteria, fungi, mycobacteria, and other organisms. Pericarditis, an inflammation of the pericardium, is most frequently idiopathic; however, it can develop as a result of bacterial, viral or fungal infections, autoimmune diseases, myocardial infarction, systemic lupus, and others.

34. Answer: B

Nursing Process: Assessment   .

Rationale: **Heart failure is the result of structural and functional impairment of ventricular filling or ejection of blood. Most patients have impairment of myocardial function, ranging from normal ventricular size and function to marked dilation and reduced function. Worsening dyspnea is a cardinal symptom of heart failure and dyspnea at rest is often mentioned by patients. The symptoms stated in the question reflect pulmonary congestion.** Pulmonary embolism occurs

with an occlusion of pulmonary blood vessels and the patient may have dyspnea, but pleuritic chest pain, pleural friction rub, and signs and symptoms of a deep vein thrombosis would also be expected; edema would not occur with a pulmonary embolism. Cardiac tamponade is the collection of blood in the pericardial sac, which limits ventricular filling and thus decreases cardiac output; signs and symptoms would include chest pain and Beck's triad: distended neck veins (JVD), distant heart sounds (muffled), and hypotension. Tension pneumothorax occurs when air enters the pleural space during inspiration and is unable to escape during exhalation. This leads to a rising intrathoracic pressure which compresses the lungs, heart, and great vessels in the chest. It is preceded by blunt or penetrating trauma and causes severe respiratory distress and absent breath sounds on the affected side.

35. Answer: B

Nursing Process: Analysis

Rationale: **Raynaud's disease, by definition, severely reduces blood flow by vasospasm following a stimulus, such as extreme cold, stress, or smoking. This causes pallor, cyanosis, coldness, numbness, and tingling in the affected hand.** Peripheral artery disease is a narrowing or occlusion of arteries outside the heart as a result of thickening of the intimal wall, caused primarily by atherosclerosis. Buerger's disease is an occlusive, chronic, inflammatory disorder of the arteries, veins, and surrounding nerves; decreased blood flow in the hands and feet leads to ischemia and pain initially, intermittent claudication, and decreased or absent peripheral pulses later. This may lead to infection, skin ulcers, and gangrene. Atherosclerosis is a type of hardening caused by the accumulation of fats and cholesterol that creates plaque in the arteries and reduces blood flow.

 CENsational Pearl of Wisdom!

Raynaud's disease is one of the processes where a formerly "male-only" medication is finding indications for use. Sildenafil (Viagra) can be used to treat this malady due to its vasodilatory effects. So be sure to ask both genders about the use Viagra before administration of nitroglycerin during episodes of chest pain! Nitroglycerin can also be used on the fingertips to heal skin ulcers that can develop after multiple episodes. Other vasodilators such as losartan (Cozaar) can also be used, as well as prostaglandins. Repeated episodes of Raynaud's disease can cause gangrene. Other treatment options that can be help are to avoid smoking, decrease stress, exercise, and try to avoid rapid, extreme changes in temperature.

36. Answer: A

Nursing Process: Analysis

Rationale: **Hypovolemia and hypoxia are the two most common underlying and potentially reversible causes of pulseless electrical activity (PEA) in the trauma patient. Uncontrolled bleeding and resultant hypovolemia may occur after a crash of an unrestrained driver at high speeds.** Although thrombosis, toxins, acidosis, and hypothermia are causes of pulseless electrical activity according to the American Heart Association, they are not necessarily implicated in a car crash at high speeds. Hypoglycemia and syncope are not common causes of pulseless electrical activity according to the American Heart Association.

37. Answer: A

Nursing Process: Analysis

Rationale: **Most patients who present with cardiogenic shock do so in conjunction with a myocardial infarction. Clinical manifestations of cardiogenic shock reflect heart failure and inadequate tissue perfusion, that is, tachypnea, crackles, hypotension, and pale, clammy skin.** Anaphylactic shock from allergic reaction presents with dyspnea, stridor, wheezing, bronchospasm, and erythema. Neurogenic shock includes signs/symptoms of bradycardia, hypotension, and warm, dry skin. Tachycardia, altered level of consciousness, and uncontrolled external bleeding are signs of hypovolemic shock.

 CENsational Pearl of Wisdom!

Hypovolemic shock can occur for an absolute loss of volume as listed earlier with uncontrolled external bleeding and with a relative loss of fluid such as with burns and ascites. The fluid is present in the body, but it is not useful at this time. Third spacing can be another cause of hypovolemic shock.

38. Answer: D

Nursing Process: Analysis

Rationale: **Obstructive shock results from an inadequate circulating blood volume because of an obstruction or compression of the great veins, aorta, pulmonary arteries, or the heart itself. Cardiac tamponade compresses the heart so that the atria cannot fill, leading to a decrease in stroke volume and then circulating blood volume. Tension pneumothorax may displace the inferior vena cava and obstruct venous return to the right atrium, also decreasing circulating blood volume.** Hypovolemic shock is a decrease in

circulating blood volume, from hemorrhage after trauma, extensive burns, or gastrointestinal bleeding. Cardiogenic shock results from ineffective perfusion caused by inadequate contractility of the heart from myocardial infarction, blunt cardiac injury, mitral valve insufficiency, dysrhythmias, and cardiac failure. Neurogenic shock results from injury to the spinal cord in the cervical or upper thoracic region.

39. Answer: A

Nursing Process: Analysis

Rationale: **SCAD is a disease process that usually occurs in young women—many times associated with peripartum women. However, this can present in women younger than age 50 and has been seen in postmenopausal women as well.** SCAD stands for spontaneous coronary artery dissection and involves the tearing and separation of two layers of a coronary artery, which then develops a hematoma within the wall of the artery causing subsequent compression of the lumen. Atherosclerosis is not present. The myocardial infarction occurs during episodes of extreme exercise, severe coughing/vomiting, or intense stress. It can also occur during the delivery process and has been seen with illicit drug use, such as cocaine and amphetamines. Thrombolytic therapy is contraindicated in the treatment of SCAD.

 CENsational Pearl of Wisdom!

Yes! This one was a bit unfair, wasn't it! Sorry about that! But now you know what SCAD is— an sudden cardiac death event for mostly young women that has recently come to the forefront.

40. Answer: A

Nursing Process: Intervention

Rationale: **Motor vehicle crashes and falls are the most common causes of aortic injury. When the aorta is subjected to accelerating, decelerating, horizontal, or vertical traumatic forces, it may tear. Signs and symptoms include decreased level of consciousness, hypotension, tachycardia, tachypnea, chest wall ecchymosis, and paraplegia. Paraplegia can occur due to the ischemia of the anterior spinal artery which is fed by branches of the aorta. Diagnosis is suspected by the history of rapid deceleration forces and chest radiograph, and confirmed by arteriography,** transesophageal echo, or computed tomography (CT) scan. Surgical intervention is indicated. Pericardial tamponade occurs most often with penetrating injury; classic signs are hypotension, distended neck veins, and muffled heart sounds, and is treated with pericardiocentesis or pericardial window. Hemothorax is an accumulation of blood in the pleural space and signs/symptoms are dyspnea, tachypnea, chest pain, signs of shock, and decreased breath sounds on the affected side; treatment is chest tube insertion and closed chest drainage system. Tension pneumothorax would present with severe respiratory distress, diminished or absent breath sounds, hypotension, distended neck veins, and tracheal deviation. Treatment is immediately preparing for a needle thoracentesis.

41. Answer: A

Nursing Process: Assessment

Rationale: **The signs of acute arterial occlusion are referred as the "5 Ps": Pain, Pallor, Pulselessness, Paresthesia, and Paralysis.** Chest pain, tachycardia, tachypnea, and elevated temperature may be seen in pericarditis. Severe pain, blood pressure variations in the arm and peripheral cyanosis are seen in aortic injuries. Chest pain, dyspnea, nausea, diaphoresis, and fatigue are seen in myocardial infarctions.

42. Answer: A

Nursing Process: Analysis

Rationale: **The long QT syndrome is a disorder of myocardial repolarization characterized by a prolonged QT interval on the electrocardiogram. This syndrome is associated with an increased risk of polymorphic ventricular tachycardia, a characteristic life-threatening cardiac dysrhythmia also known as torsades de pointes. The primary symptoms include palpitations, syncope, seizures, and sudden cardiac death.** Atrial fibrillation, complete heart block, and supraventricular tachycardia are not precipitated by long QT syndrome.

43. Answer: C

Nursing Process: Analysis

Rationale: **Cardiac output (CO) is defined as a product of heart rate (HR) times stroke volume (SV) (CO = HR × SV).** Preload is the passive stretching force of the ventricles during diastole; afterload is the resistance of the system that the ventricles must overcome to eject blood. Zone 1 and Zone 2 are anatomic landmarks of the neck and serve to identify structures in each zone. (Age in years)/4 + 4 is the formula to estimate pediatric endotracheal tube size.

CENsational Pearl of Wisdom!

Children have a fixed stroke volume. Because the stroke volume cannot change, they can only compensate by increasing their heart rates to augment their cardiac output. Tachycardia is often the first manifestation that something is wrong!

44. Answer: B

Nursing Process: Analysis

Rationale: **Commotio cordis causes sudden cardiac death from blunt trauma to the left anterior chest wall, usually from a thrown or batted ball and occurs predominantly in young, male athletes.** The cause of death is ventricular fibrillation due to the blow to the chest ocurring during a critical point in the cardiac cycle. The long QT syndrome (LQTS) is a disorder of myocardial repolarization characterized by a prolonged QT interval on the electrocardiogram and results from many things, including medications, electrolyte disorders, and congenital defects. The point of maximal impulse (PMI) is located in the fifth intercostal space at the midclavicular line. PMI is where the cardiac impulse can be best palpated. The PMI may be displaced with increased right ventricular pressure (large right pleural effusion, right tension pneumothorax) and volume overload (heart failure). Kawasaki disease affects children younger than 5 years with vasculitis that affects medium and small arteries, notably the coronary arteries. It is self-limiting and resolves within 1 to 2 months, although the mortality rate is 1% to 2%.

CENsational Pearl of Wisdom!

Advocate for automatic external defibrillators (AED) at school ball games! Commotio cordis (which means "commotion of the heart") causes ventricular fibrillation in these young athletes. Immediate defibrillation can save their lives!

45. Answer: C

Nursing Process: Assessment

Rationale: **Blunt cardiac injury or ischemia to myocardial tissue or the conduction system could cause dysrhythmias and affect cardiac output. This is the most common cause of trauma-related cardiogenic shock, and goal-directed therapy includes inotropic support, antidysrhythmic medications, and correction of the underlying cause.** Uncontrolled external hemorrhage would result in hypovolemic shock. Pneumothorax and cardiac tamponade would cause obstructive shock. Spinal cord injury and loss of vascular tone would result in neurogenic shock.

46. Answer: D

Nursing Process: Evaluation

Rationale: **An Osborn wave, also called a J wave, is an extra positive deflection between the QRS and the ST segment that accompanies hypothermia. It has nothing to do with cardiac reperfusion status post thrombolytic administration.** Patients who have a successful reperfusion will have relief of chest pain and ST-segment normalization. The most common reperfusion dysrhythmia is accelerated idioventricular.

47. Answer: C

Nursing Process: Assessment

Rationale: **Peripheral venous thrombosis (also known as deep vein thrombosis or DVT) is an occlusion of a vein by a thrombus restricting blood outflow. The majority of DVTs involves the lower extremities and triggers include hypercoagulable/immobility states such as cancer, pregnancy, sepsis, surgery, and/or trauma. Signs and symptoms vary, but include swelling, pain, tenderness, and warm, red, or discolored skin.** Post-thrombotic syndrome is considered the most common long-term complication of a DVT and manifests up to 2 years later as chronic venous insufficiency varying from minor leg discomfort or swelling up to venous claudication and skin ulcerations. Thromboangiitis obliterans or Buerger's disease is an occlusive, chronic, inflammatory disorder of the arteries, veins, and surrounding nerves that triggers decreased blood flow in the hands and feet, resulting in ischemia and pain. Intermittent claudication and decreased or absent peripheral pulses lead to ulcers, and gangrene may develop. Raynaud's disease produces vasospasms that reduce blood flow to the arteries of the hands and feet in response to a trigger such as cold temperatures or smoking; symptoms are pallor and numbness/tingling that returns to normal after the stimulus is removed.

CENsational Pearl of Wisdom!

Lack of arterial blood flow results in a unique absence of hair on the toes of those who have this disease process!!

48. Answer: A

Nursing Process: Assessment

Rationale: **Signs and symptoms of diaphragmatic injury may not be evident initially. This rarely occurs alone and concurrent chest, abdomen, or long-bone fractures may be present; a high index of suspicion for diaphragmatic tear should be maintained along with** these other injuries so that it is not missed. Abdominal contents may herniate into the chest cavity and cause compression of the lungs and mediastinum. Although the patient may present with many signs, **Kehr's sign referred pain to the left shoulder or sub-clavicular area and dyspnea are symptoms associated with diaphragmatic injury.** Impending doom, severe chest pain, and severe dyspnea are signs and symptoms of a tension pneumothorax. Increasing restlessness, tachycardia, tachypnea, and hypoxia may occur with a pulmonary contusion. Hemothorax signs and symptoms include altered level of consciousness along with signs of shock, hypotension, tachycardia, tachypnea, and decreased breath sounds on the affected side.

49. Answer: B

Nursing Process: Intervention

Rationale: **Administration of beta-blockers will decrease heart rate and mean arterial pressure to decrease the risk of extending the injury and rupture. Calcium channel blockers and antihypertensive medications can also be used with a goal of maintaining systolic blood pressure around 100 mm Hg and a pulse rate of less than 100 beats/minute.** Vasopressors to increase blood pressure would be contraindicated. Antiarrythmics would not be necessary as prophylaxis for potential rhythm disturbances; and although antibiotics might be given, they would not be an emergent intervention.

50. Answer: C

Nursing Process: Intervention

Rationale: **The accumulation of blood or fluid in the mostly nondistensible pericardial sac compresses the heart and leads to a decrease in stroke volume and cardiac output, as well as decreased venous return and cardiac filling. A pericardiocentesis may be done to temporarily decompress the heart and allow for transfer to the operating room for definitive treatment.** A needle thoracentesis is treatment for a tension pneumothorax. Chest tube insertion is indicated for a loss of negative intrapleural pressure and subsequent collapse of a lung. Although a thoracotomy could be done to temporarily repair an open wound in the heart, a pericardiocentesis would be attempted first.

51. Answer: C

Nursing Process: Intervention

Rationale: **The mainstay of therapy for deep vein thrombosis (DVT) is anticoagulation. Following initial anticoagulation, patients with DVT are anticoagulated further; the primary objective of anticoagulation is the prevention of further thrombosis and of early and late complications** including further clot extension, acute pulmonary embolus, major bleeding, and death. Calcium channel blockers or adrenergic blocking agents and nonnarcotic analgesia is treatment for peripheral vascular disease. Inotropic support with dobutamine if 1 to 2 L of fluid does not improve blood pressure is treatment for right ventricular infarction. Anti-inflammatory agents, antipyretics, antibiotics, and colchicine are recommended treatments for pericarditis.

52. Answer: A

Nursing Process: Intervention

Rationale: **The management of an unstable narrow-complex tachycardia is immediate synchronized cardioversion at 50 to 100 joules. The American Heart Association cautions that if the symptoms are caused by the tachycardia, it is unstable and therefore requires immediate synchronized cardioversion.** Vagal maneuvers, adenosine, beta-blockers, or calcium channel blockers are recommended for stable narrow-complex tachycardias. Amiodarone 150 mg over 10 minutes is indicated for stable wide-QRS tachycardia.

53. Answer: D

Nursing Process: Intervention

Rationale: **Synchronized cardioversion uses a sensor to deliver a shock that avoids delivery during cardiac repolarization, a period of vulnerability during which a shock can precipitate ventricular fibrillation. There will likely be a delay before the defibrillator delivers a synchronized shock because the device will look for the peak of the R wave in the QRS complex and avoid cardiac repolarization, represented by the T wave on the electrocardiogram (ECG).** With unsynchronized shocks, the shock will be delivered as soon as the operator pushes the shock button, and these shocks should use higher energy levels. Unsynchronized shocks are recommended when polymorphic ventricular fibrillation is present. Remember to read your questions very carefully. There is a huge difference between synchronized and unsynchronized shocks! Read every word in both the stem and the options! Also, when delivering synchronized shocks, the nurse must hold the buttons down until the shock is actually delivered.

 CENsational Pearl of Wisdom!

Remember to read your questions very carefully. There is a huge difference between synchronized and unsynchronized shocks! Read every word in both the stem and the options! Also, when delivering synchronized shocks, the nurse must hold the buttons down until the shock is actually delivered.

54. Answer: A

Nursing Process: Intervention

Rationale: **The American Heart Association recommends elevating the head of the bed to reduce cerebral edema, aspiration, and ventilator-associated pneumonia immediately after return of spontaneous circulation (ROSC).** Although 100% oxygen may have been used during the initial resuscitation, the lowest oxygen level needed to achieve an arterial oxygen saturation of 94% to 99% is recommended to avoid potential oxygen toxicity. Avoidance of hyperventilation is recommended by the American Heart Association standards. Targeted temperature management (TTM) is the only intervention demonstrated to improve neurologic recovery, and administration of cold fluids may be helpful for initial induction of hypothermia.

55. Answer: B

Nursing Process: Analysis

Rationale: **Common causes of supraventricular tachycardia include hypoxia, ischemia, heart failure, myocardial infarction, mitral valve prolapse, caffeine, alcohol, recreational drugs, and hyperthyroidism.** Digoxin, beta-blockers, calcium channel blockers, increased vagal tone on the sinoatrial node, and myocardial ischemia or infarction (depending on the vessel occluded) are common causes of sinus pause or sinus arrest. Hypertension, atherosclerosis, chronic cocaine use, and cardiac surgery may lead to aortic aneurysm. Thrombosis, vasospasm, cocaine use, and chemotherapeutic agents, as well as serotonin receptor agonists are risk factors for ST-elevation myocardial infarction.

56. Answer: B

Nursing Process: Assessment

Rationale: **Fatigue, dyspnea on exertion, orthopnea, and edema are symptoms of dilated cardiomyopathy and reflect the left ventricle's inability to pump blood effectively, causing reduced cardiac output. Common current or preexisting conditions include hypertension, angina, coronary artery disease, anemia, thyroid dysfunction, or breast cancer.** Hypertensive emergency presents with symptoms indicating organ damage such as ischemic stroke (with symptoms such as aphasia or loss of sensation or power of an extremity), encephalopathy, signs of myocardial infarction such as chest pain and changes on the electrocardiogram, or pulmonary edema. Fever, night sweats, arthralgia, dyspnea, cough, and chest pain are symptoms of infective endocarditis. The clinical triad of hypotension, clear lung sounds, and increased jugular venous pressure are suggestive of right ventricular infarction and indicates the right ventricle's inability to pump venous blood efficiently into the pulmonary vasculature, thereby reducing blood flow to the left ventricle.

57. Answer: C

Nursing Process: Intervention

Rationale: **In acute arterial occlusion, the objectives are to preserve limb and life, and prevent recurrent thrombosis or embolism. Anticoagulation may prevent clot extension, recurrent embolization, venous thrombosis, microthrombi distal to the obstruction, and reocclusion after reperfusion. The vascular surgeon will choose between catheter-directed intra-arterial thrombolysis, percutaneous mechanical thrombectomy, and revascularization with percutaneous transluminal angioplasty or standard surgery for definitive treatment.** Lifestyle changes such as smoking cessation, daily exercise, health diet, and control of blood pressure would be important teaching before discharge, but not first-line treatment. Compression leg garments, exercise, and preventing tissue injury are treatments for chronic venous insufficiency. Anticoagulation, ambulation, rest, and D-dimer and other laboratory studies would be indicated for venous thromboembolism treatment.

58. Answer: D

Nursing Process: Evaluation

Rationale: **The drug of choice for stable narrow-complex tachycardia is Adenocard (adenosine). This medication will cause a short period of asystole before conversion to normal sinus rhythm.** The other options are not expected outcomes.

 CENsational Pearl of Wisdom!

When giving Adenocard (adenosine), be sure to place the intravenous access in the AC space. Adenocard has a very short half-life and must be given extremely fast. Two nurses are needed to push this medication, one to push the Adenocard quickly at the closest port and one to push 20–30 mL of normal saline behind it to get it into the circulation as soon as possible. Raise the arm and run normal saline fluids wide open after the administration. Inform the patient (and any family members in the room) that there will be a short period of uncomfortableness. Be present for the patient. Hold the patient's hand because this period of asystole is very distressing. Normal sinus rhythm should occur after a brief—about 6 seconds—period of time. Family members can become very upset if they are not prepared for the aystolic period.

59. Answer: C

Nursing Process: Assessment

Rationale: **Cardiac resynchronization therapy (CRT) uses biventricular pacemakers to treat the conduction defects or ventricular dyssynchrony that cause uncoordinated contraction of the ventricles, thereby increasing cardiac output. Studies have shown that CRT is safe and effective, with patients demonstrating significant improvement in clinical symptoms, functional status, exercise capacity, quality of life, and reduction of sudden cardiac death.** Pacemakers are electronic devices that deliver low-voltage electrical stimuli to relieve or prevent symptomatic bradycardia. Ventricular assist devices (VADs) are extracorporeal mechanical pumps implanted to either assist or replace the function of either the right or left ventricle either as temporary placement as a bridge-to-transplant until a heart becomes available or as long-term support (destination therapy). An implantable cardioverter defibrillator (ICD) delivers shocks to terminate ventricular fibrillation or to convert ventricular tachycardia.

60. Answer: A

Nursing Process: Intervention

Rationale: **The standard of care, initially set by the American Heart Association, recommends door-to-needle time of 30 minutes for fibrinolytic therapy and door-to-balloon time of 90 minutes for percutaneous coronary perfusion in recognition that reperfusion therapy reduces mortality and saves heart muscle; the shorter the time to reperfusion, the greater the benefit. A 47% reduction in mortality was noted when fibrinolytic therapy was provided in the first hour after onset of symptoms.** The time limit for fibrinolytic administration is onset of symptoms within 12 hours, not 24. Percutaneous coronary intervention (PCI) can be offered to patients presenting to non–PCI-capable centers if PCI can be initiated within 2 hours of first medical contact, not 3 hours. Fibrinolytics are generally not recommended for patients presenting more than 12 hours after onset of symptoms.

 CENsational Pearl of Wisdom!

Remember that troponin stays elevated for a longer period of time—up to 10 days—when considering the cardiac biomarkers. CK-MB (creatinine kinase-muscle/brain) is also used, but troponin has greater specificity and sensitivity.

61. Answer: C

Nursing Process: Analysis

Rationale: **ST elevation myocardial infarction (STEMI) is characterized by ST-segment elevation in two or more contiguous leads and threshold values of J-point elevation greater than 2 mm in leads V_2 and V_3 and 1 mm or more in all other leads.** This is ST elevation, not peaked or inverted waves; tall T waves can signify hyperkalemia, cerebrovascular injury, and left ventricular volume loads resulting from mitral or aortic regurgitation. T-wave inversion can have various causes including ischemia or evolving myocardial infarction or cerebrovascular accidents. Pathologic Q waves appear within 24 hours of infarct at greater than 0.04 seconds in duration or greater than 25% of the R wave in depth. These indicate necrosis in the heart muscle and can be permanent.

62. Answer: C

Nursing Process: Analysis

Rationale: **An abrupt and transient loss of consciousness might indicate long QT syndrome in young people.** Symptoms in the young athlete that are suggestive of QT prolongation include exercise-induced palpitations, chest pains, syncope, and dizziness. Intense exercise can trigger arrhythmogenic sudden cardiac death (SCD) in student-athletes with occult cardiac disease. Risk assessment guidelines from the American Heart Association and American College of Cardiology advocate the use of a 14-point pre-participation history and physical examination, including eliciting information regarding unexplained syncope or near-syncope. Arteriosclerotic changes in the aorta may make it difficult to palpate pulses in the aging population but not in the young athlete.

63. Answer: B

Nursing Process: Assessment

Rationale: **Pulsus paradoxus, a fall in systolic pressure of more than 10 mm Hg during inspiration, is considered pathologic and caused by decreased venous return. Pulses paradoxus is detected by noting the difference between the systolic blood pressure at which the Korotkoff sounds are first heard during expiration and the systolic blood pressure at which the Korotkoff sounds are heard with each beat, independent of the respiratory phase. Pulsus paradoxus is a sign of pericardial tamponade, but it also may be present with pulmonary embolus, hemorrhagic shock, severe obstructive lung disease, or tension pneumothorax.** Pulsus alternans is defined by the beat-to-beat variability of the pulse amplitude and occurs in severe aortic regurgitation, hypertension, and hypovolemic states. A difference of less than 10 mm Hg between simultaneous BP measurements in both arms is a normal finding. A fall in blood pressure of more than 20 mm Hg systolic when moving from supine to standing position is the definition of orthostatic hypotension and may occur in patients with diabetes and Parkinson's disease and depends on age, hydration, medications, food, conditioning, and ambient temperature and humidity.

64. Answer: B

Nursing Process: Assessment

Rationale: **Myocarditis is characterized by inflammation and destruction of myocardial tissue with viruses being the predominant cause in North America. Fever, myalgias, headache, sinus tachycardia, and electrocardiogram (ECG) changes including nonspecific ST–T-wave changes are common symptoms.** The most common symptom of acute pericarditis is sharp or stabbing precordial or retrosternal chest pain. Referral of pain to the left trapezoidal ridge is a distinguishing feature. Chest pain may be aggravated by inspiration or movement and relieved when sitting up and leaning forward. A pericardial friction rub is the most common and important physical finding in pericarditis. Bacteria are the predominant cause of endocarditis and most cases occur with a predisposing identifiable cardiac structural abnormality, prosthetic valve, or a recognized risk factor such as intravenous drug use, intravascular devices, poor dental hygiene, and hemodialysis or human immunodeficiency virus (HIV).

 CENsational Pearl of Wisdom!

Tachycardia that is disproportionate to the degree of fever should alert the clinician to the possibility of myocarditis. In severe cases, heart failure can develop. Treatment is supportive, although antibiotics are needed for myocarditis complicating rheumatic fever, diphtheria, or meningococcemia.

65. Answer: C

Nursing Process: Assessment

Rationale: **Hypertension is the primary risk factor for acute aortic dissections, seen in 72% of cases. Patients tend to be 60- to 80-year-old men and were significantly more likely to have atherosclerosis.** The incidence of aortic injury is estimated between 1.5% and 2% of patients who sustain blunt thoracic trauma. Aortic instrumentation or cardiac surgery can be complicated by aortic dissection, but is reported at 2% of patients. Cocaine use, which may cause a transient hypertension due to catecholamine release, accounted for 37% of dissections in a report of an inner-city population.

66. Answer: B

Nursing Process: Intervention

Rationale: **Labetalol (Normodyne) is a beta-blocker that is used to decrease the blood pressure in hypertensive disorders.** It is contraindicated in patients with heart failure, bradycardias, and reactive airway disease.

CENsational Pearl of Wisdom!

Some medications were meant to be given slowly. Be careful with medications that have the potential to significantly lower blood pressure and pulse rates. It is also a good practice to take vital signs during the process of administering medications such as labetalol (Normodyne) and diltiazem (Cardizem) so that every effort is taken to document that proper precautions were taken during the administration.

67. Answer: D

Nursing Process: Intervention

Rationale: **The administration of nitroprusside (Nipride) can cause cyanide toxicity. Nipride itself contains five cyanide groups and a nitrous oxide group. When placed into contact with blood, it can react with hemoglobin to produce thiocyanate and cyanide.** This usually happens with high doses or prolonged use. Nitroprusside works through the process of vasodilation to reduce blood pressure and is therefore used in hypertensive situations that require immediate attention. Nitroprusside does not have any association with asthma or restless leg syndrome.

68. Answer: A

Nursing Process: Intervention

Rationale: **Opioids and diuretics as well as nitrates should be avoided with a right ventricular infarction because of their preload reducing effects which will reduce cardiac output further and result in hypotension. Instead, these patients should be treated with volume loading with boluses of fluid and, if that fails, inotropic support with dobutamine.** Aspirin, clopidogrel, and statin therapy should be given to these patients and atropine, dopamine, or dobutamine if needed.

69. Answer: A

Nursing Process: Evaluation

Rationale: **Raynaud's phenomenon is a circulatory disease of the arteries that severely reduces blood flow as the result of episodic intense vasospasm of the digits in response to extreme cold, emotional stress, and/or smoking. Treatment is aimed at decreasing pain and vasospastic events. The patient should be advised to keep warm, wear gloves, not smoke, and avoid cold medicines and diet pills due to their vasoconstrictive effects.** Elevating the arm and applying ice would worsen the vasoconstriction. Wrist splints or applying an elastic bandage would not help and may increase vasoconstriction. Fluids and aspirin would not help.

70. Answer: C

Nursing Process: Assessment

Rationale: **ST-segment elevation in leads V_1, V_2, and V_3 are indicative of damage to the anterior aspect of the heart. These leads look directly at the anterior heart wall.** Inferior myocardial infarctions are noted with changes in leads II, III, and AVF. The lateral leads are I, AVL, V_5, and V_6. Posterior MIs are noted as reciprocal changes in the anterior leads—V_1 and V_2. To see the ST-segment elevation changes in this MI, posterior leads—V_7, V_8, and V_9 would need to be performed.

CENsational Pearl of Wisdom!

Posterior leads are accomplished by taking leads V_4, V_5, and V_6 and placing them on the left posterior aspect to create V_7, V_8, and V_9. These should be on the same plane as the original V_6. V_7 is placed at the posterior axillary line, V_8 at the tip of the scapula, and V_9 at the left spinal border. Relabel these leads as the graph paper exits the machine—V_4 is now V_7; V_5 is now V_8; V_6 is now V_9. ST-segment elevation should now be seen in these leads if a posterior MI is in progress.

71. Answer: B

Nursing Process: Analysis

Rationale: **A right-sided electrocardiogram (ECG) is performed when concern is present for a right ventricular infarct.** V_4R to V_6R are the leads that will show the ST-segment elevation, with V_4R being the best. The lead placement for V_4R is in the fifth intercostal space at the right midclavicular line. The left side is mimicked on the right side of the chest. Lead placement in the fourth intercostal space at the left sternal border and at the right sternal border would be proper placement for V_1 and V_2. A lead placed at the fifth intercostal space posterior axillary line would be correct for the posterior lead, V_7.

CENsational Pearl of Wisdom!

Be sure to label the ECG as "right sided" and label the leads as V_1R, V_2R, V_3R, V_4R, V_5R, and V_6R. Often, only V_4R is done because this lead demonstrates the ST elevation best.

72. Answer: D

Nursing Process: Analysis

Rationale: **Pericarditis occurs due to a viral infection that may have started as a respiratory infection.** The clinical cardiovascular consequences of cocaine use include hypertensive crises, acute myocardial infarction (AMI), aortic dissection, myocarditis, and stroke. Cocaine is a powerful sympathomimetic that increases heart rate, mean arterial pressure, and left ventricular contractility by stimulation of both alpha- and beta-adrenergic receptors. Cocaine use causes coronary artery vasospasm and also causes vasoconstriction, which enhances the development of hypertension.

73. Answer: D

Nursing Process: Analysis

Rationale: **The most common and concerning electrolyte abnormality associated with acute digoxin toxicity is hyperkalemia that occurs due to the binding affinity for digoxin on the Na/K pump site on each cell.** Hyponatremia, hypercalcemia, and hypomagnesemia are not electrolyte disturbances that occur with digoxin toxicity.

CENsational Pearl of Wisdom!

Digoxin has been shown to reduce mortality and hospitalization in older patients with heart failure; however, the therapeutic window is narrowed in older adults. Because of decreases in renal elimination, glomerular filtration rate, and body mass, lower doses of digoxin are generally required. The therapeutic serum concentration of digoxin is 0.5 to 0.9 ng/mL.

74. Answer: D

Nursing Process: Intervention

Rationale: **An infant with a patent ductus arteriosus can become seriously harmed with the application of high-dose oxygen in the presence of a low pulse oximetry reading. Oxygen can close the ductus arteriosus before the required surgery has been performed.** These infants become "ductal dependent" and hyperoxia can create a deadly situation. Formula and breast milk have no bearing on a patent ductus arteriosus, and all babies should be kept warm.

CENsational Pearl of Wisdom!

Always listen to parents of infants who have chronic illness or congenital anomalies! When caring for infants with congenital heart defects, ask the parents: "What is normal for your baby?" They will know! A baby with a patent ductus arteriosus may have a normal pulse oximetry reading in the 60s or 70s. If a patent ductus arteriosus becomes closed prematurely, the medication to use is PSE or prostaglandin E. This will dilate the ductus open and reestablish the patency. This is given as a continuous infusion and should not be piggybacked into another line. Maximal effects will be seen within 30 minutes.

75. Answer: C

Nursing Process: Analysis

Rationale: **Traumatic thoracic injury can cause aortic injury and the tear most commonly occurs at the ligamentum arteriosum (80% to 90%).** This is a band of tissue that forms about 3 weeks after birth and is a vestige of the fetal ductus arteriosus. It connects the aorta to the pulmonary artery and when torn has usually fatal outcomes. If a complete tear does not occur and the adventitial layer of the vessel (the outermost layer) remains intact, an aneurysm can develop.

References

Abbott. (2015, March). *Magnet use for St. Jude medical pacemakers.* Retrieved July 29, 2018 from https://professional.sjm.com/~/media/pro/resources/emi/med-dental/FL-ICD-Magnet-Placement-042013.ashx. (28)

American Heart Association. (2015). Cardiac arrest. In M. Ralston (Ed.), *Pediatric advanced life support.* Dallas, TX: Author. Retrieved July 20, 2018, from (10, 19)

American Heart Association. (2016). Advanced cardiac life support provider manual. Dallas, TX: Author. (2, 12–15, 18, 21, 24, 36, 43, 52–54, 60, 61, 66)

American Heart Association. (2017). ACLS for experienced providers: Manual and resource text. Dallas, TX: Author. (2–4, 11–15, 18, 20, 24, 28)

Berul, C. I. (2018, June 11). Acquired long QT syndrome: Clinical manifestations, diagnosis and management. UpToDate. Retrieved August 26, 2018, from https://www.uptodate.com/contents/acquired-long-qt-syndrome-clinical-manifestations-diagnosis-and-management (42, 44)

Black, J. H., III, et al. (2018, February 1). Clinical features and diagnosis of acute aortic dissection. UpToDate. Waltham, MA: Wolters Kluwer. Retrieved August 12, 2018, from https://www.uptodate.com/contents/clinical-features-and-diagnosis-of-acute-aortic-dissection (32, 65)

Braun, J. D. (2018, January 2). Embolism to the lower extremities. UpToDate. Retrieved September 2, 2018, from https://www.uptodate.com/contents/embolism-to-the-lower-extremities (57)

Chopra, A. C. (2016). Arterial occlusion. In J. E. Tintinalli (Ed.), Tintinalli's emergency medicine: A comprehensive study guide (8th ed.). New York, NY: McGraw-Hill. (14, 57, 62, 64, 68)

Claudia, D. (2017). Right ventricular infarction clinical presentation. the Heart.org, Medscape. Retrieved from https://emedicine.medscape.com/article/157961-clinical#b3 (10)

De Laby, M. (2018). Toxicologic emergencies. In V. Sweet (Ed.), Emergency nursing core curriculum (7th ed., pp. 404–436). Philadelphia, PA: Elsevier. (72, 73)

Denke, N. J. (2018). Nursing assessment and resuscitation. In V. Sweet (Ed.), Emergency nursing core curriculum (7th ed., pp. 1–22). Philadelphia, PA: Elsevier. (10, 62)

Denno, J. (2018). Invasive hemodynamic monitoring. In V. Sweet (Ed.), Emergency nursing core curriculum (7th ed., pp. 70–79). Philadelphia, PA: Elsevier. (43, 75)

DrugBank. (2018). Nitroprusside. Retrieved from https://www.drugbank.ca/drugs/DB00325 (67)

Drugs.com. (2018). Labetalol. Retrieved from https://www.drugs.com/pro/labetalol.html (66)

Emergency Nurses Association. (2013). Emergency nursing pediatric course. Des Plaines, IL: Mosby. (10, 19, 74)

Emergency Nurses Association. (2013). ENA's Transition Into Practice: Right sided and posterior electrocardiograms (ECGs). Retrieved from https://www.ena.org/docs/default-source/resource-library/practice-resources/tips/right-side-ecg.pdf?sfvrsn=836f00e6_8 (70, 71)

Emergency Nurses Association. (2013). Sheehy's manual of emergency care. St. Louis, MO: Elsevier Mosby. (3, 9, 11–14, 20, 22–26, 28, 29, 31,32, 34, 37, 38, 41, 44, 46, 48, 49, 50, 51, 57, 62, 63, 68, 70–73)

French, A., et al. (2018). Cardiac manifestations of HIV/AIDS. In G. N. Levine (Ed.), Cardiac secrets (5th ed., pp. 407–412). Philadelphia, PA: Elsevier. (72)

Gannon, S. A. (2018). Cardiovascular complications of rheumatic diseases. In G. N. Levine (Ed.), Cardiology secrets (5th ed., pp. 413–418). Philadelphia, PA: Elsevier. (72)

Goldberger, A. L. (2018, July 7). Goldbergs clinical electrocardiography (9th ed.). Philadelphia, PA: Elsevier. (7)

Habib, G. B. (2018). Hypertension. In G. N. Levine (Ed.), Cardiology secrets (5th ed., pp. 369–376). Philadelphia, PA: Elsevier. (71)

Haynes, A. (2018). Cardiovascular disorders. In L. D. Urden (Ed.), Critical care nursing diagnosis and management (8th ed., pp. 290–358). St. Louis, MO: Elsevier. (1, 29)

Holleran, R. S. (2018). Shock emergencies. In Emergency nursing core curriculum (7th ed., pp. 473–482). Philadelphia, PA: Elsevier. Retrieved September 15, 2018, from (36–38, 45, 46, 58)

Imazio, M. (2017, October 27). Acute pericarditis: Clinical presentation and diagnostic evaluation. UpToDate. Watham, MA: Wolters Kluwer. Retrieved August 12, 2018, from https://www.uptodate.com/contents/acute-pericarditis-clinical-presentation-and-diagnostic-evaluation (33)

Kane, R. L., et al. (Eds.). (2018). Cardiovascular disorders. In Essentials of clinical geriatrics (8th ed.). New York, NY: The McGraw-Hill Companies, Inc. Retrieved September 15, 2018, from (73, 74)

Kuman, A. A. (2019). Hypertensive crises. In P. E. K. Parsons (Ed.), Critical care secrets (6th ed., pp. 295–301). Philadelphia, PA: Elsevier. (71, 72)

Levin, T. (2017, October 23). Right ventricular myocardial infarction. UpToDate. Retrieved September 9, 2018, from https://www.uptodate.com/contents/right-ventricular-myocardial-infarction (68)

Lip, G. Y. (2017, October 2). Hemodynamic consequences of atrial fibrillation and cardioversion to sinus rhythm. UpToDate. Watham, MA: Wolters Kluwer. Retrieved July 22, 2018, from https://www.uptodate.com/contents/hemodynamic-consequences-of-atrial-fibrillation-and-cardioversion-to-sinus-rhythm (17, 52)

Lip, G. Y. (2018, July 23). Overview of the treatment of lower extremity deep vein thrombosis. UpToDate. Retrieved September 1, 2018, from https://www.uptodate.com/contents/overview-of-the-treatment-of-lower-extremity-deep-vein-thrombosis-dvt (51)

Livingston, D. H., et al. (2016). Thoracic wall injuries. In J. A. Asensio (Ed.), *Current therapy of trauma and surgical critical care* (2nd ed., pp. 205–228). Philadelphia, PA: Elsevier. (32)

McCaslin, L., et al. (2017). Chest trauma. In C. K. Stone, & R. L. Humphries (Eds.), *Current diagnosis & treatment: Emergency medicine* (8th ed.). New York, NY: McGraw-Hill Education. (9, 23, 25, 28, 50)

McGrath, J., et al. (Eds.). (2017). Emergency nursing certification self-assessment and exam review. New York, NY: McGraw-Hill Education. (6, 7, 13–15, 23–25, 29, 50, 51, 54, 55, 57, 58)

Michael, M. R., et al. (2014). Thoracic and neck trauma. In *TNCC trauma nursing core course provider manual* (7th ed., pp. 137–148). Des Plaines, IL: Emergency Nurses Association. (5, 9, 11, 32, 36–38, 40, 43, 45, 48, 49, 50, 51, 75)

Navarroli, J. E. (2018). Cardiovascular emergencies. In V. Sweet (Ed.), *Emergency nursing core curriculum* (7th ed., pp. 142–182). St. Louis, MO: Elsevier. (1, 5, 7, 12–14, 23–26, 28–30, 32, 34, 35, 37, 38, 40, 41, 43–57, 59, 60–65, 67–73)

Neschis, D. G. (2018, May 31). *Management of blunt thoracic aortic injury.* UpToDate. Retrieved August 31, 2018, from https://www.uptodate.com/contents/management-of-blunt-thoracic-aortic-injury (49)

Shen, T. A. (2019). Ventricular assist device. In P. E. K. Parsons (Ed.), *Critical care secrets* (6th ed., pp. 114–119). Philadelphia, PA: Elsevier. (59)

Taghavi, S., et al. (2018). Hypovolemic shock. Treasure Island, FL: StatPearls. Retrieved from https://www.ncbi.nlm.nih.gov/books/NBK513297/ (37)

The Heart.org & Medscape. (2018). *Adenocard (RX).* Retrieved from https://reference.medscape.com/drug/adenocard-adenoscan-adenosine-342295 (58)

Upadhyaya, R. C. (2015). Cardiovascular function. In S. E. Meiner, & S. E. Meiner (Eds.), *Gerontologic nursing* (5th ed., pp. 388–421). St. Louis, MO: Elsevier Mosby. (10, 22, 25)

Urden, L. D. (2018). Critical care nursing diagnosis and management (8th ed., pp. 290–358). Maryland Heights, MO: Elsevier. (28)

Virk, F. M. (2018). Cocaine and the heart. In G. N. Levine (Ed.), *Cardiology secrets* (5th ed., pp. 425–430). Philadelphia, PA: Elsevier. (72)

Walls, R., et al. (2018). Rosen's emergency medicine concepts and clinical practice (9th ed., Vol. 1). Philadelphia, PA: Elsevier. (57, 63, 64, 68, 69, 71)

Wigley, F. M. (2018). *Treatment of the Raynaud phenomenon resistant to initial therapy.* UpToDate. Retrieved from https://www.uptodate.com/contents/treatment-of-the-raynaud-phenomenon-resistant-to-initial-therapy (35)

Yip, A., et al. (2015). Spontaneous coronary artery dissection—A review. *Cardiovascular Diagnosis and Therapy, 5*(1), 37–48. Retrieved from https://www.ncbi.nlm.nih.gov/pmc/articles/PMC4329168/ (39)

Zipes, D. P. (2019). Braunwald's heart disease: A textbook of cardiovascular medicine (11th ed.). Philadelphia, PA: Elsevier. (2, 7, 10, 12–18, 22, 23, 25, 27–29, 34, 41, 44, 59, 60–64, 71, 73)

13 Gastrointestinal Emergencies

Patricia L. Clutter, RN, MEd, CEN, FAEN

On the test, gastrointestinal (GI) emergencies are included in the blueprint under "GI /GU/OB/ GYN," and this portion of the actual test will comprise 21 questions spread across the spectrum of illnesses and injuries that afflict these systems. To prepare for the test effectively, this chapter will focus on potential test items related to the GI system.

Each of the following questions will be utilized both as a testing tool *and* as a teaching tool in the answer pages! Rationales for each correct answer and untrue answers are part of the teaching process. Additional information has been supplied in various areas.

1. Which of the following assessment parameters should be accomplished last?
[ ] **A.** Auscultation
[ ] **B.** Percussion
[ ] **C.** Palpation
[ ] **D.** Inspection

2. Which of the following medications would the emergency nurse anticipate to be prescribed for a patient presenting with a potential esophageal foreign body?
[ ] **A.** Maalox
[ ] **B.** Cimetidine (Zantac)
[ ] **C.** Omeprazole (Prilosec)
[ ] **D.** Glucagon

3. A patient presents with acute onset of right upper quadrant pain and severe nausea after eating at a local fast-food restaurant. The patient also has pain to the right subclavicular area. The pain rating is 8 out of 10. Which of the following medications would the emergency nurse anticipate to **NOT** be prescribed for this patient?
[ ] **A.** Hydromorphone (Dilaudid)
[ ] **B.** Morphine sulfate
[ ] **C.** Fentanyl (Sublimaze)
[ ] **D.** Meperidine (Demerol)

4. Which of the following laboratory values would most likely be decreased in a patient diagnosed with pancreatitis?
[ ] **A.** Lipase
[ ] **B.** Amylase
[ ] **C.** Calcium
[ ] **D.** Glucose

5. A finding of free air under the diaphragm in a patient complaining of abdominal pain and fever would most likely correlate with which of the following diagnoses?
[ ] **A.** Intestinal obstruction
[ ] **B.** Acute appendicitis
[ ] **C.** Intestinal perforation
[ ] **D.** Acute cholelithiasis

6. A patient is being treated for an acute ruptured diverticulum. Which of the following interventions would **NOT** be appropriate?
[ ] **A.** Inserting a nasogastric (NG) tube
[ ] **B.** Offering oral clear liquids
[ ] **C.** Administering intravenous antibiotics
[ ] **D.** Preparation of patient for surgery

7. A diagnostic peritoneal lavage is being performed on a patient with blunt injury to the abdomen. Which of the following must be in place before this procedure?
[ ] **A.** Urinary catheter
[ ] **B.** Endotracheal tube
[ ] **C.** Intravenous access
[ ] **D.** Oxygen cannula

8. Which of the following statements made by the emergency nurse assisting with a diagnostic peritoneal lavage (DPL) would indicate an understanding of the procedure?

[ ] **A.** "If we hear a 'whoosh' of air when it's put in that means it's positive."

[ ] **B.** "If blood is coming out of the catheter then that is a positive test."

[ ] **C.** "If nothing comes out then it must mean it's negative for sure."

[ ] **D.** "If gastric contents are detected, that is a good sign of no injury."

9. A patient is being evaluated for abdominal pain and multiple episodes of coffee ground emesis. Which of the following would be the most important piece of history provided by the patient?

[ ] **A.** Recent intake of fried food

[ ] **B.** Nonsteroidal anti-inflammatory drug (NSAID) use

[ ] **C.** Oral iron supplements ingestion

[ ] **D.** Diagnosis of alcoholic hepatic disease

10. A patient with a past history of intravenous substance abuse presents with confusion, abdominal distension, and bilateral icteric conjunctiva. Lactulose (Cholac) is prescribed for this patient. Which of the following laboratory values would be monitored to determine the effect of the lactulose?

[ ] **A.** Ammonia

[ ] **B.** Magnesium

[ ] **C.** Potassium

[ ] **D.** Sodium

11. Which of the following would be a possible indicator of an underlying primary diagnosis of pancreatitis?

[ ] **A.** Amylase in thoracentesis fluid

[ ] **B.** Hypoglycemic event

[ ] **C.** Increased calcium

[ ] **D.** Coffee ground emesis

12. All of the following medications could be utilized to treat pancreatitis **EXCEPT**:

[ ] **A.** dicyclomine (Bentyl).

[ ] **B.** fentanyl (Sublimaze).

[ ] **C.** octreotide (Sandostatin).

[ ] **D.** famotidine (Pepcid).

13. Which of the following is a nonmechanical cause of a bowel obstruction?

[ ] **A.** Foreign body

[ ] **B.** Ileus

[ ] **C.** Intussusception

[ ] **D.** Volvulus

14. Which of the following is most symptomatic for appendicitis?

[ ] **A.** Presence of ecchymosis to the periumbilical area

[ ] **B.** Right lower abdominal pain during palpation of left lower abdomen

[ ] **C.** Reddish discoloration to the right flank area

[ ] **D.** Tympany noted to palpation of generalized abdominal area

15. A patient is being assessed for possible intraperitoneal bleeding after a motor vehicle crash (MVC). Which of the following would be the most sensitive for the diagnosis of pancreatic injury?

[ ] **A.** Focused Assessment with Sonography for Trauma (FAST) examination

[ ] **B.** Flat plate of abdomen and chest radiograph

[ ] **C.** Computerized Tomography (CT) of the abdomen

[ ] **D.** Diagnostic Peritoneal Lavage (DPL)

16. A patient presents to the emergency department following a fall from a porch 3 days before. He is pale and diaphoretic and states that he feels short of breath. On assessment, he has tenderness to the right lower anterior ribs. Bilateral, clear, equal breath sounds are present. Vital signs are as follows:

Blood pressure—88/62 mm Hg

Pulse—134 beats/minute

Respirations—32 breaths/minute

Pulse oximetry—92% on room air

Temperature—98.4° F (36.8° C)

Which of the following diagnoses should the emergency nurse anticipate?

[ ] **A.** Splenic injury

[ ] **B.** Colon injury

[ ] **C.** Cardiac injury

[ ] **D.** Liver injury

17. Which of the following patients would be at highest risk for dehydration?

[ ] **A.** A 30-year-old with vomiting three times in past 12 hours

[ ] **B.** A 6-month-old with report of two wet diapers in 24 hours

[ ] **C.** An 80-year-old with noted tented skin on forearms for 48 hours

[ ] **D.** A 15-year-old with 220 mL urine output in 4 hours

18. A 14-month-old infant with vomiting and diarrhea has been prescribed a fluid bolus for treatment of dehydration. The child weighs 20 pounds. Which of the following is the correct bolus amount?
[ ] **A.** 900 ml
[ ] **B.** 180 ml
[ ] **C.** 200 ml
[ ] **D.** 400 ml

19. Which of the following would be considered to be a normal finding in an abdominal assessment?
[ ] **A.** Low-pitched regular bowel sounds
[ ] **B.** Tympany on percussion
[ ] **C.** Bruit heard on auscultation
[ ] **D.** Pulsations noted on inspection

20. Which of the following is the correct type of pain that is associated with pancreatitis?
[ ] **A.** Primary
[ ] **B.** Secondary
[ ] **C.** Referred
[ ] **D.** Somatic

21. Proton pump inhibitors are used in patients with gastroesophageal reflux disease (GERD) because of which of the following actions?
[ ] **A.** Increases lower esophageal sphincter pressure
[ ] **B.** Reduces secretions in the stomach
[ ] **C.** Lowers acid present in the stomach
[ ] **D.** Decreases the production of acid

22. Which of the following is an important landmark for the diagnosis of appendicitis?
[ ] **A.** McBurney's point
[ ] **B.** Ligament of Treitz
[ ] **C.** Cardioesophageal juncture
[ ] **D.** Sphincter of Oddi

23. Glucagon can be used for all of the following disease processes **EXCEPT**:
[ ] **A.** foreign body of the esophagus.
[ ] **B.** anaphylactic shock.
[ ] **C.** beta-blocker toxicity.
[ ] **D.** pulmonary embolism.

24. A patient is bought to the emergency department with a past history of hepatitis C, cardiac stents, and hypertension. He is vomiting large amounts of bright red blood and is nauseated. No pain is present. Based on this patient's presentation and his present symptoms, which of the following medications should the emergency nurse expect to utilize?
[ ] **A.** Octreotide (Sandostatin)
[ ] **B.** Nitroprusside (Nipride)
[ ] **C.** Amiodarone (Cordarone)
[ ] **D.** Flumazenil (Romazicon)

25. Patients with a diagnosis of pancreatitis prefer which of the following positions?
[ ] **A.** Prone
[ ] **B.** Supine
[ ] **C.** Fowler's
[ ] **D.** Fetal

26. Which of the following is **NOT** a side effect of the medication octreotide (Sandostatin)?
[ ] **A.** Hypoglycemia
[ ] **B.** Hyperglycemia
[ ] **C.** Bradycardia
[ ] **D.** Tachycardia

27. Which of the following is a true statement regarding a bowel obstruction?
[ ] **A.** Hyperactive bowel sounds can be heard in a bowel obstruction in certain situations.
[ ] **B.** Large bowel obstructions usually present with a moderate amount of abdominal swelling.
[ ] **C.** All bowel obstructions will have a fecal smell to the emesis.
[ ] **D.** A small bowel obstruction usually has a lesser amount of vomiting.

28. Which of the following is **NOT** a cause of ischemic bowel disease?
[ ] **A.** Gastroenteritis
[ ] **B.** Incarcerated hernia
[ ] **C.** Volvulus
[ ] **D.** Vasospasm

29. A patient with a history of diverticula noted on prior colonoscopies is in the emergency department with acute onset of left-sided abdominal pain. Occult blood is noted in the stool. The patient relates a subjective fever at home with chilling occurring during that day. The emergency nurse caring for this patient is aware that all of the following are potential complications for this patient **EXCEPT**:
[ ] **A.** intestinal obstruction.
[ ] **B.** perforation.
[ ] **C.** abscess.
[ ] **D.** ulcerative colitis.

30. Which of the following statements made by a patient would indicate to the emergency nurse that the "melena" stools are most likely **NOT** caused by a true gastrointestinal bleed?

[ ] **A.** "I bought some black licorice and have been eating it like crazy."

[ ] **B.** "I have been taking iron tablets for some anemia for the past 2 weeks."

[ ] **C.** "My stools are black and tarry looking and they have a different odor."

[ ] **D.** "This stuff I am vomiting up looks just like my grandpa's chew!"

31. Which of the following indicates the location of the tears that occur in Boerhaave's syndrome?

[ ] **A.** Cardioesophageal juncture

[ ] **B.** Duodenojejunal flexure

[ ] **C.** Sigmoid mesocolon

[ ] **D.** Esophageal wall

32. A patient presents to the emergency department with chief complaint of feeling weak and generalized fatigue. The patient is diaphoretic with cool skin. He states persistent nausea without vomiting. Vital signs are as follows:

Blood pressure—92/64 mm Hg
Pulse—122 beats/minute
Respirations—32 breaths/minute
Pulse oximetry—91% on room air
Temperature: 98.8° F (37.1° C)

Past history reveals hypertension, chronic bronchitis, recent history of fracture of the left 11th to 12th ribs, and hypercholesteremia. Which of the following diagnoses would the emergency nurse suspect?

[ ] **A.** Pneumonia

[ ] **B.** Pancreatitis

[ ] **C.** Splenic injury

[ ] **D.** Lacerated liver

33. Which of the following situations would cause the emergency nurse to be concerned about an increased potential severity of injury?

[ ] **A.** An 13-month-old who falls when trying to walk at home.

[ ] **B.** A 2-year-old who falls off of a dressing table at home.

[ ] **C.** A 15-year-old who falls down five rungs on a ladder.

[ ] **D.** A 25-year-old who falls off the bed of a nonmoving truck.

34. A FAST (Focused Assessment with Sonography for Trauma) examination is performed on a patient involved in a motor vehicle crash. Which of the following statements made by the emergency nurse indicates an understanding of this evaluation tool?

[ ] **A.** "I heard that this tool is great and has a 90% to 100% accuracy rating for all patients."

[ ] **B.** "This is great to use! We will have our answer for sure in a few minutes!"

[ ] **C.** "This diagnostic tool is so much better for small bowel and stomach injuries."

[ ] **D.** "This test only checks for large amounts of blood in the abdomen."

35. Which of the following would decrease the chances of abdominal organ injury in children involved in motor vehicle crashes (MVC)?

[ ] **A.** Use of a booster seat in the older child

[ ] **B.** Seat belts that lie across the abdomen

[ ] **C.** Rear-facing restrained car seats for infants

[ ] **D.** Allowing the older child to sit in the front seat

36. Which of the following would be the treatment of choice for a hemodynamically stable child who has sustained a splenic injury?

[ ] **A.** Immediate surgical intervention and repair

[ ] **B.** Removal of the spleen within 4 hours of injury

[ ] **C.** Admission and careful monitoring of the child

[ ] **D.** Discharge with instructions to return for any changes

37. A patient arrives in the emergency department after a motorcycle crash and loops of bowel are noted to be emerging from the abdominal wall. Which of the following would be the correct intervention for the emergency nurse to perform?

[ ] **A.** Place a towel over it to keep it from coming into contact with possible organisms.

[ ] **B.** Cover the organ with sterile, saline-soaked abdominal pads and keep the area moist.

[ ] **C.** Gently replace the organs back into the abdominal cavity with a tight sterile dressing.

[ ] **D.** Leave the area open to the air and do not manipulate or cover it with any type of dressing.

38. Which of the following laboratory values would be present that would necessitate the administration of *N*-acetylcysteine (Mucomyst) to a patient who is undergoing a contrast-enhanced computed tomography (CT) examination?

[ ] **A.** Elevated serum creatinine

[ ] **B.** Decreased blood urea nitrogen (BUN)

[ ] **C.** Elevated hemoglobin

[ ] **D.** Decreased potassium

39. Which of the following procedures should be delayed in a patient undergoing a FAST (Focused Assessment with Sonography for Trauma) examination?
[ ] **A.** Nasogastric tube insertion
[ ] **B.** Intravenous line insertion
[ ] **C.** Urinary catheter placement
[ ] **D.** Oxygen per nasal cannula

40. Contrast is provided to patients in different ways in order to clearly identify different organs during computed tomography (CT) examinations. Oral contrast would be necessary to visualize which of the following organs during this type of test?
[ ] **A.** Stomach
[ ] **B.** Liver
[ ] **C.** Spleen
[ ] **D.** Pancreas

41. Which of the following injuries should the emergency nurse suspect in combination with the diagnosis of lumbar region Chance fractures (also known as seatbelt fractures)?
[ ] **A.** Colon
[ ] **B.** Stomach
[ ] **C.** Spleen
[ ] **D.** Small intestine

42. Patients who have undergone splenectomies are known to be at risk for which of the following problems?
[ ] **A.** Ulcerative colitis
[ ] **B.** Immune system deficiencies
[ ] **C.** Cholelithiasis
[ ] **D.** Pancreatic cancer

43. A patient has been in the emergency department for 4 hours following a four-wheeler crash and is now complaining of severe abdominal pain. The provider caring for her states that she has a positive Cullen's sign. This sign can occur in concert with another sign known as Grey-Turner's sign. Which of the following is true regarding the similarities in these two signs?
[ ] **A.** Both occur in the periumbilical area.
[ ] **B.** Both are ecchymotic areas.
[ ] **C.** Both indicate bladder injury.
[ ] **D.** Both are present within 1 hour of injury.

44. Which of the following findings regarding bowel sounds would the emergency nurse expect to find on auscultation of the abdomen in the trauma patient with an intra-abdominal injury?
[ ] **A.** Normal
[ ] **B.** Hyperactive
[ ] **C.** Hypoactive
[ ] **D.** Shrill

45. A patient is undergoing measurement for the possibility of abdominal compartment syndrome. Which of the following would be a necessary component to complete this procedure?
[ ] **A.** Nasogastric tube
[ ] **B.** Chest tube
[ ] **C.** Intravenous line
[ ] **D.** Urinary catheter

46. When assisting with a paracentesis for a patient with cirrhosis, which of the following parameters would decrease indicating that the procedure was successful as an interventional option?
[ ] **A.** Respiratory effort
[ ] **B.** Blood pressure
[ ] **C.** Temperature
[ ] **D.** Heart rate

47. A patient is seen in the emergency department following a motor vehicle crash. He is diagnosed with a perforated stomach, a pelvic fracture, upper left arm fracture, and a mild closed head injury. Which of the following complications would the emergency nurse understand to be the highest probability to occur for this patient due to the injuries sustained?
[ ] **A.** Cardiogenic shock
[ ] **B.** Pulmonary edema
[ ] **C.** Peritonitis
[ ] **D.** Paralysis

48. A trauma patient is being seen in the emergency department and has the following values reported 30 minutes after arrival—serum lactate: 1.4 mmol/L, base deficit: −2, pH: 7.36, hemoglobin: 10.4 g/dL, and urine output: 28 mL. Which of the following reported levels received 1 hour later would indicate adequate resuscitation in an adult trauma patient?
[ ] **A.** Serum lactate level of 3.2 mmol/L
[ ] **B.** Urine output of 75 mL/hour
[ ] **C.** Base deficit of −5
[ ] **D.** Hemoglobin level of 9.6 g/dL

49. Which of the following would be the best manner to check for proper gastric tube placement?
[ ] **A.** Listen for instilled air over the epigastrium
[ ] **B.** Radiograph or computed tomography (CT) to confirm placement
[ ] **C.** pH testing of gastric aspirate
[ ] **D.** Use of carbon dioxide detector

50. When utilizing the pH method of confirmation of gastric tube placement, which of the following numbers would indicate that the tube is in the stomach?

[ ] **A.** 4.0
[ ] **B.** 8.5
[ ] **C.** 10.0
[ ] **D.** 14.5

51. An 82-year-old patient presents to the emergency department with 10 episodes of watery diarrhea starting the day prior. The patient is weak and also complains of some nausea without vomiting and subjective fever. The patient is taken to a bed and placed on which of the following types of isolation?

[ ] **A.** Droplet
[ ] **B.** Reverse
[ ] **C.** Contact
[ ] **D.** Airborne

52. Which of the following is a true statement regarding caring for individuals who are diagnosed with *Clostridium difficile* infection?

[ ] **A.** The use of alcohol-based hand cleansers is extremely useful and recommended.
[ ] **B.** Patients should remain in isolation for at least 48 hours after the last diarrhea stool.
[ ] **C.** Gowns and masks are not necessary to wear when caring for these patients.
[ ] **D.** Private rooms are not necessary when these patients are admitted for inpatient care.

53. A nurse working in the cruise industry is aware that norovirus is a particularly virulent problem in their environment for all the following reasons **EXCEPT** that:

[ ] **A.** it has a very low dose that can adequately cause infection.
[ ] **B.** it transmits very easily and is able to live in both hot and cold environments.
[ ] **C.** the average incubation time for infection passage is 6 to 8 hours.
[ ] **D.** there is no vaccine available for this viral agent to assist in containment.

54. Treatment for norovirus includes all of the following **EXCEPT**:

[ ] **A.** antibiotic therapy.
[ ] **B.** rehydration.
[ ] **C.** bed rest.
[ ] **D.** strict hand washing.

55. Which of the following would be a concern for a patient involved in a major motor vehicle crash who presents with right upper quadrant pain and has a past history of hepatitis C, COPD, and hypertension?

[ ] **A.** Respiratory distress
[ ] **B.** Uncontrolled bleeding
[ ] **C.** Hypertensive crisis
[ ] **D.** Pneumonia

56. A 3-month-old infant is brought to the emergency department by his parents with complaints of diarrhea stools for the past 2 days. The child is lethargic, pale, is noted to have retractions, and does not cry during the assessment or weight process. Which of the following acid–base disturbances would the emergency nurse suspect with this patient?

[ ] **A.** Respiratory acidosis
[ ] **B.** Respiratory alkalosis
[ ] **C.** Metabolic acidosis
[ ] **D.** Metabolic alkalosis

57. A 7-month-old infant is brought to the emergency department by her parents with a 3-day history of diarrhea. The patient is cyanotic but does not appear to be in any respiratory distress. No retractions are present. Pulse oximetry is 92% on room air, and respiratory rate is 24 breaths/minute. She is slightly lethargic but responsive and cries appropriately when the emergency nurse is examining her. Blood is drawn, which appears to have the coloration of chocolate. Oxygen is applied at 15 L/minute per blow, but this does not clear the cyanosis. Which of the following medications would the emergency nurse expect to administer to this child?

[ ] **A.** Adrenaline (Epinephrine)
[ ] **B.** Atropine
[ ] **C.** Ceftriaxone (Rocephin)
[ ] **D.** Methylene blue

58. Which of the following is **NOT** a risk factor for the development of peptic ulcers?

[ ] **A.** Long-term and high use smoking
[ ] **B.** Frequent intake of alcohol
[ ] **C.** Nonsteroidal anti-inflammatory drugs
[ ] **D.** Thyroid supplemental medications

59. Which of the following organisms is the cause of the majority of peptic ulcer disease?

[ ] **A.** *Bordetella pertussis*
[ ] **B.** Varicella-zoster virus
[ ] **C.** *Helicobacter pylori*
[ ] **D.** Human papillomavirus

60. A patient is seen in the emergency department with pain to the left upper quadrant and says he often wakes up at night with the pain. He was recently in the hospital for an extended recovery from a diagnosis of sepsis secondary to open fractures of both lower legs. He has been home for 1 week. Which of the following types of peptic ulcers does this patient most likely have?
[ ] **A.** Duodenal
[ ] **B.** Stress
[ ] **C.** Gastric
[ ] **D.** Mucosal

61. A patient arrives in the emergency department with bright red, bloody emesis. He is vomiting on arrival and continues as he is placed into a room. He is pale and diaphoretic with cold extremities. Vital signs are as follows:

Blood pressure—82/46 mm Hg
Pulse—146 beats/minute
Respirations—36 breaths/ minute
Pulse oximetry—89% on room air
Temperature—99.4° F (37.4° C)

The team starts two large-bore intravenous lines and crystalloids are begun at a rapid rate. All of the following would be anticipated by the emergency nurse **EXCEPT**:
[ ] **A.** type and screen.
[ ] **B.** gastric tube placement.
[ ] **C.** contact endoscopy.
[ ] **D.** cardiac monitoring.

62. Which of the following hemoglobin readings indicates the point at which blood replacement is recommended?
[ ] **A.** 10.2 g/dL
[ ] **B.** 9.6 g/dL
[ ] **C.** 8.4 g/dL
[ ] **D.** 7.0 g/dL

63. Which of the following is the correct action for the medication Sandostatin (octreotide) used to treat bleeding esophageal varices?
[ ] **A.** Decreases portal pressure through relaxation of mesenteric vascular smooth muscle.
[ ] **B.** Causes vasodilation of the bleeding vessels to clamp down.
[ ] **C.** Improves blood supply to the gastric mucosa to heal ulcerated areas.
[ ] **D.** Assists in production of red blood cells to replace lost blood volume.

64. Which of the following is **NOT** a risk factor for the development of cholecystitis?
[ ] **A.** Pregnancy
[ ] **B.** Caucasian
[ ] **C.** Obesity
[ ] **D.** Male

65. One of the diagnostic signs of cholecystitis is a gasp or indication of pain from the patient when the right costal arch is palpated. This occurs because the fingers of the examiner have made contact with the enlarged, inflamed gallbladder. This is known as which of the following signs?
[ ] **A.** Kehr's
[ ] **B.** Murphy's
[ ] **C.** Cullen's
[ ] **D.** Rovsing's

66. Which of the following would **NOT** be appropriate care in a patient with a diagnosis of appendicitis?
[ ] **A.** Prepare the patient for emergency surgery.
[ ] **B.** Administer broad-spectrum antibiotics.
[ ] **C.** Administer H$_2$ inhibitors.
[ ] **D.** Institute nothing by mouth (NPO).

67. Which of the following is **NOT** part of the elixir known as the GI Cocktail?
[ ] **A.** Antacid
[ ] **B.** Viscous lidocaine
[ ] **C.** Milk of magnesia
[ ] **D.** Anticholinergic

68. A Sengstaken–Blakemore tube is used for which of the following disease processes?
[ ] **A.** Cholecystitis
[ ] **B.** Diverticulitis
[ ] **C.** Pancreatitis
[ ] **D.** Esophageal varices

69. A patient presents with a large amount of abdominal distention, vomiting, and generalized abdominal pain. On assessment, the emergency nurse notes that no bowel sounds are present. The patient has a history of a temporary colostomy for a ruptured colon 5 years prior, a cholecystectomy, and appendectomy. Medical history includes hypothyroidism and hypertension. The emergency nurse realizes that this patient will be prone to all of the following potential complications **EXCEPT**:
[ ] **A.** sepsis.
[ ] **B.** pneumonia.
[ ] **C.** dehydration.
[ ] **D.** perforation.

70. A 4-month-old is brought to the emergency department by his father with symptoms of crying and drawing up his legs intermittently. The father states that the baby has been having strange stools, "They look like jelly or something like that." The emergency nurse should do which of the following regarding this child's care?
[ ] **A.** Send the patient to the waiting room.
[ ] **B.** Immediately take this patient to a room.
[ ] **C.** Reassure the father that the child is fine.
[ ] **D.** Have the father check with urgent care to be seen.

71. A mother brings her 9-week-old infant to the emergency department with abdominal distention and a 1-week history of forceful vomiting that is increasingly worse. On examination, the emergency nurse notes that the child appears dehydrated and notes a palpable mass to the right of the umbilicus. The baby has not gained weight and seems to be hungry all the time. Waves of peristalsis are noted, which move from left to right. Which of the following processes should the nurse suspect?
[ ] **A.** Reflux disease
[ ] **B.** Failure to thrive
[ ] **C.** Intussusception
[ ] **D.** Pyloric stenosis

72. A 2-year-old female child is brought to the emergency department with a distended abdomen and vomiting. Assessment reveals a lethargic toddler who does not cry when examined. The child's skin is cool and slightly diaphoretic. No bowel sounds are heard. Breath sounds are clear to auscultation. Vital signs are as follows:

Blood pressure—76/42 mm Hg
Pulse—164 beats/minute
Respirations—44 breaths/minute
Pulse oximetry—84% on room air
Temperature—99.8° F (37.6° C) rectal

A KUB (kidney, ureter, and bladder) radiograph is obtained which shows air–fluid levels. Which of the following would be the highest priority for this child?
[ ] **A.** Oxygen by mask or flow-by
[ ] **B.** Intravenous line
[ ] **C.** Fluid administration
[ ] **D.** Urinary catheter

73. A 3-year-old child is brought to the emergency department after his parents saw him put a button battery in his mouth and swallow it. He is not in respiratory distress but cannot seem to swallow anything. Which of the following is a true statement regarding this ingestion?
[ ] **A.** Button batteries are not a danger when swallowed and will pass through without problems.
[ ] **B.** Button batteries must always be removed immediately by endoscopy or surgical procedure.
[ ] **C.** Button batteries that have passed beyond the esophagus can be allowed to pass on their own.
[ ] **D.** Button batteries can be removed by administering ipecac to the child and having them vomit.

74. Which of the following is a manifestation of an esophageal obstruction?
[ ] **A.** Abdominal pain
[ ] **B.** Drooling
[ ] **C.** Nausea
[ ] **D.** Abdominal distention

75. Which of the following gastrointestinal disease processes is one in which surgery is **NOT** able to correct the underlying problem?
[ ] **A.** Crohn's disease
[ ] **B.** Cholecystitis
[ ] **C.** Incarcerated hernia
[ ] **D.** Ulcerative colitis

Answers/Rationales

1. Answer: C

Nursing Process: Assessment
Rationale: **Palpation should occur after inspection and auscultation in the assessment of a patient with abdominal pain. False bowel sounds can occur due to the mechanism of palpation.** Inspection of the abdomen is done first and can provide much information, including visible pulsations, masses, symmetry, and scars which can then open the door for the attainment of history—an important piece of information! Auscultation should be done second and should involve all four quadrants. Percussion is third on the list and the normal finding would be tympany.

CENsational Pearl of Wisdom!

The proper sequence of assessment should be an easy question, but it is often the easy questions that stump the test taker. Another important aspect of inspection is the position of the patient—that is, pancreatitis patients tend to lie in curled up or fetal position because it is too painful to lie totally supine. And look at facial grimacing! That can tell you so much about their pain level!

2. Answer: D

Nursing Process: Intervention

Rationale: **Glucagon is the medication of choice for an esophageal foreign body as it can relax smooth muscle and allow the foreign body to pass.** Maalox is utilized to reduce acidity in the stomach. Cimetidine (Zantac) can help reduce secretions and is used primarily for GERD (Gastro-Esophageal Reflux Disease) and omeprazole (Prilosec) is a proton pump inhibitor also utilized in treating GERD. They work by reducing the production of stomach acids over a longer period of time.

3. Answer: B

Nursing Process: Intervention

Rationale: **This patient presents with manifestations of cholecystitis. Although there is some controversy regarding this, it is thought that morphine sulfate can cause spasm of the sphincter of Oddi and increase pain.** Hydromorphone (Dilaudid) and fentanyl (Sublimaze) are other common narcotic medications that are used to treat this type of pain. Meperidine (Demerol) is not used as much in health care today and should not be utilized for chronic pain; however, it can be used to treat acute situations such as cholecystitis.

4. Answer: C

Nursing Process: Analysis

Rationale: **Pancreatitis can cause a systemic hypocalcemia due to the available calcium in the body binding with free fatty acids that are formed from the release of lipase. This would render the calcium unable to perform its duties.** In pancreatitis, lipase and amylase values are typically elevated and are diagnostic for this disease process. Hypoglycemia would not be suspected, although an elevated blood glucose value might be present in a patient with a history of diabetes mellitus due to the stress incurred with an acute disease process.

CENsational Pearl of Wisdom!

Other laboratory values that might be present include a decreased hemoglobin and hematocrit if the pancreatitis is hemorrhagic in nature, and a decreased potassium from vomiting. Hemoglobin and hematocrit could also be elevated slightly if dehydration from vomiting is present.

5. Answer: C

Nursing Process: Analysis

Rationale: **A finding of free air under the diaphragm is associated with a diagnosis of an intestinal perforation.** An obstruction would most likely demonstrate visible air–fluid levels with dilated bowel. An ultrasound or computed tomography (CT) scan would best show an inflamed appendix. Cholelithiasis would be diagnosed with ultrasonography.

CENsational Pearl of Wisdom!

This is also known as a pneumoperitoneum. What a cool word! Free air is the presence of air or another type of gas that is not normally found in the abdomen and radiographically is best seen on an upright chest radiograph. It can also be noted on a computerized tomography (CT) scan. Surgical practices, which utilize the introduction of carbon dioxide into the abdomen in order to perform laparoscopic surgical procedures, can cause pain that is associated with pneumoperitoneum.

6. Answer: B

Nursing Process: Intervention

Rationale: **The patient with an acute abdominal emergency would not be given liquids of any kind due to the imminence of surgical repair.** A nasogastric (NG) tube would be appropriate to decompress the gastro-intestinal (GI) tract and decrease vomiting of the patient. Antibiotics should be provided intravenously as this situation is a clear setup for sepsis. Surgery is the mainstay of treatment of this kind of process, especially with an acute onset.

7. Answer: A

Nursing Process: Intervention

Rationale: **When a diagnostic peritoneal lavage is being performed, both a urinary catheter and nasogastric (NG) tube should be in place to decompress both the bladder and the stomach before the insertion of the**

lavage catheter. Patients are not always unresponsive and unable to maintain their own airway when the need arises for this test. Intravenous access is important for any critical patient, but is not mandatory for a diagnostic peritoneal lavage. Oxygen is not a necessity for this procedure. The administration of oxygen would be dependent on the patient.

CENsational Pearl of Wisdom!

Diagnostic Peritoneal Lavage (also known as a "belly tap") is not performed as often as before the advent of the computed tomography (CT) examination. However, it might be utilized in situations in which the patient is too ill to travel to the CT scanner or if the scanner were not working. It is easy, fast, and has a high level of predictability for accuracy. It is often, also, used as an incorrect answer on questions for abdominal trauma questions, so be aware of some of these "older" procedures!

8. Answer: B

Nursing Process: Evaluation

Rationale: **When a peritoneal catheter is inserted into the abdominal cavity, a positive test would be indicated if blood were to be aspirated or it flowed freely from the catheter.** Hearing a "whoosh" of air would not occur with this procedure. (That would be great to hear with attempting to treat a tension pneumothorax in the chest!) If no blood comes out of the catheter, it would not necessarily mean the test was negative as retroperitoneal blood may not manifest itself with this procedure. Organs such as the pancreas and kidneys are retroperitoneal organs. Fluid from the lavage is sent to laboratory, and if gastric contents as well as fecal material, bile, food, or bacteria are noted, the test is positive. Red and white cells are also counted in this process.

CENsational Pearl of Wisdom!

Sometimes, blood will actually spurt out of the catheter when performing a DPL and aim for the ceiling! That is a positive test! If blood does not "shoot" out of the abdomen—yes that does happen!—it's quite dramatic!—then 1 liter of warm normal saline is introduced into the peritoneal cavity and then the bag is turned upside down on the floor with the clamp open—make sure to not use tubing that has a check valve on it!—and the returned contents are sent to the laboratory.

9. Answer: B

Nursing Process: Assessment

Rationale: **Ingestion of NSAIDs (non-steroidal anti-inflammatory drugs) can cause inflammatory reactions in the stomach contributing to an active GI bleed.** Coffee ground emesis occurs when bleeding has slowed or stopped and has been converted to a brownish color—known as hematin—by the gastric acids. Intake of fried foods usually is associated with attacks of cholecystitis. Oral iron supplements can cause patients to have black looking stools, but, of course, they will be guaiac negative for occult blood. This would be a good piece of history if the stools were black in color but not coffee ground emesis. A history of liver disease, especially associated with alcoholism, would cause one to suspect bleeding varices if the bleeding was bright red, spontaneous, and painless.

10. Answer: A

Nursing Process: Evaluation

Rationale: **High ammonia levels are found in patients who are experiencing hepatic encephalopathy, which is treated with lactulose (Cholac).** This patient, with a prior history of intravenous substance abuse, is presenting with manifestations of this disease process. Other electrolytes including potassium, sodium, and magnesium are noted to be deficient in liver failure; however, lactulose (Cholac) is not utilized to treat these deficiencies.

CENsational Pearl of Wisdom!

Lactulose (Cholac) is given orally or rectally. Do not draw this up to give intravenously!!! It works in the colon to pull out the ammonia before excretion. This can improve mentation. It is also used as a laxative in the treatment of constipation.

11. Answer: A

Nursing Process: Analysis

Rationale: **One of the possible complications of pancreatitis is a pleural effusion. This is thought to occur due to increased vascular permeability and possible fistula formation. Amylase in thoracentesis fluid should create a suspicion for this.** Hyperglycemia would most likely occur with a malfunctioning pancreas, not hypoglycemia, due to lack of insulin production. Low calcium levels can occur due to the binding of calcium to free fatty acids produced by the release of lipase. The most common concern with coffee ground emesis is gastrointestinal bleeding.

12. Answer: C

Nursing Process: Intervention

Rationale: **Octreotide (Sandostatin) is used to treat esophageal varices associated with liver disease.** Dicyclomine (Bentyl) is an anticholinergic medication that hinders the release of pancreatic secretions by preventing nerve impulses from stimulating the cells. Fentanyl (Sublimaze) can be used to treat the pain associated with pancreatitis. Histamine H_2 inhibitors such as famotidine (Pepcid) prevents histamine release, which increases the pancreatic secretions.

CENsational Pearl of Wisdom!

Remember that morphine is not *the drug of choice for pancreatitis. Morphine can cause spasm of the sphincter of Oddi, increasing pain. Hydromorphone (Dilaudid) and fentanyl along with the older medication, meperidine (Demerol), are more useful in this disease process. And—contrary to what many people believe—alcohol consumption is* not *always the primary cause of pancreatitis. Biliary problems—gallstones—is another major etiology!*

13. Answer: B

Nursing Process: Assessment

Rationale: **An ileus is caused by decreased muscle activity, which then reduces the movement of the intestines.** Mechanical etiologies involve some type of blockage either inside or outside the intestinal tract that causes an actual obstruction. Examples of this are foreign bodies, intussusception (a telescoping of the intestinal tract into itself), and volvulus (twisting of the colon on itself).

14. Answer: B

Nursing Process: Assessment

Rationale: **Pain that increases in the right lower quadrant of the abdomen when the left side of the abdomen is palpated can be indicative of appendicitis. This is known as Rovsing's sign.** The presence of a reddened area (ecchymosis) to the periumbilical area of the abdomen is usually a sign of a retroperitoneal or intraperitoneal bleed or hematoma. This known as Cullen's sign. Grey-Turner's sign is indicated by ecchymosis to the flank area that can occur later in retroperitoneal bleeds. Tympany would be a normal finding on percussion of the abdomen as it is present with gas-filled areas.

CENsational Pearl of Wisdom!

Other indications of appendicitis are generalized abdominal pain (early stages) that then localizes to the right lower quadrant, nausea, vomiting, and low-grade fever. A good question to ask patients who are suspicious for appendicitis is "Did the pain increase when the car hit a rut in the road or you went over railroad tracks?" Jumping up and down in place should also create pain in the right lower quadrant.

15. Answer: C

Nursing Process: Analysis

Rationale: **The computed tomography (CT) test is the most sensitive of those listed for pancreatic injury because the pancreas is a retroperitoneal organ.** The FAST (Focused Assessment with Sonography for Trauma) examination is a valuable tool, but its sensitivity for the presence of retroperitoneal bleeding is not good. An upright chest may indicate free air, which might supply valuable information; however, a flat plate of the abdomen/chest does not usually afford positive data regarding retroperitoneal hemorrhages. The diagnostic peritoneal lavage (DPL), though a useful tool to determine bleeding in the abdominal cavity, can provide a false-negative response with retroperitoneal injuries.

CENsational Pearl of Wisdom!

Other retroperitoneal organs include the duodenum and the kidneys. The advent of the CT examination has become a great tool in the care of the trauma patient.

16. Answer: D

Nursing Process: Assessment

Rationale: **Right lower rib fractures can cause liver injury, especially with fractures from the eighth rib down. Emergency personnel should be aware of this as a mechanism of injury and be alert to the possibility.** This patient is demonstrating signs of hypovolemic shock and a major clue should be the tenderness to the right lower rib area along with the vital signs and the fall from the porch. Splenic injuries can occur with left lower rib fractures. Colonic injuries are not associated with rib fractures. Blunt cardiac injury can happen with sternal fractures.

CENsational Pearl of Wisdom!

Always remember that both the liver and the spleen can be lacerated, but the capsule surrounding it can encapsulate the injury and "tamponade" it off until it eventually breaks through and then becomes a major problem. Patients can bleed out from these injuries and they may not show up until several days later. Ears should perk up when patients say they were involved in motor vehicle crashes or other traumatic events days earlier. This is one time that orthostatic vital signs (OSVS) can be a good test when the patient does not present with altered vital signs. And yes, sitting and standing OSVS can be done in the triage area!

17. Answer: B

Nursing Process: Evaluation

Rationale: **Infants contain a large amount of water and are therefore at very high risk for dehydration. An infant who is not producing enough urine for normal diaper changes should be considered at risk.** An adult who has vomited three times over the past 12 hours does not present an urgent suspicion for dehydration. Elder patients should not have their skin turgor checked on their forearms. Loss of collagen as part of the normal aging process causes this assessment finding. Skin turgor is best checked on the forehead, the sternum, or the thigh in the older patient. It is not a good tool in the older adult. A teenager who is producing at least 30 to 50 mL of urine per hour can be considered to be maintaining their body fluid normal.

18. Answer: A

Nursing Process: Intervention

Rationale: **Fluid bolus rehydration for infants and children is based on 20 mL/kg of body weight.** For this patient weighing 20 pounds, the first step in the mathematical equation is to change the pounds to kilograms. This is the most common error in calculations. Therefore, 20 pounds is equal to 9 kg (20 divided by 2.2), 9 kg × 20 mL = 180 mL bolus. If the pounds are not changed to kilograms, then the incorrect mathematical outcome would be 400 mL. If an incorrect formula is used and 10 mL/kg is considered to be correct, then the outcome utilizing pounds is 200 mL or 900 mL if the correct conversion is made to kilograms but the incorrect formula is used.

CENsational Pearl of Wisdom!

Children who have underlying congenital heart problems may need 10 mL/kg of fluid bolus instead of the standard 20 mL/kg.

19. Answer: B

Nursing Process: Assessment

Rationale: **Air masses provide for tympany when the abdomen is percussed. Since the abdomen has many air-filled organs, tympany would be the normal.** Dullness to percussion is indicative of solid organs. Normal bowel sounds are irregular and high pitched. A bruit would be present as an indication of a vascular abnormality. Pulsations, when inspecting the abdomen, could suggest a disease process such as an aortic aneurysm.

20. Answer: A

Nursing Process: Assessment

Rationale: **Primary pain is also known as "visceral" pain. This originates within the organ itself. Appendicitis is another example of this type of pain.** Secondary or somatic pain occurs because of irritation from a bacterial or chemical etiology. Disease processes that fall into this category are peritonitis and gastroenteritis. Referred pain occurs in an area different than the organ that is affected. Cholecystitis would fall into this category as pain is referred to the subclavicular area with this problem.

21. Answer: D

Nursing Process: Analysis

Rationale: **Proton pump inhibitors such as omeprazole (Prilosec) and pantoprazole (Prevacid) decrease the production of acid in the stomach and cause a reduction of irritation of the lining of the stomach.** These also help to kill the organism *Helicobacter pylori* when used in combination with antibiotics. Medications such as metoclopramide (Reglan) help to increase lower esophageal sphincter pressure. Ranitidine (Zantac) and famotidine (Pepcid) reduce secretions and Maalox and Mylanta lowers the acid content that is present in the stomach.

22. Answer: A

Nursing Process: Analysis

Rationale: **McBurney's point lies within the iliac crest and is the point of tenderness for patients diagnosed** with appendicitis. The ligament of Treitz is a muscle that helps to suspend the stomach and is the separating point between the upper gastrointestinal (GI) tract and the lower GI tract. The cardioesophageal juncture occurs at the terminal end of the esophagus and the beginning of the stomach where they meet. The sphincter of Oddi is located between the pancreas and small intestine and functions as a valve to control the flow of bile and pancreatic secretions.

23. Answer: D

Nursing Process: Analysis

Rationale: **Of the disease processes presented as options, pulmonary embolism is the only one that does not have a use for glucagon.** Glucagon is used in foreign body of the esophagus in an attempt to relax smooth muscle and allow the foreign body to pass. In beta-blocker toxicity, glucagon can increase cardiac contractility (inotropic response) as well as heart rate (chronotropic response) and can affect electrical conduction through the atrioventricular node. In anaphylaxis, glucagon might be used if epinephrine does not work due to the patient being on beta-blockers. Epinephrine works on the beta-cells, so if they are blocked, the epinephrine may not work whereas, the glucagon can assist with positive chronotropic and inotropic effects.

24. Answer: A

Nursing Process: Intervention

Rationale: **This patient is experiencing symptoms consistent with esophageal varices, which also matches his past history of hepatitis C. Cirrhosis is a complicating factor of hepatitis C. The medication used for this is octreotide (Sandostatin).** Nitroprusside (Nipride) is an antihypertensive, which is used for emergencies in which blood pressures must be dropped. Amiodarone (Cordarone) is used for dysrhythmias, which would not match with this scenario. Flumazenil (Romazicon) is the antidote for benzodiazepine overdose.

 CENsational Pearl of Wisdom!

Nitroprusside is a good drug to use because it has such a short half-life, and if the blood pressure is dropping too fast, it can easily be recovered by slowing or turning off the drip. Another interesting tidbit about this medication is that it can cause cyanide poisoning! Patients who are on high doses or for long periods of time can actually die from the administration of this medication!

25. Answer: D

Nursing Process: Assessment

Rationale: **Pancreatitis pain is severe and unrelenting. It is sharp and knifelike and patients prefer to curl up on their sides in a fetal position. The supine position increases the pain level in these patients.** A prone position would place the patient on their abdomens and Fowler's is sitting upright in the bed.

 CENsational Pearl of Wisdom!

Remember that pancreatitis can be hemorrhagic or nonhemorrhagic. The hemorrhagic type affects the vascular compartment and the nonhemorrhagic type causes an "autolysis" where the digestive enzymes are causing the organ to "eat itself."

26. Answer: D

Nursing Process: Analysis

Rationale: **Octreotide (Sandostatin) does not cause tachycardias. Rather it is known to cause bradycardias as well as QT prolongation.** Interestingly enough, this medication can cause both hypo- and hyperglycemia! Type I diabetic patients are prone to hypoglycemia and type II diabetics tend to have hyperglycemia. This is due to its action with insulin and glucagon.

27. Answer: A

Nursing Process: Assessment

Rationale: **Bowel obstructions that are in the early stages or are partial obstructions can have hyperactive bowel sounds.** These sounds are usually high pitched. In the later stages and if there is a complete obstruction, the bowel sounds will be absent. In the early phases, the bowel is attempting to overcome the obstruction. A large bowel obstruction will present with a great deal of abdominal swelling, whereas a small bowel obstruction will carry a smaller amount of swelling. Fecal odor to the emesis is a good clue for a bowel obstruction, but it is not always present. Small bowel obstructions usually have a much greater amount of vomiting.

 CENsational Pearl of Wisdom!

There is hardly ever a situation in which the word "all" is true! If you see the word "all" or "none" in a potential answer, it is probably a wrong answer.

28. Answer: A

Nursing Process: Analysis

Rationale: **There are many causes for ischemic bowel disease, but gastroenteritis is not one of them. This disease process will cause intestinal symptoms such as nausea, vomiting, and diarrhea, but does not contribute to ischemia.** An incarcerated hernia could cause the bowel to become ischemic. Another example of an etiology for ischemic bowel is a volvulus when the bowel twists on itself. Vasospasms of the vessels feeding the bowel is also a cause for this malady, as well as a thrombus that travels to the colonic vessels or a build-up of plaque. All of these can cause a decrease in the blood flow, causing an ischemic reaction. This makes those with cardiovascular disease, hypertension, and increased lipid levels at risk.

29. Answer: D

Nursing Process: Analysis

Rationale: **Ulcerative colitis is not a complication of diverticulitis.** This patient has manifestations and history conducive to a diagnosis of diverticulitis. Ulcerative colitis occurs as an inflammatory reaction, causing "sores" on the innermost layer of the colon. This is a disease process all its own. Diverticulitis can cause intestinal obstruction, perforation, and abscesses as well as strictures and fistulas.

30. Answer: B

Nursing Process: Analysis

Rationale: **Iron tablets and bismuth-containing compounds such as Pepto-Bismol will cause stools to appear black.** Black licorice consumption can cause hypokalemia, but will not create the appearance of a gastrointestinal bleed. Black, tarry looking stools with a distinctive odor is a good definition of melena. Coffee ground emesis correlates with bleeding that has slowed or stopped for a period of time and has converted from the red hemoglobin to brown hematin by coming into contact with the gastric acid. This emesis looks very much like tobacco "chew"! A patient could have both an upper and lower gastrointestinal bleed at the same time.

31. Answer: D

Nursing Process: Assessment

Rationale: **In Boerhaave's syndrome, the patient vomits with great force and the tears that occur are in the esophagus itself.** In Mallory-Weiss syndrome, the patient vomits with normal emptying and the tear occurs at the cardioesophageal (also known as gastroesophageal) juncture. The duodenojejunal flexure and sigmoid mesocolon are anatomical features and landmarks but do have anything to do with Boerhaave's syndrome.

CENsational Pearl of Wisdom!

Boerhaave's syndrome can actually rupture the esophagus! This would be a medical emergency!

32. Answer: C

Nursing Process: Analysis

Rationale: **This patient's recent fall has probably contributed to the development of a splenic injury. Fractures of the left lower ribs can lead to spleen lacerations that become evident several days after initial injury.** Fractures of the lower right ribs are prone to cause liver injuries. This patient is not demonstrating any manifestations that should make the nurse consider pneumonia or pancreatitis. A fever and usually a cough should be present with pneumonia and pancreatitis would present with severe pain to left mid-quadrant.

CENsational Pearl of Wisdom!

Remember that both the liver and the spleen have a capsule surrounding them making them prone to manifestations several days after injury. Bleeding can occur within the capsule with subsequent tamponading at that time. When the capsule finally breaks through, the patient can develop hypovolemic shock. This is a good use of orthostatic vital signs, which would most likely (but not 100% of the time!) be positive.

33. Answer: B

Nursing Process: Analysis

Rationale: **The 2-year-old who fell off of a dressing table is most at risk because he was probably three times his height. This should raise a red flag as to the potential severity of a fall for a child.** For adults, an increased concern for severity usually occurs when they fall 12 to 20 feet. Consider the need for transfer to a tertiary trauma center for these patients.

34. Answer: D

Nursing Process: Evaluation

Rationale: **The FAST (Focused Assessment with Sonography for Trauma) examination is sensitive for large amounts of blood in the abdomen. If there is less than 400 mL fluid in the abdomen, it is not usually identified. It is most sensitive (90% to 100% of the time) if there is at least 1,000 mL present in the abdomen.** This test does not work as well as the diagnostic peritoneal lavage or the computed tomography (CT) for injuries of the stomach or small bowel. If the FAST examination is negative, it does not mean there are no injuries.

CENsational Pearl of Wisdom!

The great thing about the FAST examination is that it is not invasive and can also cut down on the amount of radiation that patients receive. A positive FAST examination would assist in obtaining prompt treatment but does not assess well for retroperitoneal bleeding or injuries to hollow organs. Unfortunately, the FAST examination also has only a moderate level of sensitivity in the child. If it is negative in a child, further investigation with computed tomography (CT) should be performed.

35. Answer: A

Nursing Process: Analysis

Rationale: **The use of booster seats in older children (up to age 12 or 36 kg in the United States) allows for proper fit of the seat belt. When children sit in the seat and use a seat belt, the lap portion is usually sitting at the abdomen instead of proper placement across the hips. With the lap belt across the abdomen, this creates a situation in which the abdominal organs are compressed increasing potential for injury. The booster seat also allows for better positioning of the shoulder harness as well.** A rear-facing restrained car seat for infants helps prevent all types of injuries in the child but mostly decreases the risk of cervical fracture at C1 to C3, which is seen at greater levels with front-sitting car seats due to the infant's head being thrown forward. Children should not be in the front seat due to potential damage from the air bag.

36. Answer: C

Nursing Process: Intervention

Rationale: **In the hemodynamically stable pediatric patient with a splenic injury, 90% to 98% of these patients are able to heal spontaneously.** If the patient was unstable or if there was a substantial disruption, then surgical intervention with possible removal would be in order. It would not be appropriate to discharge this child to home.

37. Answer: B

Nursing Process: Intervention

Rationale: **The loops of bowel should be covered immediately with a large sterile dressing such as abdominal pads that are saline-soaked. Keep the area moist until surgical repair can occur.** An unsterile towel would not maintain the sterility of the area and would increase the

potential of bacterial contamination. Do not attempt to replace the organs or create a tight dressing over the area. Leaving the area open would also increase the potential for contamination of the wound leading to peritonitis and would also dry out the eviscerated organs.

38. Answer: A

Nursing Process: Intervention

Rationale: **Utilizing a contrast-enhanced computed tomography (CT) with elevated serum creatinine level above 1.2 mg/dL could cause renal problems posttest. The addition of prophylactic *N*-acetylcysteine (Mucomyst) can decrease the potential of this process.** The blood urea nitrogen (BUN), hemoglobin level, and potassium reading would not be indicators for the use of this medication in this situation.

39. Answer: C

Nursing Process: Intervention

Rationale: **When performing a Focused Assessment with Sonography for Trauma (FAST) examination, a distended bladder increases the sensitivity of the examination by allowing for better visualization. If possible, delay this procedure until the FAST examination is completed.** Intravenous line placement is of high priority in the trauma patient, so make sure this is completed quickly. Oxygen in the early stages of trauma care is also a priority. If a nasogastric or orogastric tube needs to be inserted, it does not interfere with the FAST examination.

40. Answer: A

Nursing Process: Analysis

Rationale: **Oral contrast assists in the visualization of hollow organs; therefore, the stomach would be one of these types of organs as well as the bladder and small intestine.** One of the downsides of this type of contrast is that the patient must drink it and then wait for at least 30 minutes for the examination (time requirement to coat the small bowel). If the patient is hesitant to drink the contrast, that can delay the entire process even more. Intravenous contrast is essential for solid organ injury discovery. These organs include the liver, spleen, and pancreas.

CENsational Pearl of Wisdom!

In order to accurately diagnose injuries to the colon, a triple contrast approach is recommended—oral, intravenous, and rectal.

41. Answer: D

Nursing Process: Analysis

Rationale: **The small intestine is often injured when Chance fractures are present because of the amount of force and energy necessary to create these vertebral fractures.** Injuries to the small bowel are often insidious and so there is a delay in diagnosis. Injuries to the colon, stomach, or spleen are not necessarily associated with Chance fractures.

 CENsational Pearl of Wisdom!

Always be aware of possible concomitant injuries in trauma-related events. Remember mechanism of injury to make sure that injuries are not missed!

42. Answer: B

Nursing Process: Analysis

Rationale: **When injuries to the spleen are extreme or the patient is unable to be stabilized, splenectomies do occur. When this happens, patients are at risk for infectious disease processes because of lowered immunity and must receive appropriate immunizations at proper times for different bacteria.** These include *Streptococcus pneumoniae*, *Neisseria meningitides*, and *Hemophilus influenzae*. The patients are not at any higher risk for ulcerative colitis, cholelithiasis, or pancreatic cancer.

43. Answer: B

Nursing Process: Assessment

Rationale: **Cullen's and Grey-Turner's signs are ecchymotic areas and both indicate a retroperitoneal hemorrhage.** Cullen's sign presents as ecchymosis to the periumbilical area and Grey-Turner's sign is ecchymosis to the flank area. These usually occur well after the initial injury and may not be present for up to 24 hours.

 CENsational Pearl of Wisdom!

CEN test questions may not ask outright "What is Cullen's sign?," but it is always good to know what signs are present with different disease processes and what they mean—just in case!

44. Answer: C

Nursing Process: Assessment

Rationale: **With an intra-abdominal injury, the bowel sounds are absent or hypoactive.** This may be due to

the irritation from the blood in the abdomen and should at the least be cause for concern. Normal bowel sounds would be present if there was no injury. Hyperactive and shrill bowel sounds would not be expected in this situation.

45. Answer: D

Nursing Process: Assessment

Rationale: **In order to perform a measurement for the diagnosis of compartment syndrome of the abdomen, the patient must have a urinary catheter in place.** The side port that is normally used for specimen sampling is accessed with a needle that is set up with a manometer hooked to it. Some of these may hook into the monitor for waveforms. Saline is introduced and then the reading is taken when the fluid level balances out or the reading appears on the screen. A nasogastric tube, chest tube, and intravenous lines may be necessary to care for the trauma patient, but they are not necessary for this procedure.

 CENsational Pearl of Wisdom!

Yes, the abdomen can be a focus of compartment syndrome—just like the extremities! Readings below 10 cm H_2O are considered normal. The patient may have elevated lactate levels with this process and end organ damage.

46. Answer: A

Nursing Process: Evaluation

Rationale: **When ascites is removed from the peritoneal cavity, the patient will usually have relief related to their respiratory effort. When the intra-abdominal pressure is relieved, the patient is able to breathe better and so the effort and rate will decrease.** Blood pressure and temperature will not be affected. The heart rate may decrease because the patient is no longer struggling to breath, but the main parameter affected is the work of the respiratory system.

47. Answer: C

Nursing Process: Analysis

Rationale: **When the stomach is torn or perforated, hydrochloric acid and enzymes escape that then causes peritonitis. There is a very high probability that peritonitis will follow for this patient.** The patient is at much higher risk for hypovolemic shock rather than cardiogenic. Pulmonary edema and paralysis would not occur in this scenario. There is no chest or spinal cord injury.

CENsational Pearl of Wisdom!

It is also important to remember that patients involved in traumatic events can be susceptible to sepsis even though we usually think about that shock situation with more medical types of patients. When the integrity of the skin is compromised, infectious processes can also enter in that way as well.

48. Answer: B

Nursing Process: Evaluation

Rationale: **Urine output is a sensitive indicator for systemic perfusion. The increase or adequacy of the urine output in this patient would be a good indication that adequate perfusion and thus resuscitation of the patient was occurring.** The increased base deficit demonstrates a greater amount of cellular hypoxia. The patient arrived with a base deficit in the normal range of −2 to +2 and with a base deficit of −5 this would indicate a worsening situation for the patient. The serum lactate in this question is also increasing, which would indicate inadequate perfusion. A drop in the hemoglobin level would also not indicate good progress for the patient, but rather that bleeding was occurring and the source would need to be explored.

CENsational Pearl of Wisdom!

"The kidney is the window to the viscera" is an old saying that simply means the urine output tells us a lot about how the organs in the "gut" or abdominal cavity are being perfused. (Sorry! My "old nurse" is showing!) Watch urine output closely in your patients—it will tell you a great deal!

49. Answer: B

Nursing Process: Evaluation

Rationale: **The method now recommended to achieve the highest level of certainty of proper placement of a nasogastric tube is to have radiograph or computed tomography (CT) evidence.** The next recommended method is to utilize pH testing of the gastric aspirate. The use of a carbon dioxide detector to determine it is not in the lungs is the third highest recommendation, although it is considered to be weak. The common practice of listening over the stomach area for the sound of instilled air is not recommended anymore. This is an unreliable method.

50. Answer: A

Nursing Process: Evaluation

Rationale: **The pH of gastric contents should be acidic, which would correlate with an acid pH of 1 to 5.5.** Any number above 5.5 must have a radiograph to confirm placement. (Radiograph is the preferred method.)

51. Answer: C

Nursing Process: Intervention

Rationale: **Patients with the potential of infection with *Clostridium difficile* should be placed in contact isolation.** *Clostridium difficile* is passed in the stool but has the potential to be acquired from any surface that might have come in contact with the spores of the infecting agent such as surfaces in rooms, toilet seats, and medical equipment that might have been used on the patient.

52. Answer: B

Nursing Process: Intervention

Rationale: **Patients can continue to shed the *Clostridium difficile* spores for several days after the last diarrheal stool. Therefore, it would be advantageous for them to remain in isolation even after their diarrhea has stopped.** *Clostridium difficile* is not killed by alcohol. Alcohol-based hand cleansers are not adequate for the health care providers to use during the care of these patients. Soap and water are the best hand cleanser agents to use. Gloves are actually best as even hand washing cannot always adequately prevent the spread of this organism. Gowns should be worn when caring for these individuals. Private rooms are necessary or at least room the patient with another patient who is diagnosed with *Clostridium difficile*. This is known as "cohorting."

53. Answer: C

Nursing Process: Analysis

Rationale: **The average incubation time of norovirus is 12 to 48 hours. So, it is short, but not as short as 6 to 8 hours.** The dose that can actually transmit this virus to another person is as low 18 virus particles. The virus is very stable in all types of hot or cold situations, being able to survive both freezing and high temperatures. There is presently no vaccine available.

CENsational Pearl of Wisdom!

Norovirus is an extreme problem in areas where large groups of people are in a confined space. This is why cruise ships are particularly at high risk for an outbreak of epidemic proportions. It is taken very seriously on board the ships. Other areas of high risk include tour buses, day care centers, and long-term care facilities. This virus can also be passed in the vomitus as well as the fecal-oral route.

54. Answer: A

Nursing Process: Intervention

Rationale: **Viruses are not treated with antibiotics.** Treatment for norovirus is supportive care, which includes rehydration through intravenous fluids if necessary, rest which usually includes bed rest for a day or two, and strict hand washing to prevent further contamination.

55. Answer: B

Nursing Process: Analysis

Rationale: **The liver is the major involved organ in hepatitis C, and in a motor vehicle crash the emergency nurse should be concerned about the patient's ability to clot. The liver is extremely involved in the clotting process as most of the necessary clotting factors are produced here. In these traumatic situations, the clotting cascade may not work appropriately.** The liver is located in the right upper quadrant and the liver also receives a large amount of cardiac output and has the potential to bleed copiously if damaged. Respiratory distress would be a concern, but the lack of ability to clot would take precedence. There were no symptoms of respiratory distress noted in the stem of the question. Hypertensive crisis is not a concern in this scenario. The emergency nurse should be most concerned about hypotension with the strong possibility of hypovolemic shock being present. Pneumonia may occur later but would not be a primary concern in this case.

 CENsational Pearl of Wisdom!

Remember to read the question carefully and do not "add in" information! This is a pitfall for many of us! If the question had mentioned something about respiratory distress or provided information that might lead the test taker to respiratory distress, hypertension, or pneumonia, then those might be a concern. Everything you need to know to answer the question is in the stem!

56. Answer: C

Nursing Process: Analysis

Rationale: **Diarrhea causes loss of bicarbonate in the stools. With the loss of bicarbonate, metabolic acidosis quickly occurs.** This can be a major complication especially in a child of this age. It does not take very long for an infant to develop acidosis, which can take a deadly turn very fast.

57. Answer: D

Nursing Process: Intervention

Rationale: **Methylene blue is the treatment for methemoglobinemia. The fact that this child is cyanotic-appearing but has no respiratory distress and applied oxygen does not help the cyanosis are two big hints that the child may be suffering from this disease process. In an infant, diarrhea can cause metabolic acidosis, which then can create the methemoglobinemia.** The other clues were the 3-day history of diarrhea and the fact that the blood draw appeared to look like "chocolate." Methylene blue will reverse the process. Nothing in the scenario would lead the emergency nurse to administer epinephrine or atropine and there are no signs of infection listed such as a fever to warrant an antibiotic.

58. Answer: D

Nursing Process: Analysis

Rationale: **The use of thyroid supplements is not a risk factor for the development of peptic ulcers.** Smoking, alcohol intake, and the use of NSAIDs (non-steroidal anti-inflammatory drugs) are risk factors as well as some other medications such as anticoagulants, steroids, and medications like alendronate (Fosamax). Stress and eating spicy foods are also factors in peptic ulcer disease.

59. Answer: C

Nursing Process: Analysis

Rationale: **Peptic ulcer disease is caused by the virus *Helicobacter pylori.*** *Bordetella pertussis* causes whooping cough (pertussis), varicella-zoster virus is the causative agent for chickenpox, and human papillomavirus causes cervical cancer.

 CENsational Pearl of Wisdom!

Helicobacter pylori is found in up to 90% of duodenal and gastric ulcers. It is treated with antibiotic therapy.

60. Answer: B

Nursing Process: Assessment

Rationale: **Stress ulcers occur after long hospitalizations with severe illness, injury, or physical stress. The cause of this is the actual stress response of the body, which shunts blood away from some areas in order to conserve the blood flow for more important areas. This ischemia to the mucosal lining causes ulcerations to form in the stomach.** The most common type of ulcer is the duodenal ulcer that forms due to an increase in parietal cells in the stomach thus causing an increase in acid and gastrin. Gastric ulcers are in the antral area of the stomach close to the parietal cells and tend to become a chronic issue for the patient. All ulcers are caused by problems in the mucosal layer.

 CENsational Pearl of Wisdom!

Gastric ulcers often progress to gastric cancer. The pain associated with gastric ulcers occurs after eating. Duodenal ulcers cause pain before eating and are relieved by eating or by using antacids. Be sure to get a good history from your patients!!

61. Answer: A

Nursing Process: Intervention

Rationale: **This patient is actively bleeding. A type and crossmatch is needed, not a type and screen.** Blood needs to be set up immediately and the patient may need type-specific or universal donor (O negative) blood products before the crossmatch can be completed. Gastric tube placement, contacting the endoscopy department for a potential emergent procedure, and cardiac monitoring are all important treatment interventions for this patient. The patient needs close monitoring of vital signs and cardiac rhythms.

 CENsational Pearl of Wisdom!

Ice water or room temperature lavage is no longer performed for these patients. This can actually destroy clot formations and increase the amount of bleeding. Also, this question is another good example of reading the information and options closely—paying attention to detail. It would have been very easy to think that option A was an appropriate action if the reader did not pick up on the nuances and the vital signs.

62. Answer: D

Nursing Process: Analysis

Rationale: **The newer accepted hemoglobin level for administering blood products is 7.0 g/dL and below.**

63. Answer: A

Nursing Process: Intervention

Rationale: **The correct action for the medication Sandostatin (Octreotide) is that it decreases portal pressure through the relaxation of the mesenteric vascular smooth muscle.** Vasodilation would not cause vessels to clamp down. This medication does not help improve blood supply to the ulcerated areas or assist in erythropoiesis.

64. Answer: D

Nursing Process: Analysis

Rationale: **Females are at higher risk of developing cholecystitis and pregnancy increases the chances.** It is more frequent in the Caucasian population, and obesity also increases the likelihood of developing this problem.

 CENsational Pearl of Wisdom!

There is a classic mnemonic to help remember these risk factors: Fat/Female/Forties/Fertile/Fair/Flatulent—a little "non-classy" but it works to help remember!

65. Answer: B

Nursing Process: Assessment

Rationale: **Murphy's sign is indicative of cholecystitis and occurs during palpation of the gallbladder area.** Kehr's sign occurs with splenic rupture or tear and creates pain in the left subclavicular/subscapular area. Cullen's sign is an indication of retroperitoneal hemorrhage and is noted as an ecchymotic area to the periumbilical area. Rovsing's sign is present in appendicitis when the left lower quadrant is palpated, causing pain to the right lower quadrant.

66. Answer: C

Nursing Process: Intervention

Rationale: **H$_2$ inhibitors would be used in a patient with a diagnosis of gastro-esophageal reflux disease (GERD), not appendicitis.** Proper management of the patient with a diagnosis of appendicitis would be to maintain NPO (nothing by mouth) status, prepare the patient for surgery, and administer broad-spectrum antibiotics as well as pain and nausea control before surgery.

67. Answer: C

Nursing Process: Intervention

Rationale: **Milk of magnesia is a laxative.** The "GI Cocktail" is administered to treat reflux disease. It contains a combination of an antacid such as Maalox, viscous lidocaine, and an anticholinergic such as Donnatal.

CENsational Pearl of Wisdom!

Some institutions do not use the anticholinergic portion of the GI Cocktail. Be aware that this is the "accepted" version of the GI Cocktail. Remember that questions will focus on "classic textbook" and not "the way we do it."

68. Answer: D

Nursing Process: Intervention

Rationale: **The Sengstaken–Blakemore tube is a last option for the treatment of esophageal varices. It is a form of esophagogastric tamponade to compress the bleeding varices and control bleeding.** It has a triple lumen and two balloons. Other types of balloon tubes that can be used are the Minnesota and the Linton-Nachlas tubes. These tubes are not necessary in cholecystitis, diverticulitis, or pancreatitis.

69. Answer: B

Nursing Process: Analysis

Rationale: **Pneumonia would not be a possible complication. The description of this patient in the scenario is that of bowel obstruction.** Patients with bowel obstruction will have generalized abdominal pain, vomiting, and abdominal distention. In this case, the large amount of distention would point toward a large bowel obstruction. The past history of the repair for a ruptured colon and the appendectomy could create a situation in which adhesions are present that could cause a bowel obstruction. Complications for this disease process include sepsis, dehydration due to a third spacing that occurs and the vomiting and possible perforation.

70. Answer: B

Nursing Process: Intervention

Rationale: **This child has manifestations of intussusception, which is an emergent condition. No child with this suspicion should be sent to the waiting room.** It would also be inappropriate to tell the father that the child is "fine" because that might encourage him to leave and not be seen. Urgent care would not be an appropriate place for this child to be assessed and treated.

CENsational Pearl of Wisdom!

Intussusception can cause necrosis and rupture the bowel. These patients need to be seen immediately. This is usually a diagnosis for young children up to the age of 5 years; however, though rare, it can be seen in older children and young adults. This occurs as a result of one portion of the intestine telescoping into another and can move in and out thus causing the intermittent symptoms.

71. Answer: D

Nursing Process: Assessment

Rationale: **The manifestations in the stem of this question are significant for pyloric stenosis.** This is a congenital anomaly that causes an obstruction at the pyloric sphincter arising from hypertrophy of the circular pylorus. This usually occurs in infants aged 2 to 5 months. Failure to thrive would be indicated by dehydration and a decrease in the physical growth of the infant. Intussusception is manifested by crying and pulling the legs upward intermittently and the presence of "red currant" jelly-like stools. Reflux in an infant would be noted as "colic."

72. Answer: A

Nursing Process: Intervention

Rationale: **This child is in distress, most likely with a bowel obstruction, and needs to have oxygen started immediately.** She obviously needs an intravenous line and fluid administration, but these will take time, and therefore, the fastest intervention that can be done is to start high-flow oxygen. The urinary catheter also is important but again will take time and can be done after the airway is maintained and the fluid boluses are started.

CENsational Pearl of Wisdom!

Bowel obstruction in children can often be missed and can have fatal outcomes. One of the items that children have been known to ingest over the past several years are magnets. These can attach to each other in the intestines and cause a blockage. These magnets can also cause necrosis, perforation, and the creation of fistulas. Be suspicious for objects being ingested, inhaled, or placed in orifices with children. And remember! Airway is always the first priority unless uncontrolled bleeding is present.

73. Answer: C

Nursing Process: Analysis

Rationale: **Button batteries are a major danger to children. If the ingested battery has passed through the esophagus, the child can be watched with serial radiographs to monitor its progress. If it is in the esophagus, it must be removed.** These batteries can cause permanent injuries to tissues whether it is ingested or placed as a foreign body in orifices such as the ears or nose. Never have a child attempt to vomit if they have swallowed one of these batteries. This can actually cause movement of the battery back up in to the esophagus.

 CENsational Pearl of Wisdom!

Burns occur from the electrical current that is present in the button batteries. This electrical current also creates sodium hydroxide, which contributes to the injury. Perforation has been known to occur within 6 hours of ingestion of the foreign body. The stronger the voltage, the more damage is done due to the creation of stronger currents. If the battery was successful in moving through the esophagus, it should be able to pass through the rest of the digestive system without difficulty. However, if it is in the esophagus, endoscopy must be done to retrieve it before it causes major damage to these tissues.

74. Answer: B

Nursing Process: Assessment

Rationale: **Patients who have an esophageal obstruction will not be able to swallow. Drooling is a common manifestation with this process.** Abdominal pain, distention and nausea are not usually part of the assessment picture.

 CENsational Pearl of Wisdom!

Any patient who is drooling and cannot swallow their sputum must be seen immediately. Never put these patients back in the waiting room!

75. Answer: A

Nursing Process: Analysis

Rationale: **A patient with Crohn's disease can have surgical repair of complications from the disease (strictures/fistulas) but there is no surgical procedure that is curable. Crohn's disease affects all parts of the**

entire GI tract. Cholecystitis is most often managed surgically. An incarcerated hernia can be repaired surgically if manual reduction is not successful. Ulcerative colitis is a colonic problem, and there are surgical procedures that are curative for this disease process.

References

AAC, Lab Tests Online. (2018). *Cirrhosis*. Retrieved from https://labtestsonline.org/conditions/cirrhosis (55)

Ansari, P. (2017). *Acute perforation of the GI tract*. Merck Manual. Retrieved from https://www.merckmanuals.com/professional/gastrointestinal-disorders/acute-abdomen-and-surgical-gastroenterology/acute-perforation-of-the-gi-tract#v890558 (5)

Ansari, P. (2018). *Overview of GI bleeding*. Merck Manual. Retrieved from https://www.merckmanuals.com/professional/gastrointestinal-disorders/gi-bleeding/overview-of-gi-bleeding (30)

Art and Science Clinical Skills. (2016). *How to insert a nasogastric tube and check gastric position at the bed side*. Retrieved from https://rcni.com/sites/rcn_nspace/files/ns.30.38.36.s43.pdf (49, 50)

Bajaj, J., et al. (2018). *Methods to achieve hemostasis in patients with acute variceal hemorrhage*. Retrieved from https://www.uptodate.com/contents/methods-to-achieve-hemostasis-in-patients-with-acute-variceal-hemorrhage (24)

Bjerke, H. S. (2015). *Pancreatic trauma workup*. Emedicine. Retrieved from https://emedicine.medscape.com/article/433177-workup#c4 (15)

Bloom, A. A. (2017). *Cholecystitis medication*. Retrieved from https://emedicine.medscape.com/article/171886-medication#3 (3)

Cadogan, M. (2018). *Rovsing sign*. Life in the Fast Lane. Retrieved from https://litfl.com/rovsing-sign (65)

CDC. (2018) *FAQS for Clinicians about C Diff*. Retrieved from https://www.cdc.gov/cdiff/clinicians/faq.html#anchor_1529601716735 (51, 52)

CDC. (2018). *Norovirus in healthcare facilities fact sheet*. Retrieved from https://www.cdc.gov/hai/pdfs/norovirus/229110-ANoroCaseFactSheet508.pdf (53, 54)

Chahine, A. A. (2017). *Intussusception*. Emedicine. Retrieved from https://emedicine.medscape.com/article/930708-overview (70)

Comerford, K. C. (2017). Nursing 2017 drug handbook. Philadelphia, PA: Wolters/Kluwer. (24)

Daley, B. J. (2017). *Peritonitis and abdominal sepsis*. Emedicine. Retrieved from https://emedicine.medscape.com/article/180234-overview (47)

Denshaw-Burke, M. (2017). *Methemoglobinemia treatment and management*. Emedicine. Retrieved from https://emedicine.medscape.com/article/204178-treatment (57)

Dire, D. J. (2015). *Disk battery ingestion management and treatment.* Medscape. Retrieved from https://emedicine.medscape.com/article/774838-treatment (73)

Edgington, J., et al. (2018). *Evaluation, resuscitation, and DCO.* Ortho Bullets. Retrieved from https://www.orthobullets.com/trauma/1005/evaluation-resuscitation-and-dco (48)

Emergency Nurses Association. (2012). Emergency nursing pediatric course (4th ed.). Des Plaines, IL: Emergency Nurses Association. (17, 18, 34, 35, 36, 37)

Emergency Nurses Association. (2014). Trauma nurse core course (7th ed.). Des Plaines, IL: Emergency Nurses Association. (7, 8, 32, 33, 34, 39, 40, 42, 43, 44, 48)

Emergency Nurses Association. (2015). *Clinical practice guideline, gastric tube verification.* Retrieved from https://www.ena.org/docs/default-source/resource-library/practice-resources/cpg/gastrictubecpg7b5530b71c1e49e8b155b6cca1870adc.pdf?sfvrsn=a8e9dd7a_12 (49)

Emergency Nurses Association. Core Curriculum (2017). (7th ed.). St. Louis, MO: Elsevier. (4, 7, 11, 14, 22)

Emergency Physicians Monthly. (2016). *Octreotide use in the ED.* Retrieved from http://epmonthly.com/article/octreotide-in-the-ed (26)

Hammond, B., et al. (2012). Sheehy's manual of emergency care (7th ed.). Maryland Heights, MO: Mosby. (2, 9, 17, 31, 58, 59, 60, 61, 62, 63, 64, 65, 66, 67, 68, 69, 70, 71, 74, 75)

Herrine, S. K. (2018). *Acute liver failure.* Merck Manual. Retrieved from https://www.merckmanuals.com/professional/hepatic-and-biliary-disorders/approach-to-the-patient-with-liver-disease/acute-liver-failure (10)

Howard, P. K., et al. (2010). Sheehy's emergency nursing principles and practice (6th ed.). St. Louis, MO: Elsevier. (1, 5, 6, 9, 11, 12, 13, 14, 15, 16, 17, 18, 20, 23)

Huang, L. H. (2015). *Pediatric metabolic acidosis.* Emedicine. Retrieved from https://emedicine.medscape.com/article/906440-overview#a5 (56)

Khan, A. N. (2016). *Pneumoperitoneum imaging.* Medscape Emedicine. Retrieved from https://emedicine.medscape.com/article/372053-overview (5)

Koyfman, A. (2018). *Pediatric dehydration.* Emedicine. Retrieved from https://emedicine.medscape.com/article/801012-overview#a5 (17)

Mace, S. (2017). *Images of note: Grey-Turner and Cullen signs.* Cleveland Clinic. Retrieved from https://consultqd.clevelandclinic.org/images-of-note-grey-turner-and-cullen-signs (43)

Mayeaux, E. J., Jr. (2018). *Abdominal paracentesis.* Five Minute Consult. Retrieved from https://5minuteconsult.com/collectioncontent/30-156350/procedures/abdominal-paracentesis (46)

Mayo Clinic. (2018). *Intestinal ischemia.* Retrieved from https://www.mayoclinic.org/diseases-conditions/intestinal-ischemia/symptoms-causes/syc-20373946 (28)

Mayo Clinic. (2018). *Peptic ulcer.* Retrieved from https://www.mayoclinic.org/diseases-conditions/peptic-ulcer/symptoms-causes/syc-20354223 (58)

MedicineNet. (2018). *Medical definition of esophagogastric tamponade.* Retrieved from https://www.medicinenet.com/script/main/art.asp?articlekey=7020 (68)

Mills, W. A., et al. (2015). *So your kid swallowed a little magnet . . ..* Emergency Physicians Monthly. Retrieved from http://epmonthly.com/article/what-the-buck-did-you-swallow (72)

Mustafa, S. S. (2018). *What is the role of glucagon in the treatment of anaphylaxis?* Medscape Nurses. Retrieved from https://www.medscape.com/answers/135065-52990/what-are-the-role-of-glucagon-in-the-treatment-of-anaphylaxis (23)

National Institute of Diabetes and Digestive and Kidney Diseases. (2014). *Ulcerative colitis.* Retrieved from https://www.niddk.nih.gov/health-information/digestive-diseases/ulcerative-colitis (29)

O'Brien, S., et al. (2018). *Mucosal damage.* Retrieved from https://inflammatoryboweldisease.net/symptoms/complications/mucosal-damage (29)

Patti, M. G. (2017). *Gastroesophageal reflux disease treatment and management.* Emedicine. Retrieved from https://emedicine.medscape.com/article/176595-treatment#d11 (21)

Paula, R. (2017). *Abdominal compartment syndrome work-up.* Emedicine. Retrieved from https://emedicine.medscape.com/article/829008-workup#c9 (45)

Phillips, Q., et al. (2017). *Need to know facts about ischemic colitis and seniors.* Everyday Health. Retrieved from https://www.everydayhealth.com/ulcerative-colitis/living-with/ischemic-colitis-and-seniors (28)

Poison Control, National Capital Poison Center. (2018). *Swallowed a button battery? Battery in the nose or ear?* Retrieved from https://www.poison.org/battery (73)

RXList. (2018). *Prilosec.* Retrieved from https://www.rxlist.com/prilosec-drug.htm#description (21)

Schonwald, S. (2017). *Licorice poisoning.* Medscape. Retrieved from https://emedicine.medscape.com/article/817578-overview (30)

Sharma, A. (2018). *Beta blocker toxicity treatment and management*. Emedicine. Retrieved from https://emedicine.medscape.com/article/813342-treatment#d11 (23)

Smith, D. A., et al. (2018). *Bowel, obstruction*. StatPearls. Retrieved from https://www.ncbi.nlm.nih.gov/books/NBK441975 (27)

Turner, A., et al. (2017). *Boerhaave syndrome*. StatPearls. Retrieved from https://www.ncbi.nlm.nih.gov/books/NBK430808 (31)

U.S. National Library of Medicine. (2017). *Lactulose*. Medline Plus. Retrieved from https://medlineplus.gov/druginfo/meds/a682338.html (10)

Vera, M. (2014). *8+ pancreatitis nursing care plans*. Nurseslabs. Retrieved from https://nurseslabs.com/5-pancreatitis-nursing-care-plans (12)

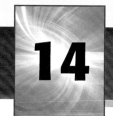

14 Genitourinary, Gynecologic, and Obstetrical Emergencies

Monta Rae Glaser, RN, CEN

Genitourinary, gynecologic, and obstetrical emergencies cover a lot of ground! This part of our patient population is included with gastrointestinal emergencies on the Certified Emergency Nurse (CEN) test. There are 21 questions on this part of the blueprint. These questions range from simple recall to patient scenarios that require the reader to determine the disease process and then choose the correct intervention. Take your time and utilize the wrong answers to learn data as well. The CENsational Pearls of Wisdom are added to enhance the learning process.

1. The emergency nurse is providing education regarding prevention of urinary tract infections. This would include all of the following **EXCEPT**:
[ ] **A.** wipe from the back to the front of the perineum.
[ ] **B.** drink plenty of fluids on a daily basis.
[ ] **C.** voiding immediately following intercourse.
[ ] **D.** avoiding bubble baths and hot tubs.

2. Which of the following is the most common etiology for urinary tract infection?
[ ] **A.** *Streptococcus*
[ ] **B.** *Neisseria gonorrhoeae*
[ ] **C.** *Escherichia coli*
[ ] **D.** *Chlamydia trachomatis*

3. A patient experiencing epididymitis may experience relief of pain by elevation of the scrotum. This is known as which of the following signs?
[ ] **A.** Kehr's
[ ] **B.** Prehn's
[ ] **C.** Kernig's
[ ] **D.** Brudzinski's

4. Priapism may be caused by all of the following disease processes **EXCEPT**:
[ ] **A.** sickle cell crisis.
[ ] **B.** spinal cord injury.
[ ] **C.** bladder cancer.
[ ] **D.** trichomonas.

5. Pain that occurs as a transient mid-cycle, sudden sharp and unilateral pain is known as:
[ ] **A.** dysmenorrhea.
[ ] **B.** endometriosis.
[ ] **C.** appendicitis.
[ ] **D.** mittelschmerz.

6. Which of the following conditions occurs when the normal bacterial flora in the vagina is replaced with "bad" bacteria due to a decrease in lactobacillus?
[ ] **A.** Bacterial vaginosis
[ ] **B.** Candidiasis
[ ] **C.** Trichomoniasis
[ ] **D.** Herpes simplex

7. In certain cases, which of the following medications may be used to medically manage an ectopic pregnancy instead of surgery?
[ ] **A.** Doxycycline (Vibramycin)
[ ] **B.** Ceftriaxone (Rocephin)
[ ] **C.** Methotrexate (Trexall)
[ ] **D.** Metronidazole (Flagyl)

8. A pregnant patient presents with complaints of heavy vaginal bleeding and severe abdominal cramping. Further diagnostic testing reveals that she has a positive pregnancy test and an open cervical os. Which of the following diagnoses would the emergency nurse expect?
[ ] **A.** Threatened abortion
[ ] **B.** Inevitable abortion
[ ] **C.** Missed abortion
[ ] **D.** Septic abortion

9. A 35-week pregnant patient presents with complaints of a headache, vision changes, and decreased urination. The emergency nurse assesses her and discovers edematous hands, legs, and feet. Her vital signs are as follows:

Blood pressure—160/100 mm Hg
Heart rate—80 beats/minute
Respirations—14 breaths/minute
Pulse oximetry—98% on room air
Temperature—98.2° F (36.7° C)

Which of the following medications would the emergency nurse expect the provider to prescribe to prevent seizure activity?
[ ] **A.** Lorazepam (Ativan)
[ ] **B.** Diazepam (Valium)
[ ] **C.** Calcium gluconate
[ ] **D.** Magnesium sulfate

10. A delivery occurs in the emergency department. The baby presents with blue limbs, pink body, heart rate of 142 beats/minute, some flexion, some motion, and a weak cry. What is this infant's APGAR score?
[ ] **A.** 10
[ ] **B.** 9
[ ] **C.** 7
[ ] **D.** 6

11. The parents of a learning impaired child report the child has been crying with urination and an odor has been noted from his penis. Which of the following diagnoses would be the highest suspicion for this child?
[ ] **A.** Urinary tract infection
[ ] **B.** Foreign body in the urethra
[ ] **C.** Hypospadias
[ ] **D.** Hyperspadias

12. An emergent urologic consult has been made for a patient with a penile amputation. Which of the following actions should the emergency nurse take to preserve the amputated penis?
[ ] **A.** Place it directly on ice.
[ ] **B.** Place it in a clean towel.
[ ] **C.** Place it in a dry gauze dressing.
[ ] **D.** Place it in a saline-soaked gauze dressing.

13. The absence of the cremasteric reflex has a high sensitivity but low specificity for which of the following conditions?
[ ] **A.** Penile foreign body
[ ] **B.** Testicular torsion
[ ] **C.** Urethral tear
[ ] **D.** Epididymitis

14. A patient is recovering from a transurethral resection of the prostate. The nurse is comfortable that the patient understood his postoperative discharge instructions when he presents to the emergency department with complaints of which of the following?
[ ] **A.** Bright red blood in the urine
[ ] **B.** Passing small blood clots in urine
[ ] **C.** Inability to urinate
[ ] **D.** Low-grade fever

15. The emergency nurse should suspect which of the following types of injury if a 22-year-old patient presents with a history of falling on to a balance beam from a standing position on the beam?
[ ] **A.** Hangman's injury
[ ] **B.** Straddle injury
[ ] **C.** Chance fracture
[ ] **D.** Salter–Harris fracture

16. Which of the following conditions is manifested by frequent sustained vomiting, often resulting in dehydration and weight loss of the pregnant patient?
[ ] **A.** Cyclical vomiting
[ ] **B.** Gastroenteritis
[ ] **C.** Hyperemesis gravidarum
[ ] **D.** Ulcerative colitis

17. Which of the following blood tests detects fetal red blood cells in the maternal circulation indicating fetal hemorrhage through the placenta?
[ ] **A.** Kleihauer–Betke test
[ ] **B.** Fecal occult blood test
[ ] **C.** Adrenal stress profile
[ ] **D.** Thromboelastogram

18. Which of the following is **NOT** a normal physiologic change that occurs in pregnancy?
[ ] **A.** Resting heart rate increases.
[ ] **B.** Peripheral resistance increases.
[ ] **C.** Circulating plasma increases.
[ ] **D.** Oxygen consumption increases.

19. Which of the following is **NOT** an indicator that the placenta is ready to deliver?
[ ] **A.** Umbilical cord advances 2″ to 3″.
[ ] **B.** Fundus rises upward.
[ ] **C.** Uterus becomes soft.
[ ] **D.** Small gush of blood noted.

20. A patient enters the emergency department complaining of nausea, vomiting, restlessness, and severe right-sided lower back pain with sudden onset 1 hour ago. The patient appears slightly pale and is diaphoretic. Vital signs are as follows:

Blood pressure—140/92 mm Hg
Pulse—120 beats/minute
Respirations—32 breaths/minute
Pulse oximetry—96% on room air
Temperature—98° F (36.7° C)

Which of the following would be subjective data supporting a diagnosis of renal calculi?
[ ] **A.** Mild flu symptoms last week
[ ] **B.** Coffee-ground emesis
[ ] **C.** Dark, scant urine output
[ ] **D.** Right upper quadrant pain

21. Which of the following laboratory values supports a diagnosis of pyelonephritis?
[ ] **A.** Myoglobinuria
[ ] **B.** Ketonuria
[ ] **C.** Pyuria
[ ] **D.** Leucopenia

22. A patient with a history of heart failure and sepsis is at risk for which of the following genitourinary complications?
[ ] **A.** Renal calculi
[ ] **B.** Urinary retention
[ ] **C.** Acute renal failure
[ ] **D.** Urethral stricture

23. Which of the following is an appropriate intervention for a patient with a renal calculus?
[ ] **A.** IV fluids at 100 mL/hour
[ ] **B.** Nonsteroidal anti-inflammatory drugs
[ ] **C.** Indwelling urinary catheter
[ ] **D.** Nasogastric tube

24. Which of the following is a virus in which there are more than 100 types and may present with tall, pinkish gray lesions or genital warts?
[ ] **A.** Bacterial vaginosis
[ ] **B.** Gonorrhea
[ ] **C.** Herpes simplex
[ ] **D.** Human papillomavirus

25. Which of the following is a gynecologic/obstetric condition that must be considered as a potentially dangerous situation for every female presenting with abdominal pain during childbearing years?
[ ] **A.** Ectopic pregnancy
[ ] **B.** Ovarian cyst
[ ] **C.** Ovarian torsion
[ ] **D.** Dysmenorrhea

26. Which of the following is **NOT** a disease process that HELLP (hemolysis, elevated liver enzymes, and low platelets) syndrome can mimic and needs to be part of the differential diagnosis?
[ ] **A.** Thrombocytopenic purpura
[ ] **B.** Pyelonephritis
[ ] **C.** Hepatitis
[ ] **D.** Crohn's disease

27. Which of the following statements made by a patient being discharged with a diagnosis of trichomonas and placed on a regimen of metronidazole (Flagyl) indicates that instructions were understood?
[ ] **A.** "I'm very glad that I don't have to tell anyone about this."
[ ] **B.** "I'm so excited that I just found out that I am pregnant."
[ ] **C.** "I should not drink alcohol while I am taking this medication."
[ ] **D.** "The doctor said this would not impact my coumadin medication."

28. A patient with scrotal pain that has been present for 2 days is admitted to the emergency department. Which of the following signs would indicate a diagnosis of epididymitis rather than testicular torsion?
[ ] **A.** Hypoperfusion on testicular scan
[ ] **B.** Leukopenia on complete blood count
[ ] **C.** Bacteriuria in urinalysis
[ ] **D.** Elevated creatinine level

29. Which of the following orthostatic vital sign readings would be of concern for a patient suspected of internal hemorrhage from a possible ruptured ectopic pregnancy?

[ ] **A.** Lying—blood pressure, 120/64 mm Hg; heart rate, 82 beats/minute
Sitting—blood pressure, 114/60 mm Hg; heart rate, 72 beats/minute
Standing—blood pressure, 132/84 mm Hg; heart rate, 92 beats/minute

[ ] **B.** Lying—blood pressure, 92/40 mm Hg; heart rate, 64 beats/minute
Sitting—blood pressure, 94/60 mm Hg; heart rate, 72 beats/minute
Standing—blood pressure, 86/54 mm Hg; heart rate, 78 beats/minute

[ ] **C.** Lying—blood pressure, 128/52 mm Hg; heart rate, 74 beats/minute
Sitting—blood pressure, 96/48 mm Hg; heart rate 94 beats/minute
Standing—blood pressure, 72/40 mm Hg; heart rate, 120 beats/minute

[ ] **D.** Lying—blood pressure, 116/80 mm Hg; heart rate, 76 beats/minute
Sitting—blood pressure, 120/76 mm Hg; heart rate, 82 beats/minute
Standing—blood pressure, 130/64 mm Hg; heart rate, 88 beats/minute

30. A patient is being treated for urinary calculi and his urine pH is reported to be 4.8. Which of the following types of renal calculi would this patient most likely have?

[ ] **A.** Magnesium
[ ] **B.** Struvite
[ ] **C.** Calcium phosphate
[ ] **D.** Uric acid

31. All of the following are possible complications of an ovarian cyst **EXCEPT**:

[ ] **A.** adhesions.
[ ] **B.** peritonitis.
[ ] **C.** ischemic ovary.
[ ] **D.** mittelschmerz.

32. Which of the following medications in the patient's medical history can increase the risk of dysfunctional uterine bleeding (DUB)?

[ ] **A.** Antibiotics
[ ] **B.** Nonsteroidal anti-inflammatory drugs
[ ] **C.** Steroids
[ ] **D.** Muscle relaxants

33. In which of the following positions should the patient be placed to achieve the most accurate diagnostic bladder ultrasound result?

[ ] **A.** Prone
[ ] **B.** Supine
[ ] **C.** Semi-Fowler's
[ ] **D.** Lithotomy

34. Zovirax (Acyclovir) is the drug of choice for the treatment of genital herpes lesions. The mechanism of action includes all of the following **EXCEPT**:

[ ] **A.** providing bactericidal functions.
[ ] **B.** relieving local and systemic pain.
[ ] **C.** diminishing the interval of viral shedding.
[ ] **D.** decreasing the formation of new lesions.

35. Which of the following is an ovarian cyst that usually contains hair and teeth?

[ ] **A.** Corpus luteum
[ ] **B.** Teratoma
[ ] **C.** Endometrioma
[ ] **D.** Chocolate cyst

36. The provider has diagnosed a patient with a hydatidiform mole. The emergency nurse will expect the human gonadotropin level to be:

[ ] **A.** zero.
[ ] **B.** very low.
[ ] **C.** very high.
[ ] **D.** normal for gestational age.

37. Which of the following test results provides information that is important immediately following a sexual assault?

[ ] **A.** Negative serologic test for syphilis
[ ] **B.** Normal complete blood count
[ ] **C.** Rhogam test for blood type
[ ] **D.** Negative pregnancy test

38. As part of the sexual assault examination, which of the following should be done with the victim's clothing?

[ ] **A.** Place it in a paper bag and seal it with evidence tape.
[ ] **B.** Return it to the patient after examining it.
[ ] **C.** Place it in a plastic bag and seal it with paper tape.
[ ] **D.** Shake it out carefully to look for hidden evidence.

39. Which of the following should **NOT** be collected during a sexual assault examination?
[ ] **A.** Fingernail scrapings
[ ] **B.** Pubic hair
[ ] **C.** Saliva specimen
[ ] **D.** Upper thigh scrapings

40. A direct blow to the male groin will most likely result in which of the following?
[ ] **A.** Right testicular injury
[ ] **B.** Left testicular injury
[ ] **C.** Penile fracture
[ ] **D.** Urethral tear

41. A trauma patient with a diagnosis of a ruptured bladder has two large-bore intravenous lines, oxygen, a nasogastric tube, and an indwelling urinary catheter in place. Initial vital signs are as follows:

Blood pressure—120/54 mm Hg
Pulse—120 beats/minute
Respirations—28 breaths/minute
Pulse oximetry—95% on room air
Temperature—98.2° F (36.7° C)

Which of the following might indicate impending hypovolemic shock?
[ ] **A.** Pulse of 100 beats/minute
[ ] **B.** Restlessness
[ ] **C.** Blood pressure of 110/64 mm Hg
[ ] **D.** Request for pain relief

42. Which of the following indicates the possibility of a urethral injury during a rectal examination of a trauma patient?
[ ] **A.** Low-riding prostate
[ ] **B.** High-riding prostate
[ ] **C.** Absent sphincter tone
[ ] **D.** Positive hemoccult test

43. Which of the following vaginal infections does **NOT** require treatment of sexual partners?
[ ] **A.** *Neisseria gonorrhoeae*
[ ] **B.** *Candida albicans*
[ ] **C.** *Trichomonas vaginalis*
[ ] **D.** *Chlamydia trachomatis*

44. A patient sustains an 8-foot fall landing on his buttocks. Along with possible spinal compression fractures, which of the following signs would be present indicating possible genitourinary vascular trauma?
[ ] **A.** Bruit at the second lumbar vertebra
[ ] **B.** Suprapubic pain on palpation
[ ] **C.** Slowly escalating hypertension
[ ] **D.** Decreased or absent bowel sounds

45. Which of the following diluents helps to decrease discomfort of an IM injection of ceftriaxone (Rocephin)?
[ ] **A.** Sterile water
[ ] **B.** Dextrose 5% in water (D_5W)
[ ] **C.** Sterile normal saline
[ ] **D.** 1% Lidocaine plain

46. A pregnant patient has been diagnosed with a chlamydial infection. Cesarean birth is usually the delivery method of choice because it decreases the infant's risk of developing which of the following disease processes?
[ ] **A.** Endocarditis
[ ] **B.** Hepatitis
[ ] **C.** Pneumonia
[ ] **D.** Encephalitis

47. A patient complains of a foul-smelling vaginal discharge and intermittent vaginal bleeding. She normally has irregular menses and does not recall the date of her last menstrual cycle. Her triage vital signs are as follows:

Blood pressure—104/62 mm Hg
Pulse—118 beats/minute
Respirations—22 breaths/minute
Pulse oximetry—99% on room air
Temperature—102.4° F (39.1° C)

Which of the following should the emergency nurse suspect?
[ ] **A.** Septic abortion
[ ] **B.** Pyelonephritis
[ ] **C.** Vaginitis
[ ] **D.** Ovarian cyst

48. A teenaged boy comes to the emergency department after waking with severe pain to his left testicle. Examination reveals the following vital signs:

Blood pressure—110/72 mm Hg
Pulse—120 beats/minute
Respirations—30 breaths/minute
Pulse oximetry—98% on room air
Temperature—98.5° F (36.9° C)

His left testicle is slightly elevated and firm. Which of the following would be the most appropriate intervention?
[ ] **A.** Send patient for ultrasound.
[ ] **B.** Apply ice packs to the scrotum.
[ ] **C.** Prepare to transfuse blood products.
[ ] **D.** Elevate scrotum to 45-degree angle.

49. A patient presents with a history of benign prostatic hyperplasia and an inability to void for 12 hours. Which medication could contribute to his urinary retention?
[ ] **A.** Ibuprofen (Motrin)
[ ] **B.** Terazosin (Hytrin)
[ ] **C.** Vitamin C
[ ] **D.** Pseudoephedrine (Sudafed)

50. Which of the following patients would the emergency nurse expect to be admitted to an inpatient area?
[ ] **A.** A 3-year-old child diagnosed with a grade I kidney contusion and microscopic hematuria
[ ] **B.** A 19-year-old woman diagnosed with her second urinary tract infection in the past year
[ ] **C.** A 45-year-old man with hypertension (150/100 mm Hg) and acute onset of urethritis
[ ] **D.** A 32-year-old woman, 30 weeks pregnant, diagnosed with fever and pyelonephritis

51. A patient arrives in the emergency department stating that she was sexually assaulted multiple times over the past 12 hours. She is tearful and accompanied by a friend. The emergency nurse knows that which of the following is the most important piece of information from this patient at this time?
[ ] **A.** She notified the police.
[ ] **B.** She uses birth control.
[ ] **C.** She has changed clothing.
[ ] **D.** She has been sexually assaulted before.

52. When caring for a sexually assaulted patient, the highest priority would be:
[ ] **A.** evidence collection and preservation.
[ ] **B.** report of the crime to the authorities.
[ ] **C.** caring for injuries sustained in the assault.
[ ] **D.** updating her family and friends.

53. Which of the following responses indicates understanding of discharge instructions by the sexual assault victim?
[ ] **A.** "I will need to have follow-up care regarding my test results for possible STDs."
[ ] **B.** "I will stay at home with my family and friends until I get my test results."
[ ] **C.** "I will return to the emergency department in a few days to get rechecked."
[ ] **D.** "This is all my fault. I am ashamed of myself."

54. A patient complains of abdominal pain. Her last menstrual period was 8 weeks ago. Which type of pain is usually associated with a ruptured ectopic pregnancy?
[ ] **A.** Lower quadrant pain radiating to the shoulder
[ ] **B.** Sharp, right upper abdominal pain
[ ] **C.** Unilateral flank pain with hematuria
[ ] **D.** Colicky, diffuse abdominal pain

55. A patient in her 34th week of pregnancy comes to the emergency department and complains of sudden onset of bright red vaginal bleeding. Her uterus is soft, and she is not experiencing any pain. Fetal heart tones are 120 beats/minute. Based on this history, the emergency nurse should suspect which of the following conditions?
[ ] **A.** Abruptio placentae
[ ] **B.** Preterm labor
[ ] **C.** Placenta previa
[ ] **D.** Threatened abortion

56. Following a fall down a flight of stairs, a patient in her 38th week of pregnancy is brought to the emergency department. Unless contraindicated, she should be placed in which position during assessment?
[ ] **A.** Trendelenburg
[ ] **B.** Supine
[ ] **C.** Left lateral recumbent
[ ] **D.** Knee-chest

57. Which of the following interventions is **NOT** considered appropriate for a patient with placenta previa?
[ ] **A.** Performing a pelvic examination to determine cervical dilatation
[ ] **B.** Maintaining strict bed rest and observing for further bleeding
[ ] **C.** Monitoring for signs of shock
[ ] **D.** Preparing the patient for ultrasound

58. Delivery of an infant is imminent in the emergency department. Meconium is noted in the amniotic fluid. Upon delivery, the neonate is limp and not responding to stimuli. Which of the following actions should be taken first?
[ ] **A.** Simulation of the neonate
[ ] **B.** Suctioning of the oropharynx and the nasopharynx
[ ] **C.** Endotracheal (ET) intubation with suction
[ ] **D.** Placement of an umbilical line

59. A patient in her 34th week of pregnancy presents to the emergency department. Her blood pressure is 180/110 mm Hg and she complains of headache and blurred vision. During treatment of this patient, the emergency nurse should be prepared for which of the following complications?
[ ] **A.** Precipitous delivery
[ ] **B.** Vaginal bleeding
[ ] **C.** Cardiac dysrhythmias
[ ] **D.** Seizure activity

60. Postpartum hemorrhage can occur immediately after delivery or can be delayed by as much as 6 weeks. Which of the following is **NOT** a cause of postpartum hemorrhage?
[ ] **A.** Retained products of conception
[ ] **B.** Vaginal or cervical tear
[ ] **C.** Failure of uterus to contract to normal
[ ] **D.** Amniotic fluid embolism

61. Which of the following indicates imminent delivery?
[ ] **A.** Need to bear down by the mother
[ ] **B.** Rupture of membranes
[ ] **C.** Loss of mucus plug
[ ] **D.** Lengthening of contractions

62. A patient has been diagnosed with pregnancy-induced hypertension. She is being transported to another facility. Which of the following measures would be important for the transport crew to follow?
[ ] **A.** Have cabin lights well lit.
[ ] **B.** Read her a story of her choice.
[ ] **C.** Dim lights and ear plugs may decrease stimulation.
[ ] **D.** Run ambulance lights and siren to facility.

63. The perineum totals approximately 1% of the total body surface area. Treatment options for a patient who has experienced a burn to this area would include which of the following?
[ ] **A.** At home after explicit discharge instructions
[ ] **B.** At a local physician's office
[ ] **C.** At a community emergency department or urgent care
[ ] **D.** At a tertiary a burn center

64. Prophylactic treatment of sexually transmitted infections for the sexually assaulted victim usually includes all of the following **EXCEPT**:
[ ] **A.** ceftriaxone (Rocephin).
[ ] **B.** metronidazole (Flagyl).
[ ] **C.** zosyn (Piperacillin).
[ ] **D.** azithromycin (Zithromax).

65. Which of the following is the most common injury associated with a pelvic fracture?
[ ] **A.** Urethral tear
[ ] **B.** Bladder rupture
[ ] **C.** Fractured penis
[ ] **D.** Fractured femur

66. The diaphragm is pushed upward by the expanding gravid uterus. Which of the following areas would be correct for chest tube placement in the pregnant patient?
[ ] **A.** First to second intercostal space
[ ] **B.** Third to fourth intercostal space
[ ] **C.** Fourth to fifth intercostal space
[ ] **D.** Sixth to seventh intercostal space

67. Increased capillary engorgement heightens the risk of bleeding with the insertion of which of the following tubes during pregnancy?
[ ] **A.** Urinary catheter
[ ] **B.** Oral endotracheal tube
[ ] **C.** Nasogastric tube
[ ] **D.** Arterial line

68. A 42-week pregnant patient arrives in active labor and will be staying in a small community emergency department until after delivery. Assessment reveals that she has been taking narcotics throughout her pregnancy and appears impaired at this time. The emergency nurse would expect to perform which of the following interventions?
[ ] **A.** Administer intravenous Narcan (Naloxone) immediately.
[ ] **B.** Observe patient's respirations and assist intubation as needed.
[ ] **C.** Allow patient to take her normal street drugs.
[ ] **D.** Keep it a secret so she does not get in trouble.

69. Which of the following heart rates indicates the point at which chest compressions should be initiated in the newborn?
[ ] **A.** 60 beats/minute
[ ] **B.** 80 beats/minute
[ ] **C.** 100 beats/minute
[ ] **D.** 110 beats/minute

70. The emergency nurse should determine an APGAR score on the neonate at 1 minute and again at 5 minutes. Which of the following parameters are assessed with this scoring?
[ ] **A.** Heart rate, muscle tone, reflexes, respiratory effort, and color
[ ] **B.** Heart rate, temperature, reflexes, respiratory effort, and color
[ ] **C.** Heart rate, muscle tone, weight, respiratory effort, and color
[ ] **D.** Heart rate, muscle tone, reflexes, respiratory effort, and swallowing ability

71. Which of the following is the most common risk factor for an ectopic pregnancy?
[ ] **A.** Pelvic inflammatory disease (PID)
[ ] **B.** Spontaneous abortion
[ ] **C.** Fertility difficulties
[ ] **D.** Multiple pregnancies

72. An emergency nurse is suctioning an infant's airway upon delivery due to respiratory distress in the infant. Which of the following is the correct procedure?
[ ] **A.** Use a bulb syringe to suction the oral pharynx first.
[ ] **B.** Use a bulb syringe to suction the nares first.
[ ] **C.** Do not suction the infant's airway.
[ ] **D.** Lower the neonate's head to assist drainage of fluid.

73. During an emergency delivery in the emergency department what should the emergency nurse do during the delivery of the neonate's head?
[ ] **A.** Instruct the mother to hold her breath until the provider arrives.
[ ] **B.** Instruct the mother to pant and apply gentle pressure to the perineum.
[ ] **C.** Instruct the mother to push for a count of 10.
[ ] **D.** Apply fundal pressure to assist with delivery.

74. A trauma patient who is 36 weeks pregnant is brought to the emergency department in full spinal immobilization. She was involved in a one-car motor vehicle crash. She was wearing her seatbelt and paramedics report minor damage to the vehicle. She has no complaints, but the paramedics report her vital signs as follows:

Blood pressure—86/50 mm Hg
Heart rate—120 beats/minute
Respirations—16 breaths/minute
Pulse oximetry—95% on room air
Temperature—98.8° F (37.1° C)

Which of the following measures should the emergency nurse perform to improve her vital signs?
[ ] **A.** Place the patient in Trendelenburg's position.
[ ] **B.** Remove the patient from spinal immobilization.
[ ] **C.** Tilt the patient to the left side.
[ ] **D.** Tilt the patient to the right side.

75. A paraplegic patient presents to the emergency department with diaphoresis, inability to urinate, and has not had a bowel movement for the past 3 days. His blood pressure reading is noted 180/96 mm Hg. Which of the following nursing interventions would the emergency nurse expect to be ordered?
[ ] **A.** Insertion of a rectal tube
[ ] **B.** Administration of intravenous hydralazine (Apresoline)
[ ] **C.** Insertion of a urinary catheter
[ ] **D.** Administration of oral magnesium citrate

Answers/Rationales

1. Answer: A

Nursing Process: Evaluation
Rationale: **Wiping after using the toilet should be done from the front to the back of the perineum.** Drinking fluids, voiding after intercourse, and avoiding bubble baths and hot tubs as well as voiding frequently, not "holding it" and being cautious with feminine products that are irritating are appropriate prevention techniques for urinary tract infections.

2. Answer: C

Nursing Process: Analysis
Rationale: ***Escherichia coli*** **(E.Coli) is the most common cause. This is due to the close proximity of the rectum and the *E. coli* that is found in the stool.** The remaining choices can also be causes of a urinary tract infection, although not as common.

3. Answer: B

Nursing Process: Intervention
Rationale: **Pain associated with epididymitis is relieved by elevation of the scrotum. This test can be used as a diagnostic tool as well and is called Prehn's sign.** Kehr's sign is diagnostic in splenic injuries and any other condition that causes irritation to the diaphragm. It causes referred pain to the left shoulder. Kernig's sign and Brudzinski's sign are both signs of meningeal irritation. They include inability to straighten the leg without pain with the hip flexed while supine (Kernig's) and involuntary flexion of arms, hips, and knee with passive flexion of the neck (Brudzinski's).

4. Answer: D

Nursing Process: Assessment
Rationale: **Priapism is a prolonged erection in the absence of stimulation. Trichomonas is a sexually transmitted disease and does not cause this. Sickle cell**

crisis, spinal cord injury, and bladder cancer can cause this symptom. Other causes include fat embolism, cauda equina, and leukemia.

5. Answer: D

Nursing Process: Analysis

Rationale: **Mittelschmerz pain occurs during ovulation and is caused by increasing ovarian capsular pressure before the follicle erupts; therefore, the unilateral pain.** Dysmenorrhea is pelvic pain during menses. Endometriosis is a condition where endometrial tissue develops outside of the uterus and causes pain during menses. Appendicitis does not occur in conjunction with menses or ovulation.

6. Answer: A

Nursing Process: Analysis

Rationale: **Bacterial vaginosis is an infection that is believed to be caused by a decrease in the organism *Lactobacillus*. This helps to maintain the acidic environment that is necessary for a healthy vagina. When the count of this organism is lowered, "bad" bacteria can grow and cause problems. Although this is not considered a sexually transmitted disease (STD), it can create a situation where the potential for STDs is increased.** Candidiasis is an airborne fungal colonization, trichomoniasis is a protozoan infection that is sexually transmitted, and herpes simplex is a viral STD.

 CENsational Pearl of Wisdom!

Symptoms of bacterial vaginosis are vaginal odor; thin, whitish discharge; and irritation to the vulva. This can be associated with recent antibiotic use, douching, the use of IUD's, and increased sexual activity. Remember that "natural or lambskin" condoms do not offer effective protection against sexually transmitted infections.

7. Answer: C

Nursing Process: Intervention

Rationale: **Methotrexate (Trexall), a cytotoxic medication, is a folic acid antagonist and inhibits further duplication of fetal cells.** Doxycycline (Vibramycin), ceftriaxone (Rocephin), and metronidazole (Flagyl) are antibiotics and not used for this condition but are used in the treatment of pelvic inflammatory disease (PID).

 CENsational Pearl of Wisdom!

Methotrexate is used on embryos that are less than 4.0 cm in diameter or greater than 3.5 cm with a

heart-beat, which makes it then a relative rather than absolute contraindication. Patients receiving this medication must have serial beta-human chorionic gonadotropins (BHCGs) drawn to make sure it is effective. Every hospital should have written policies on the administration of methotrexate.

8. Answer: B

Nursing Process: Analysis

Rationale: **An inevitable abortion would present with an open os, which indicates that there is no way to save the pregnancy.** A threatened abortion is defined as vaginal bleeding, mild cramping, and a closed or slightly opened cervical os. In a missed abortion, the fetus has not formed or has died at some point in the process but remains within the uterus along with the placenta. A septic abortion is characterized by severe abdominal cramping, high fever, and malodorous vaginal discharge after an elective abortion has occurred.

9. Answer: D

Nursing Process: Intervention

Rationale: **Magnesium sulfate is a smooth muscle relaxant and is the most effective preventive treatment for the preeclamptic patient.** Lorazepam (Ativan) and diazepam (Valium) are given to stop seizures. They would not be the first choice for seizure prevention in the preeclamptic patient. Calcium gluconate is given to counteract a magnesium sulfate toxicity.

 CENsational Pearl of Wisdom!

Continuous fetal monitoring should be done for the preeclamptic patient. Vital signs, especially respirations and deep tendon reflexes, should be checked at least every 15 minutes. Do not take responsibility for fetal monitoring unless you have been trained in this piece of equipment! Leave it to the Labor and Delivery folks!!

10. Answer: D

Nursing Process: Assessment

Rationale: **According to the APGAR scoring scale, this infant would receive 1 point for the flexion (Activity or muscle tone); 2 points for Pulse rate, which is over 100 beats/minute; 1 point for the motion activity (Grimace or reflex irritability); 1 point for the blue limb color with the pink body (Appearance); and 1 point for the weak cry (Respirations). This equals a scoring of 6.**

CENsational Pearl of Wisdom!

	Score 0	Score 1	Score 2
Appearance			
Pulse	No pulse	<100/min	>100/min
Grimace			
Activity			
Respirations	No respirations	Weak, slow	Strong cry

11. Answer: B

Nursing Process: Assessment

Rationale: **Foreign bodies are often placed in orifices as a means of exploration, especially in the developmentally impaired.** One might suspect a urinary tract infection in this patient as well, but they are less common in male patients. Hypospadias is a birth defect in which the urinary meatus is located inferior/below the glans penis and may actually be near the scrotum. Hyperspadias is also a congenital defect in which the urinary meatus is located on the superior/upper surface of the penis.

12. Answer: D

Nursing Process: Intervention

Rationale: **Proper care for an amputated part is to place it in a saline-soaked dressing, which will keep the tissue moist.** A sterile bag will keep it clean and then placing it on ice will help keep the tissue viable. Placing the amputated part directly on ice may damage the tissue. Placing it in a dry towel or gauze may dry out the edges, making it difficult to reattach.

13. Answer: B

Nursing Process: Assessment

Rationale: **The cremasteric reflex is characterized by the normal elevation of the testes that occurs when the upper medial thigh is stroked. This will not be present if there is a testicular torsion.** A penile foreign body, urethral tear, or epididymitis does not have this as a manifestation of these processes.

14. Answer: C

Nursing Process: Evaluation

Rationale: **Patients are told to seek attention if an inability to urinate occurs, as there may be a clot obstructing the flow.** Discharge instructions for this surgical procedure should direct the patient to expect the urine to be bloody and have some small clots. He may even expect to run a low-grade fever, but should contact the physician for a fever above 102° F (38.9° C).

CENsational Pearl of Wisdom!

Urologists should instruct their postoperative TURP (transurethral resection of the prostate) patients to drink more water if their urine becomes the consistency of ketchup.

15. Answer: B

Nursing Process: Assessment

Rationale: **Straddle injuries occur when patients fall onto objects while their legs are apart. Serious injuries can occur to the perineum. Among these are urethral tears, vulvar hematomas, and extensive ecchymosis to the perineum. Surgical intervention may be required to repair tears or evacuate hematomas.** A hangman's injury is a fracture of the second cervical vertebrae or subluxation of C_2 on C_3 caused by an accidental or violence-related hanging. A chance fracture is a spinal fracture that extends through all three spinal columns (anterior, middle, and posterior) and is very unstable requiring surgical intervention. Salter–Harris is a classification that is associated with fractures that extend through the epiphysis (growth plate).

16. Answer: C

Nursing Process: Assessment

Rationale: **Hyperemesis gravidarum is more extreme than morning sickness and is experienced by 70% to 80% of women early in their pregnancy. This condition often continues throughout pregnancy and is thought to be caused by the rise of hormone levels. It may lead to hospitalization for rehydration.** Cyclical vomiting occurs as sudden and repeated episodes of vomiting but is not associated with pregnancy. Gastroenteritis is inflammation of the stomach and intestine, and ulcerative colitis is inflammation of the colon with ulcers.

17. Answer: A

Nursing Process: Analysis

Rationale: **The Kleihauer–Betke assay is a necessary test anytime a pregnant patient is involved in a trauma situation because it detects a disruption in the feto-maternal circulation. The presence of fetal red cells in the maternal circulation is a positive test.** The fecal occult blood test would check for blood in the stool. An adrenal stress profile would check for adrenal hormone levels assisting in the diagnosis of adrenal insults. Cortisol and dehydroepiandrosterone (DHEA) hormones are measured in this test. A thromboelastogram test deals with the recognition of acute coagulopathies and also assists with the use of blood products during resuscitative events.

18. Answer: B

Nursing Process: Assessment

Rationale: **Peripheral resistance decreases during pregnancy causing a slight decrease in systolic and diastolic blood pressure.** The resting heart rate actually increases 10 to 20 beats/minute and the circulating blood volume increases by 30% to 50%. Respirations increase to help accommodate for the increased oxygen consumption during pregnancy.

CENsational Pearl of Wisdom!

Cardiac output increases during pregnancy and can elevate to 50% greater than prepregnancy by the 16th to 20th week. Increases in stroke volume and heart rate are also present. Remember that the formula for cardiac output is: CO = SV × HR (cardiac output = stroke volume × heart rate).

19. Answer: C

Nursing Process: Analysis

Rationale: **Delivery of the placenta may take some time after the baby appears. Evidence that delivery of the placenta is imminent includes the uterus becoming firm and globular in nature.** The umbilical cord will advance a few inches, the fundus will rise, and a gush of blood will occur.

CENsational Pearl of Wisdom!

It is important when the placenta is delivering to not pull or tug on it too hard. Just exert a small amount of traction on it and have the mother bear down. Countertraction is important in this part of the delivery process. Pulling too hard could pull the uterus inside out (uterine inversion) causing the necessity of an emergent hysterectomy.

20. Answer: C

Nursing Process: Assessment

Rationale: **Most patients with renal calculi have blood in the urine from the stone's passing. The urine is dark, tests hemoccult positive (which would be objective data), and is usually scant.** Coffee-ground emesis refers to an upper gastrointestinal bleed. Right upper quadrant pain is a manifestation of cholecystitis. Mild flu symptoms are not a precipitating factor related to renal calculi.

21. Answer: C

Nursing Process: Analysis

Rationale: **Pyelonephritis is diagnosed by the presence of leukocytosis (increased white blood cell count), hematuria, pyuria, and bacteriuria.** Myoglobinuria indicates the muscle protein, myoglobin, is being released in the process of rhabdomyolysis; ketonuria is present in diabetics; and leukopenia indicates a decrease in white blood cell counts.

 CENsational Pearl of Wisdom!

Pyelonephritis can often develop into sepsis. It is important to make sure that if these patients arrive and cannot be bedded immediately, they understand the importance of waiting for treatment. Treating pyelonephritis early can help decrease their chances of the greater worry of a septic event.

22. Answer: C

Nursing Process: Assessment

Rationale: **Heart failure and sepsis can decrease cardiac output. Decreased perfusion to the kidney can lead to acute renal failure.** Renal calculi, urinary retention, and urethral strictures are urinary disease processes dealing with obstruction in the renal urine collection system.

23. Answer: B

Nursing Process: Intervention

Rationale: **The medication of choice to treat the pain associated with kidney stones are the NSAIDS. Ketorolac (Toradol) can be used intravenously and is often used with great success for this disease process.** Opioids can be used but, the movement, of course, is away from opioid use. Intravenous fluids are important as well, but the rate is wrong in the option. Some believe that increased fluids would be needed to encourage passage of the stone. There is some controversy on this aspect, but the general train of thought is hydration with intravenous fluids. Indwelling urinary catheter and nasogastric tubes are not necessary.

24. Answer: D

Nursing Process: Analysis

Rationale: **Human papillomavirus is part of a family that contains more than 100 different types. Each of these types can cause different processes. Types 6 and 11 are associated with genital warts, whereas types 16, 18, 31, 33, and 35 are seen with cervical neoplasms.** Bacterial vaginosis is an infectious process due to a depletion of normal vaginal flora. Gonorrhea is a sexually transmitted disease that is one of the main causes of pelvic inflammatory disease. Herpes simplex has two strains—HSV-1 causes oral herpes (cold sores) and HSV-2 causes genital herpes. The sores associated with genital herpes appear as blisters.

25. Answer: A

Nursing Process: Assessment

Rationale: **Ectopic pregnancy (pregnancy occurring outside of the uterus) usually manifests before 12 weeks' gestation, produces pelvic pain, and shock if ruptured. It is considered a true emergency and is a major cause of maternal death.** An ovarian cyst is a fluid-filled sac in the ovary that may be painful, is usually self-limiting, but may develop hypovolemia when it ruptures. Ovarian torsion occurs when the ovary twists itself around the stalk, that contains the blood vessels feeding the ovary and the fallopian tube. Pain is due to ischemia and requires surgical intervention. Dysmenorrhea is defined as painful menstruation in the absence of any other pelvic condition.

 CENsational Pearl of Wisdom!

If an ectopic pregnancy is suspected, be sure to initiate a large-bore intravenous line. It is much easier to obtain this before the pregnancy ruptures and the patient is hypovolemic and in shock! And be sure to be suspicious of this in every woman of childbearing age with lower abdominal pain. Do not lower your concern for this potentially fatal process!

26. Answer: D

Nursing Process: Analysis

Rationale: **HELLP syndrome is a potentially life-threatening form of preeclampsia that occurs when the patient develops multisystem organ failure. Symptoms of Crohn's disease are not part of the picture of HELLP syndrome.** Thrombocytopenic purpura, pyelonephritis, and hepatitis are all part of the differential diagnosis that must be done because the symptoms are similar with HELLP syndrome.

CENsational Pearl of Wisdom!

HELLP stands for Hemolysis, Elevated Liver Enzymes, and Low Platelets. One of the most important things to remember is that this syndrome, as well as preeclampsia, can occur in the postpartum period!

27. Answer: C

Nursing Process: Evaluation

Rationale: **Alcohol should not be used while the patient is taking metronidazole (Flagyl). It will cause extreme vomiting, headaches, and flushing.** Patients who are diagnosed with trichomonas must share this information with their sexual partners and they should be treated as well. Patients who are in the first trimester of pregnancy should not take metronidazole (Flagyl). Metronidazole (Flagyl) can potentiate the effects of warfarin (Coumadin), resulting in a prolonged prothrombin time.

28. Answer: C

Nursing Process: Analysis

Rationale: **Epididymitis is suggested by hyperperfusion on the testicular scan, an elevated white blood cell count, and the presence of bacteria in the urine.** Hypoperfusion or no perfusion would indicate testicular torsion. Leukopenia indicates a decrease in white blood cell count. An elevated creatinine level is an indicator of renal, not scrotal disease.

CENsational Pearl of Wisdom!

Epididymitis, an inflammation of the epididymis, can be seen in any age group but is more common in those aged 14 to 35 years. Testicular torsion is a disease process seen more in prepubertal and pubertal aged boys. Never leave a young boy with complaints of scrotal pain in the waiting room! Request an ultrasound if no beds are available.

29. Answer: C

Nursing Process: Evaluation

Rationale: **Orthostatic hypotension can be a sign of hemorrhage and a precursor to hypovolemic shock. An increase in the pulse of 20 beats/minute or a systolic drop of 10 to 20 mm Hg is a positive indicator of occult blood loss.** A negative orthostatic test does not rule out

the possibility of bleeding. The other options do not indicate these changes.

CENsational Pearl of Wisdom!

A newer method of orthostatic vital signs has been presented that recommends the measurement of vital signs in supine and then standing at 1 minute and 3 minutes. Positive indicators are: systolic change—decrease of 20 mm Hg; diastolic change—decrease of 10 mm Hg; heart rate—increase by 20 beats/minute. Most clinicians adhere to the older version of orthostatic vital signs. Be aware that negative readings do not mean that the patient is "OK." One of the best types of patients to perform this easy test on is the one who arrives to the emergency department days after a traumatic event with vague symptoms of "not feeling well" along with possible diaphoresis and nausea or vomiting.

30. Answer: D

Nursing Process: Analysis

Rationale: **Uric acid crystals precipitate in a pH condition less than 5.5, leading to stone formation.** Magnesium, ammonia, and phosphate stones (also called triple phosphate, struvite or infection stones) develop when the urine pH is higher than 7.2 and ammonia is present in the urine. Calcium phosphate stones also develop in alkaline urine (pH greater than 7.2).

CENsational Pearl of Wisdom!

When discharging a patient with a kidney stone, be sure to send them home with a strainer to catch the offending stone. If no strainer is available, a coffee filter can be substituted.

31. Answer: D

Nursing Process: Analysis

Rationale: **An ovarian cyst can cause adhesions and peritonitis from leakage of cystic contents. An ovary can become ischemic from torsion that occurs when a cyst is twisted on its pedicle. Mittelschmerz occurs in the form of abdominal pain at ovulation; it needs to be considered in the differential diagnosis of an ovarian cyst.**

32. Answer: C

Nursing Process: Assessment

Rationale: **Dysfunctional uterine bleeding can be caused by hormone replacement therapy, steroids, androgens, digitalis, and anticoagulants.** Nonsteroidals may increase bleeding after it has started. Antibiotics and muscle relaxants are not known to cause dysfunctional uterine bleeding.

33. Answer: B

Nursing Process: Assessment

Rationale: **A diagnostic bladder ultrasound is performed to determine bladder volume. The bladder is most easily accessed with the patient in a supine position.** Accurate determination of bladder volumes can guide the need for bladder aspiration or catheterization. The prone (lying on the abdomen), semi-Fowler's (sitting up at a 30- to 45-degree position), and lithotomy (pelvic examination position) positions will not achieve accurate results.

34. Answer: A

Nursing Process: Analysis

Rationale: **Herpes is a viral, not bacterial, infection (although a secondary bacterial infection can occur), and acyclovir is not bactericidal.** Acyclovir relieves systemic pain, diminishes the interval of viral shedding, and decreases the formation of new lesions.

35. Answer: B

Nursing Process: Analysis

Rationale: **A teratoma, or dermoid cyst, is produced from all three germ layers and usually contains hair and teeth, although it can contain tissue from any body structure. Teratoma cysts usually occur during the active reproductive years.** A corpus luteum cyst is caused by cystic changes in an ovary from hemorrhage in a mature corpus luteum. It can cause bleeding and hemorrhage. An ovarian endometrioma is a chocolate cyst and occurs when endometrial tissue in an ovary cyclically bleeds with monthly periods and collects blood and blood clots.

36. Answer: C

Nursing Process: Assessment

Rationale: **A hydatidiform mole or gestational trophoblastic tumor demonstrates an extremely elevated human chorionic gonadotropin level.** Other signs include snowstorm pattern on ultrasound, early preeclampsia, absence of fetal heart tones, bleeding or spotting, and enlarged uterus.

37. Answer: D

Nursing Process: Analysis

Rationale: **It is important to know if the patient was pregnant when the attack occurred. If she is not pregnant, the appropriate "morning after" medication (ethinyl estradiol and norgestrel) can be given within 72 hours.** If the patient chooses to use plan B (morning after pill), they will need a prescription for an antiemetic as the medication can cause nausea. Other treatments for the patient would include prophylactic antibiotic therapy. Cultures and tests for syphilis will not be resulted for several days. A complete blood count does not provide vital information unless the patient is injured and hypovolemia is suspected. Rhogam will provide information regarding the Rh of the mother. This test is not indicated in this situation.

38. Answer: A

Nursing Process: Intervention

Rationale: **Clothing that was worn by the patient and obtained during the sexual assault examination should be placed in a paper bag and secured with evidence tape to ensure that no tampering occurs.** When performing a sexual assault examination and collecting the clothing, each piece of clothing should be placed in a separate paper bag. Also, the patient should stand on a sheet and then that sheet should also be sent as evidence. The emergency nurse should also put their name or initials across the fold of the bag to assist with knowledge of nontampering as well. The patient's clothing should be carefully removed, but not shaken out; microscopic evidence may be lost. All clothing should be given to the police; it is their responsibility to determine if evidence is present. Clothing should not be placed in plastic bags, which can cause mildew and moisture retention, both of which can cause loss of evidence. All evidence collected should be labeled with the victim's name, site of collection, date and time of collection, and the name of the person collecting the evidence.

 CENsational Pearl of Wisdom!

The nurse collecting the evidence should be sure to follow chain of custody to the "T"! All individuals touching the evidence must be documented with great care and the exchange to law enforcement of the kit must be clearly represented in the charting.

39. Answer: D

Nursing Process: Intervention

Rationale: **Any potential foreign material, such as suspected semen, blood, or saliva, should be collected with a cotton swab moistened with sterile water, not by scraping.** However, evidence under the fingernails must be obtained by scraping or clipping. Pubic hair samples and saliva specimens are all part of routine evidence collection.

 CENsational Pearl of Wisdom!

Never chart subjective information! Always remain objective. Never chart anything like, "No evidence of sexual assault." Be prepared for sexual assault questions on the test! They are always there!

40. Answer: A

Nursing Process: Assessment

Rationale: **Possibly due to its higher position, the right testicle is more prone to injury following a blow to the male groin. Penile fracture occurs following trauma while engorged. Urethral tear is more likely with a shearing-type injury as opposed to a direct blow.**

41. Answer: B

Nursing Process: Evaluation

Rationale: **Restlessness is typically the first sign of impending hypovolemic shock or hypoxia.** A pulse rate of 100 beats/minute is actually a decrease compared with the original 120 beats/minute, and the blood pressure has not dropped significantly. Requests for pain relief are normal for a trauma patient.

 CENsational Pearl of Wisdom!

If you are caring for a patient who is constantly pulling on or trying to remove their oxygen cannula or mask, they are probably hypoxic and confused. These are the patients who need their oxygen the most. Be ready to intubate this patient!

42. Answer: B

Nursing Process: Assessment

Rationale: **When the urethra is torn, a hematoma or collection of blood separates the two sections of the urethra. This may feel like a boggy mass on rectal**

examination and the prostate becomes "high riding." A palpable prostate gland usually indicates an intact urethra. Absent sphincter tone would refer to a spinal cord injury. The presence of blood in the rectum would probably correlate with a GI bleed or colon injury.

43. Answer: B

Nursing Process: Intervention

Rationale: **Candida albicans is a yeast (fungal infection) treated with Mycostatin (nystatin) and does not require sexual partner treatment.** *Neisseria gonorrhoeae, Trichomonas vaginalis,* and *Chlamydia trachomatis* all are sexually transmitted diseases that necessitate partner treatment and thorough patient education.

44. Answer: A

Nursing Process: Assessment

Rationale: **A contrecoup injury can occur to the kidney after a fall that exerts force above the kidney. The force tears the renal pedicle and causes a bruit that can be auscultated at the first or second lumbar vertebra.** Suprapubic pain accompanies a bladder injury, not a vascular disruption. Hypertension may occur after a renal injury has been repaired. Decreased or absent bowel sounds would occur with an abdominal insult that created an ileus.

45. Answer: D

Nursing Process: Analysis

Rationale: **Ceftriaxone (Rocephin) injections are very painful. Lidocaine is recommended as the diluent of choice.** Sterile water, D_5W, and sterile saline do not have any numbing properties.

 CENsational Pearl of Wisdom!

Do not use intravenous ceftriaxone (Rocephin) with lactated ringers or other solutions that contain calcium as a precipitate can occur. Do not use this medication in infants under 28 days of life with high bilirubin levels. Ceftriaxone (Rocephin) can displace the bilirubin from binding sites, adding to the disease process and producing encephalopathy.

46. Answer: C

Nursing Process: Analysis

Rationale: **A mother infected with Chlamydia can pass the organism to her infant during its passage through** the cervix. Potential complications for the infant include conjunctivitis and chlamydial pneumonia. Endocarditis, hepatitis, and encephalitis are not passed through *Chlamydia*.

47. Answer: A

Nursing Process: Assessment

Rationale: **A patient with a septic abortion will present with prolonged retained products of conception, resulting in foul-smelling vaginal bleeding or discharge, abdominal pain, and fever.** Pyelonephritis does not produce a foul-smelling discharge. Vaginitis is not generally associated with bleeding and the discharge is typically frothy or curd-like. Ovarian cysts are not generally associated with discharge.

CENsational Pearl of Wisdom!

Many times, patients who have had a recent abortion will not share this information readily. The emergency nurse must be able to ask important questions without making the patient feel uncomfortable. The emergency nurse should also understand the signs and symptoms so that suspicion can lead the nurse down the right pathway.

48. Answer: A

Nursing Process: Intervention

Rationale: **This patient has signs and symptoms of testicular torsion. Testicular torsion results from congenital maldevelopment between the testis and the posterior scrotal wall. This is an emergency situation and an emergent ultrasound must be done.** Twisting of the spermatic cord compromises the circulation causing severe pain that is not relieved by ice or elevation. There is no blood loss associated with testicular torsion, so blood products are not indicated.

CENsational Pearl of Wisdom!

Young boys may not want to tell nurses that they have testicular pain. They may describe the pain as being in the lower abdomen. Also, the testicle in testicular torsion can cause an upwardly retracted testicle, making the pain seem to be in the lower abdomen. Be suspicious with pubertal and prepubertal boys! No fever is usually present with this process.

49. Answer: D

Nursing Process: Analysis

Rationale: **Pseudoephedrine (Sudafed) is an alpha-adrenergic agonist that increases urinary resistance. The effect is minimal but can contribute to urinary retention in combination with bladder outlet obstruction (enlarged prostate gland).** Nonsteroidal anti-inflammatory drugs such as Ibuprofen (Motrin) are associated with hematuria and acute renal failure, but not urinary retention. Terazosin is an alpha-adrenergic blocker used to improve bladder neck dyssynergia (improve bladder outlet). Adverse effects of vitamin C include acidic urine, oxaluria, and renal stones.

50. Answer: D

Nursing Process: Analysis

Rationale: **A pregnant patient with pyelonephritis requires aggressive treatment. She could quickly develop acute renal failure or sepsis.** Children with renal injury can usually be managed as an outpatient. A young patient with an uncomplicated urinary tract infection can be discharged with thorough discharge instructions and treatment. Urethritis in a male patient is likely caused by a sexually transmitted disease and can be treated orally or intramuscularly.

51. Answer: C

Nursing Process: Assessment

Rationale: **Whether the patient has changed her clothes, or even brushed her teeth since the attack, is critical to evidence collection and preservation.** It is also helpful if the patient has not showered, urinated, or defecated. Determining if the patient has notified the police is also important, but does not affect the assessment. It is not relevant to know if she has been previously sexually assaulted or if she is using a method of birth control at this time.

52. Answer: C

Nursing Process: Analysis

Rationale: **The patient's well-being is always the priority.** Evidence collection and preservation and encouraging police involvement are important, but is not the priority. Notifying family and friends is up to the discretion of the patient.

53. Answer: A

Nursing Process: Evaluation

Rationale: **Sexual assault patients typically receive prophylaxis for sexually transmitted diseases and pregnancy when undergoing treatment. To ensure the treatment was adequate, follow-up with either the local**

health department or the patient's primary care physician is necessary. A return visit to the emergency department would not be warranted for follow-up care. While some sexual assault victims blame themselves for the attack, this certainly is not a healthy coping mechanism. Secluding herself in her home is also not a healthy option.

 CENsational Pearl of Wisdom!

When caring for sexual assault victims, encourage the use of local rape crisis departments. These individuals can help the victim through the entire process. Also, encourage reporting to the proper authorities. Even if the patient does not want to file charges, it can help identify the perpetrator if subsequent events occur.

54. Answer: A

Nursing Process: Assessment

Rationale: **Ectopic pregnancies that are leaking or have ruptured result in referred pain to the shoulder from blood irritating the diaphragm. Pain with an ectopic pregnancy occurs in either the left or right lower abdominal area.** Sharp upper abdominal pain is too high for pain caused by an ectopic pregnancy. Flank pain and hematuria may be caused by a kidney infection or kidney stones. Colicky, diffuse abdominal pain is commonly associated with intestinal disorders.

55. Answer: C

Nursing Process: Analysis

Rationale: **Placenta previa is associated with painless vaginal bleeding that occurs when the placenta, or a portion of the placenta, covers the cervical os. Serious hemorrhage can occur.** In abruptio placentae, the placenta tears away from the wall of the uterus before delivery. The patient usually has pain and a board-like uterus. Preterm labor is associated with contractions and should not involve bright red bleeding. By definition, threatened abortion occurs during the first 20 weeks of gestation.

56. Answer: C

Nursing Process: Intervention

Rationale: **The left lateral recumbent position avoids compression of the inferior vena cava; compressing the vessel may result in decreased uterine blood flow, fetal hypoxia, and maternal hypotension.** Trendelenburg or supine position would compress this vessel. If a pregnant patient must lie flat on a backboard for spinal evaluation, a wedge may be placed under the back board to tilt it, or manual manipulation of the uterus may also be done by

a provider. The knee-chest position is used to avoid compressing the umbilical cord when it is prolapsed.

 CENsational Pearl of Wisdom!

Vena cava syndrome, when the fetus is lying on the vena cava, can reduce maternal cardiac output by 30% causing hypotension. The uteroplacental bed is already vasoconstricted, which then places the fetus in danger as well.

57. Answer: A

Nursing Process: Intervention

Rationale: **A pelvic examination should not be performed on a pregnant patient with vaginal bleeding in the third trimester. This can cause further bleeding and damage the placenta.** The patient should be placed on bed rest, monitor a pad count, and be admitted if bleeding is heavy and persists. A pelvic ultrasound is useful for detecting placenta previa.

58. Answer: C

Nursing Process: Intervention

Rationale: **Meconium-stained amniotic fluid can be an emergency for the neonate; therefore, endotracheal (ET) intubation with suction applied to the ET tube should be performed.** Stimulating the neonate will cause more amniotic-stained fluid to enter the lungs. It is no longer recommended to routinely perform oropharynx and nasopharynx suctioning for neonates born to mothers with meconium-stained fluid. Placing an umbilical line is not necessary at this time.

59. Answer: D

Nursing Process: Evaluation

Rationale: **This scenario provides information for symptoms associated with pregnancy-associated hypertension; the patient has a potential for seizure activity because of central nervous system irritability.** Seizure precautions should be instituted. Precipitous delivery, vaginal bleeding, and cardiac dysrhythmias are not complications of pregnancy-associated hypertension.

60. Answer: D

Nursing Process: Analysis

Rationale: **Postpartum hemorrhage is defined as blood loss greater than 500 mL and is a common complication of labor and delivery. Amniotic fluid embolism, a complication experienced by the mother, is caused when amniotic fluid leaks into the mother's venous** circulation during labor and delivery. It does not cause postpartum hemorrhage. Retained products of conception or placental fragments can interfere with involution or return of the uterus to normal size. Vaginal or cervical tears can be a cause of postpartum bleeding.

61. Answer: A

Nursing Process: Assessment

Rationale: **The desire to bear down or push usually indicates that delivery is near (especially in the multiparous mother).** Other signs of imminent delivery are heavy bloody show and a bulging perineum. Rupture of membranes may occur before labor begins. Loss of the mucus plug is likely to occur up to a month before delivery. Lengthening of contractions does not necessarily indicate that delivery is imminent.

62. Answer: C

Nursing Process: Intervention

Rationale: **Dimming lights and wearing earplugs may decrease stimulation, which would help to decrease the potential for seizures.** Noise, vibration, and light may increase blood pressure. Reading her a story would be nice, but it may or may not lower her blood pressure. Even watching TV is sometimes considered too much stimulation. Having the cabin lights lit and the siren on would cause overstimulation.

63. Answer: D

Nursing Process: Analysis

Rationale: **Burns that involve the face, eyes, ears, hands, feet, major joints, genitalia, or perineum should be transferred to a burn center. These patients need special attention to prevent infection, scarring, and contractures.** Care at home, with a local physician or in the emergency department, is not adequate.

64. Answer: C

Nursing Process: Intervention

Rationale: **Although Zosyn (Pipericillin) is a wide-spectrum antibiotic, ceftriaxone (Rocephin), metronidazole (Flagyl), and azithromycin (Zithromax) are usually prescribed prophylactically for possible sexually transmitted diseases. Remember that metronidazole (Flagyl) should not be taken with alcohol. This medication may be needed to be started the next day depending on the circumstances.**

65. Answer: A

Nursing Process: Analysis

Rationale: **A urethral tear is more common in males because the urethra is longer with more exposure.**

Bladder rupture can occur with a pelvic fracture, but is less common. A fractured penis usually derives from a direct blow or injury during an erection, not necessarily a pelvic fracture. Femur fractures may occur depending on the mechanism of injury.

 CENsational Pearl of Wisdom!

Suspect urethral tears early in the trauma assessment to avoid further injury by insertion of a urethral catheter. Blood found at the urinary meatus along with an abnormal prostate examination is indicative of this injury. A cystogram can be done to rule out injury in the acute setting.

66. Answer: B

Nursing Process: Intervention

Rationale: **The gravid uterus will push the diaphragm upward, the lungs will shorten, and the functional reserve decreases. The chest tube should be placed one to two intercostal spaces higher than the standard fourth to fifth intercostal space.** The first and second intercostal space would be too high. Anything distal would be too low.

67. Answer: C

Nursing Process: Intervention

Rationale: **Capillary engorgement of the upper respiratory passages increases the risk of nasopharyngeal bleeding and airway obstruction.** This does not increase bleeding upon insertion of the urinary catheter, oral endotracheal tube, or arterial line.

68. Answer: B

Nursing Process: Intervention

Rationale: **Observation of the patient's respiratory status is of highest importance. Narcotics suppress respiratory effort and the patient may need to be intubated.** Administering Narcan to this patient may lead to rapid withdrawal and seizures in the newborn. Not reporting the situation and allowing the patient to continue her normal activity with illicit drug use are not appropriate interventions.

69. Answer: A

Nursing Process: Intervention

Rationale: **The normal neonatal heart rate is 120 to 160 beats/minute. Heart rates below 60 beats/minute necessitate chest compressions and ventilatory support.**

70. Answer: A

Nursing Process: Assessment

Rationale: **The APGAR score should be determined at 1 and 5 minutes and should include assessment of heart rate, muscle tone, reflexes, respiratory effort, and color.** A score of 7 to 10 is favorable.

71. Answer: A

Nursing Process: Analysis

Rationale: **Ectopic pregnancies are typically related to scarring of the fallopian tubes secondary to pelvic inflammatory disease (PID).** Spontaneous abortion and multiple pregnancies are not associated with this condition. Scarring from PID may also result in fertility difficulties.

 CENsational Pearl of Wisdom!

Another complication of pelvic inflammatory disease is called Fitz-Hugh-Curtis syndrome. This is also known as gonococcal perihepatitis, which causes an inflammatory disease process on the lining of the liver. Other organs that can be affected are the peritoneal lining and the diaphragm.

72. Answer: A

Nursing Process: Intervention

Rationale: **Although more recent information shows that all infants should not be routinely suctioned at birth, if the situation arose that suctioning was necessary, it is important to suction the mouth first, followed by the nose. Infants are obligate nose breathers, which means they prefer breathing through their nose.** This will help clear the oral airway, before the infant takes their first breath through the nose. The neonate's head should be kept level with the rest of the body.

73. Answer: B

Nursing Process: Intervention

Rationale: **Risk of perineal tears is increased if the mother pushes at the moment of delivery. Having the mother pant while applying gentle pressure to the perineum decreases the risk of tears.** Fundal pressure is not necessary and may cause damage to the uterus. The mother should not attempt to not push when the baby is ready to deliver.

 CENsational Pearl of Wisdom!

When delivering an infant be sure to place two clamps! And cut in between!

74. Answer: C

Nursing Process: Intervention

Rationale: **The patient should be tilted on her left side to relieve pressure on the vena cava by the gravid uterus.** Trendelenburg's position is contraindicated for this patient. Tilting to the right side is preferable to lying flat, but is not as beneficial as tilting to the left. It will be appropriate to remove spinal immobilization as soon as possible, but must be under the direction of the provider. The preferable position would be on her left side or sitting as soon as the backboard is removed.

75. Answer: C

Nursing Process: Intervention

Rationale: **Early insertion of a urinary catheter is essential for this patient. These are symptoms of autonomic dysreflexia. The increase of sympathetic responses causes cutaneous vasodilatation above the cord lesion (diaphoresis and flushing) and cutaneous vasoconstriction below the lesion (blanching, coolness, and elevated blood pressure). A distended bladder is one of the most common precursors and can be caused by pressure from stool in the rectal vault.** Insertion of a rectal tube will not remove the fecal impaction. Administration of hydralazine (or any antihypertensive) is not the cure for the problem. Laxatives may stimulate a bowel movement, but is not really the treatment for this patient.

 CENsational Pearl of Wisdom!

Autonomic dysreflexia is usually caused by GI or GU problems and these issues must be rectified before the hypertensive episode will resolve. While constipation and impaction are common problems, urinary retention, renal calculi, and catheter malfunction are also very common. Most patients with spinal cord injuries are aware of this possibility and understand the importance of "fixing" the underlying problem immediately.

References

Al-qudah, H. S. (2016). *Priapism*. Emedicine. Retrieved from https://emedicine.medscape.com/article/437237-overview#a4 (4)

Chang, A. K. (2015). *Pregnancy trauma treatment and management*. Emedicine. Retrieved from https://emedicine.medscape.com/article/796979-treatment (56)

Cummings, J. M. (2017). *Urethral trauma workup*. Emedicine. Retrieved from https://emedicine.medscape.com/article/451797-workup (65)

Dave, C. N. (2018). *Nephrolithiasis treatment and management*. Emedicine. Retrieved from https://emedicine.medscape.com/article/437096-treatment-d7#d7 (23, 30)

DiMare, M. (2018). *Acute epididymitis*. Medscape. Retrieved from https://emedicine.medscape.com/article/777181-overview (28)

Emergency Nurses Association. (2017). Emergency nursing pediatric course (5th ed.). Des Plaines, IL: Emergency Nurses Association. (69, 72)

Emergency Nurses Association. (2014). Trauma nurse core course (7th ed.). Des Plaines, IL: Emergency Nurses Association. (12, 19, 41, 42, 44, 64, 67)

Emergency Nurses Association. (2017). Emergency nursing core curriculum (7th ed.). Philadelphia, PA: W. B. Saunders. (2, 3, 8, 10, 11, 20, 27, 32, 50–53, 55, 57, 73–75)

Fryhofer, S. A. (2014). *Can vitamin C cause kidney stones?* Medscape for Nurses. Retrieved from https://www.medscape.com/viewarticle/825349 (49)

Genetics Home Reference. (2018). *Cyclic vomiting syndrome*. Retrieved from https://ghr.nlm.nih.gov/condition/cyclic-vomiting-syndrome (16)

Girerd, P. H. (2018). *Bacterial vaginosis*. Emedicine. Retrieved from https://emedicine.medscape.com/article/254342-overview#a5 (6, 24)

Grabosch, S. M. (2018). *Ovarian cysts*. Emedicine. Retrieved from https://emedicine.medscape.com/article/255865-overview (35)

Hall, M. E., et al. (2013). *The heart during pregnancy*. Retrieved from https://www.ncbi.nlm.nih.gov/pmc/articles/PMC3802121 (18)

Hamilton, C. A. (2018). *Cystic teratoma*. Emedicine. Retrieved from https://emedicine.medscape.com/article/281850-overview (35)

Hammond, B., et al. (2013). Sheehy's manual of emergency care (7th ed.). St. Louis, MO: Mosby Elsevier. (13)

Howard, P., et al. (2010). Sheehy's emergency nursing principles and practice (6th ed.). St. Louis, MO: Mosby Elsevier. (1, 5, 9, 15, 21, 25, 26. 29, 31, 34, 36–39, 43, 47, 54, 58–61, 64, 70)

Jarra-Almonte, G. (2015). *Resuscitation of the pregnant trauma patient*. emDocs. Retrieved from http://www.emdocs.net/resuscitation-of-the-pregnant-trauma-patient-pearls-pitfalls (66)

Kaye, K. M. (2018). *Herpes simplex virus (HSV) infections*. Merck Manual. Retrieved from https://www.merckmanuals.com/home/infections/herpesvirus-infections/herpes-simplex-virus-hsv-infections (24)

Luciano, R., et al. (2018). *NSAIDS: Acute kidney injury (acute renal failure)*. UpToDate. Retrieved from https://www.uptodate.com/contents/nsaids-acute-kidney-injury-acute-renal-failure (49)

Mayo Clinic. (2018). *HPV infection*. Retrieved from https://www.mayoclinic.org/diseases-conditions/hpv-infection/symptoms-causes/syc-20351596 (24)

Mevorach, R. A. (2015). *Scrotal trauma*. Emedicine. Retrieved from https://emedicine.medscape.com/article/441272-overview#a7 (40)

National Institute of Diabetes and Digestive and Kidney Diseases. (2014). *Urinary retention*. Retrieved from https://www.niddk.nih.gov/health-information/urologic-diseases/urinary-retention (49)

Paushter, D. (2015). *Testicular torsion imaging*. Emedicine. Retrieved from https://emedicine.medscape.com/article/381204-overview (28)

RXList. (2017). *Terazosin*. Retrieved from https://www.rxlist.com/consumer_terazosin_hytrin/drugs-condition.htm (49)

RXList. (2018). *Flagyl*. Retrieved from https://www.rxlist.com/flagyl-drug.htm#description (7, 27)

RXList. (2018). *Rocephin*. Retrieved from https://www.rxlist.com/rocephin-drug.htm#description (45)

Sepillian, V. P. (2017). *Ectopic pregnancy treatment and management*. Emedicine. Retrieved from https://emedicine.medscape.com/article/2041923-treatment#d11 (7)

Shenot, P. J. (2018). *Testicular torsion*. Merck Manual. Retrieved from https://www.merckmanuals.com/professional/genitourinary-disorders/penile-and-scrotal-disorders/testicular-torsion (48)

Shepherd, S. M. (2017). *Pelvic inflammatory disease*. Emedicine. Retrieved from https://emedicine.medscape.com/article/256448-overview (71)

Sobol, J. (2017). *Transurethral resection of the prostate—discharge*. U.S. National Library of Medicine. Retrieved from https://medlineplus.gov/ency/patientinstructions/000300.htm (14)

WebMD. (2018). *What is HPV?* Retrieved from https://www.webmd.com/sexual-conditions/hpv-genital-warts/hpv-virus-information-about-human-papillomavirus#1 (24)

WEM. (2018). *Thromboelastography (TEG)*. Retrieved from https://wikem.org/wiki/Thromboelastography_(TEG) (17)

wikiHow. (2018). *How to use a bladder scanner*. Retrieved from https://www.wikihow.com/Use-a-Bladder-Scanner (33)

Part II
Sample Tests and Appendices

Sample Test 1

Patricia L. Clutter, RN, MEd, CEN, FAEN

This test has been created according to the Blueprint found on the BCEN website for the CEN test.

Remember that the actual test will have 175 questions as it will have 25 pretest questions–to test the question itself–not you!!

Good Luck!

Questions

1. An unrestrained passenger is thrown 20 feet (6 m) from a car that hit an embankment. On arrival to the emergency department, the patient is conscious and complains of shortness of breath. His vital signs are as follows: blood pressure 108/66 mm Hg, pulse 116 beats/minute with weak radial pulses, and respirations 26 breaths/minute and shallow. Capillary refill is delayed. The lungs are clear bilaterally with diminished breath sounds on the right. Paradoxical chest movement is noted on the right side. A chest radiograph shows a right pneumothorax and multiple rib fractures on the right (fourth to seventh). Which of the following potential injuries would be the trauma nurse's primary concern for this patient?
[ ] **A.** Flail chest
[ ] **B.** Tension pneumothorax
[ ] **C.** Ruptured diaphragm
[ ] **D.** Massive hemothorax

2. A 24-year-old patient is in the early stage of an acute asthma attack. Knowing the pathology of asthma and the progression of an asthma attack and its correlation with arterial blood gases (ABGs), the emergency nurse anticipates which of the following ABG results on this patient?
[ ] **A.** Normal pH, normal $PaCO_2$, and normal PaO_2
[ ] **B.** Elevated pH, decreased $PaCO_2$, and decreased PaO_2
[ ] **C.** Decreased pH, increased $PaCO_2$, and decreased PaO_2
[ ] **D.** Normal pH, normal $PaCO_2$, and decreased PaO_2

3. Which of the following is the most common area of rupture in traumatic cardiac injury?
[ ] **A.** Aortic arch
[ ] **B.** Pulmonary vein
[ ] **C.** Ligamentum arteriosum
[ ] **D.** Right coronary artery

4. A patient arrives with a history of surgery 3 weeks ago and now has complaints of leg swelling, redness, warmth, and tenderness. The emergency nurse suspects which of the following?
[ ] **A.** Postthrombotic syndrome (PTS)
[ ] **B.** Thromboangiitis obliterans (Buerger disease)
[ ] **C.** Peripheral venous thrombosis
[ ] **D.** Raynaud's disease

5. A patient presents to the emergency department following a fall from a porch 3 days before. He is pale and diaphoretic and states that he feels short of breath. On assessment, he has tenderness to the right lower anterior ribs. Bilateral, clear, equal breath sounds are present. Vital signs are as follows:

Blood pressure—88/62 mm Hg
Pulse—134 beats/minute
Respirations— 32 breaths/minute
Pulse oximetry—92% on room air
Temperature—98.4° F (36.8° C)

Which of the following diagnoses should the emergency nurse anticipate?
[ ] **A.** Splenic injury
[ ] **B.** Colon injury
[ ] **C.** Cardiac injury
[ ] **D.** Liver injury

6. A patient presents with a large amount of abdominal distention, vomiting, and generalized abdominal pain. On assessment, the emergency nurse notes that no bowel sounds are present. The patient has a history of a temporary colostomy for a ruptured colon 5 years before, a cholecystectomy, and appendectomy. Medical history includes hypothyroidism and hypertension. The emergency nurse realizes that this patient will be prone to all of the following potential complications **EXCEPT**:

[ ] **A.** sepsis.

[ ] **B.** pneumonia.

[ ] **C.** dehydration.

[ ] **D.** perforation.

7. Signs and symptoms of acute arterial occlusion include which of the following symptoms?

[ ] **A.** Pain, pallor, pulselessness, paresthesia, and paralysis

[ ] **B.** Chest pain, tachycardia, tachypnea, and elevated temperature

[ ] **C.** Severe pain, blood pressure variation in arms, and peripheral cyanosis

[ ] **D.** Chest pain, dyspnea, nausea, diaphoresis, and fatigue

8. A patient presents with a narrow-complex tachycardia. Vital signs are as follows:

Blood pressure—110/82 mm Hg
Pulse—180 beats/minute
Respirations—20 breaths/minute
Pulse oximetry—95% on room air
Temperature—98.6° F (37° C)

Which of the following initial outcomes will be expected with the successful use of the proper medication to treat this patient?

[ ] **A.** Third-degree AV block

[ ] **B.** Burst of atrial fibrillation

[ ] **C.** Ventricular tachycardia

[ ] **D.** Period of asystole

9. Which of the following is the primary goal in the treatment of a patient with acute respiratory distress syndrome (ARDS)?

[ ] **A.** Treating the underlying condition

[ ] **B.** Maintaining nutritional requirements

[ ] **C.** Maintaining adequate tissue oxygenation

[ ] **D.** Preventing secondary infection

10. A FAST (Focused Assessment with Sonography for Trauma) examination is performed on a patient involved in a motor vehicle crash. Which of the following statements made by the emergency nurse indicates an understanding of this evaluation tool?

[ ] **A.** "I heard that this tool is great and has a 90% to 100% accuracy rating for all patients."

[ ] **B.** "This is great to use! We will have our answer for sure in a few minutes!"

[ ] **C.** "This diagnostic tool is so much better for small bowel and stomach injuries."

[ ] **D.** "This test only checks for large amounts of blood in the abdomen."

11. The level of anxiety at which a patient loses their ability to think logically is:

[ ] **A.** level I: mild.

[ ] **B.** level II: moderate.

[ ] **C.** level III: severe.

[ ] **D.** level IV: panic.

12. Which of the following statements made by the wife of a patient who was an unsuccessful resuscitation attempt would most indicate that her presence during the attempt was a positive experience?

[ ] **A.** "I wonder if more medicine would have helped?"

[ ] **B.** "I will never get over seeing the screen show that flat line."

[ ] **C.** "I feel like nothing more could have been done."

[ ] **D.** "I wish I had had someone to explain things to me."

13. Which of the following is the most critical intervention during the first minutes of ventricular fibrillation?

[ ] **A.** Advanced airway

[ ] **B.** Epinephrine 0.1 mg IV/IO

[ ] **C.** Immediate cardiac compressions

[ ] **D.** Electrical defibrillation

14. All of the following would indicate reperfusion after thrombolytic therapy **EXCEPT**:

[ ] **A.** relief of chest pain.

[ ] **B.** onset of dysrhythmia.

[ ] **C.** ST-segment normalization.

[ ] **D.** Osborn wave.

15. Which of the following statements made by a patient being discharged with a diagnosis of Raynaud's phenomenon would indicate that the discharge instructions were understood?

[ ] **A.** "I will wear gloves to keep warm and work hard on stopping smoking."

[ ] **B.** "I will keep my arm elevated on a pillow and apply ice to my hand."

[ ] **C.** "I have an elastic bandage at home that I can wear when I am on the computer."

[ ] **D.** "I will drink plenty of fluids and take aspirin for the pain."

16. A 14-month-old infant with vomiting and diarrhea has been prescribed a fluid bolus for treatment of dehydration. The child weighs 20 pounds. Which of the following is the correct bolus amount?

[ ] **A.** 180 mL

[ ] **B.** 200 mL

[ ] **C.** 400 mL

[ ] **D.** 900 mL

17. During a manic episode, a patient with bipolar disorder may:

[ ] **A.** present withdrawn and depressed.

[ ] **B.** present unkempt with poor hygiene.

[ ] **C.** display poor social judgment.

[ ] **D.** refuse to answer questions.

18. Which level trauma center must have a trauma surgeon, trauma director, operating suite, and in-house operating room staff on duty 24 hours per day?

[ ] **A.** Level I trauma center only

[ ] **B.** Level I, II, and III trauma centers

[ ] **C.** Level I and II trauma centers

[ ] **D.** Level IV trauma center

19. Which of the following is a manager allowed to do in response to a collective bargaining initiative?

[ ] **A.** Prevent employees from engaging in recruiting activities during nonworking hours.

[ ] **B.** Prevent employees from participating in informal union activities in patient care areas.

[ ] **C.** Withhold desirable assignments from those nurses who are union organizers.

[ ] **D.** Provide special considerations to discourage employees from joining the union.

20. A patient arrives in the emergency department with the following signs and symptoms: worsening dyspnea, tachypnea, cough, edema, fatigue, and distended neck veins. The emergency nurse suspects which of the following as a primary diagnosis?

[ ] **A.** Pulmonary embolism

[ ] **B.** Heart failure

[ ] **C.** Cardiac tamponade

[ ] **D.** Tension pneumothorax

21. Which of the following would the emergency nurse anticipate for a patient with an aortic dissection?

[ ] **A.** Emergent surgery

[ ] **B.** Chest tube insertion

[ ] **C.** Immediate intubation

[ ] **D.** Pericardial decompression

22. A patient with a previous medical history of stroke is brought to the emergency department with altered mental status. The patient's baseline mental status is alert and oriented to person, place, time, and event; however, at this time, the patient is responsive to painful stimuli only. Examination reveals hot, moist skin with a tympanic temperature of 102.2° F (39° C), adventitious lung sounds, and tachycardia. The emergency nurse suspects which of the following as a possible reason for these signs?

[ ] **A.** Congestive heart failure

[ ] **B.** Meningitis

[ ] **C.** Aspiration pneumonia

[ ] **D.** Stroke

23. The Joint Commission in 2018 released a Quick Safety alert on "identifying Human Trafficking Victims" and pinpointed several red flags of a potential victim. All of the following would be examples of human trafficking victims **EXCEPT**:

[ ] **A.** acting fearful, anxious, depressed, submissive, tense, nervous or paranoid, and avoiding eye contact.

[ ] **B.** requesting additional follow-up treatment at a separate appointment in order to see another provider.

[ ] **C.** showing reluctance or refusing to change into a gown and/or to cooperate with the physical examination.

[ ] **D.** exhibiting behavior or demeanor not in alignment with injury or complaint (i.e., acts like it is "no big deal").

24. An elderly patient with stroke-like symptoms has an active DNR (Do Not Resuscitate) order. In caring for this patient, the understanding would be which of the following options?

[ ] **A.** Should not initiate labs or an IV line as the patient does not want further treatment.

[ ] **B.** May not provide care for this patient until family arrives and gives consent.

[ ] **C.** An intravenous line may be established, but no medications should be given.

[ ] **D.** Should initiate care for this patient's stroke symptoms regardless of the DNR wishes.

25. A patient presents to the emergency department with chief complaint of feeling weak and generalized fatigue. The patient is diaphoretic with cool skin. He states persistent nausea without vomiting. Vital signs are as follows:

Blood pressure—92/64 mm Hg
Pulse—122 beats/minute
Respirations—32 breaths/minute
Pulse oximetry—91% on room air
Temperature—98.8° F (37.1° C)

Past history reveals hypertension, chronic bronchitis, recent history of fracture of the left 11th to 12th ribs, and hypercholesteremia. Which of the following diagnoses would the emergency nurse suspect?
[ ] **A.** Pneumonia
[ ] **B.** Pancreatitis
[ ] **C.** Splenic injury
[ ] **D.** Lacerated liver

26. The psychiatric condition with the highest mortality rate is:
[ ] **A.** anorexia nervosa.
[ ] **B.** bipolar disorder.
[ ] **C.** dementia.
[ ] **D.** psychotic depression.

27. All of the following medications could be utilized to treat pancreatitis **EXCEPT**:
[ ] **A.** dicyclomine (Bentyl).
[ ] **B.** fentanyl (Sublimaze).
[ ] **C.** octreotide (Sandostatin).
[ ] **D.** famotidine (Pepcid).

28. A patient is seen in the emergency department following a motor vehicle crash. He is diagnosed with a perforated stomach, a pelvic fracture, upper left arm fracture, and a mild closed head injury. Which of the following complications would the emergency nurse understand to be the highest probability to occur for this patient due to the injuries sustained?
[ ] **A.** Cardiogenic shock
[ ] **B.** Pulmonary edema
[ ] **C.** Peritonitis
[ ] **D.** Paralysis

29. Research that aims to examine the feelings and perceptions of emergency nurses working with battered female patients is which of the following types of study?
[ ] **A.** Qualitative
[ ] **B.** Quasi-scientific
[ ] **C.** Quantitative
[ ] **D.** Experimental

30. An 11-month-old child is brought to the emergency department by his parents. His parents tell the emergency nurse he has been coughing and has had a runny nose for 1 day. He has a red rash on his face, a rectal temperature of 102.5° F (39.2° C), and bluish-white spots on his buccal mucosa. Which of the following conditions are these symptoms associated with?
[ ] **A.** Mumps
[ ] **B.** Measles (Rubeola)
[ ] **C.** Allergic reaction
[ ] **D.** Varicella (chicken pox)

31. Sickle cell crisis is associated with a number of precipitants. Which of the following is **NOT** one of these precipitants?
[ ] **A.** Cold ambient temperature
[ ] **B.** Infection
[ ] **C.** Metabolic or respiratory alkalosis
[ ] **D.** High altitude

32. Objective assessment of an acute aortic dissection would include which of the following?
[ ] **A.** Manual blood pressure taken in both arms
[ ] **B.** Inspection for petechial rash to extremities
[ ] **C.** Inspection for extremity edema, anasarca, and ascites
[ ] **D.** Auscultation of heart sounds for prominent apical pulse/S3 and S4

33. A patient arrives with a gunshot wound to the left chest. The patient is alert, complaining of pain and difficulty breathing. Objective data include hypotension, muffled heart sounds, jugular vein distention (JVD), tachycardia, tachypnea, and an open wound to the left chest. Oxygen via non-rebreather and two large-bore intravenous catheters have been placed. Vital signs on arrival were as follows:

Blood pressure—80/50 mm Hg
Pulse—125 beats/minute
Respirations—32 breaths/minute
Pulse oximetry—80% on room air
Temperature—98.6° F (37° C)

Which of the following should the emergency nurse anticipate to prepare for next?
[ ] **A.** Assist with a resuscitative thoracotomy.
[ ] **B.** Prepare for massive blood transfusion.
[ ] **C.** Assist with a pericardiocentesis.
[ ] **D.** Prepare for aggressive ventilatory support.

34. A nonresponsive 64-year-old patient has the following findings in the emergency department: blood glucose 340 mg/dL, serum osmolality 320 mOsm/kg, and pH 7.2. The patient is taking deep, gasping respirations. The emergency nurse should suspect which of the following disease processes?

[ ] **A.** Hyperthyroid crisis (Storm)
[ ] **B.** Hyperosmolar hyperglycemic syndrome (HHS)
[ ] **C.** Syndrome of inappropriate antidiuretic hormone (SIADH)
[ ] **D.** Diabetic ketoacidosis (DKA)

35. A mother brings her 3-year-old to the emergency department because of blood in the child's underwear. The examination by the sexual assault nurse examiner (SANE nurse) reveals sexual assault and felonious penetration. The mother wants to leave. Which action should the nurse take?

[ ] **A.** No action is necessary because the mother is the child's legal guardian and her decisions are final.
[ ] **B.** Immediately report the findings to Child Protective Services and the police.
[ ] **C.** Encourage the mother to reconsider her decision and refer her to a child psychologist.
[ ] **D.** Have the emergency department physician talk to the mother and try to persuade her to stay.

36. A 2-year-old female child is brought to the emergency department with a distended abdomen and vomiting. Assessment reveals a lethargic toddler who does not cry when examined. The child's skin is cool and slightly diaphoretic. No bowel sounds are heard. Breath sounds are clear to auscultation. Vital signs are as follows:

Blood pressure—76/42 mm Hg
Pulse—164 beats/minute
Respirations—44 breaths/minute
Pulse oximetry—84% on room air
Temperature—99.8° F (37.6° C) rectal

A KUB (kidney, ureter, bladder) radiograph is obtained that shows air–fluid levels. Which of the following would be the highest priority for this child?

[ ] **A.** Oxygen by mask or flow-by
[ ] **B.** Intravenous line
[ ] **C.** Fluid administration
[ ] **D.** Urinary catheter

37. Potential nonpsychiatric causes of acute agitation and behavior changes include all of the following **EXCEPT**:

[ ] **A.** hypoxia.
[ ] **B.** thyroid disorders.
[ ] **C.** stroke.
[ ] **D.** dementia.

38. A patient arrives in the emergency department with bright red, bloody emesis. He is vomiting on arrival and continues as he is placed into a room. He is pale and diaphoretic with cold extremities. Vital signs are as follows:

Blood pressure—82/46 mm Hg
Pulse—146 beats/minute
Respirations—36 breaths/minute
Pulse oximetry—89% on room air
Temperature—99.4° F (37.4° C)

The team starts two large-bore intravenous lines and crystalloids are begun at a rapid rate. All of the following would be anticipated by the emergency nurse **EXCEPT**:

[ ] **A.** type and screen.
[ ] **B.** gastric tube placement.
[ ] **C.** contact endoscopy.
[ ] **D.** cardiac monitoring.

39.

The emergency nurse recognizes the above rhythm as:

[ ] **A.** first-degree heart block.
[ ] **B.** second-degree heart block, type I.
[ ] **C.** second-degree heart block, type II.
[ ] **D.** third-degree heart block.

40. Which of the following is the most common and concerning electrolyte imbalance associated with digoxin toxicity?

[ ] **A.** Hyponatremia
[ ] **B.** Hypercalcemia
[ ] **C.** Hypomagnesemia
[ ] **D.** Hyperkalemia

41. After teaching the patient with asthma about inhalers, which of the following statements indicates the need for further instruction?

[ ] **A.** "I should hold the inhaler upright and shake it well."
[ ] **B.** "I should hold my breath for 5 to 10 seconds after each puff."
[ ] **C.** "I should hold the inhaler in my mouth with a good seal."
[ ] **D.** "I should hold my head back and forcefully exhale."

42. Which of the following is the most likely intervention for a patient with a suspected diaphragmatic rupture?
[ ] **A.** Needle thoracostomy
[ ] **B.** Chest tube insertion
[ ] **C.** Preparation for surgery
[ ] **D.** Transfer to unit for observation

43. Which of the following statements would suggest that the patient diagnosed with mononucleosis understands their condition?
[ ] **A.** "I can share eating utensils with others as long as I don't have a fever."
[ ] **B.** "I need to avoid strenuous activity and contact sports for a month."
[ ] **C.** "A vaccination would have prevented me from contracting this."
[ ] **D.** "This is an inherited disease and there is nothing I can do about it."

44. When caring for a patient who is acutely agitated and presenting a risk to self and others, which of the following is an appropriate intervention?
[ ] **A.** Administer enough medication to get them to sleep.
[ ] **B.** Place them in a seclusion room with a sitter or status checks every 15 minutes.
[ ] **C.** Immediately implement four-point leather restraints.
[ ] **D.** Begin with the least restrictive means necessary to keep them and others safe.

45. "The protective privilege ends where the public peril begins" indicates the duty of the emergency nurse when a patient threatens another person with bodily injury or harm. What does the quoted statement mean?
[ ] **A.** Confidentiality between patient and nurse does not relieve staff of the duty to warn the threatened person and authorities.
[ ] **B.** Confidentiality between nurse and patient is as sacred as the attorney–client privilege and is never broken.
[ ] **C.** The emergency nurse must weigh the seriousness of the threat before breaking the confidentiality of that patient.
[ ] **D.** Warning the patient not to commit a felony covers the emergency nurse as duty to warn and is sufficient.

46. An elderly patient has decided to discontinue treatment. It would be recognized that the patient is competent to make this decision and support the decision based on which of the following ethical principles?
[ ] **A.** Justice
[ ] **B.** Fidelity
[ ] **C.** Autonomy
[ ] **D.** Confidentiality

47. A patient is being seen in the emergency department with Herpes Zoster. The appropriate staff member to care for this patient would be a nurse who has never had:
[ ] **A.** pertussis.
[ ] **B.** chickenpox.
[ ] **C.** mumps.
[ ] **D.** measles.

48. Which of the following is **NOT** a component of the transfer system between facilities?
[ ] **A.** Communications with the receiving hospital
[ ] **B.** Following your hospital's policies and procedures
[ ] **C.** Available transportation resources in the community
[ ] **D.** Cost of the transfer to the appropriate location

49. An 86-year-old patient is being prepared for surgery. Which of the following approaches best ensures he will understand the risks and benefits?
[ ] **A.** Give him enough time to process the information.
[ ] **B.** Ask family members to make these decisions.
[ ] **C.** Ask patient to respond immediately so he does not forget.
[ ] **D.** Give the patient reading material to review postoperatively.

50. Disseminated Intravascular Coagulation (DIC) is characterized by all of the following **EXCEPT**:
[ ] **A.** microvascular clots.
[ ] **B.** increased clotting factors.
[ ] **C.** decreased platelets.
[ ] **D.** impaired hemostasis.

51. Which of the following is the major cause of anaphylaxis?
[ ] **A.** Food products
[ ] **B.** Latex
[ ] **C.** Insect stings
[ ] **D.** Exercise

52. Which of the following would be the proper lead placement to definitively diagnosis a right ventricular infarct?

[ ] **A.** Fourth intercostal space left sternal border
[ ] **B.** Fifth intercostal space right midclavicular line
[ ] **C.** Fifth intercostal space posterior axillary line
[ ] **D.** Fourth intercostal space right sternal border

53. Which of the following findings indicate that a chest tube is **NOT** effective in the management of a pneumothorax?

[ ] **A.** Patient resting, pulse oximetry 96% on 2 L/nasal cannula
[ ] **B.** Breath sounds equal bilaterally, equal chest excursion
[ ] **C.** Patient anxious, respirations 36 breaths/minute
[ ] **D.** Trachea midline, jugular veins not distended

54. Which of the following would indicate successful use of thrombolytic therapy?

[ ] **A.** T-wave inversion
[ ] **B.** Decreased ST segment
[ ] **C.** Prolonged QT intervals
[ ] **D.** Pathologic Q waves

55. A patient arrives in the emergency department with a potential anaphylactic reaction after eating peanuts. The patient has edematous lips, urticaria, and inspiratory stridor. Vital signs are as follows:

Blood pressure—86/60 mm Hg
Heart rate—116 beats/minute
Respirations—24 breaths/minute
Pulse oximetry—94% on room air
Temperature—98.4° F (36.8° C)

After administering epinephrine (Adrenaline), the nurse can anticipate an order for which of the following types of medication?

[ ] **A.** Corticosteroid
[ ] **B.** Beta-blocker
[ ] **C.** Histamine-2 blocker
[ ] **D.** Antibiotic

56. Priority interventions for a patient with acute adrenal insufficiency (Addison's disease) include all of the following **EXCEPT**:

[ ] **A.** administration of intravenous (IV) antibiotics.
[ ] **B.** rapid infusion of a crystalloid solution.
[ ] **C.** continuous vital sign monitoring.
[ ] **D.** administration of intravenous (IV) hydrocortisone (Solu-Cortef).

57. A patient being discharged from the emergency department after treatment for hemophilia demonstrates understanding of his condition with which of the following statements?

[ ] **A.** "I can tell the gang that I can play touch football next weekend."
[ ] **B.** "If I need to I can take aspirin for my pain."
[ ] **C.** "I will arrange for prophylactic care prior to having dental treatments."
[ ] **D.** "I will avoid extremes of hot and cold weather."

58. Which of the following is a true statement regarding restraining a patient when necessary?

[ ] **A.** Utilize a trained and coordinated team approach.
[ ] **B.** Have the strongest members of the staff overpower the patient.
[ ] **C.** Direct the patient to cooperate or law enforcement will be called.
[ ] **D.** Engage family members to physically assist.

59. The Health Insurance Portability and Accountability Act (HIPAA) includes protected information in public venues. However, protected health information can be shared without patient consent in which of the following situations?

[ ] **A.** Insurance companies for billing purposes
[ ] **B.** To an ex-spouse for legal recovery of information
[ ] **C.** EMS to determine patient's marital status
[ ] **D.** To share with neighbors or friends who call

60. When caring for a case involving forensics, which of the following is an important concept?

[ ] **A.** Cut off clothing through holes and stains.
[ ] **B.** Place all clothing together in one neat pile.
[ ] **C.** Package each piece of clothing in a plastic airtight bag.
[ ] **D.** Use paper bags with tamper-resistant seal for evidence.

61.

Which of the following identifies the significance of the above rhythm?

[ ] **A.** Hyperkalemia; tall, peaked T waves; and early hyperacute sign
[ ] **B.** T-wave inversion, ischemia, and T wave appears deep and symmetrical
[ ] **C.** Injury pattern and elevation above the isoelectric line indicates acuteness of injury
[ ] **D.** Pathologic Q wave appears within 24 hours of infarct and may remain permanent

62. A patient is transported via EMS to the emergency department after having fallen from a roof. On assessment, the nurse notes lack of breath sounds on the left side. A chest tube is inserted in the left chest, but instead of releasing air, the catheter expels blood. Which of the following might be the reason for this?

[ ] **A.** Tension pneumothorax
[ ] **B.** Open pneumothorax
[ ] **C.** Hemothorax
[ ] **D.** Simple pneumothorax

63. Which of the following is a true statement regarding emphysema?

[ ] **A.** Emphysema creates increased dead space in the lung fields.
[ ] **B.** An emphysemic patient is one who develops cor pulmonale.
[ ] **C.** A stocky build is a normal body shape for emphysemic patients.
[ ] **D.** Respiratory infections are dominant in the patient with emphysema.

64. Allergic stings are most commonly caused by which of the following?

[ ] **A.** Hornets
[ ] **B.** Scabies
[ ] **C.** Bumble bees
[ ] **D.** Bed bugs

65. A patient in the triage area is yelling and becoming increasingly agitated; he throws his bottle of water on the floor. The family states this agitated and aggressive behavior is new over the past few hours. Which of the following is the best response for the triage nurse at this time?

[ ] **A.** Approach the patient and directly confront him to control him through authority.
[ ] **B.** Inform the patient that this is not an acceptable behavior in the emergency department.
[ ] **C.** Reassure the patient that the nurse is here to help him.
[ ] **D.** Shout for security to call the police immediately.

66. The emergency nurse recognizes which of the following as common causes or precipitants of supraventricular tachycardia?

[ ] **A.** Digoxin, beta-blockers, and calcium channel blockers
[ ] **B.** Hypoxia, ischemia, heart failure, myocardial infarction, caffeine, and alcohol
[ ] **C.** Hypertension, atherosclerosis, chronic cocaine use, and cardiac surgery
[ ] **D.** Thrombosis, vasospasm, cocaine use, and chemotherapeutic agents

67. Which of the following arterial blood gas (ABG) readings is correct for the following results?

pH—7.52
pCO_2—22 mm Hg
HCO_3—26 mEq/L
PaO_2—92 mm Hg

[ ] **A.** Respiratory acidosis
[ ] **B.** Respiratory alkalosis
[ ] **C.** Metabolic acidosis
[ ] **D.** Metabolic alkalosis

68. A patient without human immunodeficiency virus (HIV) infection has a tuberculin skin test (purified protein derivative [PPD]). Which of the following is considered a positive result?

[ ] **A.** Redness >10 mm
[ ] **B.** Induration >10 mm
[ ] **C.** Redness of 5 mm
[ ] **D.** Induration of 5 mm

69. A delivery occurs in the emergency department. The baby presents with blue limbs, pink body, heart rate of 142 beats/minute, some flexion, some motion, and a weak cry. What is this infant's APGAR score?

[ ] **A.** 10
[ ] **B.** 9
[ ] **C.** 7
[ ] **D.** 6

70. A patient in her 34th week of pregnancy presents to the emergency department. Her blood pressure is 180/110 mm Hg and she complains of headache and blurred vision. During treatment of this patient, the emergency nurse should be prepared for which of the following complications?

[ ] **A.** Precipitous delivery
[ ] **B.** Vaginal bleeding
[ ] **C.** Cardiac dysrhythmias
[ ] **D.** Seizure activity

71. Neurotoxin released by the black widow spider can lead to:

[ ] **A.** hypotension and tachycardia.
[ ] **B.** urticaria and necrosis.
[ ] **C.** tingling and muscle fasciculation.
[ ] **D.** hemolysis and renal failure.

72. Which of the following is the primary physiologic reason for hypotension and bradycardia in neurogenic shock?
[ ] **A.** Third spacing of intracellular fluid
[ ] **B.** Disruption in sympathetic nervous system
[ ] **C.** Hypersensitivity to allergen
[ ] **D.** Left ventricular hypertrophy

73. Screening questions to identify human trafficking must be brief and limited because the perpetrator will not leave the victim alone for long. Simple screening questions include all of the following **EXCEPT**:
[ ] **A.** "Are the doors and windows locked so you cannot leave?"
[ ] **B.** "Has your ID or documentation been taken from you?"
[ ] **C.** "Have you been denied food, water, sleep, or medical care?"
[ ] **D.** "What is your cell phone number so we can reach you?"

74. A registered nurse reads a journal's research study. The study taught fever control measures to first-time parents. Which of the following is most important to determine before attempting to apply the same project in the nurse's emergency department?
[ ] **A.** Was the study approved by an Institutional Review Board (IRB)?
[ ] **B.** What was the actual content that the researcher taught to the parents?
[ ] **C.** Are the researcher's and nurse's settings similar enough for transferability?
[ ] **D.** Did the researcher statistically verify the data results with an analysis of variance (ANOVA)?

75. A patient has fever, gingival pain, bleeding gums, and foul breath. The patient is suspected of having trench mouth. Which of the following of the following is another term for this disorder?
[ ] **A.** Ludwig's angina
[ ] **B.** Vincent's angina
[ ] **C.** Pericoronitis
[ ] **D.** Dental abscess

76. Which of the following areas of the brain controls the respiratory and cardiac systems?
[ ] **A.** Medulla
[ ] **B.** Frontal lobe
[ ] **C.** Diencephalon
[ ] **D.** Hypothalamus

77. Which of the following statements made by a patient indicates the need for further instruction about the treatment of bacterial conjunctivitis?
[ ] **A.** "I can use disposable daily contact lenses since starting antibiotic ointment."
[ ] **B.** "I will discard all of my old eye makeup and clean my makeup brushes."
[ ] **C.** "I will avoid use of eye makeup until the infection is gone."
[ ] **D.** "Warm compresses will help to remove discharge from my eyelids."

78. When treating an acutely psychotic patient, all of the following are appropriate **EXCEPT**:
[ ] **A.** reorienting them back to reality as frequently as necessary.
[ ] **B.** policy requirement of mandatory seclusion or four-point restraints.
[ ] **C.** comprehensive assessment for potential medical causes of their psychosis.
[ ] **D.** escalation of restrictive intervention to protect them and others from harm.

79. The absence of the cremasteric reflex has a high sensitivity but low specificity for which of the following conditions?
[ ] **A.** Penile foreign body
[ ] **B.** Testicular torsion
[ ] **C.** Urethral tear
[ ] **D.** Epididymitis

80. A paraplegic patient presents to the emergency department complaining of a headache. He is noted to be flushed and is sweating profusely. Which of the following should be the first action for this patient?
[ ] **A.** Apply compression stockings.
[ ] **B.** Lower his head to increase cerebral circulation.
[ ] **C.** Massage lower extremities to cause vasodilation.
[ ] **D.** Assess for a blocked urinary catheter.

81. Causes of disseminated intravascular coagulopathy (DIC) include all of the following **EXCEPT**:
[ ] **A.** sepsis.
[ ] **B.** hemolytic transfusion reaction.
[ ] **C.** idiopathic thrombocytopenia.
[ ] **D.** transplant rejection.

82. Which of the following symptoms would be indicative of the compensatory stage in hypovolemic shock?
[ ] **A.** Narrowing pulse pressure
[ ] **B.** Severe hypotension
[ ] **C.** Increasing lactic acid level
[ ] **D.** Increasing urine output

83. A patient presents with high fever and the following signs and symptoms affecting the right ear: swelling, erythema and pain to the pinna, otorrhea, and decreased hearing. The emergency nurse prepares interventions for which of the following?
[ ] **A.** Ruptured tympanic membrane
[ ] **B.** Parotitis
[ ] **C.** Otitis externa
[ ] **D.** Mastoiditis

84. The Emergency Medical Treatment and Active Labor Act (EMTALA) requires that a patient with no insurance:
[ ] **A.** should be transferred to a teaching hospital that receives federal funds.
[ ] **B.** must be transferred to a Level I trauma center as soon as possible.
[ ] **C.** should be transferred if the receiving hospital can provide additional care.
[ ] **D.** cannot be transferred to another facility, as defined by the COBRA law.

85. When caring for a sexually assaulted patient, the highest priority would be:
[ ] **A.** evidence collection and preservation.
[ ] **B.** report of the crime to authorities.
[ ] **C.** caring for injuries sustained in the assault.
[ ] **D.** updating her family and friends.

86. Which of the following should be performed by the emergency nurse caring for a patient with suspected Herpes Zoster (shingles)?
[ ] **A.** Place the patient in a negative-pressure room
[ ] **B.** Administer postexposure prophylaxis
[ ] **C.** Place the patient on contact precautions
[ ] **D.** Wear an N-95 respiratory mask

87. Which of the following would be most concerning regarding a patient diagnosed with heat stroke?
[ ] **A.** Persistent lack of shivering
[ ] **B.** Pink/reddish-colored urine
[ ] **C.** Sinus tachycardia on the monitor
[ ] **D.** Presence of a Lichtenberg Figure

88. A patient presents with an ingestion of an unknown substance. The emergency nurse notes the patient to have bradycardia, diminished bowel sounds, miosis, and cool, dry skin. Which of the following agents did the patient most likely ingest?
[ ] **A.** Opioid
[ ] **B.** Anticholinergic
[ ] **C.** Sedative-hypnotic
[ ] **D.** Sympathomimetic

89. Which of the following would indicate an improvement in a patient experiencing neurogenic shock associated with a spinal cord injury?
[ ] **A.** Heart rate of 46 beats/minute
[ ] **B.** Blood pressure of 90/62 mm Hg
[ ] **C.** Temperature of 98.6° F (37° C)
[ ] **D.** Respiratory rate of 28 breaths/minute

90. Which of the following does the emergency nurse prepare the patient for in the treatment of iritis?
[ ] **A.** Instillation of antibiotic ophthalmic ointment
[ ] **B.** Eye flush with normal saline
[ ] **C.** Cold compress to the eye
[ ] **D.** Instillation of ophthalmic steroids

91. Which of the following is an indication for an emergency resuscitative thoracotomy?
[ ] **A.** Patients sustaining penetrating abdominal injuries
[ ] **B.** Blunt trauma with no signs of life
[ ] **C.** Penetrating thoracic wound with recent loss of vital signs
[ ] **D.** Qualified trauma surgeon is not available.

92. Which of the following is **NOT** an appropriate intervention for the child with suspected epiglottitis?
[ ] **A.** Obtaining a throat culture
[ ] **B.** Providing supplemental oxygen
[ ] **C.** No invasive procedures
[ ] **D.** Lateral neck radiograph

93. Assessment of an unrestrained patient from a motor vehicle crash reveals hypotension, warm, dry skin, and bradycardia. Which of the following is the most likely cause?
[ ] **A.** Cardiogenic shock
[ ] **B.** Neurogenic shock
[ ] **C.** Hypovolemic shock
[ ] **D.** Septic shock

94. On assessment of a patient with a suspected single-drug intentional overdose, the emergency nurse notes dilated pupils, hypoactive bowel sounds, and hot, dry, and flushed skin. Which of the following medications would be the most likely source of the overdose based on the symptoms present?
[ ] **A.** Alprazolam (Xanax)
[ ] **B.** Amitriptyline (Elavil)
[ ] **C.** Methylphenidate (Ritalin)
[ ] **D.** Morphine sulfate (Roxanol)

95. A group of nursing friends are attending a nursing conference in a mountainous area. On arrival, several of the group members become irritable and are complaining of persistent headache, nausea, and extreme fatigue. There is a planned event that afternoon to the summit of one of the near mountains. Which of the following would be the best recommendation for those feeling ill?

[ ] **A.** Take 1,000 mg acetaminophen, increase fluids, and attend the trip.

[ ] **B.** Drink two large glasses of nonalcoholic fluids, rest, and decline the trip.

[ ] **C.** Increase noncaffeinated fluids, eat some protein, and attend the trip.

[ ] **D.** Eat and drink normally, go on the trip, but decline the hike.

96. Two hours after taking an overdose of acetaminophen (Tylenol), a patient arrives in the emergency department. Based on the nomogram for acute ingestion, when can emergency the nurse expect to draw a blood acetaminophen level?

[ ] **A.** Immediately

[ ] **B.** In 1 hour

[ ] **C.** In 2 hours

[ ] **D.** In 4 hours

97. A patient with a diagnosis of ischemic stroke is being prepped for the initiation of TPA (tissue plasminogen activator). The patient is on the cardiac monitor. Oxygen has been applied at 2 L/nasal cannula. Labetalol (Normodyne) 5 mg intravenous was administered. A light, warm blanket has been applied. Which of the following would indicate that proper interventions have been completed that allow for the administration of this medication?

[ ] **A.** Pulse rate of 120 beats/minute

[ ] **B.** Blood pressure of 168/98 mm Hg

[ ] **C.** Pulse oximetry reading of 94%

[ ] **D.** Temperature of 98.6° F (37° C)

98. Which of the following two extracellular substances work together to regulate pH?

[ ] **A.** Sodium bicarbonate and acetic acid

[ ] **B.** Sodium bicarbonate and carbonic acid

[ ] **C.** Sodium bicarbonate and sodium hydroxide

[ ] **D.** Sodium bicarbonate and carbon dioxide

99. A patient in her 34th week of pregnancy comes to the emergency department and complains of sudden onset of bright red vaginal bleeding. Her uterus is soft, and she is not experiencing any pain. Fetal heart tones are 120 beats/minute. Based on this history, the emergency nurse should suspect which of the following conditions?

[ ] **A.** Abruptio placentae

[ ] **B.** Preterm labor

[ ] **C.** Placenta previa

[ ] **D.** Threatened abortion

100. Which of the following is the drug of choice for the treatment of cardiogenic shock?

[ ] **A.** Dopamine (Intropin)

[ ] **B.** Dobutamine (Dobutrex)

[ ] **C.** Nitroglycerin (Trinitrate)

[ ] **D.** Vasopressin

101. Septic shock in a pediatric patient often has which of the following associated clinical assessment findings?

[ ] **A.** Projectile vomiting

[ ] **B.** Pulmonary edema

[ ] **C.** Petechial rash

[ ] **D.** Jugular venous distention

102. A patient presents to the emergency department complaining of pain in her jaw. The emergency nurse notes facial drooping to the corner of the mouth on the left side. Which of the following cranial nerves (CNs) is affected?

[ ] **A.** Cranial Nerve VI (Abducens)

[ ] **B.** Cranial Nerve VIII (Acoustic)

[ ] **C.** Cranial Nerve V (Trigeminal)

[ ] **D.** Cranial Nerve III (Oculomotor)

103. Which of the following is the priority intervention for a child with epiglottitis?

[ ] **A.** Providing oxygen by nasal cannula

[ ] **B.** Administering antibiotics

[ ] **C.** Assisting with intubation

[ ] **D.** Monitoring for dysrhythmias

104. Which of the following would indicate treatment for pertussis (whooping cough) has been effective?

[ ] **A.** Resolution of characteristic "whooping" cough and fever

[ ] **B.** Completion of the prescribed antibiotic treatment

[ ] **C.** Negative nasopharyngeal swap for *Bordetella pertussis*

[ ] **D.** Negative reading of chest radiograph

105. A patient is brought to the emergency department 15 minutes after ingesting a full bottle of the tricyclic antidepressant amitriptyline (Elavil). Which of the following interventions would **NOT** be utilized in this scenario?
[ ] **A.** Gastric lavage
[ ] **B.** Syrup of ipecac
[ ] **C.** Activated charcoal
[ ] **D.** Electrocardiogram (ECG)

106. A 1-year-old girl has experienced a febrile seizure. Which of the following statements made by the parents would indicate that they understood the discharge instructions regarding temperature control?
[ ] **A.** "We will use alcohol baths if her temperature gets too high."
[ ] **B.** "We will keep her temperature down with tepid sponge baths and acetaminophen (Tylenol)."
[ ] **C.** "We will give her the phenobarbital when the temperature is above 101° F (38.3° C)."
[ ] **D.** "We will use ice baths if her temperature goes up and we cannot get it to come down."

107. Which of the following is the best treatment for high-altitude pulmonary edema (HAPE)?
[ ] **A.** Acclimatization
[ ] **B.** Antibiotics
[ ] **C.** Decrease in altitude
[ ] **D.** No specific treatment exists

108. A pediatric patient is unstable with poor perfusion, hypotension, and supraventricular tachycardia with a rate of 300 beats/minute. Immediate treatment would include which of the following?
[ ] **A.** Administer adenosine intravenously using the port closest to the infusion site.
[ ] **B.** Apply ice to the child's face for 10-15 seconds.
[ ] **C.** If the child is older, consider vagal maneuvers, such as coughing.
[ ] **D.** Initiate synchronized cardioversion with 0.5 to 1 J/kg.

109. An infant with a high-pitched cry, irritability, and fever is being prepped for a lumbar puncture (LP). Which of the following is an appropriate position for this patient during this procedure?
[ ] **A.** Lateral with knees to chest and chin to chest
[ ] **B.** Lateral with legs extended and arms above the head
[ ] **C.** Placing the patient in the prone position
[ ] **D.** Placing the patient in the supine position

110. A patient was involved in a fire inside a backyard shed and sustained deep partial-thickness burns to his face, head, and neck with singed nasal hair. He arrives with a hoarse voice. Which of the following is the priority nursing management for this patient's airway?
[ ] **A.** Deliver high-flow oxygen by rebreather mask
[ ] **B.** Monitor for increasing hoarseness of voice
[ ] **C.** Prepare for emergent intubation
[ ] **D.** Obtain equipment for emergency cricothyrotomy

111. Which of the following eye complaints stated by a patient does the triage nurse recognize as emergent?
[ ] **A.** Facial numbness and inability to look upward
[ ] **B.** Bloody appearance to the sclera
[ ] **C.** Perception of five to six floaters in the eye
[ ] **D.** Pain on the surface of the eye and excessive tearing

112. A patient is treated for a cholinergic exposure. Which of the following manifestations would indicate successful treatment?
[ ] **A.** Miosis
[ ] **B.** Dry skin
[ ] **C.** Tachycardia
[ ] **D.** Hypotension

113. A patient with a history of poor dental hygiene and recent completion of chemotherapy presents with fever, mouth pain, swelling and bleeding to the gums, and malodorous breath. Which of the following actions would **NOT** be appropriate?
[ ] **A.** Initiate dental consult
[ ] **B.** Suction the oropharynx
[ ] **C.** Intravenous access
[ ] **D.** Antibiotic administration

114. A tennis player presents at triage with a swollen and painful elbow joint. The emergency nurse suspects which of the following types of joint effusion?
[ ] **A.** Septic arthritis
[ ] **B.** Gout
[ ] **C.** Blood
[ ] **D.** Bursitis

115. A patient comes to the emergency department with complaints of burning and itching pain and intermittent numbness in the palm of the hand. The patient reports that it is usually worse upon awakening in the morning. The emergency nurse notes decreased grip strength to the affected hand. Which of the following is the nerve most often responsible for this problem?

[ ] **A.** Ulnar
[ ] **B.** Median
[ ] **C.** Peroneal
[ ] **D.** Radial

116. A 4-month-old presents with decreased feeding and increased somnolence. He has had two episodes of vomiting in the last 3 hours. Vital signs are as follows:

Blood pressure—108/38 mm Hg
Pulse—66 beats/minute
Respirations—30 breaths/minute
Temperature—97° F (36.1° C)

Which of the following is the most likely cause of these symptoms?

[ ] **A.** Dehydration
[ ] **B.** Increased intracranial pressure
[ ] **C.** Autonomic dysreflexia
[ ] **D.** Increased intra-abdominal pressure

117. A patient has profuse bleeding from the nose that has persisted despite application of firm pressure to the nostrils. Which of the following diagnostic evaluations is the priority test?

[ ] **A.** Activated partial thromboplastin time (aPTT)
[ ] **B.** Complete blood count (CBC) and prothrombin time (PT)
[ ] **C.** International normalized ratio (INR)
[ ] **D.** Hematocrit count and type and crossmatch

118. Thirty minutes after a patient is admitted to the emergency department, the emergency nurse performs a repeat neurologic examination. The patient does not follow commands, but after several attempts by the nurse to apply noxious stimuli, he opens his eyes and moves the nurse's hand. The patient utters a one-word response to the nurse. Which of the following is the correct Glasgow Coma Scale for this patient?

[ ] **A.** 5
[ ] **B.** 7
[ ] **C.** 10
[ ] **D.** 12

119. Which of the following conditions is manifested by frequent sustained vomiting, often resulting in dehydration and weight loss of the pregnant patient?

[ ] **A.** Cyclical vomiting
[ ] **B.** Gastroenteritis
[ ] **C.** Hyperemesis gravidarum
[ ] **D.** Ulcerative colitis

120. When assessing a patient with an eyelid laceration, the emergency nurse concludes that the patient has a deep laceration with injury to the levator muscle due to which of the following alterations?

[ ] **A.** Inability to close the eyelid
[ ] **B.** Inability to open the eyelid
[ ] **C.** Bleeding to the lid
[ ] **D.** Visual disturbance

121. Which of the following statements made by a patient being discharged with a tick bite indicates the need for further instructions?

[ ] **A.** "I need to get antibiotics every time I find a tick walking on me."
[ ] **B.** "When I go walking I will wear my pants tucked into my socks."
[ ] **C.** "To remove a tick—grab the head with tweezers and twist it off."
[ ] **D.** "I will use tick repellant when walking in areas with known ticks."

122. While caring for a patient with a ventriculostomy, the nurse notices that the intracranial pressure (ICP) reading is 30 mm Hg. The nurse assesses the patient and the ICP monitor and determines that the drain is open. Which of the following would be the appropriate immediate intervention for this patient?

[ ] **A.** Move the head from a rotated position to the midline.
[ ] **B.** Lower the head of the bed to the Trendelenburg position.
[ ] **C.** Close the stopcock on the ventriculostomy.
[ ] **D.** Elevate the head of the bed to high Fowler's position.

123. A patient is diagnosed with a knee dislocation after a sporting event. The emergency nurse should consider which of the following additional injuries that is common with this primary injury?

[ ] **A.** Fibula fracture
[ ] **B.** Saphenous vein injury
[ ] **C.** Popliteal artery injury
[ ] **D.** Tibial nerve injury

124. Postpartum hemorrhage can occur immediately after delivery or can be delayed by as much as 6 weeks. Which of the following is **NOT** a cause of postpartum hemorrhage?

[ ] **A.** Retained products of conception
[ ] **B.** Vaginal or cervical tear
[ ] **C.** Failure of uterus to contract to normal
[ ] **D.** Amniotic fluid embolism

125. A patient presents after being hit in the face with a baseball. The patient states he has "bloody vision" and assessment reveals decreased visual acuity. What other assessment data confirms the presence of a hyphema?

[ ] **A.** Patient describes perception of a curtain coming down over his eye
[ ] **B.** Visualization of blood covering the lower half of the iris
[ ] **C.** Limitation in extraocular eye movements
[ ] **D.** Severe pain when blinking the eye

126. Which of the following tests is frequently used to diagnose myasthenia gravis?

[ ] **A.** Lumbar puncture
[ ] **B.** Tensilon test
[ ] **C.** Allen's test
[ ] **D.** Magnetic resonance imaging (MRI)

127. When administering intravenous magnesium, the emergency nurse should take which of the following actions?

[ ] **A.** Administer the infusion slowly
[ ] **B.** Dilute the solution with normal saline only
[ ] **C.** Administer narcotics at routine dose strength
[ ] **D.** Monitor pulse and blood pressure every 4 hours

128. Which of the following is **NOT** a normal physiologic change that occurs in pregnancy?

[ ] **A.** Resting heart rate increases
[ ] **B.** Peripheral resistance increases
[ ] **C.** Circulating plasma increases
[ ] **D.** Oxygen consumption increases

129. A patient receiving pharmacologic medications for combativeness associated with a head injury responds to noxious stimuli only. Which of the following scores on the Ramsay Score for Sedation (RASS) would be documented?

[ ] **A.** 1
[ ] **B.** 3
[ ] **C.** 5
[ ] **D.** 15

130. As part of the sexual assault examination, which of the following should be done with the victim's clothing?

[ ] **A.** Place it in a paper bag and seal it with evidence tape.
[ ] **B.** Return it to the patient after examining it.
[ ] **C.** Place it in a plastic bag and seal it with paper tape.
[ ] **D.** Shake it out carefully to look for hidden evidence.

131. Which of the following is a potential complication after manipulation of a long-bone fracture?

[ ] **A.** Deep vein thrombosis
[ ] **B.** Pulmonary embolism
[ ] **C.** Acute respiratory distress syndrome
[ ] **D.** Fat embolism

132. A patient has the appearance of bright red blood to the lateral portion of the sclera. The patient states he noticed the redness after continuous harsh coughing yet denies recent trauma and pain. The emergency nurse suspects this patient will be diagnosed with which of the following?

[ ] **A.** Retinal hemorrhage
[ ] **B.** Ultraviolet keratitis
[ ] **C.** Subconjunctival hemorrhage
[ ] **D.** Eight-ball hyphema

133. Which of the following would be the priority action if an ischemic stroke patient receiving tissue plasminogen activator (TPA) infusion begins to vomit bright red blood?

[ ] **A.** Notify the physician
[ ] **B.** Place a nasogastric tube
[ ] **C.** Decrease the infusion
[ ] **D.** Stop the infusion

134. A patient comes to the emergency department complaining of a nosebleed, which began 2 hours before her arrival, and has not subsided, despite direct pressure. She has generalized ecchymosis and states she has a history of idiopathic thrombocytopenia (ITP). Replacement therapy is indicated based on the diagnostic workup. Which of the following is the appropriate treatment?

[ ] **A.** Desmopressin (DDAVP)
[ ] **B.** IVIg (intravenous immunoglobulin)
[ ] **C.** Thrombin injection
[ ] **D.** Factor VIII

135. Which of the following vaginal infections does **NOT** require treatment of sexual partners?

[ ] **A.** *Neisseria gonorrhoeae*
[ ] **B.** *Candida albicans*
[ ] **C.** *Trichomonas vaginalis*
[ ] **D.** *Chlamydia trachomatis*

136. A patient presents with unilateral painless loss of vision and is being evaluated for central retinal artery occlusion. Priority intervention by the emergency nurse includes which of the following?

[ ] **A.** Digital ocular massage
[ ] **B.** Patch the affected eye
[ ] **C.** Facilitate mild hyperventilation
[ ] **D.** Assist the patient to supine position

137. A patient presents to triage several hours after having a cast placed complaining of severe pain uncontrolled by pain medication. Which of the following would be the priority intervention for this patient?

[ ] **A.** Provide pain medication
[ ] **B.** Ultrasound for deep vein thrombosis
[ ] **C.** Bivalve the cast immediately
[ ] **D.** Check compartmental pressure

138. Goal-directed initial resuscitation measures for septic shock include which of the following?

[ ] **A.** Treating a state of hypoperfusion
[ ] **B.** Decreasing systemic vascular resistance (SVR)
[ ] **C.** Administrating epinephrine subcutaneously
[ ] **D.** Utilizing intravenous diuretic therapy

139. Which of the following does the emergency nurse expect to be in the treatment plan for a patient with Meniere's disease, yet not for labyrinthitis?

[ ] **A.** Administration of antiemetic medication
[ ] **B.** Instructions to change positions slowly
[ ] **C.** Instructions to avoid operation of heavy machinery
[ ] **D.** Administration of diuretic medication

140. Which of the following statements made by a patient being discharged with a new prescription for phenytoin (Dilantin) indicates that the patient understands their instructions?

[ ] **A.** "I know that if I miss a routine dose I cannot easily make it up."
[ ] **B.** "I am glad to know that I won't have to have routine lab tests."
[ ] **C.** "I am aware that if I stop taking this medication I am at risk for status epilepticus."
[ ] **D.** "It's good that I don't have to worry about a bunch of adverse effects from this drug."

141. Which of the following statements made by a patient diagnosed with Vincent's angina indicates the need for further instruction?

[ ] **A.** "I will eat a well-balanced diet."
[ ] **B.** "I know to take all the antibiotics as directed."
[ ] **C.** "I should rinse my mouth with antiseptic mouthwash."
[ ] **D.** "I will brush my teeth with a hard-bristle toothbrush."

142. A patient with an amputation of the hand from being caught in a machine at work presents with ongoing bleeding despite direct pressure and elevation of the extremity. Which of the following is the next appropriate interventional step?

[ ] **A.** Apply pressure dressing
[ ] **B.** Insert an intravenous catheter
[ ] **C.** Notify the physician
[ ] **D.** Apply a tourniquet

143. A patient reports acute onset of loss of partial vision described as a cloudy veil over the top portion of the eye. The patient denies pain. The emergency nurse prepares for which of the following diagnostic evaluations that will confirm the diagnosis?

[ ] **A.** Tonometry for intraocular pressure measurement
[ ] **B.** Fluorescein stain for examination of the cornea
[ ] **C.** Pupil dilation for fundal examination
[ ] **D.** Computed tomography (CT) of the orbits

144. A teenaged boy comes to the emergency department after waking with severe pain to his left testicle. Examination reveals the following vital signs:

Blood pressure—110/72 mm Hg
Pulse—120 beats/minute
Respirations—30 breaths/minute
Pulse oximetry—98% on room air
Temperature—98.5° F (36.9° C)

His left testicle is slightly elevated and firm. Which of the following would be the most appropriate intervention?

[ ] **A.** Send the patient for ultrasound.
[ ] **B.** Apply ice packs to the scrotum.
[ ] **C.** Prepare to transfuse blood products.
[ ] **D.** Elevate scrotum to 45-degree angle.

145. Which of the following electrolyte abnormalities is commonly experienced by a patient in adrenal crisis?

[ ] **A.** Hypocalcemia
[ ] **B.** Hypernatremia
[ ] **C.** Hyperglycemia
[ ] **D.** Hyperkalemia

146. An immunocompromised patient presents to the emergency department on the advice of their primary physician based on which of the following physiologic criteria?

[ ] **A.** Elevated neutrophil count
[ ] **B.** Wound with purulent drainage
[ ] **C.** Warm, red, swollen insect bite
[ ] **D.** Temperature >100.4° F (38° C)

147. A trauma patient with a diagnosis of a ruptured bladder has two large-bore intravenous lines, oxygen, a nasogastric tube, and an indwelling urinary catheter in place. Initial vital signs are as follows:

Blood pressure—120/54 mm Hg
Pulse—120 beats/minute
Respirations—28 breaths/minute
Pulse oximetry—95% on room air
Temperature—98.2° F (36.7° C)

Which of the following might indicate impending hypovolemic shock?
[ ] A. Pulse of 100 beats/minute
[ ] B. Restlessness
[ ] C. Blood pressure of 110/64 mm Hg
[ ] D. Request for pain relief

148. A parent presents with their infant requesting a "rabies shot" because they saw a bat flying in the child's bedroom. The emergency nurse would anticipate:
[ ] A. reassuring the parent that unless a wound is found, there is no risk of rabies.
[ ] B. administering Rabies Immune Globulin and first dose of Rabies vaccine.
[ ] C. setting up appointments for the series of rabies injections twice a day for 21 days.
[ ] D. initiating prophylactic intravenous antibiotics as soon as possible.

149. Which of the following interventions is most appropriate for a patient with a pulmonary contusion?
[ ] A. Restrict intravenous fluid administration
[ ] B. Provide supplemental humidified oxygen
[ ] C. Position the patient to facilitate breathing
[ ] D. Assist with removal of secretions

150. Which of the following is the most important treatment for the patient with tension pneumothorax?
[ ] A. Elevate the head of the patient's bed.
[ ] B. Administer 100% oxygen.
[ ] C. Infuse intravenous normal saline slowly.
[ ] D. Assist with needle decompression.

Answer Sheet

	A B C D		A B C D		A B C D		A B C D
1.	○ ○ ○ ○	26.	○ ○ ○ ○	51.	○ ○ ○ ○	76.	○ ○ ○ ○
2.	○ ○ ○ ○	27.	○ ○ ○ ○	52.	○ ○ ○ ○	77.	○ ○ ○ ○
3.	○ ○ ○ ○	28.	○ ○ ○ ○	53.	○ ○ ○ ○	78.	○ ○ ○ ○
4.	○ ○ ○ ○	29.	○ ○ ○ ○	54.	○ ○ ○ ○	79.	○ ○ ○ ○
5.	○ ○ ○ ○	30.	○ ○ ○ ○	55.	○ ○ ○ ○	80.	○ ○ ○ ○
6.	○ ○ ○ ○	31.	○ ○ ○ ○	56.	○ ○ ○ ○	81.	○ ○ ○ ○
7.	○ ○ ○ ○	32.	○ ○ ○ ○	57.	○ ○ ○ ○	82.	○ ○ ○ ○
8.	○ ○ ○ ○	33.	○ ○ ○ ○	58.	○ ○ ○ ○	83.	○ ○ ○ ○
9.	○ ○ ○ ○	34.	○ ○ ○ ○	59.	○ ○ ○ ○	84.	○ ○ ○ ○
10.	○ ○ ○ ○	35.	○ ○ ○ ○	60.	○ ○ ○ ○	85.	○ ○ ○ ○
11.	○ ○ ○ ○	36.	○ ○ ○ ○	61.	○ ○ ○ ○	86.	○ ○ ○ ○
12.	○ ○ ○ ○	37.	○ ○ ○ ○	62.	○ ○ ○ ○	87.	○ ○ ○ ○
13.	○ ○ ○ ○	38.	○ ○ ○ ○	63.	○ ○ ○ ○	88.	○ ○ ○ ○
14.	○ ○ ○ ○	39.	○ ○ ○ ○	64.	○ ○ ○ ○	89.	○ ○ ○ ○
15.	○ ○ ○ ○	40.	○ ○ ○ ○	65.	○ ○ ○ ○	90.	○ ○ ○ ○
16.	○ ○ ○ ○	41.	○ ○ ○ ○	66.	○ ○ ○ ○	91.	○ ○ ○ ○
17.	○ ○ ○ ○	42.	○ ○ ○ ○	67.	○ ○ ○ ○	92.	○ ○ ○ ○
18.	○ ○ ○ ○	43.	○ ○ ○ ○	68.	○ ○ ○ ○	93.	○ ○ ○ ○
19.	○ ○ ○ ○	44.	○ ○ ○ ○	69.	○ ○ ○ ○	94.	○ ○ ○ ○
20.	○ ○ ○ ○	45.	○ ○ ○ ○	70.	○ ○ ○ ○	95.	○ ○ ○ ○
21.	○ ○ ○ ○	46.	○ ○ ○ ○	71.	○ ○ ○ ○	96.	○ ○ ○ ○
22.	○ ○ ○ ○	47.	○ ○ ○ ○	72.	○ ○ ○ ○	97.	○ ○ ○ ○
23.	○ ○ ○ ○	48.	○ ○ ○ ○	73.	○ ○ ○ ○	98.	○ ○ ○ ○
24.	○ ○ ○ ○	49.	○ ○ ○ ○	74.	○ ○ ○ ○	99.	○ ○ ○ ○
25.	○ ○ ○ ○	50.	○ ○ ○ ○	75.	○ ○ ○ ○	100.	○ ○ ○ ○

	A	B	C	D			A	B	C	D
101.	○	○	○	○		126.	○	○	○	○
102.	○	○	○	○		127.	○	○	○	○
103.	○	○	○	○		128.	○	○	○	○
104.	○	○	○	○		129.	○	○	○	○
105.	○	○	○	○		130.	○	○	○	○
106.	○	○	○	○		131.	○	○	○	○
107.	○	○	○	○		132.	○	○	○	○
108.	○	○	○	○		133.	○	○	○	○
109.	○	○	○	○		134.	○	○	○	○
110.	○	○	○	○		135.	○	○	○	○
111.	○	○	○	○		136.	○	○	○	○
112.	○	○	○	○		137.	○	○	○	○
113.	○	○	○	○		138.	○	○	○	○
114.	○	○	○	○		139.	○	○	○	○
115.	○	○	○	○		140.	○	○	○	○
116.	○	○	○	○		141.	○	○	○	○
117.	○	○	○	○		142.	○	○	○	○
118.	○	○	○	○		143.	○	○	○	○
119.	○	○	○	○		144.	○	○	○	○
120.	○	○	○	○		145.	○	○	○	○
121.	○	○	○	○		146.	○	○	○	○
122.	○	○	○	○		147.	○	○	○	○
123.	○	○	○	○		148.	○	○	○	○
124.	○	○	○	○		149.	○	○	○	○
125.	○	○	○	○		150.	○	○	○	○

Sample Test 1

Answers and Rationales

1. Answer: A

Nursing Process: Assessment/Respiratory

Rationale: **Fail chest is caused by two or more fractures of two to three or more adjacent ribs. These fractures do not move with the chest wall during respiration. Signs include paradoxical movement of the chest wall during inspiration and expiration, ineffective ventilation, and dyspnea.** Although flail chest can also cause a tension pneumothorax, this is not the primary concern for the trauma nurse. Classic signs of a tension pneumothorax include tracheal deviation, cyanosis, severe dyspnea, absent breath sounds on the affected side, distended jugular veins, and shock. The patient with a ruptured diaphragm will present with hypotension, dyspnea, dysphagia, shifted heart sounds, and bowel sounds in the lower to middle chest. A patient with a massive hemothorax will show signs of shock (tachycardia and hypotension), dullness on percussion on the injured side, decreased breath sounds on the injured side, respiratory distress, and, possibly, a mediastinal shift.

2. Answer: B

Nursing Process: Analysis/Respiratory

Rationale: **Early in an acute asthma attack, respiratory alkalosis should be present, which should be evident with a pH greater than 7.45 and a decreased $PaCO_2$ (hypocarbia) because the carbon dioxide is being blown off at an increased rate. A low PaO_2 (hypoxemia) should be present if a true asthmatic event is occurring.** Acidosis indicated by a decreased pH (lower than 7.35) would be present in a patient with hypoventilation, which would be demonstrated by an increased $PaCO_2$. Normal readings on the arterial blood gas report would not indicate an asthma attack.

3. Answer: C

Nursing Process: Analysis/Cardiovascular

Rationale: **Traumatic thoracic injury can cause aortic injury and the tear most commonly occurs at the ligamentum arteriosum (80% to 90%).** This is a band of tissue that forms about 3 weeks after birth and is a vestige of the fetal ductus arteriosus. It connects the aorta to the pulmonary artery and when torn has usually fatal outcomes. If a complete tear does not occur and the adventitial layer of the vessel (the outermost layer) remains intact, an aneurysm can develop.

4. Answer: C

Nursing Process: Assessment/Cardiovascular

Rationale: **Peripheral venous thrombosis (also known as deep vein thrombosis or DVT) is an occlusion of a vein by a thrombus restricting blood outflow. The majority of DVTs involves the lower extremities and triggers include hypercoagulable/immobile states such as cancer, pregnancy, sepsis, surgery, and/or trauma. Signs and symptoms vary, but include swelling, pain, tenderness, and warm, red, or discolored skin.** Postthrombotic syndrome is considered the most common long-term complication of a DVT and manifests up to 2 years later as chronic venous insufficiency varying from minor leg discomfort or swelling up to venous claudication and skin ulcerations. Thromboangiitis obliterans or Buerger's disease is an occlusive, chronic, inflammatory disorder of the arteries, veins, and surrounding nerves that trigger decreased blood flow in the hands and feet resulting in ischemia and pain. Intermittent claudication and decreased or absent peripheral pulses lead to ulcers and gangrene may develop. Raynaud's disease produces vasospasms that reduce blood flow to the arteries of the hands and feet in response to a trigger such as cold temperatures or smoking; symptoms are pallor and numbness/tingling that returns to normal after the stimulus is removed.

5. Answer: D

Nursing Process: Assessment/Gastrointestinal

Rationale: **Right lower rib fractures can cause liver injury, especially with fractures from the eighth rib down. Emergency personnel should be aware of this as a mechanism of injury and be alert to the possibility.** This patient is demonstrating signs of hypovolemic shock and a major clue should be the tenderness to the right lower rib area along with the vital signs and the fall from the porch. Splenic injuries can occur with left lower rib fractures. Colonic injuries are not associated with rib fractures. Blunt cardiac injury can happen with sternal fractures.

6. Answer: B

Nursing Process: Analysis/Gastrointestinal

Rationale: **Pneumonia would not be a possible complication. The description of this patient in the scenario is that of bowel obstruction.** Patients with bowel obstruction will have generalized abdominal pain, vomiting, and abdominal distention. In this case, the large amount of distention would point toward a large bowel obstruction. The past history of the repair for a ruptured colon and the appendectomy could create a situation in which adhesions are present that could cause a bowel obstruction. Complications for this disease process include sepsis, dehydration due to a third spacing that occurs and the vomiting and possible perforation.

7. Answer: A

Nursing Process: Assessment/Cardiovascular

Rationale: **The signs of acute arterial occlusion are referred as the "5Ps": Pain, Pallor, Pulselessness, Paresthesia, and Paralysis.** Chest pain, tachycardia, tachypnea, and elevated temperature may be seen in pericarditis. Severe pain, blood pressure variation in arm, and peripheral cyanosis are seen in aortic injuries. Chest pain, dyspnea, nausea, diaphoresis, and fatigue are seen in myocardial infarctions.

8. Answer: D

Nursing Process: Evaluation/Cardiovascular

Rationale: **The drug of choice for stable narrow-complex tachycardia is Adenocard (adenosine). This medication will cause a short period of asystole before conversion to normal sinus rhythm.** The other options are not expected outcomes.

9. Answer: A

Nursing Process: Analysis/Respiratory

Rationale: **Identifying and treating the underlying condition is the *primary* goal.** If the condition causing acute respiratory distress syndrome (ARDS) is not treated, injury to the lung will continue, preventing adequate tissue oxygenation and predisposing the patient to a secondary infection. Later, the nurse should also provide adequate nutritional support in the form of increased protein and calories and limited carbohydrate intake.

10. Answer: D

Nursing Process: Evaluation/Gastrointestinal

Rationale: **The FAST (Focused Assessment with Sonography for Trauma) examination is sensitive for large amounts of blood in the abdomen. If there is less than 400 mL of fluid in the abdomen, it is not usually identified. It is most sensitive (90% to 100% of the time) if there is at least 1,000 mL present in the abdomen.** This test does not work as well as the diagnostic peritoneal lavage or the computed tomography (CT) for injuries of the stomach or small bowel. If the FAST examination is negative, it does not mean there are no injuries.

11. Answer: D

Nursing Process: Assessment/Psychosocial

Rationale: **Level IV anxiety is typified by an inability to solve problems or think logically and obligates the nurse to identify safety plans for the patient and others as the patient may experience changes in their personality.** Patients with Level I anxiety are aware of their environmental stimuli and can rationally problem-solve. Level II is associated with a heightened focus on immediate concerns while the patient remains cooperative with care providers. Level III anxiety patients do not engage with the full spectrum of their situation and demonstrate regressive behaviors while often needing repetitive direction.

12. Answer: C

Nursing Process: Evaluation/Psychosocial

Rationale: **The Emergency Nurses Association (ENA) as well as other international emergency nurse associations (and national emergency care organizations) support family presence during resuscitation. Family members who are in the room can see all of the things that are being done for their loved one. This is a positive outcome for those who are left behind.** It is difficult for them to see the reality of the death but it can help the grieving process to begin. Staff members should always be present when this is done. That staff member's total responsibility is the family member. Family members should have this support or they should not be allowed into the resuscitation room.

13. Answer: C

Nursing Process: Intervention/Cardiovascular

Rationale: **CPR performed early can double or triple survival from witnessed sudden cardiac arrest. For every minute that passes between collapse and defibrillation, the chance of survival from a witnessed ventricular fibrillation declines by 7% to 10% per minute if no bystander cardiopulmonary resuscitation is provided.** A major emphasis of the 2015 American Heart Association (AHA) Guidelines Update for Cardiopulmonary Resuscitation (CPR) and Emergency Cardiac Care (ECC) is high-quality chest compressions with minimal interruption and a decreased emphasis on early placement of an advanced airway; providers may defer insertion of an advanced airway until the patient fails to respond to initial CPR and defibrillation attempts or demonstrates return of spontaneous circulation (ROSC). The optimal number of cycles of CPR and shocks required before starting pharmacologic therapy remains unknown; however, epinephrine should be given when IV/IO access is accomplished. Defibrillation should be performed as soon as it can be accomplished and immediate CPR should be performed while waiting to shock.

14. Answer: D

Nursing Process: Evaluation/Cardiovascular

Rationale: **An Osborn wave, also called a J wave, is an extra positive deflection between the QRS and the ST segment that accompanies hypothermia. It has nothing to do with cardiac reperfusion status post thrombolytic administration.** Patients who have a successful reperfusion will have relief of chest pain and ST-segment normalization. The most common reperfusion dysrhythmia is accelerated idioventricular.

15. Answer: A

Nursing Process: Evaluation/Cardiovascular

Rationale: **Raynaud's phenomenon is a circulatory disease of the arteries that severely reduces blood flow as the result of episodic intense vasospasm of the digits in response to extreme cold, emotional stress, and/or smoking.** Treatment is aimed at decreasing pain and vasospastic events. **The patient should be advised to keep warm, wear gloves, not smoke, and avoid cold medicines and diet pills because of their vasoconstrictive effects.** Elevating the arm and applying ice would worsen the vasoconstriction. Wrist splints or applying an elastic bandage would not help and may increase vasoconstriction. Fluids and aspirin would not help.

16. Answer: A

Nursing Process: Intervention/Gastrointestinal

Rationale: **Fluid bolus rehydration for infants and children is based on 20 mL/kg of body weight.** For this patient weighing 20 pounds, the first step in the mathematical equation is to change the pounds to kilograms. This is the most common error in calculations. Therefore, 20 pounds is equal to 9 kg (20 divided by 2.2), 9 kg × 20 mL = 180 mL bolus. If the pounds are not changed to kilograms, then the incorrect mathematical outcome would be 400 mL. If an incorrect formula is used and 10 mL/kg is considered to be correct, then the outcome utilizing pounds is 200 mL or 900 mL if the correct conversion is made to kilograms but the incorrect formula is used.

17. Answer: C

Nursing Process: Assessment/Psychosocial

Rationale: **During a manic phase, the patient with bipolar disorder often has poor social judgment, which can manifest as sexual inappropriateness, become hypersocial, with rapid, verbose speech without allowing opportunity for reciprocal communication, and/or display grandiosity of thought and ideas.** The manic phase is the opposite of the depressed phase, which may manifest with social withdrawal. The manic patient is more likely to display flamboyant personal style and dress rather than be unkempt. Patients in a manic episode will usually be more than willing to answer questions—often providing long and rambling explanations to questions. It will be difficult to keep them on task and to elicit appropriate answers from them.

18. Answer: C

Cognitive Level: Recall/Professional Issues

Rationale: **Level I and Level II trauma centers must have a trauma surgeon, trauma director, and staffed operating room available around the clock.** Level III trauma centers are excused from the staffed operating room requirement. Level IV trauma centers are excused from all the above requirements.

19. Answer: B

Cognitive Level: Application/Professional Issues

Rationale: **Federal laws allow management to prevent employees from engaging in collective bargaining in patient care areas.** The same laws prohibit managers from preventing union activities during nonworking hours, from withholding desirable assignments from staff engaging in union activities, and from providing special favors to discourage union activity or membership.

20. Answer: B

Nursing Process: Assessment/Cardiovascular

Rationale: **Heart failure is the result of structural and functional impairment of ventricular filling or ejection of blood. Most patients have impairment of myocardial function, ranging from normal ventricular size and function to marked dilation and reduced function. Worsening dyspnea is a cardinal symptom of heart failure and dyspnea at rest is often mentioned by patients. The symptoms stated in the question reflect pulmonary congestion.** Pulmonary embolism occurs with an occlusion of pulmonary blood vessels and the patient may have dyspnea, but pleuritic chest pain, pleural friction rub, and signs and symptoms of a deep vein thrombosis would also be expected; edema would not occur with a pulmonary embolism. Cardiac tamponade is the collection of blood in the pericardial sac, which limits ventricular filling and thus decreases cardiac output; signs and symptoms would include chest pain and Beck's triad: distended neck veins (JVD), distant heart sounds (muffled), and hypotension. Tension pneumothorax occurs when air enters the pleural space during inspiration and is unable to escape during exhalation. This leads to a rising intrathoracic pressure, which compresses the lungs, heart, and great vessels in the chest. It is preceded by blunt or penetrating trauma and causes severe respiratory distress and absent breath sounds on the affected side.

21. Answer: A

Nursing Process: Intervention/Cardiovascular

Rationale: **Definitive treatment of an acute aortic dissection consists of surgical repair of the rupture.** Chest tube placement is indicated for pneumothoraces or hemothorax. The priority is to move the patient to definitive care; intubation can be accomplished in the operating room. Pericardial decompression is indicated for pericardial tamponade.

22. Answer: C

Nursing Process: Assessment/Respiratory

Rationale: **Because a patient who has had a stroke may be at high risk for aspiration, the combination of warm, moist skin, and adventitious lung sounds most likely results from aspiration pneumonia.** An acute onset of altered mental status may indicate a new stroke; however, the presence of a fever suggests an infectious process, ruling out congestive heart failure and a stroke. The adventitious lung sounds do not correlate with meningitis.

23. Answer: B

Cognitive Level: Recall/Professional Issues

Rationale: **Option B is the exception to behaviors related to human trafficking victims because the patient will not request additional follow-up or treatment; the patient will most likely refuse any follow-up if provided.** Each of the other answers describe behaviors that may indicate the patient is a victim of trafficking.

24. Answer: D

Cognitive Level: Analysis/Professional Issues

Rationale: **The DNR order is meant to inform health care providers that the patient does not want life-saving techniques performed at the time of cardiac/respiratory arrest.** It does not allow the nurse to assume the patient does not want care for his current condition. Care should be provided to this patient following the standards of care for a stroke patient.

25. Answer: C

Nursing Process: Analysis/Gastrointestinal

Rationale: **This patient's recent fall has probably contributed to the development of a splenic injury. Fractures of the left lower ribs can lead to spleen lacerations that become evident several days after initial injury.** Fractures of the lower right ribs are prone to causing liver injuries. This patient is not demonstrating any manifestations that should make the nurse consider pneumonia or pancreatitis. A fever and usually a cough should be present with pneumonia, and pancreatitis would present with severe pain to left mid-quadrant.

26. Answer: A

Nursing Process: Analysis/Psychosocial

Rationale: **Anorexia nervosa has the highest mortality rate due to metabolic complications and concomitant risk of suicidal ideation.** Although all other mentioned diagnoses have mortality risks, anorexia has the highest risk of all psychiatric diagnoses.

27. Answer: C

Nursing Process: Intervention/Gastrointestinal

Rationale: **Octreotide (Sandostatin) is used to treat esophageal varices associated with liver disease.** Dicyclomine (Bentyl) is an anticholinergic medication that hinders the release of pancreatic secretions by preventing nerve impulses from stimulating the cells. Fentanyl (Sublimaze) can be used to treat the pain associated with pancreatitis. Histamine H_2-inhibitors such as famotidine (Pepcid) prevents histamine release that increases the pancreatic secretions.

28. Answer: C

Nursing Process: Analysis/Gastrointestinal

Rationale: **When the stomach is torn or perforated, hydrochloric acid and enzymes escape that then causes peritonitis. There is a very high probability that peritonitis will follow for this patient.** The patient is at much higher risk for hypovolemic shock rather than cardiogenic. Pulmonary edema and paralysis would not occur in this scenario. There is no chest or spinal cord injury.

29. Answer: A

Cognitive Level: Application/Professional Issues

Rationale: **A study that examines thoughts and perceptions is one that lends itself to a qualitative design. Qualitative research is concerned with understanding human beings and the nature of their transactions with themselves and their surroundings.** The process is not quasi-scientific, rather a well-accepted mode of rigorous, systematic inquiry used in the social sciences. Quantitative research methods analyze data statistically while striving for precision and control over external variables. Experimental research involves doing something to some of the subjects and not doing something to others; in it, subjects are randomly assigned to either group.

30. Answer: B

Nursing Process: Assessment/Communicable

Rationale: **The CDC immunization schedule for children is a first dose at age 12 to 15 months, followed by a second dose between ages 4 to 6 years, before the child enters school. An 11-month-old would not have had the vaccine. Koplik spots, small, red specks with a bluish-white center on the buccal mucosa, are a diagnostic lesion of measles. They appear approximately 2 days before the rash and disappear within 48 hours after the rash.** There is a difference between rubella (also known as 3 day measles) and rubeola (commonly known as measles). Mumps cause glandular enlargement of the parotid and salivary glands. There is no rash associated with mumps. In postpuberty males, the testes may be involved, producing orchitis and a risk of infertility. An allergic reaction may produce urticaria, hives, and a disseminated rash. The characteristic symptom of varicella is a vesicular rash that begins on the trunk and becomes generalized.

31. Answer: C

Nursing Process: Assessment/Medical

Rationale: **A state of acidosis, not alkalosis, can precipitate a sickle cell crisis. Acidosis results in a shift to the right on the oxyhemoglobin dissociation curve (Bohr effect), causing hemoglobin to desaturate (release oxygen) more readily.** Cold ambient temperature, infection, and high altitude are well-documented triggers of sickle cell crisis, and patients with this disease are instructed to take appropriate actions to avoid exposure to these triggers.

32. Answer: A

Nursing Process: Assessment/Cardiovascular

Rationale: **Manual blood pressures taken in both arms would be the correct objective assessment parameter. The primary event in an aortic dissection is a tear in the aortic intima, which allows blood to pass into the aortic media, thereby creating a false lumen; pressure within this false channel can compress the true aortic lumen and reduce blood flow. A considerable variation greater than 20 mm Hg systolic may be seen when comparing the blood pressure in the arms with this diagnosis.** Inspection for petechiae related to microemboli is performed for a suspected acute arterial occlusion. Edema of the extremities, anasarca (generalized swelling), or ascites would be assessed for heart failure and cardiogenic pulmonary edema. Prominent apical pulse, S3 or S4 are found in hypertensive crises cases.

33. Answer: C

Nursing Process: Intervention/Cardiovascular

Rationale: **Beck's triad, which consists of hypotension, muffled heart sounds, and jugular vein distension, along with tachycardia, dyspnea, cyanosis and a history of penetrating trauma, are signs of a pericardial tamponade, a collection of blood in the pericardial sac. As blood accumulates in the noncompliant pericardial sac, it exerts pressure on the heart, inhibiting ventricular filling and, therefore, cardiac output. A pericardiocentesis will aspirate the blood out of the sac and relieve the pressure on the heart.** A resuscitative thoracotomy is indicated with a traumatic cardiac arrest. Massive blood transfusion is not indicated at this point. Ventilatory support may be necessary when the patient goes for surgical repair, but the first priority is relieving pressure on the heart to improve cardiac output.

34. Answer: D

Nursing Process: Assessment/Medical

Rationale: **Most hyperglycemic emergencies are due to diabetic ketoacidosis (DKA). A decrease in available insulin increases the blood glucose level because it cannot be transported into cells. To meet the body's energy needs, the liver metabolizes fatty acids which break down into ketone bodies. Dehydration, electrolyte losses, acidosis, and ketonuria ensues. Kussmaul respirations (deep, rapid breathing) are a compensatory mechanism to buffer the acidosis by reducing serum carbon dioxide levels.** Patients in thyroid storm will appear in a hyperdynamic state, with elevated heart rate, blood pressure, and temperature. Metabolic changes are not common. Hyperosmolar hyperglycemic syndrome (HHS) is characterized by blood glucose levels more than 600 mg/dL and an absence of acidosis. Syndrome of inappropriate antidiuretic syndrome, due to oversecretion of the antidiuretic hormone, is characterized by decreased urinary output and sodium levels, lethargy, and confusion.

35. Answer: B

Cognitive Level: Application/Professional Issues

Rationale: **The nurse has a duty of care to the patient and to the public and must report the crime to the authorities.** Regardless of the mother's wishes, the child has been harmed and a report to the authorities is necessary. Even though the emergency physician may talk to the mother and the mother may be encouraged to reconsider her wishes, the fact remains that the crime must be reported and evidence must be collected.

36. Answer: A

Nursing Process: Intervention/Gastrointestinal

Rationale: **This child is in distress, most likely with a bowel obstruction, and needs to have oxygen started immediately.** She obviously needs an intravenous line and fluid administration, but these will take time and, therefore, the fastest intervention that can be done is to start high-flow oxygen. The urinary catheter is also important but again will take time and can be done after the airway is maintained and the fluid bolus is started.

37. Answer: D

Nursing Process: Analysis/Psychosocial

Rationale: **Dementia can result in acute agitation related to confusion and amplified sensory stimulation in the emergency department but is not the cause of the initial presenting symptom.** All the other conditions are considerations for medical causes of agitation that may be part of the decision making before a patient is "medically cleared" for psychiatric treatment. Both hypothyroidism and hyperthyroidism are causes of behavioral issues that can appear to be psychiatric in nature.

38. Answer: A

Nursing Process: Intervention/Gastrointestinal

Rationale: **This patient is actively bleeding. A type and crossmatch is needed, not a type and screen.** Blood needs to be set up immediately and the patient may need type-specific or universal donor (O negative) blood products before the crossmatch can be completed. Gastric tube placement, contacting the endoscopy department for a potential emergent procedure, and cardiac monitoring are all important treatment interventions for this patient. The patient needs close monitoring of vital signs and cardiac rhythms.

39. Answer: C

Nursing Process: Assessment/Cardiovascular

Rationale: **Second-degree heart block, type II, is characterized by a constant PR interval that is followed by a nonconducted P wave.** First-degree heart block is the most common conduction disturbance and is characterized by a PR interval that is greater than 0.20 seconds and rarely requires treatment. Type I second-degree heart block (Mobitz I or Wenckebach) is slower and slower impulse conduction through the AV node and is seen as gradual prolongation of the PR interval until one depolarization from the atria is completely blocked. Third-degree heart block results from injury to the cardiac conduction system so that no impulses are conducted from the atria to the ventricles; the atrial contractions are faster and independent of the slower beating ventricles.

40. Answer: D

Nursing Process: Analysis/Cardiovascular

Rationale: **The most common and concerning electrolyte abnormality associated with acute digoxin toxicity is hyperkalemia that occurs due to the binding affinity for digoxin on the Na/K pump site on each cell.** Hyponatremia, hypercalcemia, and hypomagnesemia are not electrolyte disturbances that occur with digoxin toxicity.

41. Answer: D

Nursing Process: Evaluation/Respiratory

Rationale: **A forced exhalation is not recommended during inhaler use because coughing, small-airway closure, and air trapping may result.** The correct technique for using an inhaler is as follows: the inhaler must be held upright and shook to ensure it is mixed thoroughly before administration. After inhalation of the medication, the patient should then hold his/her breath for 5 to 10 seconds to allow the medication to reach as far as possible into the lungs. If the patient has difficulty with this technique, a spacer device may be added to the inhaler. A good seal should also be part of the process.

42. Answer: C

Nursing Process: Intervention/Respiratory

Rationale: **Preparing a patient for surgical repair is the most important intervention for a ruptured diaphragm.** Needle thoracostomy and chest tube insertion are contraindicated in this patient because of the risk of puncturing the bowel and releasing its contents into the chest cavity. The potential for serious complications contraindicates transfer for observation. Intravenous (IV) fluids may become necessary if the bowel compresses large vessels, causing a decrease in preload.

43. Answer: B

Nursing Process: Evaluation/Medical

Rationale: **Splenomegaly occurs frequently in mononucleosis. Because of the risk of injury to an enlarged spleen, strenuous activity and contact sports should be avoided for at least 4 weeks.** The virus is shared primarily via saliva and oropharyngeal route. Sharing eating utensils or food, kissing, and similar actions should be avoided during the incubation period of up to 60 days. There is no vaccine to prevent mononucleosis. It is a communicable virus, not a hereditary disorder.

44. Answer: D

Nursing Process: Intervention/Psychosocial

Rationale: **Keeping the patient and others safe during a period of crisis is the priority and should be achieved using the least restrictive yet effective means.** This may include a combination of medications and changes to the physical environment and their mobility, but it must be implemented in a measured fashion that may involve escalating restriction and medication modalities with the goal of being effective, not excessive and never punitive or because it is just too hard to care for them short of sedation until asleep.

45. Answer: A

Cognitive Level: Application/Professional Issues

Rationale: **Confidentiality between patient and nurse (or physician) should be breached to alleviate a threat to another person.** Medical personnel have a duty to warn the intended victim (if known) and the authorities. Warning the patient not to commit a felony or weighing the seriousness of the threat is not sufficient grounds for relief from the duty to warn.

46. Answer: C

Cognitive Level: Application/Professional Issues

Rationale: **A patient is competent to make his/her own decisions and therefore entitled by the ethical principle of autonomy, the right to make decisions regarding a patient's own body.** Autonomy is the right of the patient to retain control over his or her body. Actions that attempt to persuade or coerce the patient into making a choice are violations of this principle, whether the medical provider believes these choices are in that patient's best interest. Beneficence refers to doing all that can be done to benefit the patient in each situation. All recommended procedures and treatments should consider each patients' individual circumstances. Emergency staff members should be trained in the most current and best practices and must recognize that what is good for one patient will not necessarily benefit another. Non-maleficence means "to do no harm." This means that we must also consider whether other people or society could be harmed by a decision made, even if it is made for the benefit of an individual patient. Justice recognizes that there should be fairness in all our decisions, including equal distribution of scarce resources and new treatments.

47. Answer: B

Nursing Process: Analysis/Communicable

Rationale: **Herpes Zoster is caused by the reactivation of a dormant varicella (chickenpox) virus. Vesicular lesions develop along a nerve dermatome and contain the live virus. It is contagious to unvaccinated or susceptible hosts. A person who has not had chickenpox may be susceptible to the virus and become ill.** Pertussis is caused by the *Bordetella pertussis* organism. The measles and mumps viruses are not harbored in the body after the infection clears.

48. Answer: D

Cognitive Level: Recall/Professional Issues

Rationale: **The components of a transfer system are communications, transport resources, and policies and procedures.** Although financial issues may influence where and how the patient is transferred, it is not a component of the transfer itself.

49. Answer: A

Cognitive Level: Application/Professional Issues

Rationale: **Allowing time for the information to be processed is necessary because the aging process affects the speed with which cognitive and motor processes are performed.** This does not mean that the activities cannot be performed, but rather that they take longer. Family members should not make these decisions unless it is a situation in which the patient cannot capably process the information and make an informed decision. Reading material postoperatively will not assist in making this decision preoperatively.

50. Answer: B

Nursing Process: Assessment/Medical

Rationale: **In Disseminated Intravascular Coagulopathy (DIC), both thrombosis and fibrin degradation occur simultaneously, leading to widespread bleeding along with abnormal clotting in the microcirculation.** DIC involves inappropriate and accelerated activation of the coagulation cascade manifested by impaired hemostasis, and a depletion of platelets and clotting factors.

51. Answer: A

Nursing Process: Analysis/Medical

Rationale: **Food is implicated in the largest percentage of anaphylactic episodes, causing approximately 13% to 65% of all episodes.** Latex is the cause of between 7% and 9% of anaphylactic reactions and has been steadily decreasing with the use of latex-free products, especially in the hospital setting. Insect stings account for 1% to 7% of episodes. Exercise-induced anaphylaxis is rare, occurring in less than 1% of the population.

52. Answer: B

Nursing Process: Analysis/Cardiovascular

Rationale: **A right-sided electrocardiogram (ECG) is performed when concern is present for a right ventricular infarct.** V_4R to V_6R are the leads that will show the ST-segment elevation with V_4R being the best. The lead placement for V_4R is in the fifth intercostal space at the right midclavicular line. The left side is mimicked on the right side of the chest. Lead placement in the fourth intercostal space at the left sternal border and at the right sternal border would be proper placement for V_1 and V_2. A lead placed at the fifth intercostal space posterior axillary line would be correct for the posterior lead, V_7.

53. Answer: C

Nursing Process: Evaluation/Respiratory

Rationale: **After chest tube insertion, the patient should be calm. A patient who is anxious with rapid respirations is showing signs of respiratory distress.** If the chest tube is effective, respirations and pulse oximetry reading should be within normal limits. Breath sounds should be heard in all lobes bilaterally with equal excursion of chest. The trachea should be midline without jugular vein distention.

54. Answer: B

Nursing Process: Evaluation/Cardiovascular

Rationale: **Thrombolytic therapy should open closed coronary arteries and reperfuse the heart. Reperfusion would be indicated by ST segments falling back to normal levels. Elevated ST segments indicate injury to the heart muscle.** T-wave inversion would demonstrate ischemia. Prolonged QT intervals are a negative finding and can be a forerunner of torsade de pointes. Pathologic Q waves are indicative of necrosis in the heart wall.

55. Answer: C

Nursing Process: Intervention/Medical

Rationale: **Studies have shown the combination of an H_1-blocker such as diphenhydramine (Benadryl) and an H_2-blocker such as famotidine (Pepcid) to be superior to an H_1-blocker alone in relieving the histamine-mediated symptoms of anaphylaxis.** Corticosteroids have no immediate effect on mitigating anaphylaxis. Beta-blockers may increase the risk of anaphylaxis and inhibit the therapeutic effect of epinephrine in treating anaphylaxis. There is no value to administration of antibiotics in treating anaphylaxis because it is not an infectious process.

56. Answer: A

Nursing Process: Intervention/Medical

Rationale: **Adrenal insufficiency is an endocrine disorder and does not require antibiotic therapy unless there is evidence of an underlying infection. It is not a priority intervention.** Hypovolemic shock is a life-threatening complication of acute adrenal insufficiency and requires aggressive fluid resuscitation. Additional priority interventions include administration of exogenous corticoids such as hydrocortisone (Solu-Cortef) or dexamethasone (Decadron). Vital signs should be continually monitored during the initial treatment phase.

57. Answer: C

Nursing Process: Evaluation/Medical

Rationale: **Hemophiliac patients should prepare for dental procedures such as extractions by consulting both the dentist and their hematologist for clotting factor replacement therapy, antifibrinolytic agents, and local hemostatic measures.** Patients with hemophilia should avoid contact sports. Over-the-counter medications containing aspirin or NSAIDs, which can precipitate or prolong bleeding, should be avoided. Temperature extremes do not influence hemophilia.

58. Answer: A

Nursing Process: Intervention/Psychosocial

Rationale: **This is a high-risk situation for both the patient and staff. A trained team approach that has been practiced outside of emergent circumstances is indicated.** Attempting to use the strongest staff approach is likely to harm both the patient and the provider. Threatening the patient with police intervention is abusive and not likely to result in a therapeutic result. Family should not be allowed to participate in such an intervention.

59. Answer: A

Cognitive Level: Application/Professional Issues

Rationale: **Insurance companies are included in the transmission of protected health information.** It would not be appropriate to give the information to individuals (such as the ex-wife/husband or friends who call in). EMS personnel would already have the patient's consent because they brought the patient in to the hospital. The Privacy Rule protects all "individually identifiable health information" held or transmitted by a covered entity (i.e., hospital) or its business associate, in any form or media (whether electronic, paper, or oral). The hospital may share protected health information (PHI) during the course of treatment, payment, and health care operations.

60. Answer: D

Cognitive Level: Analysis/Professional Issues

Rationale: **Paper allows the evidence to breathe, whereas plastic could destroy the evidence with mold and other issues. Applying and initialing the seals ensures the safety of the evidence as the tape is designed to fracture easily to indicate tampering.** When cutting the clothing off a patient, never cut through any cuts, holes, or other marks that may be entrance/exit wounds or contain evidence. It is important these areas be left unaltered. Each piece of evidence should be gathered separately to avoid cross-contamination, not piled on top of each other.

61. Answer: C

Nursing Process: Analysis/Cardiovascular

Rationale: **ST-elevation myocardial infarction (STEMI) is characterized by ST-segment elevation in two or more contiguous leads and threshold values of J-point elevation greater than 2 mm in leads V_2 and V_3 and 1 mm or more in all other leads.** This is ST elevation, not peaked or inverted waves; tall T waves can signify hyperkalemia, cerebrovascular injury, and left ventricular volume loads, resulting from mitral or aortic regurgitation. T-wave inversion can have various causes, including ischemia or evolving myocardial infarction or cerebrovascular accidents. Pathologic Q waves appear within 24 hours of infarct at greater than 0.04 seconds in duration or greater than 25% of the R wave in depth. These indicate necrosis in the heart muscle and can be permanent.

62. Answer: C

Nursing Process: Analysis/Respiratory

Rationale: **A hemothorax is caused by free blood in the pleural space, usually caused by trauma, which will result in diminished or absent breath sounds on the affected side.** A tension pneumothorax or simple pneumothorax will not expel blood through the chest tube. An open pneumothorax will present with a bubbling, sucking noise at the site of injury but will not usually be associated with loss of blood.

63. Answer: A

Nursing Process: Analysis/Respiratory

Rationale: **An increase in dead space occurs with emphysema because of destruction of alveolar walls and overdistention of the alveoli.** When this happens, these alveoli are no longer functional because they cannot participate in diffusion of gases. This increases dead space— a space where air is transported but does not assist with the work of the pulmonary system such as with the trachea. Cor pulmonale, right-sided heart failure caused by a pulmonary issue, is associated with chronic bronchitis. Chronic bronchitis patients usually have a stocky build as opposed to the thin extremities and barrel chest of the emphysema patient and respiratory infections are more prone in the chronic bronchitis patient due to the increase in secretions.

64. Answer: A

Nursing Process: Analysis/Medical

Rationale: **Hornets, yellow jackets, and wasps are the leading cause of allergic stings. They are aggressive and can sting repeatedly with minimal provocation.** Scabies is an intensely itchy skin infestation caused by a mite. It does not produce an allergic reaction. Bumble bees can produce an allergic reaction but are much less aggressive and sting with much lower frequency. Bed bugs are parasitic insects that feed on blood. The bite produces a painless, pruritic lesion. Urticaria may develop from repeated exposure.

65. Answer: C

Cognitive Level: Application/Professional Issues

Rationale: **The patient is exhibiting excessive agitation, which has a potential for violence; therefore, reassuring the patient and his family is the most therapeutic response.** The nurse should avoid being within the patient's physical reach to reduce the risk of being hit. Taking an authoritative stance is likely to further agitate the patient. He may not be able to cognitively take verbal cueing or instructions because of an underlying pathologic process. Shouting that outside authorities should be called will also likely incite further agitation.

66. Answer: B

Nursing Process: Analysis/Cardiovascular

Rationale: **Common causes of supraventricular tachycardia include hypoxia, ischemia, heart failure, myocardial infarction, mitral valve prolapse, caffeine, alcohol, recreational drugs, and hyperthyroidism.** Digoxin, beta-blockers, calcium channel blockers, increased vagal tone on the sinoatrial node, and myocardial ischemia or infarction (depending on the vessel occluded) are common causes of sinus pause or sinus arrest. Hypertension, atherosclerosis, chronic cocaine use, and cardiac surgery may lead to aortic aneurysm. Thrombosis, vasospasm, cocaine use, chemotherapeutic agents, and serotonin receptor agonists are risk factors for ST-elevation myocardial infarction.

67. Answer: B

Nursing Process: Analysis/Respiratory

Rationale: **Correct interpretation of these blood gas values is respiratory alkalosis.** The pH determines whether the reading is acidotic or alkalotic, and because this is greater than 7.45, the patient is alkalotic. Normal pH is 7.35 to 7.45. The next determination is whether the problem is related to carbon dioxide or bicarbonate. The parameter that is not normal is the pCO_2 level with the bicarbonate level being within normal limits. Also, the pH and the respiratory components are opposite each other, that is, the pH is "up" and the CO_2 is "down." This meets criteria for a diagnosis of respiratory alkalosis. A common problem that creates this blood gas reading is hyperventilation. Metabolic problems are directly related to each other, thus, a metabolic alkalosis would show an increase in both the pH and the HCO_3. The PaO_2 is normal.

68. Answer: B

Nursing Process: Evaluation / Communicable

Rationale: **If a patient has HIV infection, induration of 5 mm or more is considered a positive result. Induration 10 mm or more is considered a positive PPD result in the absence of HIV infection.** Redness may be related to an allergic process but is not considered a positive PPD finding. If a patient has HIV infection, induration of 5 mm or more is considered a positive result.

69. Answer: D

Nursing Process: Assessment/GU/GYN/OB

Rationale: **According to the APGAR scoring scale, this infant would receive 1 point for the flexion (Activity or muscle tone); 2 points for Pulse rate, which is over 100 beats/minute; 1 point for the motion activity (Grimace or reflex irritability); 1 point for the blue limb color with the pink body (Appearance); and 1 point for the weak cry (Respirations). This equals a scoring of 6.**

70. Answer: D

Nursing Process: Evaluation/GU/GYN/OB

Rationale: **This scenario provides information for symptoms associated with pregnancy-associated hypertension; the patient has a potential for seizure activity because of central nervous system irritability.** Seizure precautions should be instituted. Precipitous delivery, vaginal bleeding, and cardiac dysrhythmias are not complications of pregnancy-associated hypertension.

71. Answer: C

Nursing Process: Assessment/Environmental

Rationale: **Black widow spider neurotoxin causes nausea and weakness as well as hypertension and tachycardia. Other symptoms include muscle fasciculations, spasm, tingling, altered mental status, and potentially seizures.** Renal failure from hemolysis can occur with brown recluse bites. Brown recluse bites, not black widow, can demonstrate urticaria and a necrotic wound.

72. Answer: B

Nursing Process: Assessment/Neurologic/Shock

Rationale: **Neurogenic shock occurs when there is a disruption in the sympathetic nervous system, allowing the parasympathetic nervous system to take over, which causes hypotension and bradycardia.** No other form of shock causes these connected symptoms. Third spacing of intracellular fluid leads to hypovolemia. Left ventricular hypertrophy may be a contributing factor for cardiogenic shock. A hypersensitivity reaction would involve anaphylactic shock.

73. Answer: D

Cognitive Level: Analysis/Professional Issues

Rationale: **Asking for a cell phone number may trigger fear in the victim that the perpetrator will find out and/or that the victim "said too much."** All the other questions are brief, appropriate, and can be answered quickly.

74. Answer: C

Cognitive Level: Application/Professional Issues

Rationale: **To apply the study, the two settings need to be similar enough to allow transferability.** It would not be as effective, for instance, if the emergency department in the study was an inner-city teaching facility treating 200 patients a day and the nurse reading the study worked at a small community hospital with 20 patients a day. An institutional review board (IRB) is a type of committee that applies research ethics by reviewing the methods proposed for research to ensure that they are ethical. They also ensure the rights of the subjects. Such boards are formally designated to approve (or reject), monitor, and review biomedical and behavioral research involving humans. It is essential to know the content of the teaching so it can be implemented, but transferability needs to be determined first. ANOVA is one statistical option for testing differences among three or more group means.

75. Answer: B

Nursing Process: Assessment/Maxillofacial/Ocular

Rationale: **Vincent's angina, also referred to as acute necrotizing ulcerative gingivitis or trench mouth is a bacterial infection of the gums.** Classic presentation of Vincent's angina includes bleeding, painful, swollen gums, fever, halitosis, and gray pseudomembranous ulcers on the pharynx. Ludwig's angina is bacterial invasion of the submandibular structures. Pericoronitis is inflammation of the gingival tissue around the crown of an erupting or impacted tooth. Dental abscess is the localized accumulation of pus in various regions of the tooth and gum. Dental abscess can lead to complications of Vincent's or Ludwig's angina.

76. Answer: A

Nursing Process: Analysis/Neurologic

Rationale: **The medulla controls the arterioles, the blood pressure, and the rate and depth of respirations. Severe injury to this area generally results in death.** The medulla also controls yawning, coughing, vomiting, and hiccoughing. The frontal lobe of the cerebrum controls personality, judgment, thought, and logic. The diencephalon contains the thalamus, which is the sensory pathway between the spinal cord and the cortex of the brain. The hypothalamus regulates body temperature, appetite, and sleep.

77. Answer: A

Nursing Process: Evaluation/Maxillofacial/Ocular

Rationale: **Contact lenses should not be worn at all during a bout with conjunctivitis.** Bacterial conjunctivitis is highly contagious. Infection control measures include handwashing, instillation of antibiotic ophthalmic ointment, eye cleansing procedure, avoiding use of eye makeup, and discarding previously used eye makeup.

78. Answer: B

Nursing Process: Intervention/Psychosocial

Rationale: **Policy requirement of mandatory seclusion or restraints for a diagnosis is not appropriate.** The acutely psychotic patient may require frequent reorientation to reality. Ruling out medical causes of psychosis is a standard of care. The decision for the level of restraint necessary should be borne in assessment and should progress from the least restrictive to the level necessary to protect the patient and others.

79. Answer: B

Nursing Process: Assessment/GU/GYN/OB

Rationale: **The cremasteric reflex is characterized by the normal elevation of the testes that occurs when the upper medial thigh is stroked. This will not be present if there is a testicular torsion.** A penile foreign body, urethral tear, or epididymitis does not have this as a manifestation of these processes.

80. Answer: D

Nursing Process: Intervention/Neurologic

Rationale: **This patient is demonstrating manifestations of autonomic dysreflexia. This is the sudden onset of an abnormal sympathetic nervous system response to a noxious stimuli such as a full bladder, full rectum, or pressure on an ulcer. The symptoms include bradycardia, hypertension, headache, flushing, and excessive sweating.** Emergency treatment involves raising the head of the bed and loosening any constricting clothing. If compression stockings are present on the patient, they should be removed to encourage venous pooling. The most important intervention for this response is to resolve the offending stimulus. Assess for G-I-related or G-U-related situations. Often irrigation of a urinary catheter or unkinking the tubing may relieve the sympathetic response. Enemas or removal of an impaction may be necessary. Antihypertensives can be given but the hypertension will not resolve until the stimulus has been removed.

81. Answer: C

Nursing Process: Analysis/Medical

Rationale: **Idiopathic thrombocytopenia is a disease of increased peripheral platelet destruction, commonly seen in children several weeks after a viral infection such as chickenpox or rubella.** DIC is a thrombohemorrhagic disorder involving inappropriate and accelerated stimulation of the clotting cascade. Common causes include sepsis, a hemolytic transfusion reaction, transplant rejection as well as massive blood transfusions, major trauma, and obstetrical complications such as abruptio placentae and retained placenta.

82. Answer: D

Nursing Process: Evaluation/Ortho/Shock

Rationale: **Increasing urine output indicates that renal perfusion is maintained and is a sign of compensated hypovolemic shock.** A narrowing pulse pressure, severe hypotension, and increased lactic acid levels are indicative of uncompensated forms of shock.

83. Answer: D

Nursing Process: Assessment/Maxillofacial/Ocular

Rationale: **Acute mastoiditis is an inflammatory process secondary to bacterial infection of the mastoid air cells of the temporal bone. It may occur with an associated otitis media. Presentation includes fever, inflammation, and erythema to the mastoid and auricle, otorrhea, hearing loss, and deep, localized pain behind the ear.** Ruptured tympanic membrane may result in impaired hearing, vertigo, and drainage (blood) from the ear. Parotitis is inflammation of the parotid gland and presents with unilateral swelling below the ear and jaw. Otitis externa is an infection and inflammation of the auditory canal and may present with itching of the ear canal and external ear, pain with movement of the ear, and swelling of the ear canal. Fever is not a classic symptom of otitis externa.

84. Answer: C

Cognitive Level: Application/Professional Issues

Rationale: **EMTALA is a federal law that requires hospital emergency departments to medically screen every patient who seeks emergency care and to stabilize or transfer those with medical emergencies, regardless of health insurance status or ability to pay.** This law has been an unfunded mandate since it was enacted in 1986. Transferring to a teaching hospital is not part of the process. Patients should be transferred to an appropriate hospital relative to the illness or injury and must be stabilized before the transfer.

85. Answer: C

Nursing Process: Analysis/GU/GYN/OB

Rationale: **The patient's well-being is always the priority.** Evidence collection and preservation and encouraging police involvement are important, but is not the priority. Notifying family and friends is up to the discretion of the patient.

86. Answer: C

Nursing Process: Intervention/Communicable

Rationale: **Herpes Zoster is spread via direct contact with the herpetic lesions.** Negative-pressure isolation is indicated for airborne, not contact, isolation. A patient who is already symptomatic will not benefit from postexposure prophylaxis. The N-95 respiratory mask is required for droplet infections such as tuberculosis.

87. Answer: B

Nursing Process: Analysis/Environmental

Rationale: **One of the consequences of heat exhaustion is the breakdown of skeletal muscle tissue, leading to rhabdomyolysis which presents as pinkish to dark red-colored urine.** This occurs because of the release of myoglobin into the plasma. "Rhabdo" can lead to renal failure if sufficient fluids are not flushed through the kidneys. One of the challenges when cooling a hyperthermic patient is preventing shivering because this actually creates heat. Sinus tachycardia is expected. A Lichtenberg Figure is associated with a lightning strike at the point of entry. This transient discoloration lasts for only a few hours.

88. Answer: A

Nursing Process: Assessment/Toxicology

Rationale: **The opioid toxidrome includes bradycardia, constricted pupils (miosis), hypotension, hypothermia, diminished bowel sounds, bradypnea, and no change in diaphoresis; therefore, opioid would be the most likely choice in this scenario.** Anticholinergics and sympathomimetics are known to have tachycardia, rather than bradycardia, mydriasis (dilated pupils) rather than miosis, and increased body temperature. Sedative-hypnotics are known to cause bradycardia, diminished bowel sounds, and cool, dry skin, but are not associated with miosis.

89. Answer: C

Nursing Process: Evaluation/Neurologic/Shock

Rationale: **Patients with neurogenic shock associated with spinal cord injuries have difficulty maintaining their temperature control. This is known as poikilothermia. A normalized temperature would be a positive turn for a patient with this type of shock.** A heart rate of 46 beats per minute would be part of the symptomatology for neurogenic shock as would the hypotension and the rapid breathing.

90. Answer: D

Nursing Process: Intervention/Maxillofacial/Ocular

Rationale: **Iritis is an inflammatory process that may be idiopathic or secondary to systemic inflammatory disorders. Instillation of topical ophthalmic steroids and cycloplegic agents is indicated to treat the inflammation and reduce ciliary spasms.** Warm compresses and resting the eye by darkening the environment is indicated. There is no therapeutic benefit of instilling antibiotic ointment or flushing the eyes, because neither of these interventions will directly decrease the inflammation.

91. Answer: C

Nursing Process: Intervention/Cardiovascular

Rationale: **Penetrating thoracic wounds with recent loss of vital signs is an indication for an emergency thoracotomy in order to determine the site of injury and stop persistent hemorrhage.** Penetrating abdominal injuries and blunt trauma with no signs of life are not indications for an emergency thoracotomy. A qualified surgeon who *is* available as back-up is an indication for emergency thoracotomy to take the patient to the operating room for definitive repair.

92. Answer: A

Nursing Process: Intervention/Respiratory

Rationale: **Obtaining a throat culture can lead to increased airway obstruction due to initiation of epiglottic spasm when irritated with the swab and, as such, would not be an appropriate intervention.** Epiglottitis is a true medical emergency due to the abrupt inflammation of the epiglottis causing airway obstruction. A lateral neck radiograph may indicate epiglottic and aryepiglottic swelling, referred to as the "thumbprint sign" and the "posterior triangle." The treatment goal is to maintain the airway until surgical capability in the operating room (OR) is possible. This is accomplished by providing supplemental oxygen as tolerated and performing no invasive procedures until the airway is secure.

93. Answer: B

Nursing Process: Assessment/Neurologic/Shock

Rationale: **Bradycardia is the hallmark symptom of neurogenic shock.** Spinal trauma, from a motor vehicle crash, may cause an interruption in the sympathetic nervous system integrity. Although the patient may be hypotensive, the skin is often warm and dry in neurogenic shock. Hypovolemic, septic, and cardiogenic shock would most likely have tachycardia, hypotension, and cool, moist skin.

94. Answer: B

Nursing Process: Analysis/Toxicology

Rationale: **Based on this information and findings of this patient, the only medication that fits all the criteria for this toxidrome is amitriptyline (Elavil).** The four medications listed are from the toxidromes of sedatives (alprazolam), anticholinergics (amitriptyline), sympathomimetics (methylphenidate), and opioids (morphine sulfate). The symptoms for anticholinergics include tachycardia, dilated pupils (mydriasis), hypertension, hyperthermia, decreased bowel sounds, tachypnea, and dry skin. The symptoms for opioids include bradycardia, constricted pupils (miosis), hypotension, hypothermia, decreased bowel sounds, bradypnea, and no effect on diaphoresis. The symptoms for sedatives include bradycardia, hypotension, hypothermia, decreased bowel sounds, bradypnea, and no effect on diaphoresis or pupil size. The symptoms for sympathomimetics include tachycardia, dilated pupils (mydriasis), hypertension, hyperthermia, tachypnea, and diaphoresis, and bowel sounds may be hypoactive or hyperactive.

95. Answer: B

Nursing Process: Intervention/Environmental

Rationale: **At 4,900 feet, oxygen does not attach to hemoglobin as readily, leading to symptoms of tissue hypoxia which can include headache, fatigue, nausea, weakness, irritability, and dehydration. Acute mountain sickness, the milder form of altitude sickness, typically improves with rest, fluids, and time as the body acclimates to the altitude and the patient feels better within a day or two.** Ascending higher into the mountains will increase symptoms and may progress to high-altitude cerebral edema (HACE) or high-altitude pulmonary edema (HAPE). Activities such as hiking will increase symptoms and risk. Going on the trip higher into the mountain is ill-advised.

96. Answer: C

Nursing Process: Intervention/Toxicology

Rationale: **Based on nomogram for acute ingestion, serum acetaminophen levels should be drawn 4 hours after ingestion. Since the ingestion occurred 2 hours before arrival, the level should be drawn 2 hours after arrival to reach the 4-hour level.** Levels drawn sooner or later would not reflect the peak acetaminophen level. An acetaminophen level greater than 150 g/mL 4 hours after ingestion indicates toxicity.

97. Answer: B

Nursing Process: Evaluation/Neurologic

Rationale: **According to the stroke guidelines for care, a systolic blood pressure above 180 mm Hg requires treatment before the initiation of TPA. Labetalol (Normodyne) was given prior with a blood pressure now of 168/98 mm Hg, which demonstrates that the Labetalol (Normodyne) was successful in lowering the systolic pressure below 185 mm Hg.** A systolic blood pressure that remains above 185 mm Hg is a contraindication to TPA initiation. Acceptable pressures are systolic below 185 mm Hg and diastolic below 110 mm Hg. Uncontrolled hypertension increases the risk of intracranial bleeding. Tachycardia would not necessarily contraindicate the administration unless it was associated with bleeding/hypovolemia. The pulse oximetry reading and temperature are not included in the criteria, although it is recommended to supplement for SaO_2 below 94%. Hyperthermia can increase the morbidity rate, but in this scenario, the temperature is normal and a light, warm blanket was applied for patient comfort.

98. Answer: B

Nursing Process: Analysis/Medical

Rationale: **Sodium bicarbonate and carbonic acid are the two primary extracellular regulators of pH. pH is also further regulated by electrolyte composition within the intra- and extracellular compartments.** Acetic acid is commonly known as vinegar and is not an extracellular substance in the human body. Carbon dioxide combines with water to form carbonic acid. Sodium hydroxide is lye or caustic acid and is not found in the body.

99. Answer: C

Nursing Process: Analysis/GU/GYN/OB

Rationale: **Placenta previa is associated with painless vaginal bleeding that occurs when the placenta, or a portion of the placenta, covers the cervical os. Serious hemorrhage can occur.** In abruptio placentae, the placenta tears away from the wall of the uterus before delivery. The patient usually has pain and a board-like uterus. Preterm labor is associated with contractions and should not involve bright red bleeding. By definition, threatened abortion occurs during the first 20 weeks of gestation.

100. Answer: B

Nursing Process: Intervention/Cardiovascular/Shock

Rationale: **Dobutamine is a potent vasopressor but has less of a tendency to increase the heart rate as opposed to dopamine.** Tachycardia is a dangerous side effect of Dopamine and can worsen cardiogenic shock due to to the increased myocardial demands. Therefore, Dobutamine is the preferred drug for cardiogenic shock. Vasopressin is used to treat hypotension in patients who are suffering from a vasodilatory type of shock. It is used for these patients after no response from fluid boluses and catecholamine infusions. Nitroglycerin is a nitrate utilized in the treatment of angina and congestive heart failure associated with a myocardial infarction and renal failure. Nitroglycerin would bring blood pressures down due to its vasodilatory effects. It would be contraindicated in hypotension.

101. Answer: C

Nursing Process: Assessment/Medical/Shock

Rationale: **Sepsis in a pediatric patient is often accompanied by a petechial rash, usually secondary to an overwhelming infectious process, such as meningococcemia.** Projectile vomiting may be a sign of increased intracranial pressure. Pulmonary edema and jugular venous distension are associated with cardiogenic shock.

102. Answer: C

Nursing Process: Analysis/Neurologic

Rationale: **Cranial Nerve V (Trigeminal) deals with facial, cheek, and chin movement.** Cranial Nerve III (Oculomotor) constricts the pupil and is responsible for helping with eyeball movement. Cranial Nerve VI (Abducens) rotates your eyeball outward, and Cranial Nerve VIII (Acoustic) deals with hearing and balance.

103. Answer: C

Nursing Process: Intervention/Respiratory

Rationale: **Because children are at high risk for developing abrupt airway obstruction, the most important intervention for a child with epiglottitis is airway management. Intubation should be performed as soon as possible in a controlled environment.** Children need supplemental oxygen, but most are so anxious that they will not allow nasal cannula to stay in place. Provide humidified "blow-by" oxygen administered by the parent, if possible. The child needs antibiotics; however, the priority is airway management. The most common rhythm in this patient is sinus tachycardia related to compensation and, although important, cardiac monitoring is not a priority.

104. Answer: C

Nursing Process: Evaluation/Communicable

Rationale: **A negative swab is the only definitive evidence that treatment has been effective.** Despite resolution of fever and cough, pertussis infection may still be present in the body. Pertussis requires an extensive course of antibiotics, often up to 3 weeks. Pertussis is not detected on a chest radiograph.

105. Answer: B

Nursing Process: Intervention/Toxicology

Rationale: **Syrup of ipecac is contraindicated in tricyclic antidepressant overdose. Because rapid deterioration with cardiovascular collapse and seizures can occur, inducing emesis may lead to airway compromise from aspiration.** Gastric lavage could be ordered with endotracheal intubation with proper cuff inflation and mechanical ventilation. Administration of activated charcoal may be delayed. A baseline ECG may be ordered. The patient should be placed on a cardiac monitor because dysrhythmias and cardiac conduction delays are common.

106. Answer: B

Nursing Process: Evaluation/Neurologic

Rationale: **Between 25% and 30% of children who have suffered a febrile seizure may have reoccurrences. Keeping the temperature from increasing rapidly may contribute to the prevention of febrile seizures. Tepid sponge bath, administering antipyretics, and increasing fluid intake during febrile illnesses are key to preventing febrile seizures.** An ice bath is too cool to bring the temperature down and the temperature should be brought down slowly by using tepid water between 60° F to 100° F (16° C to 38° C). Alcohol baths was an accepted form of temperature control in years past, but it was then realized that the alcohol could be absorbed through the skin causing alcohol poisoning. Phenobarbital does not affect temperature.

107. Answer: C

Nursing Process: Intervention/Respiratory

Rationale: **A decrease in altitude is the best therapy for high-altitude pulmonary edema (HAPE) because it allows the body to initiate "self-correction" of many altitude-related physiologic processes, but acclimatization will rarely be sufficient without adjunctive therapy.** Getting "down off the mountain" is the most beneficial treatment option along with providing oxygen to the patient. The mechanisms of HAPE are not borne by bacteria and thus are not treated as pneumonia. There are several treatments that can be used for high-altitude sickness.

108. Answer: D

Nursing Process: Intervention/Cardiovascular

Rationale: **Initiating synchronized cardioversion with 0.5 to 1 J/kg is initial treatment for unstable infants or children with supraventricular tachycardia. The patient in this scenario is hypotensive and has evidence of poor perfusion.** Adenosine, application of ice to the face, and vagal maneuvers are attempted in children (and adults) who are hemodynamically stable.

109. Answer: A

Nursing Process: Intervention/Neurologic

Rationale: **Optimal positioning for a lumbar puncture in an infant is sitting upright or on their side with knees flexed and chin to chest.** Older children or adults may be sitting on the side of the bed leaning over a bedside table. A prone position is not appropriate and the supine position would not provide access to the spinal area. The child or infant would have to be in a curled position in order to access the proper location for needle insertion.

110. Answer: C

Nursing Process: Intervention/Respiratory

Rationale: **The priority for inhalation burn injury is to secure the airway with intubation.** Burns of the face may indicate burns to the large and small airways. Although they initially appear stable, a burn will quickly swell and loss of the airway can occur rapidly. Waiting for the situation to worsen may delay intubation to the point at which intubation or even emergency cricothyrotomy is very difficult or impossible. Delivery of high-flow oxygen is appropriate but a rebreather mask does not secure an airway.

111. Answer: A

Nursing Process: Analysis/Maxillofacial/Ocular

Rationale: **Facial numbness and inability to look upward are consistent with fracture to the orbital floor, also referred to as a blow-out fracture. The signs and symptoms are consistent with entrapment of extraocular muscles and the infraorbital nerve indicating a blow-out fracture.** Subconjunctival hemorrhage results in bloody appearance of the sclera and is typically a benign uncomplicated presentation. Floaters in the eye may be seen with retinal detachment, yet when the patient can count the number of floaters, it is usually benign and not associated with retinal hemorrhage. Corneal abrasion results in significant eye irritation and pain with excessive tearing, yet is not considered an emergent presentation.

112. Answer: B

Nursing Process: Evaluation/Toxicology

Rationale: **Drying of the skin would be an indication that the cholinergic toxicity effect has been resolved.** This toxidrome often causes lability, as either elevated or decreased, heart rate, respirations, and blood pressure, and is not known to directly change body temperature. Miosis is a symptom of cholinergic exposure; therefore, its presence would not indicate successful treatment. Tachycardia and hypotension may be symptoms of cholinergic crisis; however, the treatment of cholinergic exposure would not intentionally create an abnormally high heart rate or an abnormally low blood pressure. Tachycardia and hypotension in this case would indicate that patient was overtreated and a new problem, potentially anticholinergic crisis, was created.

113. Answer: B

Nursing Process: Intervention/Maxillofacial/Ocular

Rationale: **Airway compromise is not an expected finding and there is no indication that the airway is not patent, therefore suctioning is not indicated.** Vincent's angina, also referred to as acute necrotizing ulcerative gingivitis or trench mouth, is a bacterial infection of the gums. History typically includes immunosuppression, malnourishment, and poor dental hygiene. Classic presentation of Vincent's angina includes bleeding, painful, swollen gums, fever, halitosis, and gray pseudomembranous ulcers on the pharynx. Intravenous access should be obtained for specimen collection, intravenous fluids, and antibiotic administration. The patient should be seen by a dentist for definitive management.

114. Answer: D

Nursing Process: Assessment/Orthopedic

Rationale: **Bursitis is an inflammation of the bursa sac of a joint from overuse.** Blood in the joint occurs with trauma or surgery. Gout arises from an alteration in the production of uric acid. Septic arthritis is sudden in onset and occurs from bacteria entering the joint through the bloodstream, tissue, or a puncture wound.

115. Answer: B

Nursing Process: Analysis/Orthopedic

Rationale: **The median nerve is responsible for movement of the small muscles of the hand and sensation in the palm. This is the nerve involved in carpal tunnel syndrome. This nerve runs through the middle of the wrist into the hand. The space available for it in the carpal tunnel becomes minimized and symptoms then appear.** The ulnar nerve allows for abduction of the fingers and supplies sensation to the little finger. The radial nerve provides the ability to extend the thumb and delivers sensation to the dorsum of the thumb. Both of these nerves can be involved in carpal tunnel syndrome, but are not the cause. The peroneal nerve is located in the foot and causes extension of the foot and great toe and sensation to the first web space.

116. Answer: B

Nursing Process: Analysis/Neurologic

Rationale: **Increased intracranial pressure produces observable signs and symptoms depending on the stage of increased pressure. Early signs include headache, nausea and vomiting, altered level of consciousness, and drowsiness.** Late signs include increased systolic blood pressure, bradycardia, widening pulse pressures, and dilated nonreactive pupils. Hypothermia, bradycardia, and a widened pulse pressure are indicative of increased intracranial pressure. Two episodes of vomiting in 3 hours should not cause these symptoms. Autonomic dysreflexia is a hypertensive emergency and occurs in patients who have a history of spinal cord injuries. There is no indication in the stem of the question to indicate increased intra-abdominal pressure.

117. Answer: D

Nursing Process: Analysis/Maxillofacial/Ocular

Rationale: **The priority is to maintain a patent airway and ensure hemodynamic stability. Monitoring the amount of blood loss and preparing for blood replacement are interventions that meet those priorities. Type and crossmatch are essential to prepare for blood volume replacement, should it be needed.** Complete blood count (CBC), international normalized ratio (INR), partial Thromboplastin Time (aPTT), and protime (PT) are all important to determine clotting status and blood loss; however, the hematocrit and type and crossmatch are the priority tests.

118. Answer: C

Nursing Process: Evaluation/Neurologic

Rationale: **This patient is given 5 points for purposeful movement to pain (motor), 3 points for inappropriate words (verbal), and 2 points for eye opening in response to painful stimuli. The total score is 10.** Remember! The lowest score on a Glasgow Coma Scale is 3—not 0! Highest potential scoring is 15.

119. Answer: C

Nursing Process: Assessment/GU/GYN/OB

Rationale: **Hyperemesis gravidarum is more extreme than morning sickness and is experienced by 70% to 80% of women early in their pregnancy. This condition often continues throughout pregnancy and is thought to be caused by the rise of hormone levels. It may lead to hospitalization for rehydration.** Cyclical vomiting occurs as sudden and repeated episodes of vomiting but is not associated with pregnancy. Gastroenteritis is inflammation of the stomach and intestine and ulcerative colitis is inflammation of the colon with ulcers.

120. Answer: B

Nursing Process: Assessment/Maxillofacial/Ocular

Rationale: **Ptosis occurs with eyelid lacerations affecting the levator muscle that is located under the upper lid, above the globe.** This muscle is responsible for raising the upper lid. Bleeding may occur with any laceration and should be controlled. Visual disturbances may occur with eyelid lacerations with concurrent injury such as hyphema or globe disruption.

121. Answer: A

Nursing Process: Evaluation/Environmental

Rationale: **A walking tick has not latched on, sucked blood, or transmitted a tick-borne disease to the patient. Additionally, most patients with a tick exposure will not be prophylactically treated, but the provider will treat based on disease risk in area and type of disease risk.** It is appropriate to tuck pants legs into socks to keep ticks and other insects off of the ankle areas. Removing ticks can be accomplished by using tweezers and a twisting motion and tick repellant would be correct.

122. Answer: A

Nursing Process: Intervention/Neurologic

Rationale: **A rotated head position will prevent venous outflow via the jugular veins and contribute to increased intracranial pressure (ICP). The head of the bed should be maintained at 30 degrees, and hyperextension, flexion, and rotation of the head should be avoided.** Placing the patient in Trendelenburg by lowering the head of the bed would increase the pressure on the brain. Closing the stopcock on the ventriculostomy causes the ICP to rise because there is no longer an outlet for the cerebrospinal fluid (CSF).

123. Answer: C

Nursing Process: Assessment/Orthopedic

Rationale: **Popliteal artery injury is a frequent and significant high-risk complication with a dislocated knee. All patients including those who relocate spontaneously before arrival to the emergency department should be assessed for this event. Some can maintain pulse for a time due to collateral flow.** Fibula fracture and tibial nerve injuries are not usually associated with knee dislocation. The saphenous vein is in the lower leg away from the knee.

124. Answer: D

Nursing Process: Analysis/GU/GYN/OB

Rationale: **Postpartum hemorrhage is defined as blood loss greater than 500 mL and is a common complication of labor and delivery. Amniotic fluid embolism, a complication experienced by the mother, is caused when amniotic fluid leaks into the mother's venous circulation during labor and delivery. It does not cause postpartum hemorrhage.** Retained products of conception or placental fragments can interfere with involution or return of the uterus to normal size. Vaginal or cervical tears can be a cause of postpartum bleeding.

125. Answer: B

Nursing Process: Assessment/Maxillofacial/Ocular

Rationale: **Visualization of blood in the anterior chamber of the eye is the definition of a hyphema.** Hyphema may occur secondary to blunt or penetrating trauma, and any portion of the anterior chamber of the eye may be affected, evidenced by a blood fluid line across the iris or blacked-out appearance in an eight-ball hyphema. The patient will experience blurry vision, blood-tinged vision, pain, and decreased visual acuity. Retinal detachment gives the perception of floaters, flashing lights, or a veil or curtain across a visual field. Orbital fractures, leading to entrapment of the extraocular muscles results in the inability to move the eye. Corneal abrasion results in pain with lid or globe movement.

126. Answer: B

Nursing Process: Analysis/Neurologic

Rationale: **In the Tensilon test, edrophonium (Tensilon) is administered by intravenous infusion to a patient exhibiting signs of muscle weakness. Significant improvement, lasting approximately 4 to 5 minutes, in the patient's muscle tone indicates a positive diagnosis for myasthenia gravis.** A lumbar puncture (LP) is frequently performed to assist in diagnosing meningitis. Allen's test is performed to evaluate the circulatory function of the ulnar artery before obtaining arterial blood gases ABGs to verify collateral circulation before accessing the radial artery. An MRI is effective in detecting degenerative central nervous system diseases, malignant tumors, and oxygen-deprived tissue, but none of these findings are associated with myasthenia gravis.

127. Answer: A

Nursing Process: Intervention/Medical

Rationale: **Magnesium sulfate must be infused slowly at a rate not to exceed 125 mg/kg/hour to avoid potential cardiac or respiratory arrest.** Normal saline or 5% dextrose should be used to dilute the infusion. Caution should be used when administering CNS depressants such as narcotics and barbiturates because they potentiate the central nervous system depressant effect of magnesium. Patients being treated with intravenous magnesium sulfate should be placed on continuous cardiac/respiratory monitoring.

128. Answer: B

Nursing Process: Assessment/GU/GYN/OB

Rationale: **Peripheral resistance decreases during pregnancy, causing a slight decrease in systolic and diastolic blood pressure.** The resting heart rate actually increases 10 to 20 beats/minute and the circulating blood volume increases by 30% to 50%. Respirations increase to help accommodate for the increased oxygen consumption during pregnancy.

129. Answer: C

Nursing Process: Evaluation/Neurologic

Rationale: **The modified Ramsay Score for Sedation measures the level of sedation achieved with pharmacologic agents. A Ramsay score of 5 suggests that the patient responds only to noxious stimuli.** A patient who is anxious, agitated, or restless has a Ramsay score of 1. A patient who is cooperative, tranquil, and oriented has a score of 2. A patient who responds to voice and verbal commands has a Ramsay score of 3. A patient who responds to gentle shaking scores a 4. A patient who shows no response to noxious stimuli is considered a 6 on the scale. The scale ranges from 1 to 6 only.

130. Answer: A

Nursing Process: Intervention/GU/GYN/OB

Rationale: **Clothing that was worn by the patient and obtained during the sexual assault examination should be placed in a paper bag and secured with evidence tape to ensure that no tampering occurs.** When performing a sexual assault examination and collecting the clothing, each piece of clothing should be placed in a separate paper bag. Also, the patient should stand on a sheet and then that sheet should be also be sent as evidence. The emergency nurse should also put their name or initials across the fold of the bag to assist with knowledge of nontampering as well. The patient's clothing should be carefully removed, but not shaken out; microscopic evidence may be lost. All clothing should be given to the police; it is their responsibility to determine if evidence is present. Clothing should not be placed in plastic bags, which can cause mildew and moisture retention, both of which can cause loss of evidence. All evidence collected should be labeled with the victim's name, site of collection, date and time of collection, and the name of the person collecting the evidence.

131. Answer: D

Nursing Process: Analysis/Orthopedic

Rationale: **Fat embolism is a potential complication when long-bone fractures are manipulated. This complication may occur within 12 hours.** This is why immediate immobilization is so important. Deep vein thrombosis develops from immobility, which may then lead to pulmonary embolism. This can then progress to acute respiratory distress syndrome.

132. Answer: C

Nursing Process: Assessment/Maxillofacial/Ocular

Rationale: **Subconjunctival hemorrhage is a benign condition that occurs when blood vessels of the conjunctiva rupture and blood is trapped between the subconjunctiva and the sclera. Some cases are idiopathic, yet it frequently occurs due to increased pressure to the area secondary to coughing, straining, forceful vomiting, or vigorous rubbing of the eye. Subconjunctival hemorrhage occurs suddenly, and other than the appearance, the patient is usually asymptomatic.** Hyphema indicates blood in the anterior chamber of the eye resulting from trauma. An eight-ball hyphema occurs when the entire anterior chamber is covered in blood. Retinal hemorrhage occurs in association with other eye injuries and/or head trauma. Both hyphema and retinal hemorrhage results in visual disturbances. Ultraviolet keratitis is a type of corneal burn that may have delayed onset of symptom from the time of the exposure to ultraviolet light.

133. Answer: D

Nursing Process: Intervention/Neurologic

Rationale: **Tissue plasminogen activator (TPA) is a fibrinolytic medication that decreases the patient's ability to clot. The infusion should be stopped immediately.** While a patient is receiving TPA, all invasive procedures should be avoided due to the increased risk of bleeding; therefore, a nasogastric tube should not be placed. The physician should be notified, but the priority is to stop the infusion.

134. Answer: B

Nursing Process: Intervention/Medical

Rationale: **In the patient with known idiopathic thrombocytopenia (ITP), an intravenous infusion of immunoglobulin is a first-line intervention, because it causes a rapid rise in the platelet levels. Platelet transfusion can also be considered if the count is less than 50,000 and in the presence of severe hemorrhage.** Desmopressin is a synthetic version of vasopressin that increases the levels of factor VIIIc in the treatment of mild-to-moderate hemophilia. Factor VIII would be utilized in patients with hemophilia A. Thrombin causes blood coagulation by converting fibrinogen to fibrin. Thrombin is indicated for epistaxis but is not a treatment for ITP.

135. Answer: B

Nursing Process: Intervention/GU/GYN/OB

Rationale: ***Candida albicans* is a yeast (fungal infection) treated with Mycostatin (nystatin) and does not require sexual partner treatment.** *Neisseria gonorrhoeae, Trichomonas vaginalis,* and *Chlamydia trachomatis* all are sexually transmitted diseases that necessitate partner treatment and thorough patient education.

136. Answer: D

Nursing Process: Intervention/Maxillofacial/Ocular

Rationale: **Central retinal artery occlusion results from an embolus lodged in the retinal artery. Vision loss is sudden and painless. Priority interventions are geared toward restoring circulation within 90 minutes of symptom onset to prevent permanent blindness. Supine position optimizes circulation.** A temporary measure of having the patient rebreathe carbon dioxide (brown bag or administration of carbogen gas) may facilitate mild vasodilation. Ocular massage should be reserved for a provider and may increase circulation or dislodge a clot. An eye patch is indicated in conditions in which eye movement is prohibited to promote healing and decrease pain. Hyperventilation will result in loss of carbon dioxide that may result in vasoconstriction.

137. Answer: C

Nursing Process: Intervention/Orthopedic

Rationale: **The most important priority intervention for this patient is to bivalve the cast. Nothing can be done until the area can be visualized.** Sometimes just removing the cast can take care of the pain. Compartment syndrome is a major concern, but the pressure cannot be checked until the cast is removed. This can be caused by an external force such as a cast, and pain disproportionate to injury is an indication of this complication. Deep vein thrombus is painful but not disproportionate. Pain control may be an issue, but again the hallmark symptom in this scenario is the report of disproportionate pain to injury.

138. Answer: A

Nursing Process: Intervention/Medical

Rationale: **Because septic shock is associated with a high mortality rate due to a state of severe hypoperfusion, early goal-directed resuscitation measures include treating the state of hypoperfusion. This includes fluid boluses, increasing the systemic vascular resistance (SVR) with vasopressor agents, and/or administering packed red blood cells (PRBCs), if needed.** These measures will decrease the risk of end-organ damage often seen in cases of septic shock. Systemic vascular resistance is lowered in septic shock and treatment is aimed at increasing resistance. International guidelines recommend dopamine or norepinephrine as first-line vasopressor agents in septic shock, whereas epinephrine and vasopressin are considered second-line agents. The effect of vasopressors will improve renal output; thus, there is no indication for diuretic therapy.

139. Answer: D

Nursing Process: Intervention/Maxillofacial/Ocular

Rationale: **Diuretics and low sodium diet are part of the treatment plan for the patient with Meniere's disease to decrease the fluid and pressure build up in the endolymphatic system.** Labyrinthitis is due to viral or bacterial infections leading to inflammation of the labyrinth. Nausea and vertigo are experienced in both disorders. Hence, the need for antiemetics and instructions to manage vertigo and maintain safety.

140. Answer: C

Nursing Process: Evaluation/Neurologic

Rationale: **One of the most common causes of seizures in a patient taking phenytoin (Dilantin) is discontinuation of the medication.** Because of the slow absorption of phenytoin from the GI tract, daily drug routines can be easily adjusted when a dose is missed. The patient also needs to be made aware of possible adverse effects of his medications. Phenytoin is metabolized in the liver, and both the inactive metabolites and unchanged drug are excreted in the urine. Because phenytoin has many hematopoietic adverse effects, blood work (including complete blood count, liver, and renal function studies) should be obtained on a regular basis. Serum levels should also be monitored because serum concentrations increase disproportionately to dosing regimens.

141. Answer: D

Nursing Process: Evaluation/Maxillofacial/Ocular

Rationale: **Vincent's angina is a bacterial infection of the gums resulting in bleeding, painful, swollen gums. Once brushing can be tolerated, a soft-bristle toothbrush should be used or the patient can gently wipe the gums.** The patient should be instructed to eat nutritious food, take antibiotics as prescribed, and rinse the mouth with an antiseptic mouthwash in the acute phase of the infection.

142. Answer: D

Nursing Process: Intervention/Orthopedic

Rationale: **Controlling the hemorrhage is the highest priority. Application of a tourniquet would be the next step because direct pressure and elevation of the extremity has not stopped the bleeding.** Application of a pressure dressing would most likely not help because direct pressure has not worked. Starting an intravenous catheter and notifying the physician are important, but hemorrhage control is the priority.

143. Answer: C

Nursing Process: Analysis/Maxillofacial/Ocular

Rationale: **Painless loss of vision accompanied by the perception of floaters, flashing lights, cloudy smoky vision, or a veil or curtain over the vision are classic presentations for retinal detachment. Retinal detachment is separation of the layers of the retinal and subsequent fluid or blood pooling between the retinal layers. Retinal detachment can occur spontaneously or secondary to trauma. The condition is diagnosed by dilated posterior eye examination of the fundus.** Tonometry is indicated for glaucoma and iritis. Fluorescein stain is indicated for assessment of corneal irregularities such as abrasions or ulcerations. Computed tomography (CT) is indicated in orbital fracture, sinusitis, and associated facial trauma.

144. Answer: A

Nursing Process: Intervention/GU/GYN/OB

Rationale: **This patient has signs and symptoms of testicular torsion. Testicular torsion results from congenital maldevelopment between the testis and the posterior scrotal wall. This is an emergency situation and an emergent ultrasound must be done.** Twisting of the spermatic cord compromises the circulation, causing severe pain that is not relieved by ice or elevation. There is no blood loss associated with testicular torsion, so blood products are not indicated.

145. Answer: D

Nursing Process: Assessment/Medical

Rationale: **Potassium elevation occurs in adrenal crisis because of an inability to regulate aldosterone, resulting in sodium and water depletion and retention of potassium. These patients frequently have hyponatremia in conjunction with hyperkalemia.** Patients with Addison's disease also have low cortisol production, inhibiting the breakdown of sugar into glucose, resulting in hypoglycemia. Hypocalcemia is related to low levels of mineralocorticoids, unrelated to aldosterone production.

146. Answer: D

Nursing Process: Assessment/Medical

Rationale: **The most significant indicator of infection in an immunocompromised person is fever. Thus, this population is instructed to seek medical care whenever the body temperature reaches 100.4° F (38° C).** Immunocompromised patients become neutropenic (decreased neutrophils) and leukemic (decreased total white blood cell count). The body's phagocytic response is suppressed, because the body does not recognize the presence of an infection by typical symptoms such as heat, redness, swelling, and pus at the site of infection.

147. Answer: B

Nursing Process: Evaluation/GU/GYN/OB

Rationale: **Restlessness is typically the first sign of impending hypovolemic shock or hypoxia.** A pulse rate of 100 beats/minute is actually a decrease compared with the original 120 beats/minute, and the blood pressure has not dropped significantly. Requests for pain relief are normal for a trauma patient.

148. Answer: B

Nursing Process: Intervention/Environmental

Rationale: **Because the bite of a rabid bat is so small, difficult to find, generally unfelt during sleep, and the high risk that the bat could have rabies, the recommendation is that if a bat is seen in a room where someone was sleeping they should receive the rabies series. Initial treatment is with Rabies Immune Globulin (RIG) and the first dose of Rabies vaccine if the patient has not been vaccinated previously.** Antibiotics will not help. Rabies vaccine is no longer administered twice a day for 21 days and there is a high risk for this patient per the CDC because this is a child. Other high-risk patients include someone found altered due to alcohol or drugs, the elderly, or sound sleepers.

149. Answer: A

Nursing Process: Intervention/Respiratory

Rationale: **If the patient is not exhibiting symptoms of hypovolemic shock, intravenous fluids should be restricted during initial care.** While providing supplemental oxygen, positioning the patient to facilitate breathing, and assisting with removal of secretions are all treatments for pulmonary contusion, limiting intravenous fluid administration is associated with the best outcome for the patient.

150. Answer: D

Nursing Process: Intervention/Respiratory

Rationale: **All the options listed are important in the treatment of tension pneumothorax, but the most important is needle decompression.** A 14-G needle is inserted into the second intercostal space at the midclavicular line on the affected side is appropriate. A chest tube insertion should follow needle decompression.

Patricia L. Clutter, RN, MEd, CEN, FAEN

This test has been created according to the Blueprint found on the BCEN website for the CEN test.

Remember that the actual test will have 175 questions as it will have 25 pretest questions–to test the question itself–not you!!

Good Luck!

Questions

1. A 45-year-old patient arrives in the emergency department complaining of fever for the past 2 days. He is awake, alert, and oriented with the following vital signs:

Blood pressure—124/74 mm Hg
Heart rate—120 beats/minute
Respirations—22 breaths/minute
Pulse oximetry—94% on room air
Temperature—101.6° F (38.7° C)

He reports that he is HIV positive and taking antiviral medications. The emergency nurse should triage him at which acuity level using a 5-level system?
[ ] **A.** Level 1 (resuscitation or life-threatening)
[ ] **B.** Level 2 (high risk and/or emergent)
[ ] **C.** Level 3 (urgent)
[ ] **D.** Level 4/5 (nonurgent/nonemergent)

2. Which of the following parenteral solutions should be used in the initial treatment of intracellular fluid deficit of a patient with hyperosmolar hyperglycemic syndrome?
[ ] **A.** D_5W with 0.9% normal saline (NS)
[ ] **B.** D_5W with 0.45% normal saline (NS)
[ ] **C.** 0.9% NS with 20 mEq potassium chloride
[ ] **D.** 0.9% normal saline (NS)

3. Which of the following is a gynecological/obstetric condition that must be considered as a potentially dangerous situation for every female presenting with abdominal pain during child-bearing years?
[ ] **A.** Ectopic pregnancy
[ ] **B.** Ovarian cyst
[ ] **C.** Ovarian torsion
[ ] **D.** Dysmenorrhea

4. A patient complains of acute shortness of breath, frothy pink-tinged sputum, and chest pain. Crackles and wheezes are present. Past medical history includes diabetes, hypertension, and heart failure. The emergency nurse suspects which of the following disease processes?
[ ] **A.** Pericardial tamponade
[ ] **B.** Pneumothorax
[ ] **C.** Pulmonary embolus
[ ] **D.** Pulmonary edema

5. A patient has extensive burns to his head, face, neck, and chest with much of his hair, including his eyebrows, burned off from an ignited flammable liquid. He is conscious, breathing, and is in significant pain. He is noted to have a mildly hoarse voice. A baseline physical assessment has been completed. The most reliable additional assessment of the patient's breathing status would include:
[ ] **A.** arterial blood gases (ABGs).
[ ] **B.** complete blood count (CBC).
[ ] **C.** mixed venous blood gases.
[ ] **D.** oxygen saturation monitoring.

6. The Joint Commission sentinel event alert related to preventing restraint deaths identified all of the following risks **EXCEPT**:
[ ] **A.** placing a restrained patient in a supine position could increase aspiration risk.
[ ] **B.** placing a restrained patient in a prone position could increase suffocation risk.
[ ] **C.** a restraint may cause further psychological trauma or traumatic memories.
[ ] **D.** appropriate alternatives to restraints are to be used only as a last resort.

7. A dangerous side effect of Monoamine Oxidase Inhibitor (MAOI) antidepressant overdose is:
[ ] **A.** hypotension.
[ ] **B.** hypertension.
[ ] **C.** sedation.
[ ] **D.** severe agitation.

8. The emergency nurse identifies a condition that precipitates sudden cardiac death from blunt trauma to the left anterior chest wall that occurs predominantly in young, healthy, male athletes as:
[ ] **A.** long QT syndrome.
[ ] **B.** commotio cordis.
[ ] **C.** point of maximal impulse.
[ ] **D.** Kawasaki disease.

9. Which of the following is **NOT** a cause of noncardiac pulmonary edema?
[ ] **A.** Trauma
[ ] **B.** Aspiration
[ ] **C.** High altitude
[ ] **D.** Pneumothorax

10. Which of the following is the initial treatment for a patient with a tracheobronchial injury?
[ ] **A.** Suctioning to maintain airway patency
[ ] **B.** Preparing for chest tube insertion
[ ] **C.** Intubating and providing mechanical ventilation
[ ] **D.** Preparing for surgical intervention

11. Immediate postcardiac arrest care in comatose patients after return of spontaneous circulation (ROSC) includes which of the following?
[ ] **A.** Maintaining a ventilatory $PETCO_2$ between 55 and 60 mm Hg
[ ] **B.** Maintaining a minimum systolic blood pressure of 80 mm Hg
[ ] **C.** Maintaining a target temperature of 32° C to 36° C (89.6° F to 96.8° F)
[ ] **D.** Maintaining arterial oxygen saturation of 90% or greater

12. Which of the following is a true statement regarding a bowel obstruction?
[ ] **A.** Hyperactive bowel sounds can be heard in a bowel obstruction in certain situations.
[ ] **B.** Large bowel obstructions usually present with a moderate amount of abdominal swelling.
[ ] **C.** All bowel obstructions will have a fecal smell to the emesis.
[ ] **D.** A small bowel obstruction usually has a lesser amount of vomiting.

13. Which of the following test results provides information that is important immediately following a sexual assault?
[ ] **A.** Negative serologic test for syphilis
[ ] **B.** Normal complete blood count
[ ] **C.** Rhogam test for blood type
[ ] **D.** Negative pregnancy test

14. The classic presentation of thyroid storm includes all of the following **EXCEPT**:
[ ] **A.** fever.
[ ] **B.** tachycardia.
[ ] **C.** hot, dry skin.
[ ] **D.** mentation changes.

15. When discharging a patient with sickle cell disease, which of the following statements indicates the patient understands how to avoid precipitating a sickle cell crisis?
[ ] **A.** "I will self-manage flu-like symptoms for 48 hours before calling my physician."
[ ] **B.** "I can continue to participate in cold weather sporting events."
[ ] **C.** "When I am angry, I will keep my feelings to myself."
[ ] **D.** "I will drink at least 64 oz of water every day."

16. Common physical manifestations of eating disorders include all of the following **EXCEPT**:
[ ] **A.** dehydration/nutritional imbalances.
[ ] **B.** cardiac dysrhythmias/electrolyte imbalances.
[ ] **C.** acute renal or hepatic failure.
[ ] **D.** progressive vision loss/diplopia.

17. Following a fall down a flight of stairs, a patient in her 38th week of pregnancy is brought to the emergency department. Unless contraindicated, she should be placed in which position during assessment?
[ ] **A.** Trendelenburg
[ ] **B.** Supine
[ ] **C.** Left lateral recumbent
[ ] **D.** Knee-chest

18. The dementia patient is most likely at risk of receiving suboptimal emergency care for an acute hip fracture because:
[ ] **A.** their vascular sufficiency may be compromised and impede healing.
[ ] **B.** their ability to interpret and communicate pain may be compromised.
[ ] **C.** they are not competent to consent to a surgical treatment.
[ ] **D.** it is impossible to keep them in the bed for a thorough evaluation.

19. Which of the following would be a concern for a patient involved in a major motor vehicle crash who presents with right upper quadrant pain and has a past history of hepatitis C, COPD, and hypertension?
[ ] **A.** Respiratory distress
[ ] **B.** Uncontrolled bleeding
[ ] **C.** Hypertensive crisis
[ ] **D.** Pneumonia

20. Which of the following is another sign of burn inhalation injury besides hoarseness?
[ ] **A.** Rapid easing of the work of respiration
[ ] **B.** Carbonaceous or black-tinged sputum
[ ] **C.** Persistent wet and productive cough
[ ] **D.** Moist mucous membranes

21. Cardiac output (CO) is a product of which of the following formulas?
[ ] **A.** Preload × Afterload
[ ] **B.** Zone 1 × Zone 2
[ ] **C.** Heart rate × Stroke volume
[ ] **D.** (Age in years)/4 + 4

22. Proton pump inhibitors are used in patients with gastroesophageal reflux disease (GERD) because of which of the following actions?
[ ] **A.** Increases lower esophageal sphincter pressure
[ ] **B.** Reduces secretions in the stomach
[ ] **C.** Lowers acid present in the stomach
[ ] **D.** Decreases the production of acid

23. It is the plaintiff's responsibility to prove certain elements in a negligence lawsuit. Which of the following is **NOT** one of these elements?
[ ] **A.** A duty was owed to the patient.
[ ] **B.** The defendant breached the duty.
[ ] **C.** This breach of duty was the cause of the plaintiff's injury.
[ ] **D.** The plaintiff was at risk for an injury because of the breach of duty.

24. Which of the following would indicate an improvement in a patient with a diagnosis of serotonin syndrome?
[ ] **A.** Increased heart rate
[ ] **B.** Normothermia
[ ] **C.** Mydriasis
[ ] **D.** Dry mucous membranes

25. Treatment for norovirus includes all of the following **EXCEPT**:
[ ] **A.** antibiotic therapy.
[ ] **B.** rehydration.
[ ] **C.** bed rest.
[ ] **D.** strict handwashing.

26. Which of the following statements made by a patient being discharged with a diagnosis of trichomonas and placed on a regimen of metronidazole (Flagyl) indicates that instructions were understood?
[ ] **A.** "I'm very glad that I don't have to tell anyone about this."
[ ] **B.** "I'm so excited that I just found out that I am pregnant."
[ ] **C.** "I should not drink alcohol while I am taking this medication."
[ ] **D.** "The doctor said this would not impact my Coumadin medication."

27. A patient is complaining of chest pain unrelieved with rest. The electrocardiogram shows T-wave inversion and there is no elevation in troponin. The emergency nurse suspects which of the following disease entities?
[ ] **A.** Stable angina
[ ] **B.** Unstable angina
[ ] **C.** Non-ST elevation myocardial infarction (Non-STEMI)
[ ] **D.** ST elevation myocardial infarction (STEMI)

28. A patient has a history of heart failure and has been diagnosed with pneumonia. Audible, adventitious lung sounds are present. Which of the following sounds would the nurse **NOT** expect to hear?
[ ] **A.** Stridor
[ ] **B.** Crackles
[ ] **C.** Wheezing
[ ] **D.** Rhonchi
[ ] **E.**

29. Atypical antipsychotic drugs affect the dopamine and serotonin receptors and have lower _____ compared with typical antipsychotic medications.
[ ] **A.** daily compliance
[ ] **B.** extrapyramidal syndromes
[ ] **C.** financial burden
[ ] **D.** therapeutic benefits

30. When utilizing the pH method of confirmation of gastric tube placement, which of the following numbers would indicate that the tube is in the stomach?

[ ] **A.** 4.0
[ ] **B.** 8.5
[ ] **C.** 10.0
[ ] **D.** 14.5

31. Which of the following changes on the electrocardiogram would the emergency nurse recognize as being indicative of an acute myocardial infarction?

[ ] **A.** ST-segment depression.
[ ] **B.** Dynamic T-wave inversion.
[ ] **C.** Nondiagnostic changes in ST segment.
[ ] **D.** ST-segment elevation.

32. The provider has diagnosed a patient with a hydatidiform mole. The emergency nurse will expect the human gonadotropin level to be:

[ ] **A.** zero.
[ ] **B.** very low.
[ ] **C.** very high.
[ ] **D.** normal for gestational age.

33. Which of the following is a true statement regarding breach of duty?

[ ] **A.** Willful violation of an oath or code of ethics regarding patient care
[ ] **B.** Failure to meet accepted standards in providing care for a patient
[ ] **C.** Threatening a patient with withholding pain medication
[ ] **D.** Confining a patient to a psychiatric unit without a physician's order

34. A vesicular rash and fever are indicative of which of the following infectious diseases?

[ ] **A.** Kawasaki disease
[ ] **B.** Varicella zoster
[ ] **C.** Lyme disease
[ ] **D.** Meningococcemia

35. In certain cases, which of the following medications may be used to medically manage an ectopic pregnancy instead of surgery?

[ ] **A.** Doxycycline (Vibramycin)
[ ] **B.** Ceftriaxone (Rocephin)
[ ] **C.** Methotrexate (Trexall)
[ ] **D.** Metronidazole (Flagyl)

36. Which of the following classes of medications would most likely **NOT** be prescribed in an emergency care environment due to their slow onset of effectiveness?

[ ] **A.** Typical antipsychotic
[ ] **B.** Atypical antipsychotic
[ ] **C.** Benzodiazepine
[ ] **D.** Selective serotonin reuptake inhibitor (SSRI)

37. A patient in the emergency department is being evaluated for acute kidney injury (AKI) and appears very ill. A urinalysis and CBC have been ordered. Which of the following additional tests would be most beneficial to determine the severity and acuity of renal failure and would require immediate life-saving interventions?

[ ] **A.** Intravenous pyelogram (IVP)
[ ] **B.** Blood urea nitrogen (BUN)
[ ] **C.** Renal arteriogram
[ ] **D.** Serum potassium

38. Which of the following is the expected primary treatment outcome of postrenal acute kidney injury?

[ ] **A.** Increase outflow of urine from the kidney
[ ] **B.** Increase renal artery perfusion
[ ] **C.** Increase systemic blood pressure
[ ] **D.** Decrease systemic blood pressure

39. Which of the following is a true statement regarding caring for individuals who are diagnosed with *Clostridium difficile* infection?

[ ] **A.** The use of alcohol-based hand cleansers is extremely useful and recommended.
[ ] **B.** Patients should remain in isolation for at least 48 hours after the last diarrhea stool.
[ ] **C.** Gowns and masks are not necessary to wear when caring for these patients.
[ ] **D.** Private rooms are not necessary when these patients are admitted for inpatient care.

40. A patient is brought to the emergency department with mild respiratory distress. His oxygen saturation is 95% on 3 liters of oxygen via nasal cannula, respiratory rate is 28 breaths/minute, and temperature is 101° F (38.3° C). He has decreased breath sounds over the base of the right lung and complains of a nonproductive cough. He has a history of tuberculosis. Based on these assessment findings, which of the following should the nurse suspect?

[ ] **A.** Empyema
[ ] **B.** Transudative effusion
[ ] **C.** Exudative effusion
[ ] **D.** Pulmonary embolus

41. The patient with chronic bronchitis requires careful monitoring when receiving which of the following treatments?

[ ] **A.** Oxygen therapy

[ ] **B.** Increased fluids

[ ] **C.** Humidified air

[ ] **D.** Postural drainage

42. A radiograph demonstrates a "buckle" fracture of the arm. The emergency nurse knows this fracture is also known as which of the following types of fracture?

[ ] **A.** Torus

[ ] **B.** Greenstick

[ ] **C.** Compression

[ ] **D.** Comminuted

43. On the basis of the relationship and time frame commonly available for patient education in the emergency department, which of the following kinds of learning goals are best established with a patient in this setting?

[ ] **A.** Long term

[ ] **B.** Short term

[ ] **C.** Middle range

[ ] **D.** Tertiary range

44. Cardiogenic shock is the result of myocardial pump failure, decreased cardiac output (CO), and inadequate tissue perfusion most commonly caused by myocardial infarction or ischemia. Signs and symptoms would include which of the following?

[ ] **A.** Tachypnea, crackles, hypotension, pale, and clammy skin

[ ] **B.** Dyspnea, stridor, wheezing, bronchospasm, and erythema

[ ] **C.** Bradycardia, hypotension, and warm, dry skin

[ ] **D.** Tachycardia, altered level of consciousness, and uncontrolled external bleeding

45. Which of the following would be the best manner to check for proper gastric tube placement?

[ ] **A.** Listen for instilled air over the epigastrium

[ ] **B.** Radiograph or computed tomography (CT) to confirm placement

[ ] **C.** pH testing of gastric aspirate

[ ] **D.** Use of carbon dioxide detector

46. Which of the following indicates the possibility of a urethral injury during a rectal examination of a trauma patient?

[ ] **A.** Low-riding prostate

[ ] **B.** High-riding prostate

[ ] **C.** Absent sphincter tone

[ ] **D.** Positive hemoccult test

47. Which of the following is the normal range for arterial blood pH?

[ ] **A.** 7.38 to 7.46

[ ] **B.** 7.40 to 7.52

[ ] **C.** 7.35 to 7.45

[ ] **D.** 7.28 to 7.38

48. Which of the following is the main route of transmission for infectious mononucleosis?

[ ] **A.** Blood

[ ] **B.** Skin lesions

[ ] **C.** Stool

[ ] **D.** Saliva

49. An unrestrained driver arrives in the emergency department after a roll-over crash at 80 miles/hour. Which of the following are the most common causes of pulseless electrical activity (PEA) rhythm for this patient?

[ ] **A.** Hypovolemia and hypoxia

[ ] **B.** Thrombosis and toxins

[ ] **C.** Hydrogen ion acidosis and hypothermia

[ ] **D.** Hypoglycemia and syncope

50. Which of the following is the most serious injury associated with a fracture of the first or second rib?

[ ] **A.** Cervical spine injury

[ ] **B.** Aortic rupture

[ ] **C.** Tracheal tear

[ ] **D.** Clavicular fracture

51. The emergency nurse realizes that the student nurse understands premature atrial contractions when the student makes which of the following statements?

[ ] **A.** "Premature atrial complexes may precede supraventricular tachycardia, atrial flutter, or atrial fibrillation."

[ ] **B.** "Premature atrial complexes may occur in a saw-toothed pattern and are called flutter waves."

[ ] **C.** "Premature atrial complexes are characterized by a chaotic atrial rhythm and an irregular ventricular response."

[ ] **D.** "Premature atrial complexes occur with accessory conduction system pathways that predispose to reentrant rhythms."

52. A patient arrives in the emergency department with complaints of chest pain for the last 30 minutes after mowing the lawn. He also reports nausea, dyspnea, and dizziness. The 12-lead electrocardiogram shows greater than 2 mm ST elevation in leads V_1, V_2, and V_3. This indicates injury to which of the following areas of the heart?
[ ] **A.** Inferior
[ ] **B.** Lateral
[ ] **C.** Anterior
[ ] **D.** Posterior

53. An unrestrained patient is brought to the emergency department after a motor vehicle crash. He is alert and oriented with the following vital signs:

Blood pressure—88/40 mm Hg
Pulse—42 beats/minute
Respirations—22 breaths/minute
Pulse oximetry—95% on room air
Temperature—99.2° F (37.3° C)

This is most likely due to which of the following types of shock?
[ ] **A.** Hypovolemic
[ ] **B.** Neurogenic
[ ] **C.** Anaphylactic
[ ] **D.** Septic

54. Which of the following is **NOT** a common sign or symptom of a pulmonary embolus (PE)?
[ ] **A.** Acute respiratory distress
[ ] **B.** Nonproductive cough
[ ] **C.** Bradycardia
[ ] **D.** Sudden chest pain

55. A patient arrives in the emergency department stating that she was sexually assaulted multiple times over the past 12 hours. She is tearful and accompanied by a friend. The emergency nurse knows that which of the following is the most important piece of information from this patient at this time?
[ ] **A.** She notified the police.
[ ] **B.** She uses birth control.
[ ] **C.** She has changed clothing.
[ ] **D.** She has been sexually assaulted before.

56. Which of the following interventions is **NOT** considered appropriate for a patient with placenta previa?
[ ] **A.** Performing a pelvic examination to determine cervical dilatation
[ ] **B.** Maintaining strict bed rest and observing for further bleeding
[ ] **C.** Monitoring for signs of shock
[ ] **D.** Preparing the patient for ultrasound

57. A provider has just asked the patient "How many fingers do you see?" This question is assessing which of the following cranial nerves?
[ ] **A.** Cranial nerve II (Optic)
[ ] **B.** Cranial nerve III (Oculomotor)
[ ] **C.** Cranial nerve IV (Trochlear)
[ ] **D.** Cranial nerve VI (Abducens)

58. A patient is brought to the emergency department by emergency medical services after being crushed while standing between a loading dock and a truck. The emergency nurse can anticipate which of the following injuries?
[ ] **A.** Humeral head fracture
[ ] **B.** Closed pelvic fracture
[ ] **C.** Humeral shaft fracture
[ ] **D.** Open-book pelvic fracture

59. Which of the following are the earliest signs of hypovolemic shock?
[ ] **A.** Tachycardia, restlessness, and thirst
[ ] **B.** Hypoxia, dysrhythmias, and tremors
[ ] **C.** Hypotension, flushed extremities, and anxiety
[ ] **D.** Oliguria, cyanosis, and confusion

60. The peak frequency of onset and diagnosis of schizophrenia is in which of the following age groups?
[ ] **A.** 5 to 14 years
[ ] **B.** 15 to 24 years
[ ] **C.** 25 to 34 years
[ ] **D.** 35 to 44 years

61. Upon initial interaction with the agitated patient, the most appropriate response would include which of the following?
[ ] **A.** Medication intervention
[ ] **B.** Isolation initiation
[ ] **C.** Restraint preparation
[ ] **D.** Verbal de-escalation

62. A patient is brought to the emergency department by ambulance with a chief complaint of lethargy. Two days before, the patient was in a high-speed motor vehicle accident and refused care. Since that time, she has complained of headaches and drowsiness. Her friend states that it has now become difficult to wake her up. Assessment reveals a right pupil that is fixed and dilated with papilledema present. The Glasgow Coma Scale score is 8. Which of the following types of injury does this patient exhibit?
[ ] **A.** Subdural hematoma
[ ] **B.** Epidural hematoma
[ ] **C.** Diffuse axonal injury
[ ] **D.** Post-concussion syndrome

63. A patient is bought to the emergency department with a past history of hepatitis C, cardiac stents, and hypertension. He is vomiting large amounts of bright red blood and is nauseated. No pain is present. Based on this patient's presentation and his present symptoms, which of the following medications should the emergency nurse expect to utilize?
[ ] **A.** Octreotide (Sandostatin)
[ ] **B.** Nitroprusside (Nipride)
[ ] **C.** Amiodarone (Cordarone)
[ ] **D.** Flumazenil (Romazicon)

64. A patient with a past history of intravenous substance abuse presents with confusion, abdominal distension, and bilateral icteric conjunctiva. Lactulose (Cholac) is prescribed for this patient. Which of the following laboratory values would be monitored to determine the effect of the lactulose?
[ ] **A.** Ammonia
[ ] **B.** Magnesium
[ ] **C.** Potassium
[ ] **D.** Sodium

65. A patient arrives at the emergency department with signs and symptoms consistent with a non-ST elevation myocardial infarction (NSTEMI). His vital signs are as follows: blood pressure, 100/68 mm Hg; pulse, 46 beats/minute; and respirations, 24 breaths/minute. The physician decides to transfer him to another facility by air. After stabilizing the patient with oxygen, an arterial line, intravenous line placement, and appropriate medication therapy, which of the following should be considered before transport via aircraft?
[ ] **A.** Nothing; the patient is ready to be transported.
[ ] **B.** The effect of air transport on the arterial line pressure bag
[ ] **C.** The ability of the patient's family to accompany the patient
[ ] **D.** Ensuring that vital signs are documented just before departure

66. Tricyclic antidepressant overdoses have three main toxic features. These features are cardiotoxicity, adrenergic blocking, and:
[ ] **A.** anticoagulation.
[ ] **B.** anticholinergic effects.
[ ] **C.** sympathomimetic effects.
[ ] **D.** central nervous system excitation.

67. A patient is brought to the emergency department with burns sustained when he fell backward into a fire pit. The palms of his hands have linear charred markings and are leathery to palpation. His lower back and upper posterior thighs have reddened, blistered areas and his nylon shorts are melted into his skin. When the shorts are pulled away, the underlying skin is patchy white or charred-looking. The patient complains of pain to his back and thighs, but not his buttocks or hands. Which of the following would be the suspected depth of burn associated with his hands and buttocks?
[ ] **A.** Superficial epidermal—first degree
[ ] **B.** Superficial partial thickness—second degree
[ ] **C.** Deep partial thickness—second degree
[ ] **D.** Full thickness—third degree

68. The National Institutes for Health Stroke Scale (NIHSS) can be linked to outcomes. Which of the following indicates the meaning of the higher scoring?
[ ] **A.** Better outcome
[ ] **B.** Better orientation
[ ] **C.** Increased risk factors
[ ] **D.** Poorer outcome

69. A patient was punched in the jaw. Which of the following assessment findings is consistent with mandibular fracture?
[ ] **A.** Numbness to the cheek
[ ] **B.** Sublingual hematoma
[ ] **C.** Avulsed tooth
[ ] **D.** Blow-out fracture

70. A 3-year-old patient is brought to the emergency department by his parents. He fell down several steps and has a fracture of the forearm. Which of the following types of fractures would be the most concerning?
[ ] **A.** Epiphyseal
[ ] **B.** Transverse
[ ] **C.** Greenstick
[ ] **D.** Displaced

71. The emergency nurse is completing an assessment for a patient with sinusitis. Which of the following is a predisposing factor for sinusitis?
[ ] **A.** Recurrent episodes of epistaxis
[ ] **B.** Recent viral upper respiratory infection
[ ] **C.** Recent fitting for dentures
[ ] **D.** Recurrent migraine headache

72. A patient presents with swelling of their lips, face, and mouth; generalized hives and itching; and tachycardia, hypotension, and generalized weakness. The history reveals that the patient was at the beach when symptoms started. Which of the following is the most likely etiology for these symptoms?
[ ] **A.** A venom-specific reaction
[ ] **B.** Anaphylactic reaction to venom
[ ] **C.** Overexposure to the sun
[ ] **D.** Extracellular fluid dehydration

73. Quantitative studies are important in nursing research and utilize numeric findings for quantification. Which of the following is a true statement regarding quantitative studies?
[ ] **A.** These studies compare the results of one form of treatment against a control group.
[ ] **B.** This type of research gathers insight into a person's motivations and opinions.
[ ] **C.** This particular research study follows subjects with a particular disease process.
[ ] **D.** This study examines relationships and determines cause and effect of variables.

74. A patient presents with a known history of migraine headaches. The emergency nurse prepares for which of the following treatment regimens?
[ ] **A.** IV fluid bolus, antiemetic, and Morphine
[ ] **B.** IV fluid bolus, hydromorphone (Dilaudid), and antiemetic
[ ] **C.** Antihistamine, antiemetic, and IV fluid bolus
[ ] **D.** Antihistamine, nitroglycerin sublingual, and IV fluid bolus

75. Which of the following symptoms are indicative of measles?
[ ] **A.** Pruritic rash to the chest
[ ] **B.** Bluish-gray spots on the buccal mucosa
[ ] **C.** Parotid gland enlargement
[ ] **D.** Petechiae in the folds of the axilla

76. Which of the following is the appropriate therapeutic response in a threatening situation?
[ ] **A.** Aggression
[ ] **B.** Passivity
[ ] **C.** Assertiveness
[ ] **D.** Indifference

77. Zovirax (Acyclovir) is the drug of choice for the treatment of genital herpes lesions. The mechanism of action includes all of the following **EXCEPT**:
[ ] **A.** providing bactericidal functions.
[ ] **B.** relieving local and systemic pain.
[ ] **C.** diminishing the interval of viral shedding.
[ ] **D.** decreasing the formation of new lesions.

78. Which of the following statements is **NOT** true regarding respiratory anatomical and physiologic differences in the pediatric patient?
[ ] **A.** The diaphragm is flatter and is the primary muscle for ventilation.
[ ] **B.** Pediatric alveoli are larger and result in increased surface area for gas exchange.
[ ] **C.** Abdominal muscles play a larger role in respiration.
[ ] **D.** Children have faster and deeper respiratory rates.

79. Which of the following statements made by a patient being discharged with a diagnosis of Raynaud's phenomenon would indicate that the discharge instructions were understood?
[ ] **A.** "I will wear gloves to keep warm and work hard on stopping smoking."
[ ] **B.** "I will keep my arm elevated on a pillow and apply ice to my hand."
[ ] **C.** "I have an elastic bandage at home that I can wear when I am on the computer."
[ ] **D.** "I will drink plenty of fluids and take aspirin for the pain."

80. Which of the following interventions would **NOT** indicate to the emergency nurse that obstructive shock symptoms have been mitigated?
[ ] **A.** Successful pericardiocentesis performed
[ ] **B.** A 36-week gestation patient turned to left side
[ ] **C.** 14-G cathlon inserted into second intercostal space
[ ] **D.** Bilateral normal saline boluses infusing

81. Which of the following is the treatment of choice for a patient with a pneumothorax?
[ ] **A.** Chest tube insertion
[ ] **B.** Emergency thoracotomy
[ ] **C.** Needle thoracostomy
[ ] **D.** Emergent intubation

82. The emergency nurse is discharging a patient with a probable diagnosis of Alzheimer's versus dementia. Which of the following statements made by the family indicates an understanding of the explanations provided to them?
[ ] **A.** "We understand that hallucinations and delusions are not as common as with other forms of dementia."
[ ] **B.** "We know that he is losing his mental abilities and this will interfere with his daily activities and social interactions."
[ ] **C.** "We are glad to know that there are medications out there that we will discuss with his doctor that will cure him."
[ ] **D.** "We understand that this disease called Alzheimer's is not very common for dementia patients."

83. A patient with chronic renal failure requires multiple units of packed red blood cells. The emergency nurse should monitor the patient for:
[ ] **A.** hypocalcemia.
[ ] **B.** hypokalemia.
[ ] **C.** increased white blood cell count.
[ ] **D.** decreased clotting time.

84. A patient presents with postauricular pain, drooling, inability to blink one eye, and unilateral facial paralysis. Which of the following will be used to confirm the diagnosis?
[ ] **A.** Facial radiograph
[ ] **B.** Electromyography (EMG)
[ ] **C.** Computed tomography (CT)
[ ] **D.** Clinical presentation

85. A patient presents to triage after splashing drain cleaner in the eyes. The priority intervention for the emergency nurse is to:
[ ] **A.** assess visual acuity.
[ ] **B.** patch the affected eye(s).
[ ] **C.** initiate eye flushing.
[ ] **D.** initiate ophthalmology consult.

86. A patient with an open fracture of the elbow is now experiencing a fever of 101.6° F (38.7° C) and has yellowish drainage from the site. Which of the following organisms would be expected for this type of infectious process?
[ ] **A.** *Staphylococcus aureus*
[ ] **B.** *Escherichia coli*
[ ] **C.** *Streptococcus agalactiae*
[ ] **D.** *Serratia marcescens*

87. Which of the following is the most appropriate treatment for a stable patient with an open pneumothorax?
[ ] **A.** Immediate chest tube insertion
[ ] **B.** Emergency thoracotomy
[ ] **C.** Autotransfusion
[ ] **D.** Intravenous dextrose 5% in water

88. A patient is pacing and agitated with rapid speech and is becoming belligerent. Which of the following should be the first priority?
[ ] **A.** Provide immediate safety for the patient
[ ] **B.** Offer the patient a less stimulated area to calm down
[ ] **C.** Change the subject by offering the patient food
[ ] **D.** Assist the staff in caring for the other patients' safety

89. A dopamine (Intropin) infusion has been ordered for a patient in cardiogenic shock. Which of the following is **NOT** a precaution for the use of this medication?
[ ] **A.** Close observations for the development of tachydysrhythmias
[ ] **B.** Using a patent central line for drug administration
[ ] **C.** Regular measurements to check for QRS-complex prolongation
[ ] **D.** Frequent monitoring of vital signs and urine output

90. Which of the following head injuries results in a collection of blood between the skull and the dura mater?
[ ] **A.** Subdural hematoma
[ ] **B.** Subarachnoid hemorrhage
[ ] **C.** Epidural hematoma
[ ] **D.** Contusion

91. A store clerk was stocking cleaning supplies when the box cutter sliced open several bottles of the cleaner. The fluid splashed over the clerk's hands, arms, and legs. The cleaner contains hydrofluoric acid. Which of the following orders would the emergency nurse expect to be prescribed for this patient?
[ ] **A.** Flush area with a prepared solution of calcium gluconate.
[ ] **B.** Irrigate area with 1 liter warmed saline and report pH.
[ ] **C.** Wash area with mixture of sodium bicarbonate and ringer's lactate.
[ ] **D.** Apply thin layer of water-based ointment (bacitracin) to the area.

92. A patient is brought to the emergency department after a suspected overdose. The patient has altered perceptions of reality, shallow respirations, dysarthria, and ataxia. The emergency nurse suspects which of the following to be the causative substance?
[ ] A. Phencyclidine (PCP)
[ ] B. Cannabis (marijuana)
[ ] C. Gamma-hydroxybutyrate (GHB)
[ ] D. Lysergic acid diethylamide (LSD)

93. A patient with scrotal pain that has been present for 2 days is admitted to the emergency department. Which of the following signs would indicate a diagnosis of epididymitis rather than testicular torsion?
[ ] A. Hypoperfusion on testicular scan
[ ] B. Leukopenia on complete blood count
[ ] C. Bacteriuria in urinalysis
[ ] D. Elevated creatinine level

94. A patient's laboratory results indicate a sodium value of 106 mEq/mL. Which of the following would be the primary complication for the emergency nurse to anticipate?
[ ] A. Tetany
[ ] B. Seizure activity
[ ] C. Decreased urinary output
[ ] D. Profound bradycardia

95. Which of the following heart rates indicate the point at which chest compressions should be initiated in the newborn?
[ ] A. 60 beats/minute
[ ] B. 80 beats/minute
[ ] C. 100 beats/minute
[ ] D. 110 beats/minute

96. Which of the following is an intrarenal cause of acute kidney injury (AKI)?
[ ] A. Episode of hypovolemia
[ ] B. Development of neurogenic bladder
[ ] C. Onset of renal calculi
[ ] D. Nonsteroidal anti-inflammatory drugs (NSAIDs)

97. A patient presents with hemiplegia that started 1 hour before arrival. A computed tomography (CT) scan of the head is negative and the physician has ordered administration of tissue plasminogen activator (TPA/Activase). The emergency nurse knows that which of the following is the maximum dose of TPA?
[ ] A. 80 mg
[ ] B. 90 mg
[ ] C. 120 mg
[ ] D. No maximum as the dosage is based on weight

98. Which of the following indicates that a family member has understood instructions and education regarding their father's situation with cardiogenic shock?
[ ] A. "I understand that my father needs to get to the cath laboratory immediately."
[ ] B. "I was told that it is good that his blood pressure is so low."
[ ] C. "We should still be able to go on our planned cruise in 10 days."
[ ] D. "I heard that dad had a problem with too much oxygen getting to his cells?"

99. Urine alkalization is most likely to be considered in patients who overdose on which of the following types of medications?
[ ] A. Sulfonylureas
[ ] B. Cephalosporins
[ ] C. Calcium channel blockers
[ ] D. Phosphodiesterase inhibitors

100. Treatment for a patient with a rib fracture includes which of the following?
[ ] A. Placing the patient in the supine position
[ ] B. Taping the chest circumferentially to relieve pain
[ ] C. Controlling pain to assist with breathing
[ ] D. Forcing fluids to prevent dehydration

101. A patient presents to the triage desk and states, "This is the worst headache of my life." The patient is well known by the staff with a past history of migraine headaches and hypertension. He is vomiting on arrival. He requests to have the lights off in his room, and on assessment, the emergency nurse notes that his speech is abnormal. The patient is rubbing the back of his neck and he states that it "just hurts so much when I move my head down." All of the following make this person high risk for a catastrophic event **EXCEPT**:
[ ] A. intensity of the headache.
[ ] B. pain to the posterior neck area.
[ ] C. history of migraine headaches.
[ ] D. speech abnormalities.

102. A patient with an open pneumothorax is admitted to the emergency department. A nonporous dressing was placed in the field. Which of the following findings suggests worsening of this patient's condition?
[ ] A. Respiratory rate of 24 breaths/minute
[ ] B. Decreased breath sounds on the affected side
[ ] C. Tracheal shift with jugular vein distension (JVD)
[ ] D. Blood pressure of 120/80 mm Hg

103. Femoral head necrosis is a complication of hip dislocation. To prevent this complication, reduction of the dislocation should occur within which of the following hours?
[ ] **A.** 6
[ ] **B.** 8
[ ] **C.** 10
[ ] **D.** 12

104. Which of the following medications is most commonly used to treat anticholinergic delirium?
[ ] **A.** Naloxone (Narcan)
[ ] **B.** Lithium
[ ] **C.** Physostigmine (Antilirium)
[ ] **D.** Atropine

105. A 5-week-old is brought in by his parents for concern of fever and being inconsolable at home. On assessment, the emergency nurse notes that the infant is irritable, exhibits a high-pitched cry, has areas of purpura on his extremities, and has a rectal temperature of 102° F (38.9° C). Which of the following are these signs and symptoms most consistent with?
[ ] **A.** Henoch–Schönlein purpura
[ ] **B.** Meningococcemia
[ ] **C.** Idiopathic thrombocytopenic purpura
[ ] **D.** Kawasaki disease

106. A patient is being treated for an intentional overdose of metformin (Glucophage). Which of the following would indicate that treatment has been successfully completed?
[ ] **A.** Venous pH of 7.29
[ ] **B.** Blood glucose of 60 mg/dL
[ ] **C.** Lactate level of 1.1 mmol/L
[ ] **D.** Urine output of 3.5 mL/kg/hour

107. A little league player collapses after a light pole he was standing next to was hit by lightning. Which of the following actions would be an appropriate measure after maintaining scene safety?
[ ] **A.** Check immediately for long-bone fractures that need immobilization
[ ] **B.** Worry about cervical spine injury when attempting to resuscitate
[ ] **C.** Immediately tilt the head back opening the airway to ventilate
[ ] **D.** Begin chest compressions assuming ventricular fibrillation is present

108. A patient in the triage area is yelling and becoming increasingly agitated; he throws his bottle of water on the floor. The family states this agitated and aggressive behavior is new over the past few hours. Which of the following is the best response for the triage nurse at this time?
[ ] **A.** Approach the patient and directly confront him to control him through authority.
[ ] **B.** Inform the patient that this is not acceptable behavior in the emergency department.
[ ] **C.** Reassure the patient that the nurse is here to help him.
[ ] **D.** Shout for security to call the police immediately.

109. When evaluating parameters which of the following would have the most negative impact on a patient with a closed head injury?
[ ] **A.** Blood pressure—90/42 mm Hg
[ ] **B.** Cerebral perfusion pressure—85 mm Hg
[ ] **C.** Urine output—48 mL in 1 hour
[ ] **D.** Serum osmolality—280 mOsm

110. A patient presents with acute onset of right upper quadrant pain and severe nausea after eating at a local fast-food restaurant. The patient also has pain to the right subclavicular area. The pain rating is 8 out of 10. Which of the following medications would the emergency nurse anticipate to **NOT** be prescribed for this patient?
[ ] **A.** Hydromorphone (Dilaudid)
[ ] **B.** Morphine sulfate
[ ] **C.** Fentanyl (Sublimaze)
[ ] **D.** Meperidine (Demerol)

111. Hemophilia A is characterized by a genetic deficiency of which clotting factor?
[ ] **A.** Factor IX
[ ] **B.** Factor VIII
[ ] **C.** Factor XI
[ ] **D.** Factor IV

112. A patient presents to the emergency department complaining of pain in her jaw. The emergency nurse notes facial drooping to the corner of the mouth on the left side. Which of the following cranial nerves (CNs) is affected?
[ ] **A.** Cranial nerve VI (Abducens)
[ ] **B.** Cranial nerve VIII (Acoustic)
[ ] **C.** Cranial nerve V (Ttrigeminal)
[ ] **D.** Cranial nerve III (Oculomotor)

113. Benzodiazepines such as lorazepam (Ativan) are no longer considered a first-line treatment for insomnia, agitation, and delirium in older adults. According to guidelines published in 2013, "elderly patients are significantly more sensitive to the sedative effects of benzodiazepines." Emergency nurses know that benzodiazepines can cause which of the following?

[ ] A. Respiratory depression
[ ] B. Hypoxemia
[ ] C. Delirium
[ ] D. Alcohol withdrawal

114. A 75-year-old patient arrives with symptoms of dizziness, near syncope, shortness of breath, and chest pain. There is a history of an Implantable Electronic Device. The emergency nurse should prepare for immediate:

[ ] A. Stat 12-lead electrocardiogram.
[ ] B. magnet application.
[ ] C. interrogation of the pacemaker.
[ ] D. cardiology consult.

115. Ninety percent of acute aortic dissections occur in the ascending aorta. The emergency nurse knows that the most important predisposing risk factor for this process is which of the following?

[ ] A. Trauma
[ ] B. Cardiac surgery
[ ] C. Hypertension
[ ] D. Cocaine use

116. A patient with a ventriculostomy in place is noted to have an increasing intracranial pressure. Which of the following corrections would help remedy this situation?

[ ] A. Turn the head to the right
[ ] B. Place the patient supine
[ ] C. Remove C-Collar on neck
[ ] D. Increase activity in the room

117. Which of the following observations would indicate that a depressed patient is becoming suicidal?

[ ] A. The patient slams the phone after speaking to a loved one.
[ ] B. The patient refuses to eat a turkey sandwich.
[ ] C. The patient spits on the security officer.
[ ] D. The patient gives the nurse her favorite watch.

118. The PICO acronym is often used in quantitative studies to help researchers ask focused clinical questions. The "P" in PICO refers to the "Population" or "Problem" being considered. What do the "I" and "C" represent?

[ ] A. Intervention and Control group
[ ] B. Intervention and Comparison
[ ] C. Implementation and Considerations
[ ] D. Implementation and Consultation

119. An adult patient with significant deep partial-thickness burns is being stabilized and the calculated amount of warmed fluid has been administered. Which of the following is the best indicator that the correct amount of fluid has been administered?

[ ] A. The respiratory rate is 32 breaths/minute.
[ ] B. The mean arterial pressure is 45 mm Hg.
[ ] C. The urine output is 58 mL/hour.
[ ] D. The pulse rate is 136 beats/minute.

120. Alzheimer's disease is characterized by profound impairment of cognitive functions. Which of the following is the cause of this disorder?

[ ] A. Destruction of motor cells in the pyramidal tracts
[ ] B. Metabolic disorder involving the adrenal glands
[ ] C. Cerebral atrophy and cellular degeneration
[ ] D. Degeneration of the basal ganglia

121. Which of the following would **NOT** be an appropriate treatment regimen for a patient with a shoulder dislocation?

[ ] A. Application of ice
[ ] B. Immobilization
[ ] C. Neurovascular assessment
[ ] D. Application of traction splint

122. A construction worker fell from the 10th floor at work. He arrives restless with severe chest discomfort, hypotension, tachycardia, tachypnea, chest wall ecchymosis, and paraplegia. The emergency nurse anticipates which of the following plans for appropriate tests and subsequent intervention?

[ ] A. Transesophageal echo, computed tomography (CT) scan, and surgery
[ ] B. Echocardiography, pericardiocentesis, or pericardial window
[ ] C. Chest radiograph, chest tube insertion, and closed-chest drainage system
[ ] D. Chest radiograph, cover open wound, and needle thoracentesis

123. Which of the following interventions will decrease elevated intracranial pressure (ICP)?
[ ] **A.** Frequent suctioning of the airway
[ ] **B.** Administering morphine for pain
[ ] **C.** Maintaining the patient in trendelenburg position
[ ] **D.** Administering mannitol (Osmitrol)

124. Cardiac tamponade occurs when blood or fluid accumulates in the pericardial sac. The emergency nurse would anticipate assisting with which of the following interventions?
[ ] **A.** Needle thoracentesis
[ ] **B.** Chest tube insertion
[ ] **C.** Pericardiocentesis
[ ] **D.** Thoracotomy

125. An elderly patient has an elevated temperature, restlessness, confusion, and weakness after a radioactive iodine treatment. The physician suspects thyroid storm. Which treatment option should the emergency nurse anticipate?
[ ] **A.** Acetylsalicylic acid (Aspirin)
[ ] **B.** Propranolol (Inderal)
[ ] **C.** Atropine sulfate
[ ] **D.** Sodium bicarbonate

126. A patient presents with sudden onset of deep unilateral eye pain, blurry vision, halos around lights, and nausea. The emergency nurse recognizes this ocular emergency as:
[ ] **A.** ultraviolet keratitis.
[ ] **B.** closed-angle glaucoma.
[ ] **C.** central retinal artery occlusion.
[ ] **D.** retinal detachment.

127. Nursing care of a patient with disseminated intravascular coagulopathy (DIC) includes all of the following **EXCEPT**:
[ ] **A.** administration of medication via intramuscular route.
[ ] **B.** pressure dressings to active bleeding sites.
[ ] **C.** administration of intravenous heparin.
[ ] **D.** limiting the number of venipunctures.

128. Child Protective Services has decided to remove a child from the mother's care pending further investigation of a sexual assault on the child. The mother becomes upset and is afraid the child's father will beat her. The nurse can refer the mother to several social service agencies. Which one of the following agencies would be most appropriate in this situation?
[ ] **A.** Local women's shelter
[ ] **B.** The welfare bureau
[ ] **C.** A homeless shelter
[ ] **D.** A soup kitchen

129. Immunotherapy for anaphylaxis can be given to people with allergies to which of the following agents?
[ ] **A.** Peanuts
[ ] **B.** Insect stings
[ ] **C.** Milk
[ ] **D.** Latex

130. A patient has a suspected zygomatic fracture. The emergency nurse prepares the patient for which of the following diagnostic tests that will confirm this diagnosis?
[ ] **A.** Facial ultrasound
[ ] **B.** Lateral facial radiograph
[ ] **C.** Water's view radiograph
[ ] **D.** Facial computed tomography (CT)

131. Several victims have arrived from a chemical plant after a bomb exploded. The victims are covered with a strong-smelling liquid and have labored respirations. Which of the following actions should the emergency nurse responding take first?
[ ] **A.** Prioritize patients based on the degree of respiratory distress
[ ] **B.** Assess identity of chemicals the victims were exposed to
[ ] **C.** Don personal protective garments
[ ] **D.** Remove the victims' clothing

132. Which of the following is the definitive therapy for a patient with a massive hemothorax?
[ ] **A.** Emergency thoracotomy
[ ] **B.** Chest tube insertion
[ ] **C.** Fluid resuscitation
[ ] **D.** Supplemental oxygenation

133. A patient arrives with a persistent narrow, regular tachyarrhythmia causing hypotension, altered mental status, signs of shock, and ischemic chest discomfort. Which of the following is the recommended intervention?
[ ] **A.** Synchronized cardioversion starting at 50 to 100 J
[ ] **B.** Vagal maneuvers, adenosine, beta-blocker, or calcium channel blocker
[ ] **C.** Adenosine 6 mg rapid intravenous push, followed with a 20-mL normal saline flush
[ ] **D.** Amiodarone 150 mg over 10 minutes, repeat as needed

134. Allergic stings are most commonly caused by which of the following?
[ ] **A.** Hornets
[ ] **B.** Scabies
[ ] **C.** Bumble bees
[ ] **D.** Bed bugs

135. When the emergency nurse approaches the patient to draw blood and the patient rolls up his sleeve and holds out his arm, this type of consent would be considered:

[ ] **A.** express consent.

[ ] **B.** implied consent.

[ ] **C.** involuntary consent.

[ ] **D.** informed consent.

136. Which of the following is a true statement regarding synchronized shocks?

[ ] **A.** Electrical shock will be delivered as soon as the operator pushes the shock button.

[ ] **B.** Caution is needed because these shocks use higher energy levels.

[ ] **C.** Used for an unstable patient when polymorphic ventricular fibrillation is present

[ ] **D.** The actual shock avoids delivery during cardiac repolarization.

137. Which of the following pharmacologic therapies should the emergency nurse anticipate administering to a patient with thyroid storm?

[ ] **A.** Aspirin

[ ] **B.** Propylthiouracil (PTU)

[ ] **C.** Levothyroxine (Synthroid)

[ ] **D.** Morphine sulfate

138. Which of the following is the most appropriate intervention for a patient with chronic obstructive pulmonary disease (COPD)?

[ ] **A.** Administer 100% oxygen via non-rebreather mask.

[ ] **B.** Obtain and monitor arterial blood gas (ABG) levels.

[ ] **C.** Restrict fluids to only at meal times.

[ ] **D.** Place the patient in a supine position.

139. The following four patients arrive at triage at the same time. Which patient should be taken to a treatment room first?

[ ] **A.** A 7-year-old with a history of asthma with wheezing before arrival who now has increased respiratory rate but diminished wheezing.

[ ] **B.** A 33-year-old with sickle cell anemia complaining of joint pain and lower back pain after a recent bacterial illness.

[ ] **C.** A 12-year-old with a 1″ (2.5 cm) laceration on his left foot from stepping on a piece of glass with bleeding controlled.

[ ] **D.** A 16-year-old soccer player with a tibia–fibula deformity who has pedal and posterior tibialis pulses and capillary refill of 2 seconds.

140. Which of the following disease processes would possibly place the patient at risk for a thermal burn to the globe?

[ ] **A.** Bell's palsy

[ ] **B.** Hyphema

[ ] **C.** Conjunctivitis

[ ] **D.** Ludwig's angina

141. Interventions for a post-organ transplant patient coming to the emergency department complaining of a fever include all of the following **EXCEPT**:

[ ] **A.** identification of the source of infection.

[ ] **B.** placing the patient in a private room.

[ ] **C.** restricting fluids and food.

[ ] **D.** initiating antibiotic therapy quickly.

142. While examining a patient who sustained a direct blow to the eye, the emergency nurse notes a tear-drop-shaped pupil. The nurse prepares interventions for which of the following?

[ ] **A.** Ruptured globe

[ ] **B.** Glaucoma

[ ] **C.** Hyphema

[ ] **D.** Orbital fracture

143. A research study involves asking a group of nurses questions regarding perception of the value of an ED-specific preceptor program versus a hospital-based preceptor program. This type of research is considered to be:

[ ] **A.** qualitative.

[ ] **B.** quantitative.

[ ] **C.** systematic.

[ ] **D.** retrospective.

144. Which of the following responses from a new emergency nurse on an orientation test would indicate knowledge of the neurologic problem related to difficulty in transforming sound into patterns of understandable speech?

[ ] **A.** Receptive aphasia

[ ] **B.** Dysphagia

[ ] **C.** Expressive aphasia

[ ] **D.** Apraxia

145. Which of the following objects, if lodged in a child's nose, must be removed emergently?

[ ] **A.** Plastic toy part

[ ] **B.** Small disc battery

[ ] **C.** Rubber pencil eraser

[ ] **D.** Cashew nut

146. Which of the following eye complaints stated by a patient does the triage nurse recognize as emergent?

[ ] **A.** Facial numbness and inability to look upward

[ ] **B.** Bloody appearance to the sclera

[ ] **C.** Perception of five to six floaters in the eye

[ ] **D.** Pain on the surface of the eye and excessive tearing

147. Appropriate discharge instructions for the patient diagnosed with Bell's palsy include which of the following?

[ ] **A.** Lubricant eye drops at night

[ ] **B.** Use of ophthalmic antibiotics

[ ] **C.** Prescription for antiepileptic drugs

[ ] **D.** Bed rest until symptoms resolve

148. Which of the following actions by the emergency nurse should be questioned regarding treatment for acute angle-closure glaucoma?

[ ] **A.** The nurse requests an order for an antiemetic.

[ ] **B.** A stat dose of a topical beta-blocker is administered.

[ ] **C.** Miotic eye drops such as pilocarpine are administered immediately upon arrival, before other medication.

[ ] **D.** Stat intravenous access is obtained in preparation for administration of acetazolamide (Diamox).

149. A patient is being discharged after treatment for epistaxis. Which of the following statements indicates the patient understood the instructions?

[ ] **A.** "I will take ibuprofen for pain from the nasal packing."

[ ] **B.** "I will avoid taking hot showers when possible."

[ ] **C.** "I will instill phenylephrine nose drops for 10 days."

[ ] **D.** "I will blow my nose to clear out scabs that form."

150. The emergency nurse knows that the patient understood discharge instructions for an uncomplicated orbital fracture when they state:

[ ] **A.** "The bruising around my eye should go away in a day or so."

[ ] **B.** "Antibiotics will be prescribed so I don't get an infection."

[ ] **C.** "I will use warm packs for the pain."

[ ] **D.** "I will try to avoid blowing my nose."

Answer Sheet

	A B C D		A B C D		A B C D		A B C D
1.	○ ○ ○ ○	26.	○ ○ ○ ○	51.	○ ○ ○ ○	76.	○ ○ ○ ○
2.	○ ○ ○ ○	27.	○ ○ ○ ○	52.	○ ○ ○ ○	77.	○ ○ ○ ○
3.	○ ○ ○ ○	28.	○ ○ ○ ○	53.	○ ○ ○ ○	78.	○ ○ ○ ○
4.	○ ○ ○ ○	29.	○ ○ ○ ○	54.	○ ○ ○ ○	79.	○ ○ ○ ○
5.	○ ○ ○ ○	30.	○ ○ ○ ○	55.	○ ○ ○ ○	80.	○ ○ ○ ○
6.	○ ○ ○ ○	31.	○ ○ ○ ○	56.	○ ○ ○ ○	81.	○ ○ ○ ○
7.	○ ○ ○ ○	32.	○ ○ ○ ○	57.	○ ○ ○ ○	82.	○ ○ ○ ○
8.	○ ○ ○ ○	33.	○ ○ ○ ○	58.	○ ○ ○ ○	83.	○ ○ ○ ○
9.	○ ○ ○ ○	34.	○ ○ ○ ○	59.	○ ○ ○ ○	84.	○ ○ ○ ○
10.	○ ○ ○ ○	35.	○ ○ ○ ○	60.	○ ○ ○ ○	85.	○ ○ ○ ○
11.	○ ○ ○ ○	36.	○ ○ ○ ○	61.	○ ○ ○ ○	86.	○ ○ ○ ○
12.	○ ○ ○ ○	37.	○ ○ ○ ○	62.	○ ○ ○ ○	87.	○ ○ ○ ○
13.	○ ○ ○ ○	38.	○ ○ ○ ○	63.	○ ○ ○ ○	88.	○ ○ ○ ○
14.	○ ○ ○ ○	39.	○ ○ ○ ○	64.	○ ○ ○ ○	89.	○ ○ ○ ○
15.	○ ○ ○ ○	40.	○ ○ ○ ○	65.	○ ○ ○ ○	90.	○ ○ ○ ○
16.	○ ○ ○ ○	41.	○ ○ ○ ○	66.	○ ○ ○ ○	91.	○ ○ ○ ○
17.	○ ○ ○ ○	42.	○ ○ ○ ○	67.	○ ○ ○ ○	92.	○ ○ ○ ○
18.	○ ○ ○ ○	43.	○ ○ ○ ○	68.	○ ○ ○ ○	93.	○ ○ ○ ○
19.	○ ○ ○ ○	44.	○ ○ ○ ○	69.	○ ○ ○ ○	94.	○ ○ ○ ○
20.	○ ○ ○ ○	45.	○ ○ ○ ○	70.	○ ○ ○ ○	95.	○ ○ ○ ○
21.	○ ○ ○ ○	46.	○ ○ ○ ○	71.	○ ○ ○ ○	96.	○ ○ ○ ○
22.	○ ○ ○ ○	47.	○ ○ ○ ○	72.	○ ○ ○ ○	97.	○ ○ ○ ○
23.	○ ○ ○ ○	48.	○ ○ ○ ○	73.	○ ○ ○ ○	98.	○ ○ ○ ○
24.	○ ○ ○ ○	49.	○ ○ ○ ○	74.	○ ○ ○ ○	99.	○ ○ ○ ○
25.	○ ○ ○ ○	50.	○ ○ ○ ○	75.	○ ○ ○ ○	100.	○ ○ ○ ○

	A	B	C	D		A	B	C	D
101.	○	○	○	○	126.	○	○	○	○
102.	○	○	○	○	127.	○	○	○	○
103.	○	○	○	○	128.	○	○	○	○
104.	○	○	○	○	129.	○	○	○	○
105.	○	○	○	○	130.	○	○	○	○
106.	○	○	○	○	131.	○	○	○	○
107.	○	○	○	○	132.	○	○	○	○
108.	○	○	○	○	133.	○	○	○	○
109.	○	○	○	○	134.	○	○	○	○
110.	○	○	○	○	135.	○	○	○	○
111.	○	○	○	○	136.	○	○	○	○
112.	○	○	○	○	137.	○	○	○	○
113.	○	○	○	○	138.	○	○	○	○
114.	○	○	○	○	139.	○	○	○	○
115.	○	○	○	○	140.	○	○	○	○
116.	○	○	○	○	141.	○	○	○	○
117.	○	○	○	○	142.	○	○	○	○
118.	○	○	○	○	143.	○	○	○	○
119.	○	○	○	○	144.	○	○	○	○
120.	○	○	○	○	145.	○	○	○	○
121.	○	○	○	○	146.	○	○	○	○
122.	○	○	○	○	147.	○	○	○	○
123.	○	○	○	○	148.	○	○	○	○
124.	○	○	○	○	149.	○	○	○	○
125.	○	○	○	○	150.	○	○	○	○

Answers and Rationales

1. Answer: B

Nursing Process: Assessment/Communicable

Rationale: **Human Immunodeficiency Virus (HIV) positive patients with a fever are at high risk for deterioration and should be prioritized to an immediate open bed. The patient requires a workup to determine the source of fever and should be protected from other patients who may have a communicable infectious condition.** This patient is not unresponsive, apneic, or in need of any life-saving interventions upon arrival, thus does not meet criteria for a level 1 acuity. Level 3 patients require two or more resources according to the Emergency Severity Index (ESI) algorithm, but his immunocompromised condition escalates his acuity to level 2. Level 4 patients require only one resource and this patient will clearly need multiple resources to identify the source of, and treat, the fever. In a five-level system, level 5 requires no resources.

2. Answer: D

Nursing Process: Intervention/Medical

Rationale: **Fluid deficit can exceed 10 liters in Hyperglycemic Hyperosmolar Syndrome (HHS). Rapid rehydration with 0.9 normal saline is required to prevent circulatory collapse.** Solutions containing dextrose are not indicated in the initial treatment of HHS but may be considered once serum glucose reaches 250 to 300 mg/dL. Serum potassium levels are generally within normal limits initially but should be monitored as the serum glucose levels decrease. Supplemental potassium can be added as needed.

3. Answer: A

Nursing Process: Assessment/GU/GYN/OB

Rationale: **Ectopic pregnancy (pregnancy occurring outside of the uterus) usually manifests before 12 weeks' gestation, produces pelvic pain, and shock if ruptured. It is considered a true emergency and is a major cause of maternal death.** An ovarian cyst is a fluid-filled sac in the ovary that may be painful and is usually self-limiting, but may develop hypovolemia when it ruptures. Ovarian torsion occurs when the ovary twists itself around the stalk that contains the blood vessels feeding the ovary and the fallopian tube. Pain is due to ischemia and requires surgical intervention. Dysmenorrhea is defined as painful menstruation in the absence of any other pelvic condition.

4. Answer: D

Nursing Process: Assessment/Cardiovascular

Rationale: **The symptoms presented are typical of acute pulmonary edema related to heart failure.** Pericardial tamponade has muffled heart sounds, distended neck veins, and hypotension (Beck's triad). Breath sounds would be decreased on the affected side in a pneumothorax. Pulmonary embolus causes nonspecific signs, but dyspnea, tachypnea, syncope, and cyanosis are most common.

5. Answer: A

Nursing Process: Assessment/Respiratory

Rationale: **Arterial blood gases (ABGs) provide a specific value for the PaO_2—a much more reliable number to ascertain oxygenation status.** An oxygen saturation monitor does not differentiate among oxygen, carbon monoxide, or any other toxic substance bound to the hemoglobin. Mixed venous blood gases do not yield as useful information as an ABG. A complete blood count (CBC) will provide the hemoglobin value important in oxygen transport; however, the hemoglobin is usually reported in the ABG results.

6. Answer: D

Cognitive Level: Recall/Professional Issues

Rationale: **Appropriate alternatives are to be considered first always before the application of any type of restraints.** The goal is to use the least restrictive restraint possible and only after unsuccessful use of alternatives. Restraint use should not be part of any routine protocol. There are many risks associated with physically restraining an individual, including risk of aspiration/ suffocation and increased psychological trauma and traumatic memories. Another issue with long-term restraint use is the development of deep vein thrombosis/pulmonary embolus.

7. Answer: B

Nursing Process: Assessment/Psychosocial

Rationale: **Severe hypertension can result from monoamine oxidase inhibitors (MAOIs) overdoses, which blocks the metabolism of norepinephrine.** Hypotension, sedation, and severe agitation are not associated with MAOI overdose.

8. Answer: B

Nursing Process: Analysis/Cardiovascular

Rationale: **Commotio cordis causes sudden cardiac death from blunt trauma to the left anterior chest wall, usually from a thrown or batted ball and occurs predominantly in young, male athletes.** The cause of death is ventricular fibrillation due to the blow to the chest ocurring during a critical point in the cardiac cycle. The long QT syndrome (LQTS) is a disorder of myocardial repolarization characterized by a prolonged QT interval on the electrocardiogram and results from many things including medications, electrolyte disorders, and congenital defects. The point of maximal impulse (PMI) is located in the fifth intercostal space at the midclavicular line. PMI is where the cardiac impulse can be best palpated. The PMI may be displaced with increased right ventricular pressure (large right pleural effusion, right tension pneumothorax) and volume overload (heart failure). Kawasaki disease affects children younger than 5 years with vasculitis that affects medium and small arteries, notably the coronary arteries. It is self-limiting and resolves within 1 to 2 months, although the mortality rate is 1% to 2%.

9. Answer: D

Nursing Process: Analysis/Respiratory

Rationale: **A pneumothorax would not cause fluid accumulation in the pleural space.** Trauma may cause rib fractures or thoracic compression, which can rupture alveoli. Aspiration may contribute to a collection of nonendogenous fluids in the alveoli. Sudden movement to a higher altitude may lead to high-altitude pulmonary edema (HAPE).

10. Answer: A

Nursing Process: Intervention/Respiratory

Rationale: **The priority intervention is to maintain airway patency, which is accomplished by immediate suctioning.** Chest tube insertion and surgical intervention will be necessary after the patient is stabilized. If the patient is intubated, the end of the endotracheal tube must be positioned distal to the injury. It is also advisable to monitor for possible pneumothorax.

11. Answer: C

Nursing Process: Intervention/Cardiovascular

Rationale: **Maintaining a constant target temperature between 32° C to 36° C (89.6° F to 96.8° F) for 24 hours has been demonstrated to improve neurologic recovery.** Ventilation should be titrated to a $PETCO_2$ of 35 to 45 mm Hg or a $PaCO_2$ of 40 to 45 mm Hg. Hypotension (blood pressure of 90 mm Hg or less) should be treated with fluid bolus or vasopressor infusion. Oxygen delivery should be titrated to the lowest FiO_2 required to achieve an arterial oxygen saturation of 94% to 99% to avoid potential oxygen toxicity.

12. Answer: A

Nursing Process: Assessment/Gastrointestinal

Rationale: **Bowel obstructions that are in the early stages or are partial obstructions can have hyperactive bowel sounds.** These sounds are usually high pitched. In the later stages and if there is a complete obstruction, the bowel sounds will be absent. In the early phases, the bowel is attempting to overcome the obstruction. A large bowel obstruction will present with a great deal of abdominal swelling, whereas a small bowel obstruction will carry a smaller amount of swelling. Fecal odor to the emesis is a good clue for a bowel obstruction, but it is not always present. Small bowel obstructions usually have a much greater amount of vomiting.

13. Answer: D

Nursing Process: Analysis/GU/GYN/OB

Rationale: **It is important to know if the patient was pregnant when the attack occurred. If she is not pregnant, the appropriate "morning after" medication (ethinyl estradiol and norgestrel) can be given within 72 hours.** If the patient chooses to use plan B (morning after pill), they will need a prescription for an antiemetic as the medication can cause nausea. Other treatments for the patient would include prophylactic antibiotic therapy. Cultures and tests for syphilis will not be resulted for several days. A complete blood count does not provide vital information unless the patient is injured and hypovolemia is suspected. Rhogam will provide information regarding the Rh of the mother. This test is not indicated in this situation.

14. Answer: C

Nursing Process: Assessment/Medical

Rationale: **Patients in thyroid storm are heat-intolerant and sweat excessively, which along with vomiting and fever can exacerbate volume loss leading to hypovolemic shock.** Patients in thyroid storm typically have a core body temperature of 101.3° F (38.5° C) due to the body's increased metabolic rate. Hyperpyrexia (core temperature more than 104° F [40° C]) can occur. Mental status changes, seizures, and coma are commonly seen in this condition. Tachycardia is a classic sign of thyroid storm.

15. Answer: D

Nursing Process: Evaluation/Medical

Rationale: **Dehydration can precipitate a vaso-occlusive crisis in the capillary circulation. Microvascular occlusion leads to tissue ischemia and severe pain. Patients should ensure they have an adequate intake of fluids every day.** Infection is a precipitant of sickle cell crisis and patients should seek immediate medical attention at the first signs of malaise. Exposure to cold temperatures results in vasoconstriction of blood vessels in the skin, hands, feet, nose, and ears. This response is greatly exaggerated in the presence of sickle cell disease. Stressful events trigger the release of vasoactive hormones, which narrow blood vessels. This can lead to a vaso-occlusive crisis. Patients with sickle cell disease need strong coping mechanisms and communication skills to address stress.

16. Answer: D

Nursing Process: Assessment/Psychosocial

Rationale: **Dehydration and nutritional abnormalities are present in 47% of admissions, followed by electrolyte imbalances for 34%, cardiac dysrhythmias in 24%, and 4% presenting with renal or hepatic failure.** Visual impairment is not a complication.

17. Answer: C

Nursing Process: Intervention/GU/GYN/OB

Rationale: **The left lateral recumbent position avoids compression of the inferior vena cava; compressing the vessel may result in decreased uterine blood flow, fetal hypoxia, and maternal hypotension.** Trendelenburg or supine position would compress this vessel. If a pregnant patient must lie flat on a backboard for spinal evaluation, a wedge may be placed under the backboard to tilt it, or manual manipulation of the uterus may also be done by a provider. The knee-chest position is used to avoid compressing the umbilical cord when it is prolapsed.

18. Answer: B

Nursing Process: Analysis/Psychosocial

Rationale: **The dementia patient may have impaired ability to assess their own pain and communicate their symptoms.** It is incumbent upon the nurse to dedicate adequate attention to objective signs of discomfort such as body posture and vital sign changes. Chronic vascular pathology will not impact emergency care, but attentive monitoring of distal circulation may be a heightened concern due to communication challenges with the patient. If the patient is incompetent to consent to treatment themselves, a surrogate decision maker is indicated. Sedation and/or a bedside sitter may be necessary to ensure patient safety, and adequate pain control will facilitate safe care.

19. Answer: B

Nursing Process: Analysis/Gastrointestinal

Rationale: **The liver is the major organ involved in hepatitis C and in a motor vehicle crash the emergency nurse should be concerned about the patient's ability to clot. The liver is extremely involved in the clotting process as most of the necessary clotting factors are produced here. In these traumatic situations, the clotting cascade may not work appropriately.** The liver is located in the right upper quadrant and the liver also receives a large amount of cardiac output and has the potential to bleed copiously if damaged. Respiratory distress would be a concern, but the lack of ability to clot would take precedence. There were no symptoms of respiratory distress noted in the stem of the question. Hypertensive crisis is not a concern in this scenario. The emergency nurse should be most concerned about hypotension with the strong possibility of hypovolemic shock being present. Pneumonia may occur later but would not be a primary concern in this case.

20. Answer: B

Nursing Process: Assessment/Respiratory

Rationale: **Black-tinged (carbonaceous) sputum from smoke generated in the fire is a hallmark sign of inhalation injury.** Respirations may become increasingly difficult as the injury matures. The mucous membranes of the burn-injured patient are commonly dry. The patient may have rales and rhonchi on auscultation, but the cough is dry and generally nonproductive.

21. Answer: C

Nursing Process: Analysis/Cardiovascular

Rationale: **Cardiac output (CO) is defined as a product of heart rate (HR) and stroke volume (SV) (CO = HR × SV).** Preload is the passive stretching force of the ventricles during diastole; afterload is the resistance of the system that the ventricles must overcome in order to eject blood. Zone 1 and Zone 2 are anatomic landmarks of the neck and serve to identify structures in each zone. (Age in years)/4 + 4 is the formula to estimate pediatric endotracheal tube size.

22. Answer: D

Nursing Process: Analysis/Gastrointestinal

Rationale: **Proton pump inhibitors such as omeprazole (Prilosec) and pantoprazole (Prevacid) decrease the production of acid in the stomach and cause a reduction of irritation of the lining of the stomach.** These also help kill the organism *Helicobacter pylori* when used in combination with antibiotics. Medications such as metoclopramide (Reglan) help to increase lower esophageal sphincter pressure. Ranitidine (Zantac) and famotidine (Pepcid) reduce secretions, and maalox and mylanta lower the acid content that is present in the stomach.

23. Answer: D

Cognitive Level: Application/Professional Issues

Rationale: **The plaintiff must prove that the injuries sustained were real or actual.** The plaintiff must prove that the defendant owed him a specific duty, that the defendant breached this duty, that the plaintiff was harmed physically, mentally, emotionally, or financially, and that the defendant's breach of duty caused this harm. The plaintiff must also prove foreseeability and damages.

24. Answer: B

Nursing Process: Evaluation/Psychosocial

Rationale: **Hyperthermia is a trademark symptom of serotonin syndrome, therefore, normothermia would indicate an improvement in this patient.** Other manifestations include tachycardia, dilated pupils (mydriasis), and dry mucous membranes as well as agitation, hyperreflexia, diaphoresis, and flushed skin.

25. Answer: A

Nursing Process: Intervention/Gastrointestinal

Rationale: **Viruses are not treated with antibiotics.** Treatment for norovirus is supportive care, which includes rehydration through intravenous fluids if necessary, rest which usually includes bed rest for a day or two, and strict handwashing to prevent further contamination.

26. Answer: C

Nursing Process: Evaluation/GU/GYN/OB

Rationale: **Alcohol should not be used while the patient is taking metronidazole (Flagyl). It will cause extreme vomiting, headaches, and flushing.** Patients who are diagnosed with trichomonas must share this information with their sexual partners and they should be treated as well. Patients who are in the first trimester of pregnancy should not take metronidazole (Flagyl). Metronidazole (Flagyl) can potentiate the effects of warfarin (Coumadin), resulting in a prolonged prothrombin time.

27. Answer: B

Nursing Process: Assessment/Cardiovascular

Rationale: **Unstable angina is characterized by the classic signs of continued chest pain despite rest or nitroglycerin and no elevation of troponin.** Stable anginal pain goes away with rest. Non-STEMI is defined as ST depression or T-wave inversion with elevation of cardiac biomarkers. STEMI (ST elevation myocardial infarction) definition requires ST elevation in two or more contiguous leads or new left bundle branch block and troponin elevation beyond the 99th percentile of the upper reference limit.

28. Answer: A

Nursing Process: Assessment/Respiratory

Rationale: **Stridor is located in the upper airway and is a result of partial obstruction of the larynx or trachea.** Crackles, wheezing, and rhonchi are all possible with a patient experiencing an exacerbation of heart failure or pneumonia.

29. Answer: B

Nursing Process: Evaluation/Psychosocial

Rationale: **Extrapyramidal side effects are diminished compared with typical antipsychotics and therefore have increased compliance.** The atypicals also demonstrate benefits in reducing symptoms associated with psychosis such as hostility, violence, and suicidal behavior. This class of drug is relatively more expensive when compared with typical antipsychotic medications.

30. Answer: A

Nursing Process: Evaluation/Gastrointestinal

Rationale: **The pH of gastric contents should be acidic, which would correlate with an acid pH of 1 to 5.5.** Any number above 5.5 must have a radiograph to confirm placement. (Radiograph is the preferred method.)

31. Answer: D

Nursing Process: Assessment/Cardiovascular

Rationale: **ST-segment elevation is strongly suspicious for myocardial injury for ST-elevation myocardial infarction (STEMI).** ST-segment depression and dynamic T-wave inversion are suspicious for ischemia. Nondiagnostic changes in ST segment or T wave are low/intermediate risk for acute coronary syndrome.

32. Answer: C

Nursing Process: Assessment/GU/GYN/OB

Rationale: **A hydatidiform mole or gestational trophoblastic tumor demonstrates an extremely elevated human chorionic gonadotropin level.** Other signs include snowstorm pattern on ultrasound, early preeclampsia, absence of fetal heart tones, bleeding or spotting, and enlarged uterus.

33. Answer: B

Cognitive Level: Application/Professional Issues

Rationale: **If a patient sues a nurse for negligence, the patient must prove that the nurse owed him a specific duty and that the nurse breached this duty.** A breach of duty in this case means that the nurse did not provide care within the accepted standard. A breach is not always willful, as implied in option A. Threatening a patient is assault, more accurately described as a direct invasion of a patient's rights rather than a breach of duty. Confining a patient to a psychiatric unit without a physician's order is false imprisonment, which is another example of direct invasion of a patient's rights.

34. Answer: B

Nursing Process: Assessment/Communicable Diseases

Rationale: **Varicella zoster lesions are fluid-filled vesicles, most commonly affecting the thoracic dermatome. The patient may have flu-like symptoms with or without fever.** A petechial rash of small, pinpoint lesions progressing rapidly to purpura is the characteristic manifestation of meningococcemia. Petechial and purpuric lesions develop from bleeding under the skin and do not blanch on applying pressure. Fever has a sudden onset and rises quickly. Kawasaki disease is a rare childhood illness, which presents with a fever and rash of poorly defined spots of various sizes, often bright red that blanch when pressure is applied. The rash of Lyme disease begins at the site of a tick bite after a delay of 3 to 30 days (average is about 7 days). It expands gradually over a period of days reaching up to 12″ or more (30 cm) across. As it enlarges, the center clears, resulting in a target or "bull's-eye" appearance.

35. Answer: C

Nursing Process: Intervention/GU/GYN/OB

Rationale: **Methotrexate (Trexall), a cytotoxic medication, is a folic acid antagonist and inhibits further duplication of fetal cells.** Doxycycline (Vibramycin), ceftriaxone (Rocephin), and metronidazole (Flagyl) are antibiotics and not used for this condition but are used in the treatment of pelvic inflammatory disease (PID).

36. Answer: D

Nursing Process: Intervention/Psychosocial

Rationale: **While frequently effective after days or weeks of use, the SSRI (Selective Serotonin Reuptake Inhibitor) medications are not an acutely beneficial emergency department intervention.** All the other drugs have an onset that may be beneficial during a typical emergency department stay.

37. Answer: D

Nursing Process: Assessment/Medical

Rationale: **The most common electrolyte imbalances seen in acute renal failure are hyperkalemia, hyponatremia, hypocalcemia, and hyperphosphatemia. Hyperkalemia is a life-threatening electrolyte disturbance requiring immediate treatment.** An intravenous pyleogram visualizes abnormalities of the urinary system, including the kidneys, ureters, and bladder, and evaluates the flow of urine through the renal system. Renal angiography can be helpful in establishing the etiology of renal vascular diseases, including renal artery stenosis, but does not assist in determining the severity or acuity. An elevated blood urea nitrogen (BUN) is a hallmark of acute kidney injury but is not considered a life-threatening condition.

38. Answer: A

Nursing Process: Evaluation/Medical

Rationale: **Postrenal acute kidney injury is the result of an obstruction of the urinary collection system from the calices of the kidney to the urethral meatus. Relief of the obstruction and allowing urine to flow out of the kidney is the intention of treatment interventions.** Increasing renal artery perfusion and increasing or decreasing systemic blood pressure are interventions which influence prerenal acute kidney injury.

39. Answer: B

Nursing Process: Intervention/Communicable

Rationale: **Patients can continue to shed the *Clostridium difficile* spores for a number of days after the last diarrheal stool. Therefore, it would be advantageous for them to remain in isolation even after their diarrhea has stopped.** *Clostridium difficile* is not killed by alcohol. Alcohol-based hand cleansers are not adequate for the health care providers to use during the care of these patients. Soap and water are the best hand cleanser agents to use. Gloves are actually best as even handwashing cannot always adequately prevent the spread of this organism. Gowns should be worn when caring for these individuals. Private rooms are necessary or at least room the patient with another patient who is diagnosed with *C. difficile*. This is known as "cohorting."

40. Answer: A

Nursing Process: Analysis/Respiratory

Rationale: **An empyema contains pus and can be caused by tuberculosis.** Transudative effusion is common with heart failure, renal and liver disease, and exudative effusions are secondary to pulmonary malignancies, pulmonary embolus, and GI disease. Patients with pulmonary embolus often present with hypoxia and tachycardia and are afebrile.

41. Answer: A

Nursing Process: Evaluation/Respiratory

Rationale: **The patient with chronic bronchitis should be monitored closely when given low-flow oxygen to decrease the chances of depressing the respiratory drive because hypoxia becomes the stimulus to breathe for these patients.** Increasing fluids to liquefy secretions, humidifying the air, and performing postural drainage are also important therapies for a patient with chronic bronchitis.

42. Answer: A

Nursing Process: Analysis/Orthopedic

Rationale: **A "buckle" fracture is also known as a torus fracture.** This is demonstrated by no disruption of the cortex. In a "greenstick" fracture, the cortex does show disruption on the involved side. Both torus and greenstick fractures are breaks that involve one side of the bone, but there is a difference. In compression fractures, the bone collapses onto itself, and in comminuted fractures, the bone is splintered or fragmented with two or more fragments of bone involved. This can commonly occur with gunshot wounds, but can also be direct blunt trauma.

43. Answer: B

Cognitive Level: Application/Professional Issues

Rationale: **Short-term goals are the only ones that the emergency nurse will be able to provide in this setting.** There is no long-term, ongoing relationship in the ED setting (typically!). Middle-range goals and tertiary range goals do not exist.

44. Answer: A

Nursing Process: Analysis/Cardiovascular

Rationale: **Most patients who present with cardiogenic shock do so in conjunction with a myocardial infarction. Clinical manifestations of cardiogenic shock reflect heart failure and inadequate tissue perfusion, that is, tachypnea, crackles, hypotension, and pale, clammy skin.** Anaphylactic shock from allergic reaction presents with dyspnea, stridor, wheezing, bronchospasm, and erythema. Neurogenic shock includes signs/symptoms of bradycardia, hypotension, and warm, dry skin. Tachycardia, altered level of consciousness, and uncontrolled external bleeding are signs of hypovolemic shock.

45. Answer: B

Nursing Process: Evaluation/Gastrointestinal

Rationale: **The method now recommended to achieve the highest level of certainty of proper placement of a nasogastric tube is to have radiograph or computed tomography (CT) evidence.** The next recommended method is to utilize pH testing of the gastric aspirate. The use of a carbon dioxide detector to determine it is not in the lungs is the third highest recommendation, although it is considered to be weak. The common practice of listening over the stomach area for the sound of instilled air is not recommended anymore. This is an unreliable method.

46. Answer: B

Nursing Process: Assessment/GU/GYN/OB

Rationale: **When the urethra is torn, a hematoma or collection of blood separates the two sections of the urethra. This may feel like a boggy mass on rectal examination and the prostate becomes "high riding."** A palpable prostate gland usually indicates an intact urethra. Absent sphincter tone would refer to a spinal cord injury. The presence of blood in the rectum would probably correlate with a GI bleed or colon injury.

47. Answer: C

Nursing Process: Assessment/Medical

Rationale: **Tight regulation of $[H^+]$ is crucial for normal cellular activities. The body requires a pH of 7.35 to 7.45 to maintain homeostasis.** pH values below 7.35 are reflective of acidosis and values in excess of 7.45 represent alkalosis.

48. Answer: D

Nursing Process: Analysis/Communicable Diseases

Rationale: **The main causal agent of infectious mononucleosis is the Epstein–Barr virus. The usual route of transmission is oropharyngeal through saliva. Hence, its moniker as the "kissing disease."** The virus is not found in blood or stool. It is not passed by contact with skin lesions. Classic symptoms of mononucleosis include a flu-like prodromal period lasting 3 to 5 days followed by fever, pharyngitis, and lymphadenopathy. No rash is associated with mononucleosis.

49. Answer: A

Nursing Process: Analysis/Cardiovascular

Rationale: **Hypovolemia and hypoxia are the two most common underlying and potentially reversible causes of pulseless electrical activity in the trauma patient. Uncontrolled bleeding and resultant hypovolemia may occur after a crash of an unrestrained driver at high speeds.** Although thrombosis, toxins, acidosis, and hypothermia are causes of pulseless electrical activity according to the American Heart Association, they are not necessarily implicated in a car crash at high speeds. Hypoglycemia and syncope are not common causes of pulseless electrical activity according to the American Heart Association.

50. Answer: B

Nursing Process: Analysis/Respiratory

Rationale: **Although a cervical spine injury, tracheal tear, or clavicular fracture can be associated with a fracture of the first or second rib, the most serious injury is aortic rupture, which often results in immediate death from severe hemodynamic compromise.** Suspect an aortic rupture in a trauma patient with motor, sensory, or pulse deficits in the lower extremities. Such deficits usually result from disruption of blood flow to the spinal cord. Other symptoms include unexplained hypotension and chest or back pain. A cervical spine injury can also be serious, especially if it involves a C_3, C_4, or higher lesion, which can result in respiratory depression. Tracheal tears lead to pneumomediastinum and have the potential for tension pneumothorax if undetected. Clavicular fractures cause great pain; however, they seldom cause more severe consequences.

51. Answer: A

Nursing Process: Evaluation/Cardiovascular

Rationale: **Premature atrial complexes may precede supraventricular tachycardia, atrial flutter, or atrial fibrillation. These complexes appear on the electrocardiogram as identical to the patient's PQRST complexes but are "premature" or early in the pattern.** Flutter waves occur in atrial flutter and appear as a sawtooth pattern which can be variable. Atrial fibrillation is characterized by a chaotic atrial rhythm associated with an irregular ventricular response. Supraventricular tachycardia is common in the pediatric population, some of whom are born with accessory conduction system pathways that predispose them to reentrant rhythms.

52. Answer: C

Nursing Process: Assessment/Cardiovascular

Rationale: **ST-segment elevation in leads V_1, V_2, and V_3 are indicative of damage to the anterior aspect of the heart. These leads look directly at the anterior heart wall.** Inferior myocardial infarctions are noted with changes in leads II, III, and AVF. The lateral leads are I, AVL, V_5, and V_6. Posterior MIs are noted as reciprocal changes in the anterior leads—V_1 and V_2. To see the ST-segment elevation changes in this MI, posterior leads—V_7, V_8, and V_9—would need to be performed.

53. Answer: B

Nursing Process: Assessment/Neurologic/Shock

Rationale: **The hallmark of neurogenic shock is bradycardia. This occurs due to the loss of sympathetic responses. The parasympathetic system is in control. The vagal response associated with this system is bradycardia.** Hypovolemic, anaphylactic, and septic types of shock all have tachycardia as a predominant symptom.

54. Answer: C

Nursing Process: Assessment/Respiratory

Rationale: **Tachycardia, not bradycardia, is seen with a pulmonary embolus (PE).** Acute respiratory distress, nonproductive cough, and chest pain are all signs and symptoms of a PE.

55. Answer: C

Nursing Process: Assessment/GU/GYN/OB

Rationale: **Whether the patient has changed her clothes, or even brushed her teeth since the attack, is critical to evidence collection and preservation.** It is also helpful if the patient has not showered, urinated, or defecated. Determining if the patient has notified the police is also important, but does not affect the assessment. It is not relevant to know if she has been previously sexually assaulted or if she is using a method of birth control at this time.

56. Answer: A

Nursing Process: Intervention/GU/GYN/OB

Rationale: **A pelvic examination should not be performed on a pregnant patient with vaginal bleeding in the third trimester. This can cause further bleeding and damage the placenta.** The patient should be placed on bed rest, monitor a pad count, and be admitted if bleeding is heavy and persists. A pelvic ultrasound is useful for detecting placenta previa.

57. Answer: A

Nursing Process: Assessment/Neurologic

Rationale: **Cranial nerve II, the Optic nerve, assesses visual acuity, dark versus light, and the counting of fingers.** Cranial nerve III, Oculomotor, gives the eye the ability to constrict the pupils, move the eyeball, and open the eyelid. Cranial nerve IV, Trochlear, allows the eye to look downward and outward, and cranial nerve VI, Abducens, assists the eyeball to rotate outward.

58. Answer: D

Nursing Process: Assessment/Orthopedic

Rationale: **In this scenario, the anticipated mechanism of injury would be an open-book pelvic fracture because the patient was crushed between two objects in a standing position.** Because the patient was standing, it is unlikely his humerus or humeral head would be impacted by the crush. Closed pelvic fractures are generally caused by lateral compression from motor vehicle crashes.

59. Answer: A

Nursing Process: Assessment/Orthopedic/Shock

Rationale: **Tachycardia, restlessness, and thirst are often seen early in hypovolemic shock.** Tachycardia is due to increased epinephrine secretion in response to a decreased preload. Restlessness can occur from the epinephrine secretion as well as hypoxemia. Thirst is due to decreased extracellular fluid in mucous membranes as it is being shunted back to core circulation. This epinephrine secretion is due to the compensatory effects of the "fight-or-flight" response. The other manifestations would occur in later phases.

60. Answer: B

Nursing Process: Analysis/Psychosocial

Rationale: **The highest frequency of onset/diagnosis of schizophrenia is in the age group of 15 to 24 years.**

61. Answer: D

Nursing Process: Intervention/Psychosocial

Rationale: **It is appropriate to initiate interventions with the agitated patient with the least invasive means.** It is appropriate to escalate the level of intervention in response to ineffective therapeutic effect through isolation, medication, or as a last resort restraint.

62. Answer: A

Nursing Process: Analysis/Neurologic

Rationale: **A subdural hematoma, occurring between the dura mater and the arachnoid layer of the meninges, is bleeding that causes direct pressure to the surface of the brain. Signs and symptoms appear within 48 hours (acute) and can be delayed as long as several months (chronic).** Symptoms of an epidural hematoma include a history of momentary loss of consciousness followed by a lucid period after which the patient's mental status deteriorates rapidly due to the presence of bleeding from the middle meningeal artery. The clinical manifestations of a diffuse axonal injury are immediate and prolonged coma with decorticate or decerebrate posturing. Manifestations of postconcussion syndrome include headache, dizziness, irritability, poor judgment, and insomnia.

63. Answer: A

Nursing Process: Intervention/Gastrointestinal

Rationale: **This patient is experiencing symptoms consistent with esophageal varices, which also matches his past history of hepatitis C. Cirrhosis is a complicating factor of hepatitis C. The medication used for this is octreotide (Sandostatin).** Nitroprusside (Nipride) is an antihypertensive that is used for emergencies in which blood pressures must be dropped. Amiodarone (Cordarone) is used for dysrhythmias, which would not match with this scenario. Flumazenil (Romazicon) is the antidote for benzodiazepine overdose.

64. Answer: A

Nursing Process: Evaluation/Gastrointestinal

Rationale: **High ammonia levels are found in patients who are experiencing hepatic encephalopathy and the patients are treated with lactulose (Cholac).** This patient, with a prior history of intravenous substance abuse, is presenting with manifestations of this disease process. Other electrolytes, including potassium, sodium, and magnesium, are noted to be deficient in liver failure; however, lactulose (Cholac) is not utilized to treat these deficiencies.

65. Answer: B

Cognitive Level: Analysis/Professional Issues

Rationale: **Altitude changes will cause changes in air pressure, causing a hypobaric environment, whereby the pressure decreases as altitude increases. There will be enough of a pressure change to cause an arterial line pressure bag to lose some pressure, which may result in an inaccurate arterial blood pressure reading.** The patient is not ready to be transported as of yet. The arterial line must be considered and any other altitudinal changes that might impact the patient. Family cannot accompany the patient on board the aircraft. Documenting vital signs is important but only after the arterial line pressure bag is stabilized.

66. Answer: B

Nursing Process: Assessment/Toxicology

Rationale: **The three effects associated with tricyclic antidepressant overdoses are cardiotoxicity (prolonged PR interval, widened QRS, prolonged QT interval, heart blocks, and asystole), adrenergic blocking leading to hypotension, and anticholinergic effects (dry skin and mouth with a depressed level of consciousness).** There are no anticoagulation or sympathomimetic effects and the central nervous system is depressed rather than excited.

67. Answer: D

Nursing Process: Assessment/Environmental

Rationale: **The patient's hands and buttocks are full-thickness—often called third degree—burns because they are charred or patchy white in color and painless because nerve endings have been destroyed.** Superficial epidermal (first degree) burns are red and painful. Superficial partial-thickness and deep partial-thickness (second degree) burns are usually blistered and painful. The patient may not realize some areas do not have pain due to the pain in the areas with more superficial burns.

68. Answer: D

Nursing Process: Analysis/Neurologic

Rationale: **The higher the score, the more the deficits are present, which indicates a worse outcome for the patient. A score of 0 would indicate no deficits present for a patient with a normal examination.** The NIHSS assesses the patient's level of consciousness, orientation, response to commands, gaze, visual fields, facial movement, motor function, limb ataxia, sensation, language, articulation, and extinction.

69. Answer: B

Nursing Process: Assessment/Maxillofacial/Ocular

Rationale: **Mandibular fractures may manifest with sublingual bleeding or hematoma, trismus, malocclusion, bleeding gums, loose teeth, paresthesia of the lower lip, and ruptured tympanic membrane.** Numbness to the cheek is consistent with maxillary or zygomatic fractures. Avulsed teeth occur with direct trauma to the teeth. Blow-out fracture is a fracture to the orbital floor from direct trauma to the orbit or is seen in association with LeFort, maxillary, or zygomatic fractures.

70. Answer: A

Nursing Process: Analysis/Orthopedic

Rationale: **Fractures of the epiphyseal plate can affect healing and growth.** This area is where the bones grow; thus, major problems can be expected as the child matures. While the others would need proper care and healing, they are not as concerning as the sequelae that can occur with an epiphyseal plate injury.

71. Answer: B

Nursing Process: Assessment/Maxillofacial/Ocular

Rationale: **The most common history associated with sinusitis is recent viral upper respiratory tract infections, with up to 90% of patients having had one.** A small percentage (5% to 10%) of patients have bacterial superinfection requiring antimicrobial treatment. Invasive dental procedures such as treatment for dental abscess can be a risk factor for sinusitis; however, denture fittings are not considered to be risk factors. The patient with a migraine headache may experience sinus pain but does not constitute sinusitis. Epistaxis should be evaluated to ensure the patient does not develop a septal hematoma, which can lead to infection but is not a risk factor for sinusitis.

72. Answer: B

Nursing Process: Analysis/Environmental/Shock

Rationale: **Although hypotension and tachycardia are also signs of venom reactions, this patient is presenting with classic anaphylaxis symptoms—hives, itching, and swelling of the face, mouth, and lips.** Venom-related reactions are typically weakness and paralysis. Treatment should be aimed at the histamine reaction and circulatory collapse and should be treated as such with epinephrine, diphenhydramine (Benadryl), H_2-blockers such as famotidine (Pepcid), and fluids. Overexposure to the sun would cause more heat exhaustion or heat stroke-like symptoms, including an increased temperature. The hives, itching, and swelling would not be caused by the sun exposure nor would they be associated with dehydration, although the tachycardia, hypotension, and generalized weakness could be manifestations of this process.

73. Answer: D

Cognitive Level: Application/Professional Issues

Rationale: **Quantitative research (think *Quantity*) uses measurable data to formulate facts and uncover patterns; it examines the data to determine cause and effect.** A study that compares treatments against a control group would be classified as a randomized control study in which participants are compared with a control group. Quantitative research does not necessarily follow all subjects of a specific disease process. Cohort studies follow patients over time and qualitative research (think *Quality*) utilizes small groups and individual insights to gather greater understanding of peoples' opinions and motivations. It provides insights into the problem. *Qualitative* studies can be used to develop ideas or hypotheses for potential quantitative research.

74. Answer: C

Nursing Process: Intervention/Neurologic

Rationale: **Over 23 million patients suffer from migraine headaches. Current treatment standards for patients with migraine headaches include providing hydration (oral or intravenous); antiemetics (ondansetron hydrochloride [Zofran]) or antihistamines (intravenous diphenhydramine [Benadryl]), and NSAIDs (ibuprofen [Motrin]).** Narcotic analgesics should be avoided due to the possibility of a rebound headache and addiction. Nitroglycerin sublingual should be avoided due to the vasodilatory affect, which can increase the intensity of the headache.

75. Answer: B

Nursing Process: Assessment/Communicable Diseases

Rationale: **Bluish-gray spots (Koplik spots) appear on the inside of the cheeks after 2 to 4 days of prodromal symptoms and are visible for up to 5 days. The rash of measles is maculopapular and first appears on the face.** A pruritic rash on the chest is indicative of varicella (chickenpox). Parotid gland enlargement is characteristic of mumps. Petechiae in the skin folds of the axilla and groin are indicative of scarlet fever.

76. Answer: C

Nursing Process: Intervention/Psychosocial

Rationale: **Professional assertiveness is an appropriate and often effective response.** Aggression is not a professional response and can escalate the circumstances. Passivity is not effective and can result in increased risk for the nurse. Indifference does not facilitate a therapeutic relationship.

77. Answer: A

Nursing Process: Analysis/GU/GYN/OB

Rationale: **Herpes is a viral, not bacterial, infection (although a secondary bacterial infection can occur), and acyclovir is not bactericidal.** Acyclovir relieves systemic pain, diminishes the interval of viral shedding, and decreases the formation of new lesions.

78. Answer: B

Nursing Process: Analysis/Respiratory

Rationale: **Pediatric patients' alveoli are smaller than those of an adult and results in decreased surface area for gas exchange.** Pediatric patients also have increased respiratory rates which depletes limited reserves resulting in sudden decompensation. A pediatric patient's flatter diaphragm is the primary muscle for ventilation and their abdominal muscles play a major role in respiration, meaning that abdominal trauma can impact a child's respiratory status.

79. Answer: A

Nursing Process: Evaluation/Cardiovascular

Rationale: **Raynaud's phenomenon is a circulatory disease of the arteries that severely reduces blood flow as the result of episodic intense vasospasm of the digits in response to extreme cold, emotional stress, and/or smoking. Treatment is aimed at decreasing pain and vasospastic events. The patient should be advised to keep themselves warm, wear gloves, avoid smoking, and avoid cold medicines and diet pills due to their vasoconstrictive effects.** Elevating the arm and applying ice would worsen the vasoconstriction. Wrist splints or applying an elastic bandage would not help and may increase vasoconstriction. Fluids and aspirin would not help.

80. Answer: D

Nursing Process: Evaluation/Cardiovascular/Shock

Rationale: **Normal saline boluses would not treat an obstructive shock patient. This would be indicated in situations involving hemorrhagic or hypovolemic shock.** A patient would receive a pericardiocentesis to treat a cardiac tamponade which causes obstructive shock. A pregnant patient would need to be turned to her left side in order to keep the gravid uterus off of the inferior vena cava, thus preventing or treating hypotension associated with obstructive shock. A needle decompression would be used to treat a tension pneumothorax, which would also cause obstructive shock.

81. Answer: A

Nursing Process: Intervention/Respiratory

Rationale: **A pneumothorax is treated with the insertion of a chest tube connected to an underwater seal; the tube remains in place until reexpansion of the lung is achieved.** An emergency thoracotomy is reserved for a hemodynamically unstable patient. Needle thoracostomy is used in the treatment of tension pneumothorax. Most patients with a pneumothorax do not require emergent intubation.

82. Answer: B

Nursing Process: Evaluation/Neurologic

Rationale: **Alzheimer's disease is a type of dementia. Generally, dementia is defined as a decline in thinking, reasoning, and/or remembering. People with Alzheimer's disease have difficulty carrying out daily tasks they have performed routinely and independently throughout their lives and they can have difficulty with social interactions.** Alzheimer's disease accounts for 60% to 80% of all cases of dementia. This terminal, progressive brain disorder has no known cause or cure. Hallucinations and delusions can occur later in the disease process for these patients.

83. Answer: A

Nursing Process: Analysis/Medical

Rationale: **Each unit of packed red blood cells (PRBCs) for transfusion contains approximately 3 mg of citrate as a preservative, which accumulates in the blood where it binds to circulating calcium, thereby reducing plasma calcium concentration. Patients receiving more than 5 units of PRBCs should have serum calcium levels checked. These patients may require intravenous calcium chloride of calcium gluconate.** A patient receiving multiple transfusions of PRBCs would be at risk of hyperkalemia due to the breakdown of blood cells that releases potassium while it is being stored. White blood cell counts are not impacted with administration of packed red cells. Clotting times may be increase, because packed red cells do not contain any clotting factors. Replacement of platelets and fresh frozen plasma (FFP) should be considered when multiple units of PRBCs are infused.

84. Answer: D

Nursing Process: Analysis/Maxillofacial/Ocular

Rationale: **There is no definitive diagnostic test to confirm Bell's palsy, and diagnosis is confirmed based on clinical presentation of the hallmark signs and symptoms.** Facial radiology may confirm bone deformities and masses in the sinuses. Computed tomography (CT) is used to rule out intracranial bleed, but does not confirm the diagnosis of Bell's palsy. Electromyography (EMG) is used as part of the comprehensive evaluation to assess nerve and motor function.

85. Answer: C

Nursing Process: Intervention/Maxillofacial/Ocular

Rationale: **Immediate intervention is to irrigate the eye with normal saline or lactated ringers solution to stop the burning and minimize permanent damage to the eye.** The longer the substance remains in contact with the eye, the more damage will occur. Alkali substances may require up to 1 hour of flushing to neutralize the substance. Assessments and interventions, which may delay eye flushing, should be deferred or done concurrently with eye flushing. A detailed assessment should occur after eye flushing. There is no therapeutic value to patching the eye in the case of ocular burns. Systemic analgesics and topical cycloplegic drops may be administered, and ophthalmology will be consulted yet neither intervention should delay eye flushing.

86. Answer: A

Nursing Process: Analysis/Orthopedic

Rationale: **Osteomyelitis is an infection of the bone, most often as a result of an open fracture with direct contamination.** *Staphylococcus aureus* **is found on human skin and is the main causative bacteria.** *Escherichia coli* and *Streptococcus agalactiae* are common in the gastrointestinal tract and *Serratia marcescens* is found in water.

87. Answer: A

Nursing Process: Intervention/Respiratory

Rationale: **If the patient's vital signs are stable with no signs of shock, the most appropriate intervention is chest tube insertion for reexpansion of the lung.** If the patient is unstable, an emergency thoracotomy is the definitive therapy. Autotransfusion may be used to stabilize the unstable patient until transportation to surgery. Lactated ringers solution and normal saline are the only crystalloids acceptable for administration in traumatic emergencies.

88. Answer: A

Cognitive Level: Application/Professional Issues

Rationale: **The nurse's own and the patient's safety first is paramount.** A less stimulating environment, offering food as a distraction, and assisting other staff members in caring for other emergency patients' safety and well-being can be important; however, scene safety is the first priority.

89. Answer: C

Nursing Process: Evaluation/Cardiovascular/Shock

Rationale: **Dopamine (Intropin) does not affect prolongation of the QRS complex.** Dopamine can cause tachydysrhythmias, requires a central IV line for administration, and frequent monitoring of vital signs and urine output. Although dopamine can be used for cardiogenic shock, dobutamine (Dobutrex) is the preferred drug due to having less of a tendency to cause tachydysrhythmias.

90. Answer: C

Nursing Process: Analysis/Neurologic

Rationale: **An epidural hematoma results from blood collecting between the skull and the dura mater.** A subdural hematoma is commonly caused by trauma or violent shaking (shaken baby syndrome) and results in a collection of venous blood between the dura mater and the arachnoid mater. A subarachnoid hemorrhage is a collection of blood between the pia mater and the arachnoid membrane. A contusion is a bruise on the surface of the brain.

91. Answer: A

Nursing Process: Intervention/Environmental

Rationale: **The fluoride ion in hydrofluoric acid binds with calcium ions and will continue to "burn" until neutralized with calcium gluconate.** While waiting for the calcium gluconate, flushing with water will help dilute the pollution, but 1 liter will not be sufficient. The patient should be put in a running stream of water. Other chemicals will not help and the wound should not be covered with an ointment until the area has been completely treated with calcium chloride. Often a paste of calcium chloride is applied so it will continue to help treat this type of burn that is due to a localized hypocalcemia and will neutralize the fluoride ions found in this product.

92. Answer: C

Nursing Process: Analysis/Toxicology

Rationale: **Gamma-hydroxybutyrate (GHB) is a sedative/ hypnotic, which induces hallucinations and euphoria as well as more commonly associated sedation effects such as respiratory depression.** Phencyclidine (PCP), cannabis (marijuana), and lysergic acid diethylamide (LSD) produce hallucinations and coordination impairment but act as stimulants, rather than depressants on the respiratory drive.

93. Answer: C

Nursing Process: Analysis/GU/GYN/OB

Rationale: **Epididymitis is suggested by hyperperfusion on the testicular scan, an elevated white blood cell count, and the presence of bacteria in the urine.** Hypoperfusion or no perfusion would indicate testicular torsion. Leukopenia indicates a decrease in white blood cell count. An elevated creatinine level is an indicator of renal, not scrotal disease.

94. Answer: B

Nursing Process: Analysis/Medical

Rationale: **Normal sodium levels range between 135 and 145 mEq/mL. When serum sodium levels fall below 120 mEq/L, symptoms of hyponatremia appear. An altered level of consciousness ranging from confusion to coma and seizures are commonly seen.** Tetany is a serious complication of hypocalcemia. Decreased urinary output (less than 500 mL of urine/24 hours in an adult) is seen in both acute kidney injury and chronic renal failure. Tachycardia, not bradycardia, is seen in hyponatremia.

95. Answer: A

Nursing Process: Intervention/GU/GYN/OB

Rationale: **The normal neonatal heart rate is 120 to 160 beats/minute. Heart rates below 60 beats/minute necessitate chest compressions and ventilatory support.**

96. Answer: D

Nursing Process: Analysis/Medical

Rationale: **Intrarenal acute kidney injury (AKI) is the result of damage to the body of the kidney due to prolonged hypoperfusion and immunologic or inflammatory processes. Chronic use of NSAIDs can be directly nephrotoxic to kidney tissue.** Decreased blood flow from hypovolemia is a prerenal cause of AKI, and neurogenic bladder and renal calculi, which obstruct the flow of urine out of the bladder or kidney, are postrenal causes of AKI.

97. Answer: C

Nursing Process: Intervention/Neurologic

Rationale: **TPA is administered as a weight-based dose of 0.9 mg/kg, but with a maximum dose of 90 mg in the patient presenting with a stroke.** TPA is the only thrombolytic approved for use in stroke patients.

98. Answer: A

Nursing Process: Evaluation/Cardiovascular/Shock

Rationale: **According to the SHOCK trial, the best possible treatment for cardiogenic shock is immediate percutaneous coronary intervention (PCI) or coronary artery bypass graft (CABG). These dramatically reduce the mortality rate.** It is best to provide this option within 90 minutes but can be performed as much as 12 hours later with good results. Thinking that the patient will be well enough to travel in 10 days is not realistic on the part of the adult child. Low blood pressures do not help to perfuse the patient's body and the problem is inadequate oxygenation of the cells, not too much oxygen.

99. Answer: A

Nursing Process: Intervention/Toxicology

Rationale: **Alkalization of urine is considered effective for overdoses involving phenobarbital, sulfonylureas, formaldehyde, and salicylates.** Weak acids may become ion-trapped and excreted in the urine when urine pH is increased with controlled administration of alkalizing agents. Alkalinizing the urine does not promote excretion of cephalosporins, calcium channel blockers, or phosphodiesterase inhibitors.

100. Answer: C

Nursing Process: Intervention/Respiratory

Rationale: **Pain control for a patient with rib fractures is a priority to ensure adequate expansion of lung tissue and to facilitate turning, coughing, and deep breathing.** The patient should be placed in high Fowler's position to facilitate gas exchange and breathing. Avoid circumferential taping of the chest or rib belts because this predisposes the patient to atelectasis and pneumonia. The lung directly below the fractured rib is often bruised (pulmonary contusion). Fluids should be monitored closely to decrease the risk of acute respiratory distress syndrome (ARDS) which causes a noncardiac pulmonary edema.

101. Answer: C

Nursing Process: Evaluation/Neurologic

Rationale: **This patient is most likely experiencing a subarachnoid hemorrhage. The history of migraine headaches is not a risk factor for this catastrophic diagnosis. Patients with subarachnoid hemorrhage often state that the headache is the most severe they have ever had.** This is also a process that is a sudden onset. Often patients with cerebral aneurysms are asymptomatic until the time of bleeding. At the time of rupture, blood is forced into the subarachnoid space, causing symptoms of meningeal irritation, which would cause pain to the back of the neck when the head is moved in a forward (chin to chest) direction (nuchal rigidity). Other manifestations include nausea, vomiting, aphasia or other speech difficulties, photosensitivity, hypertension, and bradycardia. Other risk factors for this diagnosis are cocaine and amphetamine use and disease processes such as Marfan's syndrome and sickle cell disease.

102. Answer: C

Nursing Process: Evaluation/Respiratory

Rationale: **The finding that suggests a worsening of the patient's condition is a tracheal shift with jugular venous distension (JVD) which indicates a tension pneumothorax.** The respiratory rate within normal limits and blood pressure of 120/80 mm Hg are acceptable outcomes. The patient will have decreased breath sounds until reexpansion of the lung has been achieved.

103. Answer: A

Nursing Process: Intervention/Orthopedic

Rationale: **Reduction of dislocations should be done as soon as possible, and within a 6-hour timeframe.** Any time over 6 hours is incorrect as the longer the dislocation remains, the greater the risk of necrosis.

104. Answer: C

Nursing Process: Intervention/Toxicology

Rationale: **Physostigmine acts by interfering with the metabolism of acetylcholine; therefore, increasing the cholinergic effects of acetylcholine in the body and reversing anticholinergic delirium.** Remember that physostigmine must be given slowly because of the side effects! Naloxone is used in opiate overdose. Lithium is not used as an antidote in any scenario. Atropine is used in beta-adrenergic blocker, calcium channel blocker, and organophosphate and physostigmine poisonings.

105. Answer: B

Nursing Process: Analysis/Neurologic

Rationale: **Meningococcemia is a potentially life-or limb-threatening clinical entity in which the organism *Neisseria meningitidis* gains access to the bloodstream. It is characterized by rapid onset of petechiae and purpuric lesions and is spread by oral or nasal droplets. Additional signs and symptoms include irritability, fever/temperature instability, bleeding from puncture sites, tachycardia, poor perfusion, hypotension, gangrene, and tissue necrosis (late).** Henoch- Schönlein purpura (HSP) is a disease of the skin, mucous membranes, and sometimes other organs that most commonly affects children following an infectious process such as a throat infection. Palpable purpura (small, raised areas of bleeding underneath the skin), joint pain, and abdominal pain can occur. Chronic kidney disease can follow this disease process. Idiopathic thrombocytopenic purpura (ITP) is a disorder affecting both children and adults that can lead to easy or excessive bruising and bleeding. The bleeding results from unusually low levels of platelets and the cells that help blood clot. Children often develop ITP after a viral infection and usually recover fully without treatment. In adults, the disorder is often long term. Depending on the level of platelets, manifestations can range from minimal to potentially fatal with internal bleeding. Kawasaki disease affects children and includes fever, rash, swelling of the hands and feet, irritation and redness of the whites of the eyes, and swollen lymph glands in the neck with irritation and inflammation of the mouth, lips, and throat. The effects of Kawasaki disease are rarely serious. The acute phase of the condition commonly lasts 10 to 14 days or more. Most children recover fully. In some cases, Kawasaki disease can lead to long-term heart complications.

106. Answer: C

Nursing Process: Evaluation/Toxicology

Rationale: **A lactate level of 1.1 mmol/L would be in the standard reference range and indicates the lactic acidosis caused by the toxicity has been resolved.** Remember that biguanide antihyperglycemic agents, including metformin (Glucophage), act by inhibiting liver glucose production rather than, as other antidiabetic medications do, by decreasing cellular resistance of insulin. Therefore, biguanides only drop blood sugar to the euglycemic threshold of the body and are not commonly associated with hypoglycemic emergencies. They do, however, inhibit liver breakdown of lactate molecules and lead to metabolic lactic acidosis in overdoses. A venous pH of 7.29 would indicate an acidotic state and would not indicate successful treatment in this situation. Because biguanide overdose is not normally associated with hypoglycemia, a blood glucose level of 60 mg/dL would not indicate successful treatment. Although increased urine output may be present in a patient who is hyperglycemic, which is likely in a patient who has access to antidiabetic medications, it would be indicative of the condition of hyperglycemia, rather than the toxic effects of metformin (Glucophage) and would not be associated with effective treatment of the toxicity.

107. Answer: B

Nursing Process: Intervention/Environmental

Rationale: **An ever-present concern with electrical energy is muscle spasm caused when electricity courses through the body. Energy from the lighting can travel from the pole through the ground to the player and cause spasm of the heart, neck, and other muscles of the body. Due to this, a jaw-thrust maneuver that would protect the C-spine should be utilized to open this airway.** Before starting chest compressions, one should check for a pulse and respiratory effort and not assume ventricular fibrillation. Attending to the airway would take precedence over long-bone fractures or other injuries sustained.

108. Answer: C

Cognitive Level: Application/Professional Issues

Rationale: **The patient is exhibiting excessive agitation, which has a potential for violence; therefore, reassuring the patient and his family is the most therapeutic response.** The nurse should avoid being within the patient's physical reach to reduce the risk of being hit. Taking an authoritative stance is likely to further agitate the patient. He may not be able to cognitively take verbal cueing or instructions because of an underlying pathologic process. Shouting that outside authorities should be called will also likely incite further agitation.

109. Answer: A

Nursing Process: Evaluation/Neurologic

Rationale: **One episode of hypotension, which drops the mean arterial pressure (MAP) below 70 mm Hg can have devastating effects. The MAP should be maintained between 70 and 90 mm Hg. A blood pressure of 90/42 mm Hg creates an MAP of 58 mm Hg.** In a head-injured patient, the cerebral perfusion pressure (CPP) should remain above 70 mm Hg. This is the end result of the formula, CPP = MAP − ICP. The patient in this question is within normal limits for a patient with head injury. To obtain this number, an intracranial catheter must be in place. Maintaining the serum osmolality below 320 mOsm is recommended, which is noted in this question. Urine output of 48 mL/hour is adequate output.

110. Answer: B

Nursing Process: Intervention/Gastrointestinal

Rationale: **This patient presents with manifestations of cholecystitis.** Although there is some controversy regarding this, it is thought that morphine sulfate can cause spasm of the sphincter of Oddi and increase pain. Hydromorphone (Dilaudid) and fentanyl (Sublimaze) are other common narcotic medications that are used to treat this type of pain. Meperidine (Demerol) is not used much in health care today and should not be utilized for chronic pain; however, it can be used to treat acute situations such as cholecystitis.

111. Answer: B

Nursing Process: Analysis/Medical

Rationale: **Hemophilia A is caused by a deficiency of functional plasma clotting factor VIII.** An absence of factor IX results in hemophilia B, also called Christmas disease. Hemophilia C, or Rosenthal syndrome, is caused by a deficiency of factor XI. Factor IV is ionized calcium and is required in many stages of the coagulation cascade.

112. Answer: C

Nursing Process: Analysis/Neurologic

Rationale: **Cranial nerve V (Trigeminal) deals with facial, cheek, and chin movement.** Cranial nerve III (Oculomotor) constricts the pupil and is responsible for helping with eyeball movement. Cranial nerve VI (Abducens) rotates the eyeball outward, and cranial nerve VIII (Acoustic) deals with hearing and balance.

113. Answer: A

Cognitive Level: Application/Professional Issues

Rationale: **Benzodiazepines can cause respiratory depression as well as systemic hypotension in elderly adults with agitation and/or delirium.** Hypoxemia, delirium, and alcohol withdrawal are all potential causes of agitation/ delirium in elders that the emergency nurse should rule out.

114. Answer: A

Nursing Process: Intervention/Cardiovascular

Rationale: **All of the interventions may be required; however, an emergent 12-lead ECG and rhythm strip to determine whether the implantable cardioverter defibrillator (ICD) is functioning correctly should be done initially.** The magnet inactivates the sensing function so that during magnet mode, the pacemaker will pace asynchronously. Magnet application may be done later to identify battery depletion or malfunction of the ICD. Interrogation of the ICD should be done by the emergency department, cardiology, or the device manufacturer. A consult to cardiology would be needed also.

115. Answer: C

Nursing Process: Assessment/Cardiovascular

Rationale: **Hypertension is the primary risk factor for acute aortic dissections seen in 72% of cases. Patients tend to be 60- to 80-year-old men and were significantly more likely to have atherosclerosis.** The incidence of aortic injury is estimated between 1.5% and 2% of patients who sustain blunt thoracic trauma. Aortic instrumentation or cardiac surgery can be complicated by aortic dissection, but is reported at 2% of patients. Cocaine use, which may cause a transient hypertension due to catecholamine release, accounted for 37% of dissections in a report of an inner-city population.

116. Answer: C

Nursing Process: Evaluation/Neurologic

Rationale: **C-Collars can actually increase intracranial pressure (ICP). It is important to remove them as soon as possible once the C-spine has been appropriately cleared. This will help reduce the increasing intracranial pressure.** Maintaining the head in midline position, elevating the head of the bed to 30 degrees, and keeping the room quiet and dark are all ways to help keep the intracranial pressure down. Other interventions that can assist in reducing ICP are to provide pain and sedating medications and administer osmotic diuretics. Hyperventilation should only be used as a short, temporary measure when the ICP is known to be elevated. Prophylactic hyperventilation is no longer performed.

117. Answer: D

Cognitive Level: Application/Professional Issues

Rationale: **Giving away prized possessions is an indication that the person may be considering suicide.** The other options could be signs of violence, increasing hostility, or depression, but do not necessarily indicate suicidal intent.

118. Answer: B

Cognitive Level: Recall/Professional Issues

Rationale: **Evidence-based models use a framework with the acronym PICO(T). These elements include: Problem/Patient/Population, Intervention/Indicator, Comparison, Outcome, and (optional) Time element.**

119. Answer: C

Nursing Process: Evaluation/Environmental

Rationale: **Adequate fluid resuscitation is evidenced by urine output of at least 50 mL/hour. Watching urine output is considered to be the best way to monitor fluid resuscitation now.** Concern for rhabdomyolysis would increase the desired urine output to at least 100 mL/hour; however, for the adult patient an output of 50 mL or more per hour is considered adequate. The respiratory rate and pulse rate would not indicate adequate fluid resuscitation. The mean arterial pressure reading of 45 mm Hg would be present with a blood pressure of 74/30 mm Hg, which would not be a desired endpoint for fluid resuscitation.

120. Answer: C

Nursing Process: Evaluation/Neurologic

Rationale: **Alzheimer's disease is a neurologic and degenerative disorder, resulting from cerebral atrophy and cellular degeneration. Predominating symptoms are mental status changes, increased anxiety, forgetfulness, and eventually, the inability to recognize significant others and perform activities of daily living.** Destruction of motor cells in the anterior gray horns and pyramidal tracts can result in the symptoms associated with amyotrophic lateral sclerosis. Metabolic disorders may cause altered cognitive function but can be reversed by correction of the underlying problem. Degeneration of the basal ganglia is usually associated with Parkinson's disease.

121. Answer: D

Nursing Process: Intervention/Orthopedic

Rationale: **Traction splints are utilized for stabilizing long-bone fractures, most commonly the femur.** Shoulder dislocations should be immobilized with the arm close to the body with a sling. Neurovascular assessment is important for all orthopedic injuries. Ice should be applied to reduce swelling.

122. Answer: A

Nursing Process: Intervention/Cardiovascular

Rationale: **Motor vehicle crashes and falls are the most common causes of aortic injury. When the aorta is subjected to accelerating, decelerating, horizontal, or vertical traumatic forces, it may tear. Signs and symptoms include decreased level of consciousness, hypotension, tachycardia, tachypnea, chest wall ecchymosis, and paraplegia. Paraplegia can occur due to the ischemia of the anterior spinal artery which is fed by branches of the aorta. Diagnosis is suspected by history of rapid deceleration forces and chest radiograph and confirmed by arteriography, transesophageal echo, or computed tomography (CT) scan. Surgical intervention is indicated.** Pericardial tamponade occurs most often with penetrating injury; classic signs are hypotension, distended neck veins, and muffled heart sounds, and is treated with pericardiocentesis or pericardial window. Hemothorax is an accumulation of blood in the pleural space and signs/symptoms are dyspnea, tachypnea, chest pain, signs of shock, and decreased breath sounds on the affected side; treatment is chest tube insertion and closed-chest drainage system. Tension pneumothorax would present with severe respiratory distress, diminished or absent breath sounds, hypotension, distended neck veins, and tracheal deviation. Treatment is immediately preparing for a needle thoracentesis.

123. Answer: D

Nursing Process: Intervention/Neurologic

Rationale: **Mannitol is an osmotic diuretic that decreases intracranial pressure (ICP).** Suctioning the patient's airway should be minimized to prevent increased ICP. Morphine should be used cautiously in a patient with a head injury or increased ICP because the drug's respiratory depressant effects are considerably enhanced in these situations. A patient with a head injury should have his head elevated 30 degrees to promote venous drainage. Placing a patient in trendelenburg position obstructs venous return from the brain and increases ICP.

124. Answer: C

Nursing Process: Intervention/Cardiovascular

Rationale: **The accumulation of blood or fluid in the mostly nondistensible pericardial sac compresses the heart and leads to a decrease in stroke volume and cardiac output, as well as decreased venous return and cardiac filling. A pericardiocentesis may be done to temporarily decompress the heart and allow for transfer to the operating room for definitive treatment.** A needle thoracentesis is treatment for a tension pneumothorax. Chest tube insertion is indicated for a loss of negative intrapleural pressure and subsequent collapse of a lung. Although a thoracotomy could be done to temporarily repair an open wound in the heart, a pericardiocentesis would be attempted first.

125. Answer: B

Nursing Process: Intervention/Medical

Rationale: **Propranolol is the mainstay of treatment for this problem. This will decrease the heart rate and also prevents conversion of T_4 to T_3. The T_3 state is that state in which thyroid hormone is utilized in the cells.** Propranolol can be administered orally, via nasogastric tube, or intravenously. Intravenous dosing is 0.5 to 1.0 mg over a 10-minute period of time and then 1.0 to 2.0 mg every few hours depending on heart rate and blood pressure readings. Aspirin has antipyretic properties, which is usually indicated for controlling fever, but in thyroid storm, aspirin is contraindicated as it can free up more thyroid hormone in the T_3 state. Atropine would increase the heart rate. Anticholinergics such as atropine are ineffective in controlling the rapid heart rate of thyroid storm, as it is a hypermetabolic state due to excessive thyroid hormone release. Sodium bicarbonate is a buffer for the acid–base system. Acidosis may develop in the patient with thyroid storm due to their hypermetabolic condition, but sodium bicarbonate is not a primary treatment of thyroid storm.

126. Answer: B

Nursing Process: Assessment/Maxillofacial/Ocular

Rationale: **Closed-angle, also referred to as narrow-angle glaucoma, occurs when the angle between the iris and the cornea becomes blocked. The condition can lead to permanent loss of sight due to pressure on the optic nerve. Classic presentation includes painful loss of vision, blurred vision, halos around lights, photophobia, nausea, vomiting, and intense headache. The globe will feel rock hard, the cornea appears hazy, and the pupil is poorly reactive or fixed.** Ultraviolet keratitis presents with local symptoms including the sensation of something in the eye, profuse tearing, photophobia, and blurred vision, yet systemic symptoms are not usually present. Central retinal artery occlusion and retinal detachment typically present with painless loss of vision.

127. Answer: A

Nursing Process: Intervention/Medical

Rationale: **Intramuscular injections should be avoided to prevent bleeding and hematoma development at the injection site in a patient with disseminated intravascular coagulation (DIC).** Pressure dressings will slow bleeding until the coagulopathy is corrected. Heparin is the drug of choice for treatment of DIC. It acts to inhibit thrombin development, preventing clot formation in the microvasculature. Venipunctures, injections, and other interventions that may disrupt the integrity of the skin should be avoided to prevent additional bleeding.

128. Answer: A

Cognitive Levels: Analysis/Professional Issues

Rationale: **A women's shelter can provide many services that are necessary for the mother including safety for herself and her child while keeping her location confidential.** The welfare bureau is a state agency that provides funds for food, shelter, or other necessities for people who need it. Homeless shelters and soup kitchens are voluntary organizations for people in need of shelter and food. They do not necessarily have resources to accommodate patients at risk for abuse.

129. Answer: B

Nursing Process: Intervention/Medical

Rationale: **Immunotherapy can provide significant improvements in allergic symptoms and reduce the need for additional pharmacotherapy of insect stings and environmental allergens such as pollen. Immunotherapy has proven to have long-term benefits and is effective for desensitizing a person as a means of preventing reactions to subsequent stings.** There are clinical trials using immunotherapy in peanut allergies but it is not a proven therapy at this time. No specific immunological therapy has been found to desensitize milk or latex allergies.

130. Answer: D

Nursing Process: Analysis/Maxillofacial/Ocular

Rationale: **Computed tomography (CT) is the preferred diagnostic imaging for zygomatic fracture.** Water's view (occipitomental) radiographs, Caldwell's view (occipitofrontal) radiographs, and ultrasound can be used to screen (not diagnose) for zygomatic fractures. Lateral facial radiograph is not indicated for zygomatic fracture.

131. Answer: C

Cognitive Level: Application/Professional Issues

Rationale: **The emergency nurse should be donning personal protective garments for protection before caring for these patients.** All of the other answers are appropriate, but not without the nurse being safe enough to deliver care.

132. Answer: A

Nursing Process: Intervention/Respiratory

Rationale: **The definitive treatment for a patient with a massive hemothorax is emergency thoracotomy.** It is imperative to identify and repair the source of bleeding. Temporary measures to stabilize the patient include chest tube insertion and, possibly, autotransfusion, fluid resuscitation (crystalloids and colloids), and supplemental oxygenation.

133. Answer: A

Nursing Process: Intervention/Cardiovascular

Rationale: **The management of an unstable narrow-complex tachycardia is immediate synchronized cardioversion at 50 to 100 J. The American Heart Association cautions that if the symptoms are caused by the tachycardia, it is unstable and therefore, requires immediate synchronized cardioversion.** Vagal maneuvers, adenosine, beta-blockers, or calcium channel blockers are recommended for stable narrow-complex tachycardias. Amiodarone of 150 mg over 10 minutes is indicated for stable wide-QRS tachycardia.

134. Answer: A

Nursing Process: Analysis/Medical

Rationale: **Hornets, yellow jackets, and wasps are the leading cause of allergic stings. They are aggressive and can sting repeatedly with minimal provocation.** Scabies is an intensely itchy skin infestation caused by a mite. It does not produce an allergic reaction. Bumble bees can produce an allergic reaction but are much less aggressive and sting with much lower frequency. Bed bugs are parasitic insects that feed on blood. The bite produces a painless, pruritic lesion. Urticaria may develop from repeated exposure.

135. Answer: B

Cognitive Level: Application/Professional Issues

Rationale: **This voluntary physical action by the patient indicates his acceptance of the procedure and willingness to have it performed, which is considered to be implied consent.**

136. Answer: D

Nursing Process: Intervention/Cardiovascular

Rationale: **Synchronized cardioversion uses a sensor to deliver a shock that avoids delivery during cardiac repolarization, a period of vulnerability during which a shock can precipitate ventricular fibrillation. There will likely be a delay before the defibrillator delivers a synchronized shock because the device will look for the peak of the R wave in the QRS complex and avoid cardiac repolarization, represented by the T wave on the electrocardiogram (ECG).** With unsynchronized shocks, the shock will be delivered as soon as the operator pushes the shock button and these shocks should use higher energy levels. Unsynchronized shocks are recommended when polymorphic ventricular fibrillation is present. Remember to read your questions very carefully. There is a huge difference between synchronized and unsynchronized shocks! Read every word in both the stem and the options! Also, when delivering synchronized shocks, the nurse must hold the buttons down until the shock is actually delivered.

137. Answer: B

Nursing Process: Intervention/Medical

Rationale: **Thyroid storm is characterized by extremes of hyperthyroidism. Propylthiouracil (PTU) blocks thyroid hormone synthesis.** Fever is a common symptom in thyroid storm and should be treated with cooling measures and antipyretics. However, aspirin should be avoided as it can increase thyroid hormone levels. Levothyroxine (Synthroid) is a synthetic replacement for thyroid hormone to treat hypothyroidism, not thyroid storm. Morphine sulfate is an opioid analgesic and is not indicated in the treatment of thyroid storm.

138. Answer: B

Nursing Process: Intervention/Respiratory

Rationale: **Monitoring arterial blood gas (ABG) levels is the appropriate intervention for the chronic obstructive pulmonary disease (COPD) patient.** The patient with COPD has abnormal ABG levels, which may predispose him to respiratory distress. The patient is hypoxemic with hypercapnia. Oxygen should be administered at low concentrations to maintain hypoxic drive. If the PaO_2 remains inadequate at low doses, the emergency nurse should increase the oxygen while continuously monitoring the patient's respiratory status. A patient with COPD usually benefits from adequate hydration to liquefy secretions. Allow the patient to assume a position that facilitates ventilation, usually a forward-leaning high Fowler's position.

139. Answer: A

Cognitive Level: Analysis/Professional Issues

Rationale: **The asthma patient is most emergent.** This child may not be wheezing as air movement significantly decreases. Any problems in airway and breathing are considered life-threatening and should be seen immediately. In most cases, a patient presenting with sickle cell anemia is considered stable but urgent; this patient would be seen second. The 16-year-old with the fracture would most likely be seen third and a small foot laceration with controlled bleeding, fourth.

140. Answer: A

Nursing Process: Analysis/Maxillofacial/Ocular

Rationale: **Thermal burns rarely involve the actual eye globe because the eyelid protects the globe. In Bell's palsy, the patient is unable to close the eyelid, and therefore, would place the patient at risk for injury to the globe.** Exophthalmos, a bulging globe associated with Grave's disease, would also be a situation in which the globe would not be protected. A hyphema, conjunctivitis, and Ludwig's angina would not affect the ability of the eyelid to close and protect the eye.

141. Answer: C

Nursing Process: Intervention/Medical

Rationale: **Fever can result in dehydration. Oral fluids as tolerated should be encouraged, and intravenous access should be initiated for administration of crystalloid solutions and medications.** Post-transplant patients face a lifetime of taking immunosuppressant medications to prevent organ rejection. It is important to isolate the patient from others in the emergency department environment. Cultures of urine and blood and other likely sources of infection should be obtained. Antibiotics should be initiated within 1 hour of arrival in the emergency department.

142. Answer: A

Nursing Process: Assessment/Maxillofacial/Ocular

Rationale: **Globe rupture is an ophthalmic emergency caused by severe blunt or penetrating trauma to the eye and may result in permanent loss of vision. Classic presentation of ruptured globe includes a peaked or tear-drop-shaped pupil, vitreous humor leakage, enophthalmos (posterior displacement of eye due to loss of integrity), loss of vision, and pain.** Glaucoma is the result of increased intraocular pressure and distinct change in pupil shape is not a classic sign. Hyphema is blood in the anterior chamber of the eye and does not result in change in pupil shape or size. Orbital fracture is a fracture of the supporting structures of the globe and does not result in change in pupil shape or size, unless accompanied by a ruptured globe.

143. Answer: A

Cognitive Level: Recall/Professional Issues

Rationale: **Think "quality." Qualitative studies involve questions related to human responses, opinions, and motivations of the participants.** Quantitative studies review data. Systematic reviews involve extensive literature search and retrospective studies follow subjects over time.

144. Answer: C

Nursing Process: Evaluation/Neurologic

Rationale: **The new emergency nurse would provide the correct response if she/he stated that expressive aphasia is represented by the inability to speak words even though the patient is able to comprehend the spoken word. This is indicative of stroke syndromes on the left side of the brain (right-sided hemiplegia).** Receptive aphasia is an impaired ability to understand spoken words. Dysphagia refers to difficulty in swallowing, which occurs when injury affects the vertebrobasilar region. Apraxia is the inability to perform a learned movement, such as using a comb, brushing one's teeth, or waving goodbye.

145. Answer: B

Nursing Process: Intervention/Maxillofacial/Ocular

Rationale: **Any object in the nasal passage may become dislodged resulting in obstructed airway. A disc battery lodged in the ear or nose can cause tissue necrosis in as little as 4 hours.** Organic materials such as rubber, wood, or food tend to be very irritating to the mucosa, causing symptoms earlier as compared with inorganic material such as metal or plastic items.

146. Answer: A

Nursing Process: Analysis/Maxillofacial/Ocular

Rationale: **Facial numbness and inability to look upward are consistent with fracture to the orbital floor, also referred to as a blow-out fracture. The sign and symptoms are consistent with entrapment of extraocular muscles and the infraorbital nerve indicating a blow-out fracture.** Subconjunctival hemorrhage results in bloody appearance of the sclera and is typically a benign uncomplicated presentation. Floaters in the eye may be seen with retinal detachment, yet when the patient can count the number of floaters, it is usually benign and not associated with retinal hemorrhage. Corneal abrasion results in significant eye irritation and pain with excessive tearing, yet is not considered an emergent presentation.

147. Answer: A

Nursing Process: Intervention/Maxillofacial/Ocular

Rationale: **Bell's palsy is caused by damage to the Facial nerve (cranial nerve VII), often from herpes virus. Treatment includes administration of antivirals, corticosteroids, analgesics, eye lubricants, and facial massage.** Bell's palsy is not caused by bacterial infection. Antiepileptic drugs are used for treatment of trigeminal neuralgia. There is no therapeutic indication for strict bed rest.

148. Answer: C

Nursing Process: Intervention/Maxillofacial/Ocular

Rationale: **Pilocarpine is a cholinergic miotic which causes contraction of the ciliary muscle resulting in pupil constriction. The action facilitates the outflow of aqueous humor and subsequently decreases intraocular pressure. Pressure-induced ischemic paralysis of the ciliary muscle will prevent the medication from working; therefore, pilocarpine should be administered 1 hour after administration of other agents to decrease intraocular pressure.** Nausea and vomiting will result in increased intraocular pressure; therefore, an antiemetic will be helpful. Topical beta-blockers, such as Timolol and diuretics decrease aqueous humor production.

149. Answer: B

Nursing Process: Evaluation/Maxillofacial/Ocular

Rationale: **Discharge instructions for patients with epistaxis include avoiding anything that may contribute to continued bleeding or rebleed.** Specific precautions include use of saline nasal spray and a humidifier and taking warm showers to keep the nasal mucosa moist. They should also avoid hard blowing or sneezing, digital manipulation, aspirin, and nonsteroidal anti-inflammatory drugs. Phenylephrine nasal spray may be used as a vasoconstrictor, yet should not be used continuously for prolonged periods of time.

150. Answer: D

Nursing Process: Evaluation/Maxillofacial/Ocular

Rationale: **An uncomplicated orbital fracture is an isolated disruption of the orbital rim following blunt trauma to the eye. The patient should minimize any actions that place pressure on the eye, such as blowing the nose, to minimize further eye injury and prevent reinjury.** Periorbital bruising may take days to weeks to resolve. Antibiotics may not be prescribed if there is no disruption to the skin around the eye or involvement of the globe. Ice packs should be used to decrease swelling.

Appendices

Cardiac dysrhythmias

Abnormal cardiac rhythms are called arrhythmias or dysrhythmias. On the Certified Emergency Nurse (CEN) test, you may be asked to identify a cardiac rhythm in order to answer the question.

Although abnormal rhythms have basic concepts, they can appear differently on different strips and patients. Note the various features, causes, and treatments of these common cardiac dysrhythmias below.

Characteristics of normal rhythm include:

- ventricular and atrial rates of 60 to 100 beats/minute
- regular and uniform QRS complexes and P waves
- PR interval of 0.12 to 0.20 seconds
- QRS duration less than 0.12 seconds
- identical atrial and ventricular rates, with a constant PR interval

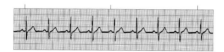

When "reading" a rhythm strip, follow a pattern:

- Is it regular?
- What is the rate?
- Is there a P wave in front of every QRS?
- What is the PR interval?
  - Normal is 0.12 to 0.20 seconds
- What does the QRS complex look like?
  - Normal width should be less than 0.12 seconds
  - Are they all the same?
- What is the QT interval?
  - Normal is 0.36 to 0.44 seconds
- What does the T wave look like?
  - Is it depressed or peaked?
- What does the ST segment look like?
  - Is it elevated or depressed?

Dysrhythmia and features	Causes	Treatment
Sinus arrhythmia 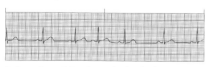 ■ Irregular atrial and ventricular rhythms ■ Rate is normal ■ Normal P wave preceding each QRS complex	■ Normal variation of normal sinus rhythm for athletes, children, and elderly people ■ Also seen in digoxin toxicity and inferior wall myocardial infarction (MI)	■ No treatment necessary unless associated with digoxin toxicity or acute MI

Dysrhythmia and features	Causes	Treatment
Sinus tachycardia 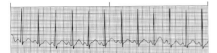 ■ Atrial and ventricular rhythms regular ■ Rate >100 beats/minute; rarely, >160 beats/minute ■ Normal P wave preceding each QRS complex	■ Normal physiologic response to fever, exercise, anxiety, pain, and dehydration; may also accompany shock, left-sided heart failure, cardiac tamponade, hyperthyroidism, anemia, hypovolemia, pulmonary embolism, and anterior wall myocardial infarction (MI) ■ May also occur with atropine, epinephrine, isoproterenol, quinidine, caffeine, alcohol, some illicit drugs, and nicotine use	■ Correction of underlying cause ■ Possible oxygen with or without normal saline infusion before Adult Cardiac Life Support (ACLS) protocol ■ Beta-adrenergic blockers or calcium channel blockers
Sinus bradycardia 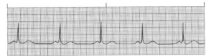 ■ Regular atrial and ventricular rhythms ■ Rate < 60 beats/minute ■ Normal P wave preceding each QRS complex	■ Normal in a well-conditioned heart, as in an athlete ■ Increased intracranial pressure; increased vagal tone due to straining during defecation, vomiting, intubation, and mechanical ventilation; sick sinus syndrome; hypothyroidism; inferior wall myocardial infarction ■ May also occur with anticholinesterase, beta-adrenergic blocker, digoxin, or morphine use ■ Any heart rate under 100 beats/minute for an infant is considered to be a bradycardic rhythm	■ Correction of underlying cause ■ For low cardiac output, dizziness, weakness, altered level of consciousness (LOC), or low blood pressure: ACLS protocol for administration of atropine ■ Temporary or permanent pacemaker ■ Dopamine ■ Epinephrine
Sinoatrial arrest or block (*sinus arrest*) 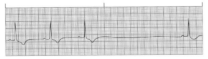 ■ Atrial and ventricular rhythms normal except for missing complex ■ Normal P wave preceding each QRS complex ■ Pause not equal to a multiple of the previous sinus rhythm	■ Acute infection ■ Coronary artery disease (CAD), degenerative heart disease, and acute inferior wall myocardial infarction (MI) ■ Vagal stimulation, Valsalva's maneuver, and carotid sinus massage ■ Digoxin, quinidine, or salicylate toxicity ■ Pesticide poisoning ■ Pharyngeal irritation caused by endotracheal (ET) intubation ■ Sick sinus syndrome ■ Hyperkalemia ■ Cardiomyopathy ■ Hypoxia	■ No treatment if asymptomatic ■ For low cardiac output, dizziness, weakness, altered level of consciousness, or low blood pressure: ACLS protocol for administration of atropine ■ Temporary or permanent pacemaker for repeated episodes
Premature atrial contraction 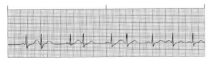 ■ Premature, abnormal-looking P waves that differ in configuration from normal P waves ■ QRS complexes after P waves ■ P wave often buried in the preceding T wave or identified in the preceding T wave	■ Coronary or valvular heart disease, atrial ischemia, coronary atherosclerosis, heart failure, acute respiratory failure, chronic obstructive pulmonary disease (COPD), electrolyte imbalance, and hypoxia ■ Digoxin toxicity; use of aminophylline, beta-adrenergic blockers, or caffeine ■ Anxiety	■ None (usually) ■ Treatment of underlying cause

Dysrhythmia and features	Causes	Treatment
Paroxysmal supraventricular tachycardia 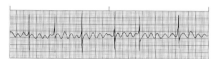 ■ Atrial and ventricular rhythms regular ■ Heart rate > 150 beats/minute; rarely exceeds 250 beats/minute ■ P waves regular but aberrant; difficult to differentiate from preceding T wave ■ P wave preceding each QRS complex ■ Sudden onset and termination of dysrhythmia	■ Intrinsic abnormality of AV conduction system ■ Physical or psychological stress, hypoxia, hypokalemia, cardiomyopathy, congenital heart disease, myocardial infarction (MI), valvular disease, Wolff-Parkinson-White syndrome, cor pulmonale, hyperthyroidism, and systemic hypertension ■ Digoxin toxicity; use of caffeine, nicotine, marijuana, or central nervous system stimulants	■ If patient is unstable: immediate cardioversion ■ If patient is stable: vagal stimulation, Valsalva's maneuver, and carotid sinus massage ■ If signs of good perfusion: ACLS priority—adenosine, calcium channel blockers, and cardioversion; if known heart failure or left ventricular failure: possible digoxin or beta-adrenergic blockers ■ If signs of poor perfusion: ACLS treatment priority—sedation then cardioversion; amiodarone or diltiazem if unresponsive to electrical therapy ■ Do not give adenosine (Adenocard), verapamil (Calan), beta-blockers, calcium channel blockers, and diltiazem (Cardizem) with Wolff-Parkinson-White (WPW) syndrome
Atrial flutter 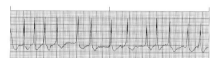 ■ Atrial rhythm regular; rate 250 to 400 beats/minute ■ Ventricular rate variable, depending on the degree of AV block (usually 60 to 100 beats/minute) ■ Sawtooth P-wave configuration possible (F waves) ■ May be hard to determine if 1:1 or 2:1 ratio ■ QRS complexes uniform in shape, but typically irregular in rate	■ Heart failure, tricuspid or mitral valve disease, pulmonary embolism, cor pulmonale, inferior wall MI, and myocarditis ■ Digoxin toxicity ■ Stress, nicotine, and increased alcohol/caffeine intake ■ Pericarditis ■ Hypoglycemia ■ Hypoxia	■ If patient is unstable with a ventricular rate more than 150 beats/minute or has signs of poor perfusion: immediate sedation and cardioversion starting at 50 J and then ACLS medication therapy, which may include calcium channel blockers, beta-adrenergic blockers, or antiarrhythmics ■ If ventricular rate is more than 150 beats/minute and no signs of poor perfusion: ACLS medication therapy is priority ■ Anticoagulation therapy, if necessary ■ Radiofrequency ablation to control rhythm
Atrial fibrillation ■ Atrial rhythm grossly irregular; rate > 400 beats/minute ■ Ventricular rate grossly irregular ■ QRS complexes of uniform configuration and duration ■ PR interval indiscernible ■ No P waves, or P waves that appear as erratic, irregular, baseline fibrillatory waves (F waves)	■ Heart failure, chronic obstructive pulmonary disease (COPD), thyrotoxicosis, constrictive pericarditis, ischemic heart disease, sepsis, pulmonary embolus, rheumatic heart disease, hypertension, mitral stenosis, atrial irritation, and complication of coronary bypass or valve replacement surgery ■ Atrial fibrillation and atrial flutter have similar etiologies	■ If patient is unstable with a ventricular rate >150 beats/minute or signs of poor perfusion: immediate sedation and cardioversion starting at 120 J biphasic or 200 J monophasic, and then ACLS medication therapy, which may include calcium channel blockers, beta-adrenergic blockers, or antiarrhythmics ■ If ventricular rate is more than 150 beats/minute and no signs of poor perfusion: ACLS medication therapy is priority ■ Anticoagulation therapy, if necessary ■ In some patients with refractory atrial fibrillation uncontrolled by drugs, radiofrequency catheter ablation

Dysrhythmia and features	Causes	Treatment
Junctional rhythm 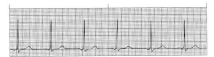 <ul><li>Atrial and ventricular rhythms regular</li><li>Atrial rate 40 to 60 beats/minute</li><li>Ventricular rate usually 40 to 60 beats/minute (60 to 100 beats/minute is accelerated junctional rhythm)</li><li>P waves preceding, hidden within (absent), or after QRS complex; usually inverted if visible</li><li>PR interval (when present) <0.12 seconds</li><li>QRS complex configuration and duration normal, except in aberrant conduction</li></ul>	<ul><li>Inferior or posterior wall myocardial infarction (MI) or ischemia, hypoxia, vagal stimulation, and sick sinus syndrome</li><li>Acute rheumatic fever</li><li>Valve surgery</li><li>Digoxin toxicity</li><li>Use of calcium channel blockers and beta-blockers</li><li>Hypokalemia</li></ul>	<ul><li>Correction of underlying cause</li><li>Atropine for symptomatic slow rate</li><li>Pacemaker insertion if patient is refractory to drugs</li><li>Discontinuation of digoxin, if appropriate</li></ul>
Premature junctional contraction 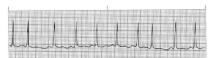 <ul><li>Atrial and ventricular rhythms irregular due to premature beat</li><li>P-waves inverted; may precede, be hidden within, or follow QRS complexes</li><li>PR interval less than 0.12 seconds if P wave precedes QRS complex</li><li>QRS complex configuration and duration normal</li></ul>	<ul><li>Inferior myocardial infarction (MI) or ischemia</li><li>Digoxin toxicity and excessive caffeine, nicotine, alcohol, or amphetamine use</li><li>Heart failure</li><li>Valvular diseases</li></ul>	<ul><li>Correction of underlying cause</li><li>None (usually)</li></ul>
Junctional tachycardia 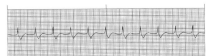 <ul><li>Atrial rate > 100 beats/minute; however, P wave may be absent, hidden in QRS complex, or preceding T wave</li><li>Ventricular rate > 100 beats/minute</li><li>P wave inverted</li><li>QRS complex configuration and duration normal</li><li>Onset of rhythm typically sudden, occurring in bursts</li></ul>	<ul><li>Myocarditis, cardiomyopathy, inferior wall myocardial infarction (MI) or ischemia, acute rheumatic fever, and complication of valve replacement surgery</li><li>Digoxin toxicity</li></ul>	<ul><li>If stable without signs of poor perfusion: ACLS guidelines for amiodarone, calcium channel blocker, or beta-adrenergic blocker</li><li>If signs of poor perfusion or known history of heart failure: ACLS guidelines for amiodarone</li></ul>

Dysrhythmia and features	Causes	Treatment
First-degree AV block 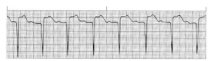 ■ Atrial and ventricular rhythms regular ■ PR interval > 0.20 seconds ■ P wave preceding each QRS complex ■ QRS complex normal	■ May be seen in a healthy person ■ Inferior wall myocardial ischemia or myocardial infarction (MI), hypothyroidism, hypokalemia, and hyperkalemia ■ Digoxin toxicity; use of quinidine, procainamide, beta-adrenergic blockers, calcium channel blockers, or amiodarone	■ Correction of underlying cause ■ Usually no treatment is necessary ■ Possibly atropine if severe bradycardia develops ■ Cautious use of digoxin, calcium channel blockers, and beta-adrenergic blockers for other pathologies
Second-degree AV block Mobitz I *(Wenckebach)* 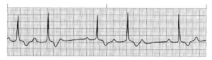 ■ Atrial rhythm regular ■ Ventricular rhythm irregular ■ Atrial rate exceeds ventricular rate ■ PR interval progressively, but only slightly longer with each cycle until QRS complex disappears (dropped beat); PR interval shorter after dropped beat	■ Inferior wall myocardial infarction (MI), cardiac surgery, acute rheumatic fever, and vagal stimulation ■ Digoxin toxicity; use of propranolol, quinidine, or procainamide	■ Treatment of underlying cause ■ Atropine or temporary pacemaker for symptomatic bradycardia ■ Discontinuation of digoxin, if appropriate
Second-degree AV block Mobitz II 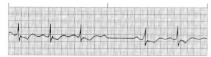 ■ Atrial rhythm regular ■ Ventricular rhythm regular or irregular, can be a regular 2:1, 3:1, 4:1, etc, block or can be a variable block throughout the rhythm strip ■ P-P interval constant ■ QRS complexes periodically absent	■ Severe coronary artery disease (CAD), anterior wall MI, acute myocarditis ■ Digoxin toxicity ■ Hodgkin's lymphoma ■ Rheumatoid arthritis and lupus	■ Temporary or permanent pacemaker ■ Atropine, dopamine, or epinephrine for symptomatic bradycardia ■ Discontinuation of digoxin or other medications such as calcium channel blockers, beta-blockers, and sodium channel blockers, if appropriate
Third-degree AV block *(complete heart block)* 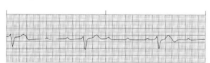 ■ Atrial rhythm regular ■ Ventricular rhythm slow and regular ■ No relation between P waves and QRS complexes ■ No constant PR interval ■ QRS interval normal (nodal pacemaker) or wide and bizarre (ventricular pacemaker)	■ Inferior or anterior wall myocardial infarction (MI), congenital abnormality, rheumatic fever, hypoxia, postoperative complication of mitral valve replacement, Lev's disease (also known as Lenegre-Lev disease this is a fibrosis and calcification that spreads from cardiac structures to the conductive tissue) ■ Digoxin toxicity	■ Immediate transcutaneous pacing for patients with symptomatic bradycardia ■ Temporary or permanent pacemaker ■ Atropine, dopamine, or epinephrine for symptomatic bradycardia ■ Discontinuation of medications that contribute to bradycardia ■ Escape beats may be present to assist with cardiac output. Be careful not to suppress these beats as they are attempting to assist the depressed cardiac output (CO). ■ Pacemaker is the definitive treatment but can be elective rather than emergent for those patients who are tolerating the bradycardia.

Dysrhythmia and features	Causes	Treatment

Premature ventricular contraction
 	
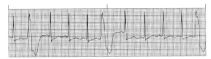
 	
■ Atrial rhythm regular
■ Underlying ventricular rhythm possibly regular except for aberrant beats
■ QRS complex premature, usually followed by a complete compensatory pause—may also be "interpolated" without a compensatory pause and does not interfere with the rate of the underlying rhythm
■ QRS complex wide and distorted, usually >0.12 seconds
■ May have bigeminy (every other beat) or trigeminy (every third beat)
■ Premature QRS complexes occurring singly, in pairs, or in threes; alternating with normal beats; focus from one or more sites causing different configurations of aberrant beats. (If the premature beats look the same, it is called unifocal. If the beats are different in configuration, it is called multifocal.)
■ Ominous when clustered, multifocal, and with R wave on T pattern
	■ Heart failure; old or acute myocardial ischemia, myocardial infarction (MI), or contusion; myocardial irritation by ventricular catheter, such as a pacemaker; hypercapnia; hypokalemia; and hypocalcemia
	■ Drug toxicity (cardiac glycosides, aminophylline, tricyclic antidepressants, beta-adrenergic blockers [isoproterenol or dopamine])
	■ Caffeine, tobacco, or alcohol use
	■ Psychological stress, anxiety, pain, and exercise
	■ Tricyclic overdose and use of street drugs such as cocaine or amphetamines
	■ Digoxin toxicity
	■ Electrolyte imbalances
		■ Usually do not need to treat unless patient is symptomatic, associated with myocardial infarction (MI), or occurring in multiples such as coupling or tripling
		■ If symptomatic: amiodarone (Pacerone), flecainide (Tambocor), or lidocaine IV
		■ Treatment of underlying cause:
		  – Bicarbonate if known acidosis
		  – Treatment for myocardial ischemia, as appropriate
		  – Discontinuation of drugs causing toxicity
		  – Potassium chloride intravenous if PVC induced by hypokalemia
		  – Intravenous magnesium sulfate if PVC induced by hypomagnesemia
		■ If symptomatic as a result of bradycardia: ACLS bradycardia algorithm (these may be escape beats in an attempt to maintain cardiac output).

|**Ventricular tachycardia** 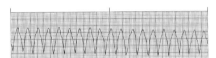 ■ Ventricular rate 140 to 220 beats/minute, regular or irregular ■ QRS complexes wide, bizarre, and independent of P waves ■ P waves not discernible ■ May start and stop suddenly ■ May have torsade de pointes if the complexes vary in their shape or configuration as well as height—torsade de pointes stands for "twisting of the points" 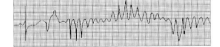	■ Myocardial infarction (MI) or aneurysm; Coronary Artery Disease (CAD); rheumatic heart disease; mitral valve prolapse; heart failure; cardiomyopathy; ventricular catheters; hypokalemia; hypercalcemia; and pulmonary embolism ■ Digoxin, procainamide, epinephrine, or quinidine toxicity ■ Tricyclic overdose ■ Cocaine overdose ■ Acid–base imbalances ■ Long QT syndrome	■ With pulse and monomorphic wide-complex QRS complexes: administer adenosine (use adenosine cautiously in the presence of an irregular pulse); can also use amiodarone, procainamide, sotalol, and lidocaine; if persistent: possible cardioversion ■ If polymorphic and hemodynamically stable with a pulse and a normal QT interval: amiodarone, procainamide, sotalol, lidocaine, over-drive pacing, and cardioversion; if obvious torsade or long baseline QT interval use magnesium sulfate ■ If with a pulse but unstable: sedation and cardioversion, and then amiodarone ■ If pulseless: cardiopulmonary resuscitation (CPR); ACLS protocol for immediate defibrillation then ACLS medication therapy, including epinephrine, amiodarone, lidocaine, bicarbonate, or magnesium sulfate as indicated; CO_2 monitor; advanced airway when available ■ If recurrent ventricular tachycardia: implantable cardioverter defibrillator ■ Do not use amiodarone with torsade de pointes

Dysrhythmia and features	Causes	Treatment
Ventricular fibrillation 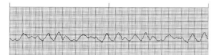 ■ Ventricular rhythm rapid and chaotic ■ QRS complexes wide and irregular; no visible P waves	■ Myocardial ischemia, myocardial infarction (MI), R-on-T phenomenon, untreated ventricular tachycardia, hypokalemia, hyperkalemia, hypercalcemia, and hypothermia ■ Digoxin, epinephrine, or quinidine toxicity ■ Electrocution ■ Acid–base imbalances ■ Hypoxia ■ Antiarrhythmic medications	■ If pulseless: CPR; ACLS protocol for immediate defibrillation; then ACLS medication therapy, including epinephrine, amiodarone, lidocaine, bicarbonate, and magnesium sulfate as indicated; CO_2 monitor; advanced airway when available ■ If recurrent ventricular tachycardia: implantable cardioverter defibrillator
Asystole 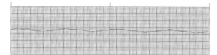 ■ No atrial or ventricular rate or rhythm ■ No discernible P waves, QRS complexes, or T waves	■ Myocardial ischemia, myocardial infarction (MI), aortic valve disease, heart failure, hypoxemia, hypokalemia, severe acidosis, electric shock, ventricular arrhythmias, AV block, pulmonary embolism, heart rupture, cardiac tamponade, hyperkalemia, and electromechanical dissociation ■ Cocaine overdose ■ Lightening strike ■ Hypoxia ■ Acid–base imbalances	■ CPR; ACLS protocol for endotracheal intubation, transcutaneous pacing, and administration of epinephrine
Idioventricular 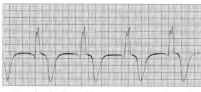 ■ Regular rhythm with rate of 20 to 40 beats/minute ■ QRS complexes are wide and bizarre ■ No P waves discernible ■ Considered accelerated if rate is >40 beats/minute. May reach higher rates up to 60 beats/minute	■ Acute myocardial infarction ■ Digoxin toxicity ■ Street drugs such as cocaine ■ Reperfusion dysrhythmia	■ Treatment may not be necessary ■ Treat underlying problem ■ May need pacemaker ■ Possible external pacing

Pulseless electrical activity
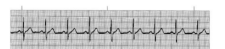
■ Any rhythm can be displayed but very often normal sinus rhythm is present without a pulse
■ No pulse is present but electrical activity is displayed on the monitor/electrocardiogram
	■ Look at the five Hs and Ts
	■ Hs
	  • Hypovolemia
	  • Hypoxia
	  • Hypo-/Hyperthermia
	  • Hypo-/Hyperkalemia
	  • Hydrogen ions (acidosis)
	■ Ts
	  • Tamponade
	  • Tension pneumothorax
	  • Thrombosis (pulmonary embolism)
	  • Thrombosis (MI)
	  • Tablets/Toxins (overdoses)
		■ Cardiopulmonary resuscitation
		■ Treatment of underlying cause

Common life-support drugs

Drug	Indication
Adenosine (Adenocard)	*Paroxysmal supraventricular tachycardia (PSVT) involving atrioventricular (AV) node reentry* ▪ Can also be used for regular, monomorphic wide-complex tachycardia now ▪ Do *not* use for irregular, wide-complex tachycardia or unstable ventricular tachycardia. ▪ May cause flushing, dyspnea, chest pain, transient periods of sinus bradycardia or asystole, transient AV block, atrial fibrillation, and ventricular ectopy ▪ Prepare patient for "bad feeling" that will occur when asystole occurs. ▪ Short half-life (<5 seconds) ▪ Do not use for Wolff–Parkinson–White syndrome-related PSVT. ▪ PSVT may recur. ▪ Dipyridamole potentiates effectiveness (can use lower dose of 3 mg instead of 6 mg). ▪ Can also use lower dose of 3 mg in heart transplant patients ▪ Patients with central line access may need lower dose of 3 mg.
Amiodarone	*Recurring ventricular fibrillation or unstable ventricular tachycardia; consider in hemodynamically stable wide-complex tachycardia* ▪ May cause hypotension and bradycardia ▪ Do *not* use with polymorphic VT associated with prolonged QT interval. ▪ Reduces the clearance of warfarin (Coumadin) and digoxin. ▪ Hypotension can occur. ▪ May be given IV push undiluted in cardiopulmonary arrest ▪ Maximum dose—2.2 g in 24 hours
Atropine (Atropen)	*Bradycardia* ▪ Lower dose (<0.5 mg) may sustain bradycardia. ▪ Higher dose (>3 mg) may cause full vagal blockage. ▪ Can increase cardiac oxygen demand ▪ Maximum dosage—3 mg in 24 hours
Beta-adrenergic blockers (atenolol [Tenormin], metoprolol tartrate [Lopressor], propranolol [Inderal], Esmolol [Brevibloc], labetalol)	*Reduced ventricular irritability after myocardial infarction (MI); for emergency antihypertensive therapy in both hemorrhagic and ischemic stroke* ▪ Can cause bradycardia, AV conduction delays, and hypotension ▪ Contraindicated with symptomatic bradycardia, second- or third-degree block ▪ The use of beta-blockers with cocaine-induced acute coronary syndrome is debated. Propranolol use can cause vasoconstriction.
Diltiazem	*Ventricular rate control in atrial fibrillation and atrial flutter; consider after adenosine for refractory supraventricular tachycardia* ▪ Blood pressure may drop from peripheral vasodilation. ▪ May drop pulse rate. ▪ Give slowly and check blood pressure and pulse rate during administration. ▪ Use with caution with beta-adrenergic blockers and calcium channel blockers.
Diuretics (furosemide [Lasix])	*Acute pulmonary edema, cerebral edema after cardiac arrest* ▪ Vasodilatory effects occur within 5 minutes; can result in hypotension. ▪ Diuresis occurs within 60 minutes. ▪ Document output.

Drug	Indication
Dobutamine	*Acute heart failure/inotropic support* <ul><li>Beta-adrenergic blockers such as propranolol can decrease the effects.</li><li>Patients with atrial fibrillation should receive digoxin first, or they can develop rapid ventricular response.</li><li>Drug is incompatible with alkaline solutions.</li><li>Infiltration may produce severe tissue damage.</li><li>Treat hypovolemic situations before administering dobutamine.</li></ul>
Dopamine	*Shock, decreased renal function, heart failure, and poor perfusion* <ul><li>Do not use for treating uncorrected tachyarrhythmias or ventricular fibrillation.</li><li>May precipitate dysrhythmias.</li><li>Drug is incompatible with alkaline solutions.</li><li>Infiltration may produce severe tissue damage.</li><li>Solution deteriorates after 24 hours.</li></ul>
Epinephrine (Adrenaclick)	*Bronchospasm, anaphylaxis, severe allergic reactions, cardiac arrest, and dysrhythmias* <ul><li>Increases perfusion pressure to heart/brain</li><li>Positive inotrope</li><li>May exacerbate heart failure, dysrhythmias, angina pectoris, hyperthyroidism, and emphysema</li><li>Can increase oxygen demands in patients with myocardial infarction (MI)</li><li>May cause headache, tremors, or palpitations</li><li>Monitor for signs of cerebral hemorrhage.</li></ul>
Lidocaine (Xylocaine)	*Ventricular dysrhythmias* <ul><li>Don't use if bradycardia is present or if patient has high-grade sinoatrial or AV block.</li><li>Don't mix with sodium bicarbonate.</li><li>May lead to central nervous system toxicity</li><li>Light-headedness and dizziness are common.</li><li>Toxicity can occur, which can lead to death—possible potentiators of this include liver problems, decreased protein, and acidotic situations.</li></ul>
Magnesium sulfate	*Hypomagnesemia and torsade de pointes* <ul><li>Serum magnesium and potassium levels should be determined.</li><li>Can precipitate hypotension</li></ul>
Nitroglycerin	*Angina and heart failure associated with myocardial infarction (MI)* <ul><li>Angina not relieved with three sublingual tablets requires emergency medical services.</li><li>May cause reflex tachycardia, hypotension, paradoxical bradycardia, and headache</li><li>Administration for >12 hours each day may produce tolerance.</li><li>Hypovolemia decreases effectiveness and worsens hypotension.</li><li>Do not use with right ventricular infarct.</li></ul>
Nitroprusside (Nitropress)	*Hypertension and increased systemic vascular resistance* <ul><li>Continuous blood pressure monitoring is required.</li><li>Deteriorates when exposed to light; wrap in opaque container.</li><li>May cause hypotension, headache, and vomiting</li><li>Cyanide toxicity may occur after 72 hours.</li></ul>
Procainamide (Pronestyl)	*Ventricular dysrhythmias, including those associated with malignant hyperthermia* <ul><li>Can cause precipitous hypotension; do not use for treating second- or third-degree heart block unless a pacemaker has been inserted.</li><li>Can cause AV block</li><li>Discontinue if PR interval or QRS complex widens or if dysrhythmias worsen.</li></ul>

(continued)

Drug	Indication
Sodium bicarbonate	*Metabolic acidosis and cardiac arrest* ■ Don't mix with epinephrine; causes epinephrine degradation. ■ Don't mix with calcium salts; forms insoluble precipitates. ■ Do not overuse—can cause rebound alkalosis. ■ Treat the underlying problem.
Thrombolytic agents (Activase [alteplase], TNKase [tenecteplase], Retavase [reteplase])	*Acute myocardial infarction and acute ischemic stroke* ■ Alteplase is the only thrombolytic agent approved for acute ischemic stroke. ■ Contraindicated in patients with a history of active internal bleeding within 2 days, history of stroke, or major surgery within 14 days. ■ Be sure the patient is a candidate—document the contraindications and relative contraindications. ■ Monitor for signs of reperfusion. ■ Monitor for signs of bleeding—may occur intracranial, intra-abdominal, in gums, etc. ■ Dosages are different for acute myocardial infarction and stroke.
Verapamil	*Supraventricular tachyarrhythmias, angina, and hypertension* ■ Contraindicated in patients with aortic stenosis, hypotension, cardiogenic shock, severe heart failure, second- or third-degree AV block, or sick sinus syndrome ■ High doses or too-rapid administration can cause a significant drop in blood pressure. ■ May increase serum digoxin levels

Holm, J., et al. (2017). The effect of amiodarone on warfarin anticoagulation: a register-based nationwide cohort study involving the Swedish population. *Journal of Thrombosis Haemostasis*, *15*(3), 446–453. Retrieved from https://www.ncbi.nlm.nih.gov/pubmed/28058824

ACLS-Algorithms.com. *Advanced cardiac life support*. Retrieved from https://acls-algorithms.com

Van Amburgh, J. A. (2016). *The ongoing debate of beta-blockers for cocaine-associated chest pain*. Medscape Nurses. Retrieved from https://www.medscape.com/viewarticle/872180_2

Triage assessment principles

Triage is a unique position in the emergency department that requires an emergency nurse to quickly and efficiently gather information about each patient presenting for care. In most instances, patients arrive in groups rather than individually, which makes it more important for the nurse functioning in this position to be experienced and able to swiftly target the chief complaint of multiple patients, while at the same time taking in the whole picture. The most experienced nurse in the department should take on the role of the triage nurse. There are many requirements that should be heeded in placing the right person in this role. Experience is at the top of the list! Having the initials CEN after their name is another privilege that is beneficial as well as denoting another educational and knowledge based milestone. This person should also be able to handle controversy, plan ahead, be flexible, and understand the workings of the department and how it interfaces with other departments, including emergency medical services (EMS). These are just a few of the qualities that are recommended.

Often a patient or family member may make a simple off-hand type of remark that markedly impacts the situation. It is important for the triage nurse to pick up on these remarks and ensure that vital aspects of care are not missed.

The main purpose of triage is to determine acuity and priority of care and place the right patient in the room/bed at the right time. Unfortunately, bed space is not always available and some patients must wait. It is imperative that the patients who are in the waiting room are appropriate and safe. This situation places a great deal of responsibility on the triage nurse. This nurse may need to initiate care in the triage area, which may be in the form of first aid or following established protocols, including ordering radiographs or laboratory tests. It also involves specialized knowledge in emergency care in order to request tests that might not be present in protocols so that patient care is optimized. For instance, a patient who fell and hit his head and who is on anticoagulant therapy but is awake, alert, and oriented at the present time with no beds available could be sent to computed tomography (CT) if the triage nurse understands the importance and knows to discuss the situation with the provider.

The Emergency Nurses Association (ENA) recommends that before performing triage activities, the emergency nurse be experienced in emergency nursing care and trained in triage concepts. Triage classes must include an understanding of both the art and science of triage. There is definitely a science involved in this position but the art of triage is another facet that should be included. Understanding the impact that triage nurses make on the outcome of patients arriving to emergency departments should not be overlooked. Other parts of the class should include an understanding of triage vital signs, both normal and abnormal (and their importance in the triage process); special patient populations such as the pediatric, geriatric, pregnant, and behavioral patients; and dealing with "frequent flyers." Presentations should also cover chief complaints and differential diagnoses including pertinent questions that must be asked for each of the chief complaints to help the triage nurse make the right decision. Legalities should also be a part of the course because the triage area is a highly litigious area. There are many legal aspects that the triage nurse should be aware of. The triage area is also potentially highly volatile with the prospect of violence a constant threat and the triage nurse should be prepared for this possibility. The triage nurse should also be educated in and have a clear and complete understanding of whichever triage acuity system is utilized.

Making triage decisions

To make triage decisions effectively, the triage nurse must gather and interpret both subjective and objective data rapidly and accurately. Follow this rule: "When in doubt, triage up." That is, if you are uncertain regarding the urgency of a patient's condition, treat it as more, rather than less, urgent.

Triage activities consist of:
- obtaining a focused history of the patient's chief complaint
- performing a limited physical examination
- considering vital signs
- classifying the patient's problem for urgency
- providing reassurance that the patient will receive definitive medical care

Obtaining a history

- Focus on the patient's chief complaint.
- Document using the patient's words; qualify the complaint as precisely as possible using the PQRST acronym (Provocative/Palliative, Quality/Quantity, Region/Radiation, Severity, Timing).
- Ask the patient if they are allergic to anything and place a band on their arm. Taking a full allergy and medication history is not necessary at triage. Pertinent pieces of these aspects are important, but the entirety of these should not be placed on the shoulders of the triage nurse.

Performing a physical examination

- Observe the patient's general appearance and assess vital signs and level of consciousness (LOC).
- Take oral, axillary, tympanic, or temporal temperatures as appropriate. Rectal temperatures are the most accurate, especially for infants; take as indicated by institution policy and ensure the patient's privacy.
- Check radial or apical pulse. Note rate, rhythm, and quality. While assessing the pulse, check skin temperature and capillary refill time.
- Note rate, depth, symmetry, and quality of respirations. Note skin color and turgor, facial expression, accessory muscle use, and any audible breath sounds. Accurately count respirations, especially in pediatric and geriatric patients.
- The pediatric patient must have their shirt removed for accurate examination. Check for retractions! This cannot be done through shirts or coats.
- Assess level of consciousness using a scale such as the Glasgow Coma Scale, or make a notation that the patient is oriented to person, place, and time.

Classifying emergency conditions

Triage acuity systems have evolved over the years and the accepted version in today's emergency world is a five-level system. There are different types, but the one used most commonly in the United States is the Emergency Severity Index (ESI).

The Emergency Nurses Association, in collaboration with the American College of Emergency Physicians, released a position statement endorsing the use of a five-level triage system in 2003 with a revision of that statement in 2010.

Highest triage priority

Regardless of the system used, the highest triage priority includes those patients needing resuscitation or other immediate medical attention. Examples of highest priority conditions include respiratory or cardiac arrest, coma, major uncontrolled bleeding, trauma-related cardiac events requiring emergency procedures such as pericardiocentesis, the need for immediate fluid or blood resuscitation, or precipitous delivery.

Emergent conditions

The next level of priority, termed "emergent," includes those conditions needing medical and nursing attention immediately, but, in these situations, the nurse and care team can initiate treatment using protocols or guidelines allowed by the facility. The patient's care requires the provider, but it is not necessary for the provider to be physically in the room on arrival such as with those in the above examples.

Some examples of this category are:
- stable chest pain
- moderate hemorrhage
- head injury
- stable poisoning or drug overdose

Triage responsibilities

Initial interventions, such as ice and elevation or pillow splints, typically need to be performed during triage when the patient cannot be taken immediately to a room. Patient teaching can begin at triage regarding the chief complaint; first aid aspects, such as treating fevers with antipyretics before arrival; safety issues, such as seat belts and infant car seat use; and hygiene concepts, such as proper hand washing. Some patients need to be educated on the necessity of coming to the emergency department earlier, such as cerebral vascular accidents (CVAs) and other chief complaints that are best treated earlier for the most optimal outcome.

Another major responsibility at triage is to keep patients in the emergency department. Reducing left without being seen patients is more about the patient and less about the numbers, but both are important. Many patients who tire of waiting either leave without telling anyone or refuse to wait longer even with explanations. Patients with possible diagnoses of orbital cellulitis or pyelonephritis, for instance, both of which can have serious complications, need to be treated but cannot always be taken to a room immediately. Performing laboratory tests that will expedite care once the patient is taken to a room will help create a feeling of being cared for in the patient's mind.

A few other actions that the triage nurse can take or keep in mind to generate an environment of caring are:
- Be a patient advocate!
- Keep patients informed in the waiting room.
- Listen to the patient or family member who is concerned.
- Recheck patients who are waiting, including vital signs.
- Intervene for problems as necessary.
- Build rapport with the patient and family members.
- Act like you care!
- Do not get defensive—deal with aggressive behavior appropriately but do not add to the violent scenarios.

The most important concept to remember is that patients trust us as nurses to care for them. Keep that in mind and always advocate for them—even those who do not seem to appreciate it!

Index